KT-211-435

PSYCHOLOGY
FOR MEDICINE
& HEALTHCARE

WITHDRAWN
BRITISH MEDICAL ASSOCIATION
FROM LIBRARY

1002517

Sara Miller McCune founded SAGE Publishing in 1965 to support the dissemination of usable knowledge and educate a global community. SAGE publishes more than 1000 journals and over 800 new books each year, spanning a wide range of subject areas. Our growing selection of library products includes archives, data, case studies and video. SAGE remains majority owned by our founder and after her lifetime will become owned by a charitable trust that secures the company's continued independence.

Los Angeles | London | New Delhi | Singapore | Washington DC | Melbourne

SUSAN AYERS AND RICHARD DE VISSER

PSYCHOLOGY FOR MEDICINE & HEALTHCARE

SECOND EDITION

WITHDRAWN FROM LIBRARY

BMA LIBRARY
BRITISH MEDICAL ASSOCIATION

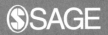

Los Angeles | London | New Delhi
Singapore | Washington DC | Melbourne

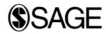

Los Angeles | London | New Delhi
Singapore | Washington DC | Melbourne

SAGE Publications Ltd
1 Oliver's Yard
55 City Road
London EC1Y 1SP

SAGE Publications Inc.
2455 Teller Road
Thousand Oaks, California 91320

SAGE Publications India Pvt Ltd
B 1/l 1 Mohan Cooperative Industrial Area
Mathura Road
New Delhi 110 044

SAGE Publications Asia-Pacific Pte Ltd
3 Church Street
#10-04 Samsung Hub
Singapore 049483

Editor: Amy Jarrold
Editorial assistant: Katie Rabot
Production editor: Imogen Roome
Copyeditor: Sarah Bury
Proofreader: Clare Weaver
Indexer: Elizabeth Ball
Marketing manager: Lucia Sweet
Cover design: Wendy Scott
Typeset by: C&M Digitals (P) Ltd, Chennai, India
Printed in the UK

© Susan Ayers & Richard de Visser 2018

First edition published 2011
Reprinted 2012, 2013, 2014 (twice), 2015 (twice), 2016 (twice), 2017

Apart from any fair dealing for the purposes of research or private study, or criticism or review, as permitted under the Copyright, Designs and Patents Act, 1988, this publication may be reproduced, stored or transmitted in any form, or by any means, only with the prior permission in writing of the publishers, or in the case of reprographic reproduction, in accordance with the terms of licences issued by the Copyright Licensing Agency. Enquiries concerning reproduction outside those terms should be sent to the publishers.

Library of Congress Control Number: 2017942556

British Library Cataloguing in Publication data

A catalogue record for this book is available from the British Library

ISBN 978-1-4739-6927-8
ISBN 978-1-4739-6928-5 (pbk)

At SAGE we take sustainability seriously. Most of our products are printed in the UK using FSC papers and boards. When we print overseas we ensure sustainable papers are used as measured by the PREPS grading system. We undertake an annual audit to monitor our sustainability.

Dedication

Susan Ayers:
For my mothers, Jane and Moira, who are my rock and counsel
and my sister, Ruth, who walks through life with me.
Richard de Visser:
For Thom, Felix, and Iris

CONTENTS

ACKNOWLEDGEMENTS

There is more to a book than its contents, and the story behind this one would make a good read in itself. The journey started because we were frustrated by the lack of a comprehensive textbook on psychology for medical students. We happened to mention this in passing to the people at SAGE who harnessed all their enthusiasm and considerable expertise into getting the first edition of this book published in 2011. SAGE started the ball rolling with the first edition and jollied us into agreeing to do this second edition, so we are grateful for their impetus and help.

This second edition has given us the opportunity to make some important changes. The first edition was used in many countries by people from medicine and other healthcare professions. We have therefore changed the language and examples throughout this edition to reflect the global community and range of healthcare professionals using this book. Some areas of research and understanding have developed rapidly since the first edition, so we've been able to include information on issues such as epigenetics, social diversity, health technology, risk, and resilience. We've also expanded important topics that we were only able to cover briefly in the previous edition, such as pain, perinatal mental health, and therapies such as mindfulness.

The real story of this book, however, is the students and medical consultants who have been so important in making it happen. With the first edition it was only really when students got involved that the book took on a life of its own. Since it was first published, our students have told us what works and what needs to change. We are truly indebted to the many amazing people who have been an integral part of both editions. Students gave up their summer vacation to help with researching literature, sourcing copyright permissions, and arranging illustrations with the requisite amount of enthusiasm and unbelievable organisational skills to make sure this book was completed. Students also read, re-read, and commented on every chapter through various drafts. They gave us their honest opinions and helped make this book what it is. When we asked for volunteers we never dreamt so many people would get involved. They told us what they liked and didn't like; where we had the tone wrong; what features were missing. The cartoons were drawn by an artist who happened to be studying medicine at the time we were writing this book. We were lucky to have excellent medical consultants advise us on chapters throughout the book – and with plenty of good humour. We laughed a lot along the way!

We have been humbled by people's enthusiasm, the amount of time they put in, and the expertise they brought to this book. We have been inspired by many of these people and are very grateful for their input. So by the time this book went to press it had already been a great experience and a testament to the combined efforts of many people who gave their considerable time and energy to get it there. This must clearly include our respective families, who put up with us being total book-bores and still supported us at every step.

RESEARCH AND ADMINISTRATIVE SUPPORT

Amalia Houlton, Clinical Psychology Department, University of Leicester

Gemima Fitzgerald, School of Psychology, University of Sussex

Lizzie Shine, School of Psychology, University of Sussex

Louise Fernay, School of Psychology, University of Sussex

Olivia Julienne, School of Psychology, University of Sussex

Shreya Badhrinarayanan, School of Psychology, University of Sussex

COPYRIGHT PERMISSIONS

Michele McKenner, School of Psychology, University of Sussex

CARTOONS

Simon Hall, Brighton & Sussex Medical School

MEDICAL ADVISOR

David Lawrence, General Practice, London

PHOTO ACKNOWLEDGMENTS

Case Study 1.3: Photo courtesy of Craig Cloutier, taken 28 March 2009, sourced: https://www.flickr.com/photos/craigcloutier/3509787315

Case Study 2.3: Photograph courtesy of: CDC/ Judy Schmidt acquired from Public Health Image Library (Website)

Research Box 3.1: Photo via Senior Airman Tristin English/Scott Air Force Base, sourced: http://www.scott.af.mil/News/Photos/igphoto/2000049812/

Research Box 3.2: U.S. Department of Defense, June 2016, sourced: https://www.defense.gov/Photos/Photo-Gallery/

Case Study 5.1, 5.2 and 5.3: Attribution-Share Alike 3.0 Unported license, Wikipedia Commons

Research Box 6.1: Unknown photographer, National Cancer Institute, August 2005, sourced: https://visualsonline.cancer.gov/details.cfm?imageid=4538

Research Box 10.1: Photo courtesy of U.S. Navy photo by Mass Communication Specialist Seaman Joseph Caballero, U.S. States Navy, sourced: http://www.navy.mil/view_image.asp?id=36338

Research Box 10.1: Photo courtesy of Leo Carbajal, February 2013, Creative Commons Attribution-Share Alike 3.0 Unported license

Case Study 10.1: Photo distributed on Creative Commons Attribution-ShareAlike 2.0, January 2003

Case Study 11.2: Photo distributed on CC0 Public Domain

Box 13.1: Photo distributed on Creative Commons Zero – CC0

Case Study 16.1: Photo distributed on CC0 Public Domain, sourced: http://maxpixel.freegreatpicture.com/Old-Sad-People-Crying-Depression-Thinking-Woman-71735

Research Box 16.2: Photo distributed on CC0 Public Domain, sourced: http://maxpixel.freegreatpicture.com/Couple-Old-Asia-Man-Taiwan-Satisfied-Woman-579172

Research Box 17.1: Photographer Rhoda Baer, National Cancer Institute, January 2013, Public Domain

Research Box 18.1: Photo courtesy of Myfuture.com, August 2011, CC BY-ND 2.0

GUIDED TOUR

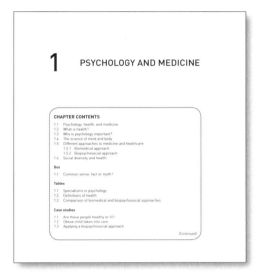

Chapter Contents Every chapter has a clear, numbered list of the contents of the chapter, including major sections, subheadings, case studies, research boxes, and other features.

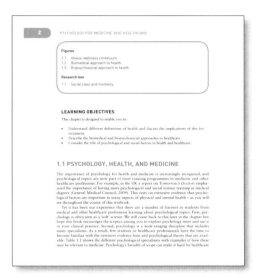

Learning Objectives Learning objectives are given at the beginning of each chapter. These state the most important things we hope you will learn from each chapter.

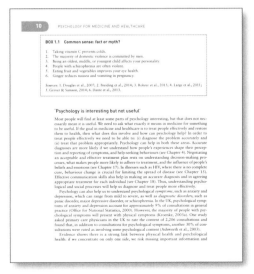

Boxes Boxes are used to illustrate key concepts described in the text. Some of these are lists of key points, some are descriptions of important issues, and others are diagrams or tables of information.

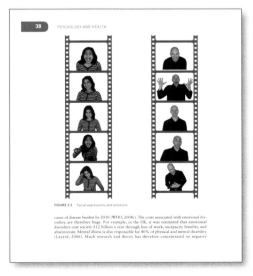

Figures A variety of figures is used to help you understand the material described in the text. These include photographs, diagrams, flowcharts, and theoretical models.

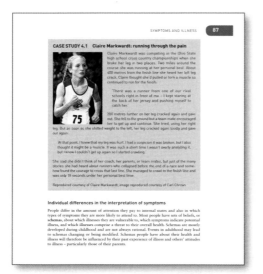

Case Studies Case studies are used to illustrate patients' experiences of the issues described in the text. They also show how psychological theories and techniques can be used in clinical practice to help patients.

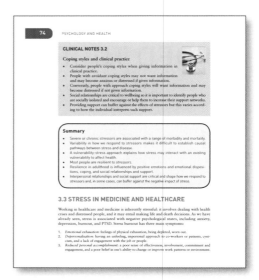

Clinical Notes Clinical notes give key recommendations and tips for healthcare practice based on the psychological principles and techniques described in the text.

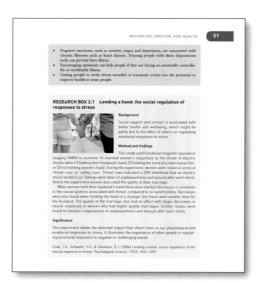

Research Boxes Each research box describes a research study that illustrates the psychological concepts or findings described in the text, and gives examples of how different research methods are applied in clinical contexts.

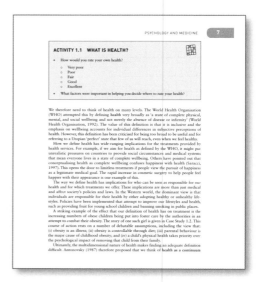

Activities Activities are designed to help you stop and think about the information contained in the text and how it might apply to your own life.

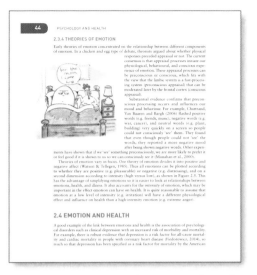

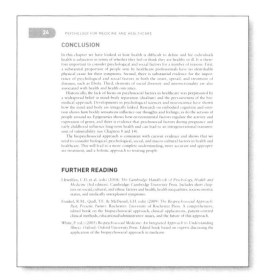

Cartoons Cartoons provide time out from the masses of words and provide a more humorous view of psychology and healthcare!

Further Reading At the end of each chapter there are suggestions for further reading, along with brief comments about each book to help you choose which ones to read.

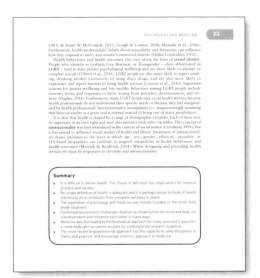

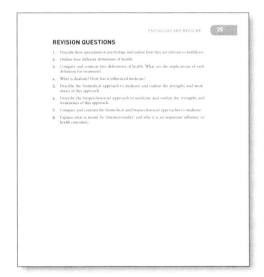

Summaries Each section concludes with a bullet-point summary of the most important psychological theories and applications covered in that section. These summaries relate to the learning objectives and revision questions so will help you learn and revise.

Revision Questions Revision questions are included at the end of every chapter to help you learn and revise for exams.

1 PSYCHOLOGY AND MEDICINE

LEARNING OBJECTIVES

This chapter is designed to enable you to:

- Understand different definitions of health and discuss the implications of this for treatment.
- Describe the biomedical and biopsychosocial approaches to healthcare.
- Consider the role of psychological and social factors in health and healthcare.

1.1 PSYCHOLOGY, HEALTH, AND MEDICINE

The importance of psychology for health and medicine is increasingly recognised, and psychological topics are now part of most training programmes in medicine and other healthcare professions. For example, in the UK a report on *Tomorrow's Doctors* emphasised the importance of having more psychological and social science training in medical degrees (General Medical Council, 2009). This rests on extensive evidence that psychological factors are important in many aspects of physical and mental health – as you will see throughout the course of this textbook.

Yet it has been our experience that there are a number of barriers to students from medical and other healthcare professions learning about psychological topics. First, psychology is often seen as a 'soft' science. We will come back to this later in the chapter but hope this book encourages the sceptics among you to explore psychology more and use it in your clinical practice. Second, psychology is a wide-ranging discipline that includes many specialisms. As a result, few students or healthcare professionals have the time to become familiar with the extensive evidence base and psychological theory that are available. Table 1.1 shows the different psychological specialisms with examples of how these may be relevant to medicine. Psychology's breadth of scope can make it hard for healthcare

TABLE 1.1   Specialisms in psychology

Specialism	Focus	Relevance to medicine
Health	Psychological factors and health	Understanding health behaviour, effective health promotion and intervention, the role of psychosocial factors in health. Resilience and protective factors.
Clinical	Psychological resilience and disorders	Understanding emotions, emotional disorders (psychopathology), and developing effective interventions.
Developmental	Development and change over the lifespan	Understanding normal and abnormal aspects of development across the lifespan.
Forensic	Criminal and judicial behaviour and systems	Understanding criminal behaviour. Medico-legal investigations and testimony.
Social	Social and group processes	Understanding how social and group processes influence our own and other people's behaviour in medical settings.
Biological and Neuropsychological	Link between physiological and mental processes or behaviour	Understanding the interaction between psychological and physiological processes.
Cognitive	Internal mental processes e.g. attention, perception, memory	Understanding risk perception and decision making. How memory processes affect treatment and adherence to medication.
Occupational	Work, the workplace, and organisations	Understanding work performance and training requirements. How medical organisations function.
Educational	Learning and education	Improving education or training for healthcare professionals. Health education.

professionals to work out which parts are most relevant to clinical practice. Third, being bombarded with psychobabble in the press makes it even more difficult to screen out evidence-based information from popular 'facts'. A further challenge is that psychological and social services are often separated from physiologically orientated services, such as acute medical wards. This makes it hard to work out where medical care stops and psychological or social care begins.

We hope this book solves this problem by providing a single, integrated overview of the psychology that is relevant to medicine and healthcare, and by considering how this can be used in healthcare practice. This is done in four sections. In this introductory chapter we examine fundamental conceptual issues of what we mean by health and illness, why psychological and social factors are important, and different approaches to medicine.

The rest of the book is divided into four sections. Section I focuses on the psychology of health and covers theories and research relevant to most areas of healthcare practice, such as emotions, stress, symptoms, and chronic illness. Section II discusses knowledge from other areas of psychology that is relevant, such as brain and behaviour, development from infancy to old age, and the effects of social factors on people's behaviour. Section III focuses on psychology that is relevant to different body systems, including the cardiovascular, respiratory, gastrointestinal, immune, genitourinary, and reproductive systems. Finally, Section IV outlines psychology that is relevant to clinical practice, such as communication skills and psychological interventions.

Throughout the book you will find clinically relevant information and tips in the clinical notes boxes. Activity boxes will encourage you to apply what you are learning to your own experiences. Case studies will also help you apply what you are learning to clinical scenarios, and help you to understand the impact of illness on individuals. Learning objectives and summary boxes provide easy guides to the main learning points that may prove useful for exams. Revision questions are given at the end of every chapter to help you revise and test yourself.

1.2 WHAT IS HEALTH?

As healthcare professionals you are embarking on careers that involve helping people to get better. But 'better', like 'health', is not the same for everyone. So how can we decide who to treat and who not to treat? Take a look at the examples in Case Study 1.1 and the definitions of health in Table 1.2.

Health operates on many levels such as the physical, subjective, behavioural, functional, and social. One survey of around 9,000 people found that people think of health in six different ways (Blaxter, 1990):

1. Not having symptoms of illness.
2. Having physical or social reserves.
3. Having healthy lifestyles.
4. Being physically fit or vital.
5. Psychological wellbeing.
6. Being able to function.

Which of these definitions we use will have implications for who receives treatment. Table 1.2 applies these to the cases of a fit young woman with a high risk of breast cancer (Jenny), a terminally ill man who is living life to the full (David), and a suicidal woman (Karen). It shows, for each one, who would be considered healthy and who would be considered ill using these different definitions. Common sense would suggest that the terminally ill man, David, and suicidal woman, Karen, are ill and need treatment. Yet David would be classified as ill by physical definitions of health but not by behavioural, functional or psychosocial definitions. In contrast, Karen would be classified as ill by behavioural, functional, and psychosocial definitions but not by physical ones. In fact, the only definition of health that would classify both of them as ill is the cultural norm for health – in other words, they are both outside the norm within our society for what is regarded as healthy.

These cases illustrate that 'health' is not easy to define and is very individual. Research shows that people with a terminal illness generally have a reduced quality of life. Yet quality of life is not a single entity and although people may report worse physical symptoms, pain, and disability, they may also report an increased appreciation of life and family and other positive benefits (as David's case illustrates). The suicidal woman may be particularly at risk, as research shows that young, divorced, or widowed women are

CASE STUDY 1.1   Are these people healthy or ill?

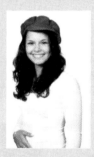

Jenny is 22 and a university student. She has a healthy diet and is a keen athlete. Her mother died of breast cancer when Jenny was 13 and Jenny's older sister has just been diagnosed with breast cancer. Screening shows that Jenny is carrying a mutation in the BRCA gene which means she is at high risk of breast cancer. She has been offered surgery to remove both breasts as a preventative measure.

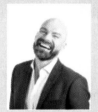

David is a businessman aged 50. He has been training to ski the 'Swiss Wall', a slope in the Alps which is notoriously difficult. David did it once when he was younger and fitter, but had to stop and inch his way down parts of it. Last week he attempted it and managed to ski all the way down without stopping. He says it was exhilarating. He has terminal liver cancer and approximately six months left to live.

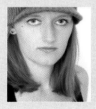

Karen is 32 and divorced with four children under the age of 7. She works part-time. Her ex-husband has remarried and has a new baby. Karen is upset about her divorce and finds it hard to maintain another steady relationship. She is depressed and smokes 30 cigarettes a day. Four weeks ago she took a large number of paracetamol with a bottle of wine and woke up in hospital.

most likely to attempt suicide, although men are more likely to succeed at completing suicide. Being depressed is a critical risk factor – in Europe, 28% of people with clinical depression will attempt suicide at some point during their lives (Bernal et al., 2007). Cases of apparently healthy people being offered interventions for genetic risk of disease are likely to become more common as screening for genetic risk becomes more widespread. Women like Jenny in the case study, who have prophylactic mastectomies, generally report a reduction in cancer-related distress afterwards, although there can be other negative impacts on their lives.

It is clear that health issues are complex and require our consideration of the individual. We need to recognise that, for individuals, health and illness are subjective states of wellbeing. In other words, does the person *feel* or *think* they are healthy or ill? Do they have physical symptoms that *they* believe mean there is a problem with their health? We also need to take account of disease in the form of underlying pathology – although research shows that a physiological basis is not found for many physical symptoms. At least a third of physical symptoms in primary care have no identifiable organic cause, and 10–15% of primary care patients have a history of multiple unexplained symptoms (Brown, 2007).

TABLE 1.2 Definitions of health

Definition	Features of definition	Are they healthy or ill?		
		Jenny	David	Karen
Physical	Absence of disease	Healthy	Ill	Healthy
	Not vulnerable to disease	Ill	Ill	Healthy
	Strong physical reserves	Healthy	Ill	Healthy
	Physically fit, has vitality	Healthy	Healthy	Ill
Subjective	No symptoms of physical illness	Healthy	Ill	Healthy
Behavioural	Living a healthy lifestyle	Healthy	Healthy	Ill
Functional	Able to function in day-to-day life	Healthy	Healthy	Ill
Psychosocial	Psychosocial wellbeing	Healthy	Healthy	Ill
Social	Able to contribute to society	Healthy	Healthy	Ill
Cultural	Matches cultural norm for health	Healthy	Ill	Ill

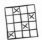

ACTIVITY 1.1   WHAT IS HEALTH?

- How would you rate your own health?

  - Very poor
  - Poor
  - Fair
  - Good
  - Excellent

- What factors were important in helping you decide where to rate your health?

We therefore need to think of health on many levels. The World Health Organisation (WHO) attempted this by defining **health** very broadly as 'a state of complete physical, mental, and social wellbeing and not merely the absence of disease or infirmity' (World Health Organisation, 1992). The value of this definition is that it is inclusive and the emphasis on wellbeing accounts for individual differences in subjective perceptions of health. However, this definition has been criticised for being too broad to be useful and for referring to a Utopian 'perfect' state that few of us will reach, even when we feel healthy.

How we define health has wide-ranging implications for the treatments provided by health services. For example, if we aim for health as defined by the WHO, it might put unrealistic pressures on countries to provide social circumstances and medical systems that mean everyone lives in a state of complete wellbeing. Others have pointed out that conceptualising health as complete wellbeing confuses happiness with health (Saracci, 1997). This opens the door to limitless treatments if people view the pursuit of happiness as a legitimate medical goal. The rapid increase in cosmetic surgery to help people feel happier with their appearance is one example of this.

The way we define health has implications for who can be seen as responsible for our health and for which treatments we offer. These implications are more than just medical and affect society's policies and laws. In the Western world, the dominant view is that individuals are responsible for their health by either adopting healthy or unhealthy lifestyles. Policies have been implemented that attempt to improve our lifestyles and health, such as providing fruit for young school children and banning smoking in public places.

A striking example of the effect that our definition of health has on treatment is the increasing numbers of obese children being put into foster care by the authorities in an attempt to combat their obesity. The story of one such girl is given in Case Study 1.2. This course of action rests on a number of debatable assumptions, including the view that: (i) obesity is an illness; (ii) obesity is controllable through diet; (iii) parental behaviour is the major cause of childhood obesity; and (iv) a child's physical health takes priority over the psychological impact of removing that child from their family.

Ultimately, the multidimensional nature of health makes finding an adequate definition difficult. Antonovsky (1987) therefore proposed that we think of **health as a continuum**

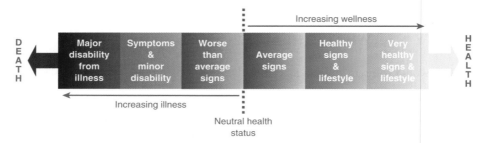

FIGURE 1.1   Illness–wellness continuum

Source: Antonovsky, 1987 – adapted from Sarafino, 2002

from optimal wellness to death, as shown in Figure 1.1. Health promotion techniques operate on the wellness side of the continuum to encourage people to choose a lifestyle that optimises their health. Medical treatment focuses on the illness side of the continuum when people show signs or symptoms of illness.

CASE STUDY 1.2   Obese child taken into care

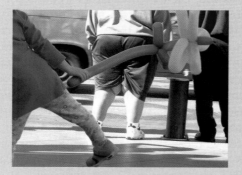

In August 2000, in a controversial case, the state of New Mexico took legal custody of a 3-year-old girl, AM, because she was morbidly obese. She was removed from her parents and put in foster care for three months. A gagging order was put on her parents so they could not talk publicly about the case for five months.

AM weighed three times more than a normal 3 year old and was 50% taller. She had undergone numerous tests to determine what was causing her increased growth but doctors could not find a medical cause.

While in foster care, AM was put on a strict diet, lost weight, and learned to walk unassisted. It is difficult to gauge the emotional impact of being taken from her parents (e.g. she stopped speaking Spanish, her father's language). After three months of legal and political wrangling, AM was returned to her parents, although the state kept legal custody of her for a while, monitoring her progress.

(Photograph reproduced courtesy of Malingering/www.flikr.com)

1.3 WHY IS PSYCHOLOGY IMPORTANT?

The importance of treating the person and not just the disease is widely recognised. Each person is a unique mix of thoughts, emotions, personality, behaviour patterns, and their own personal history and experiences. Understanding more about people will help us treat them more effectively. Psychology, however, is a subject that some students think is 'just common sense', 'interesting but I can't see how it's useful', or not 'proper medicine'. Here we will consider each of these objections in turn before looking at the science underpinning the integral nature of body and mind.

'Psychology is just common sense'

Often statements from psychological research coincide with common sense. Examples of these include 'Stress is bad for you', 'A healthy lifestyle is important', and 'People with chronic illness have a worse quality of life'. If this was all we could take from psychology, then most of us would indeed dismiss the subject as mere common sense. The value of psychological research is that:

- It *tests* common sense views empirically to confirm or disconfirm them.
- It goes *beyond* common sense.
- People don't always act according to common sense!

First, let's look at the empirical testing of common-sense views. Much common sense is in fact contradictory. For example, the proverbs 'Too many cooks spoil the broth' and 'Many hands make light work' contradict each other. In some cases psychological research has confirmed common-sense views, although in other cases it has rejected these. Examples of common-sense views that have been tested by research are given in Box 1.1 – take a look at these statements and make up your own mind about whether these are facts or myths.

In fact, statements 1, 3, and 4 in Box 1.1 have not been supported by research. In contrast, there *is* evidence that antioxidants can reduce the impact of some eye disorders (e.g. slow down age-related macular degeneration; Grover & Samson, 2014), that ginger can reduce nausea and vomiting in pregnancy (Dante et al., 2013), and that the majority of sexual violence towards women and men is carried out by men (Breiding et al., 2014). Research therefore not only challenges common sense but also examines the things that go beyond common knowledge, such as why depression puts people at a higher risk of heart disease, whether there are critical periods in development when babies are more sensitive to psychosocial or biological circumstances, and whether therapy for psychological disorders should try to change *what* people think or the *relationship* people have with their thoughts. There are many other examples of this that you will read about throughout the course of this book.

BOX 1.1   Common sense: fact or myth?

1. Taking vitamin C prevents colds.
2. The majority of domestic violence is committed by men.
3. Being an oldest, middle, or youngest child affects your personality.
4. People with schizophrenia are often violent.
5. Eating fruit and vegetables improves your eye health.
6. Ginger reduces nausea and vomiting in pregnancy.

Sources: 1. Douglas et al., 2007; 2. Breiding et al., 2014; 3. Rohrer et al., 2015; 4. Large et al., 2011; 5. Grover & Samson, 2014; 6. Dante et al., 2013.

'Psychology is interesting but not useful'

Most people will find at least some parts of psychology interesting, but that does not necessarily mean it is useful. We need to ask what exactly it means in medicine for something to be useful. If the goal in medicine and healthcare is to treat people effectively and restore them to health, then what does this involve and how can psychology help? In order to treat people effectively we need to be able to: (i) diagnose the problem accurately and (ii) treat that problem appropriately. Psychology can help in both these areas. Accurate diagnoses are more likely if we understand how people's experiences shape their perception and reporting of symptoms, and help-seeking behaviours (see Chapter 4). Negotiating an acceptable and effective treatment plan rests on understanding decision-making processes, what makes people more likely to adhere to treatment, and the influence of people's beliefs and emotions (see Chapter 17). In illnesses such as HIV, where there is no complete cure, behaviour change is crucial for limiting the spread of disease (see Chapter 15). Effective communication skills also help in making an accurate diagnosis and in agreeing appropriate treatment for each individual (see Chapter 18). Thus, understanding psychological and social processes will help us diagnose and treat people more effectively.

Psychology can also help us to understand psychological *symptoms*, such as anxiety and depression, which can range from mild to severe, as well as *diagnostic disorders*, such as panic disorder, major depressive disorder, or schizophrenia. In the UK, psychological symptoms of anxiety and depression account for approximately 9% of consultations in general practice (Office for National Statistics, 2000). However, the majority of people with psychological symptoms will present with physical symptoms (Kroenke, 2003a). One study asked primary care physicians in the UK to rate the content of 2,206 consultations and found that, in addition to consultations for psychological symptoms, another 30% of consultations were rated as involving some psychological content (Ashworth et al., 2003).

Evidence shows there is a strong link between physical health and psychological health: if we concentrate on only one side, we risk missing important information and prescribing ineffective treatments. For example, chronic illness is associated with increased rates of psychological disorders (Cooke et al., 2007). People with psychological disorders are also at an increased risk of illness. A study of 4,864 people in the USA found that anxiety, depression, psychological distress, substance use disorders, and use of healthcare services were associated with experiencing more physical symptoms, regardless of whether these symptoms had an identifiable physical cause (Escobar et al., 2010). Psychological interventions, such as cognitive behaviour therapy (CBT), can be effective in managing or treating illnesses that have physical and psychological components, such as obesity, chronic pain, irritable bowel syndrome, and addiction (see Chapters 11 to 16), as well as psychological disorders, such as bipolar disorder, personality disorder, and schizophrenia (see Chapters 16 and 19).

Although psychological knowledge can help us be more effective healthcare practitioners, many students are put off psychology because of a sense that it is 'interesting, but there's no right answer'. Psychology can appear abstract or ambiguous with many competing theories. The reasons for this are that when studying people we must deal with outcomes like behaviour that are influenced by many factors. Explanatory theories are therefore tested by using a range of research methods and statistics to try to identify which factors are the most important. This means psychology will often present students with competing theories and supporting or conflicting evidence (and this book is no exception!). The ambiguity or uncertainty this involves may contrast directly with the large amount of physiological and anatomical facts students are required to learn in the first few years of their training.

So psychology requires a different way of thinking, but this method of thinking is a useful skill in itself – and one that is essential in medical practice. A lot of medical practice is about dealing with uncertainty, often in the face of patients who want certainty. For example, people will rarely present with a clearly defined textbook set of symptoms. In trying to diagnose and treat a person, you will often have to form a hypothesis about what might be wrong, then find a way to test it, and then reformulate your hypothesis if the tests do not confirm it. Understanding the psychosocial context of a person's symptoms and concerns will help you reach a more probable diagnosis and/or provide reassurance in the face of uncertainty. For example, there are still many medical conditions that do not have suitable tests to confirm them. Examples include chronic fatigue syndrome and irritable bowel syndrome (see Chapter 13). As with psychological learning, these conditions involve a tolerance of ambiguity and an openness to alternative explanations, particularly in the early stages of diagnosis and treatment.

'Psychology is not real medicine'

Most students will come to their medical studies keen to learn about the workings of the body, how it goes wrong, and how to fix it. Learning about the heart and how to resuscitate people is much closer to the common view of what it means to be a medical doctor than learning about topics such as health behaviour and stress. This implies a mechanical view of the body and medicine. Such a view is not new: it stems from a belief in dualism, according to which the mind and body are independent. Dualism has its roots in classical philosophy and was reinforced by later thinkers, such as René Descartes (1637). Focusing on the mechanics of the body enabled rapid advances in medicine during the 18th and 19th centuries. Medical understanding grew exponentially as doctors and researchers focused on increasingly detailed physiological processes and identified the causes of pathology. Treatment also advanced: antibiotics and vaccines were developed and anaesthesia was introduced. The disadvantage of dualism is that it provided the basis for the **biomedical approach** or model, which dominated medicine for centuries. This approach, which is examined later in this chapter, is based on a separation of body and mind that is unhelpful in many ways.

1.4 THE SCIENCE OF MIND AND BODY

Science has advanced considerably since dualism and there is now increasing evidence that the mind and body are integrally linked and important in health. Throughout this book there are examples of how our mind influences physiological factors, such as fight-flight stress responses, pain, and physical symptoms. Cognitive science and neuroscience have also challenged dualism by showing that the mind (e.g. thoughts, feelings) is influenced by our body and bodily experiences. Theories of embodied cognition propose that many aspects of cognition are influenced by our bodily state. These cognitive factors include memory making and recall, tasks such as decision making and judgement, as well as higher level mental constructs such as concepts and language. Bodily factors that influence cognition include the motor system (e.g. movement, posture), perceptual system (e.g. sight, hearing), and physical interactions with others and the environment.

Theories of embodied cognition rest on research from areas like psychology, neuroscience, linguistics, and artificial intelligence. Psychological research has shown that sensorimotor feedback can influence our thoughts and emotions (Niedenthal, 2007). Many of these studies artificially place a person in a particular posture and examine the effect of this posture on thoughts, feelings, and behaviour. For example, research into feedback from facial expressions gets people to activate smile muscles by holding a pencil between their teeth and shows that when people 'smile' they are more likely to rate cartoons as funny, remember positive memories, evaluate stories more positively, and are quicker to perceive things that are congruent with a positive emotional state (Arminjon et al., 2015). Facial feedback has also been shown to reduce stress responses like heart rate and skin conductance (Lee et al., 2013), and increase recovery from stress (Kraft & Pressman, 2012).

The importance of bodily feedback in how we think and feel extends beyond an individual. Social psychologists have looked at how rapport between people is embodied through mirroring each other's posture and gestures (interpersonal synchrony). A review and meta-analysis of the research on interpersonal synchrony shows it leads to people having more prosocial attitudes and behaviours, such as perceived affiliation, cooperation, and helping behaviours (Rennung & Göritz, 2016).

Functional brain imaging has identified some of the physiological processes that under-lie this. It is now clear that other people's actions can influence neuronal activity in our brains and that animals and humans have mirror neurons which fire both when we carry out a specific act and when we see others performing the same action. So our minds respond to observed movements of others as if we were carrying out the same behaviour. Similarly, recognising someone else's facial expression of an emotion and feeling that emotion ourselves involve overlapping neural circuits in the brain (Niedenthal, 2007).

The science of mind and body has therefore moved beyond simple separation of mind and body to show that they are interdependent and influence each other in numerous ways, as does our environment and the people around us. This science has informed devel-opments in artificial intelligence and robotics, where artificial humans are being created with socio-emotional intelligence, such as virtual characters that facilitate interaction between humans and technology by interpreting and responding to nonverbal cues (Vogeley & Bente, 2010). This is also being used in healthcare interventions, such as using virtual characters to assess and train people with high-functioning autism to recognise nonverbal communication cues (Georgescu et al., 2014).

1.5 DIFFERENT APPROACHES TO MEDICINE AND HEALTHCARE

1.5.1 BIOMEDICAL APPROACH

The biomedical approach to healthcare is based on a dualistic approach to mind and body so is not consistent with current science and evidence. The biomedical approach is sum-marised in Figure 1.2. It assumes that all disease can be explained in terms of physiological processes: therefore the treatment acts on the disease and not on the person. There is a linear progression of causality from the pathogen to the person and not the other way around. Psychological and social processes are separate and incidental. The person as a whole is therefore not considered by the biomedical approach.

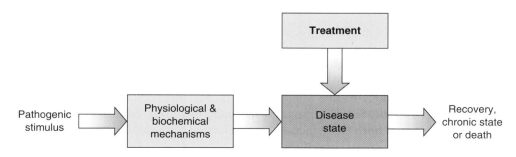

FIGURE 1.2 Biomedical approach to health (adapted from Lovallo, 2004)

Although this view has dominated medicine and led to great advances, it has been criticised for many reasons, in particular that it does not consider the influence of (i) social or (ii) psychological factors on health. Historically, the influence of social factors on population health is clear. Let us take the example of infectious diseases. The rapid decline in deaths from infectious diseases in the UK between 1859 and 1978 occurred *before* most vaccines were introduced. Some of the reason for this can be explained by more effective treatments, but a lot was due to changes in people's understanding of illness and the effect of lifestyle. For example, in the mid-1800s a physician, John Snow, noticed that patterns of cholera outbreaks clustered around particular water supplies in London. This led to a better understanding of the cause and transmission of cholera, as well as social changes such as an improved water supply and sanitation. More recently, the Ebola epidemic in Western Africa in 2014 was partly spread by burial rites that meant the Ebola virus was transmitted from the deceased person to other members of the community. A key part of the World Health Organisation's strategy was therefore to support affected communities to ensure safe burial practices (WHO, 2014a). The examples of cholera and Ebola show how social and cultural change is important and that the reduction of infectious diseases cannot be explained on a purely biomedical basis.

Social factors are just as important today. One of the most consistent findings from public health research is the influence of social class on health. People in lower social classes are at more risk of illness (**morbidity**) and death (**mortality**) from a variety of causes (see Research Box 1.1). This increased risk is partly due to differences in lifestyles. For example, people in lower social classes have a poorer diet, harder working and living conditions, and are more likely to smoke. However, studies that examine this indicate that even after these factors are taken into account, people in lower social classes still remain at an increased risk of poor health.

The role of lifestyle in illness illustrates the importance of psychosocial factors, yet these are not considered by the biomedical model. Understanding and changing health behaviour would do more than anything else to reduce morbidity and mortality in our society (see Chapter 5). For example, one in four deaths from cancer in the UK is due to unhealthy diets and obesity (Cancer Research UK, 2010). Increased alcohol use is directly related to increased rates of liver disorders and cancers of the GI tract (see Chapter 13). Smoking is directly related to lung cancer – the third highest cause of mortality in the UK (see Chapter 12).

It is not only lifestyle that is important. Individual factors such as personality, health behaviours, and beliefs also affect health. For example, individuals who are high on the personality trait of conscientiousness are less likely to engage in risky behaviours and more likely to engage in positive health behaviours. Perhaps unsurprisingly, they are therefore also more likely to live longer (Stone & McCrae, 2007). Stress and depression are strongly implicated in a range of illnesses, including cardiovascular disease: evidence suggests that both these factors are associated with the onset of heart disease (see Chapter 12).

A good example of the effect of our beliefs on health and illness is the **placebo effect**, whereby people recover because they think they are going to recover, as opposed to

RESEARCH BOX 1.1   Social class and mortality

Background

In addition to being affected by health behaviours, morbidity and mortality rates are affected by socioeconomic status. This study looked at the effect of family socioeconomic status at birth on mortality from any cause across the lifespan.

Method and findings

The Uppsala Birth Cohort is a study of 11,868 men and women born in Uppsala, Sweden, between 1915 and 1929. This study looked at death rates in this cohort up to 2009 to examine the risk of mortality according to the family's socioeconomic position and the mother's marital status.

People born in families of lower socioeconomic status and whose mothers were unmarried had an increased risk of death from any cause (hazard ratios were 1.19 and 1.18 respectively). This increased risk was still observed after adjusting for the child's sex, birth year, birth weight, gestational age, parity, and maternal age. The effect of lower socioeconomic status on mortality was found across all age groups. However, mothers' marital status had a greater effect on mortality in the first year of life and after 75 years of age.

Significance

This study shows the lifelong impact of socioeconomic status on risk of mortality from any cause.

Juárez, S.P., Goodman, A., Koupil, I. (2016) From cradle to grave: tracking socioeconomic inequalities in mortality in a cohort of 11,868 men and women born in Uppsala, Sweden, 1915–1929. *Journal of Epidemiology and Community Health, 70*(6): 569–75.

recovering because of pharmacological or physical treatment. The placebo effect is typically tested by giving one group of people a fake drug (placebo group), and comparing their recovery to another group of people given an active drug (drug group) or no drug (control). The placebo effect is the recovery that occurs in the group given the fake drug, which is over and above any recovery observed in the control group. This effect is well established and there is evidence that beliefs are responsible for a large part of it. For example, a study of surgery for osteoarthritis compared two different types of procedure (arthroscopic debridement or lavage) with placebo surgery where people were anaesthetised and skin incisions made but the arthroscope was not inserted. Those who had placebo surgery showed the same level of improvements up to two years later (Moseley et al., 2002). A review and meta-analysis of this and seven other randomised controlled trials concluded that arthroscopic debridement does not improve pain or functional status more than sham surgery or usual care (Evidence Development and Standards, 2014). The placebo effect is considered in more detail in Chapter 4.

The biomedical approach cannot account for any of these effects of social and psychological factors on health. Even when the biomedical approach dominated medicine, most healthcare professionals realised that psychological and social factors were still important. However, working within the biomedical framework meant these factors were not made explicit or used to the advantage of medicine. They therefore remained part of the *art* of medicine rather than the *science* – although ironically the term 'medicine' comes from the Latin *medici-na* (*ars*) – the (art of) healing.

CLINICAL NOTES 1.1

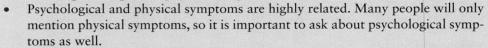

In primary care:

- At least a third of physical symptoms seen in primary care have no identifiable organic cause.
- Between 10% and 15% of primary care patients have a history of multiple unexplained physical symptoms.
- Psychological and physical symptoms are highly related. Many people will only mention physical symptoms, so it is important to ask about psychological symptoms as well.
- In treatment, a lot of the effect of drugs can be due to people believing they will recover rather than the drug itself.

1.5.2 BIOPSYCHOSOCIAL APPROACH

The **biopsychosocial approach** (Engel, 1977) is a framework that does incorporate biological, psychological, and social factors. This approach was later expanded to include such factors as ethnicity and culture (Suls & Rothman, 2004). A schematic diagram of the biopsychosocial approach is shown in Figure 1.3, which shows the personal and external factors that, according to this approach, impact on health.

External factors include the sociocultural environment, such as poverty, available support structures, access to healthcare and other facilities, and environmental factors and legislation that impact on health. External factors include pathogenic stimuli, which can range from, for example, being exposed to a virus, to passive smoking, to living in an area high in radon gas. External factors also include any treatment that the individual receives which can act on the pathogenic stimuli or the person. All of these external factors both influence the person and are influenced by the person.

Internal factors include personal history, psychosocial processes, and physiological and biochemical mechanisms. Personal history involves multiple factors such as ethnicity, genetic make-up, learned behaviour, developmental processes, and previous illnesses.

These inevitably influence psychosocial processes such as lifestyle, sociability, personality, mood, perception of symptoms, behaviour, adherence to treatment and so on. All these factors will influence, and be influenced by, physiological mechanisms.

Consider smoking, for example. Many people report that their first cigarette is fairly unpleasant, so why do people persist in smoking until they are addicted? Most people start smoking in adolescence when it is important to them to gain peer approval and fit in with group norms. In high-income countries, the prevalence of smoking is often highest in people from deprived backgrounds with a low socioeconomic status (Hiscock et al., 2012). Thus a child growing up in a deprived area may be more exposed to others who smoke and more likely to start smoking, which further reinforces the group norm. Without a motivation to quit smoking this child is also unlikely to seek help.

The pathogens in cigarettes mean that, with continued use, smokers are at increased risk of many illnesses, including lung cancer, chronic obstructive pulmonary disease, heart disease, head and neck cancer, impotence, infertility, gum disease, back pain, and type II diabetes (West & Hardy, 2007). Whether an individual develops any of these illnesses will be determined by the other aspects in the biopsychosocial approach, such as their individual vulnerability, physiological processes, other lifestyle behaviours, and exposure to other pathogens. However, to return to our example, not all children in deprived circumstances will smoke. Therefore the sociocultural environment interacts with the characteristics of each child to determine exposure to the pathogen of cigarettes, the likelihood of seeking treatment, and the risk of disease.

The biopsychosocial approach provides a clear framework that sums up what many healthcare professionals already intuitively know. It is an improvement on the biomedical approach in that it makes the links between psychological and social factors and health explicit. Illness is seen to be caused by many factors at different levels, rather than purely by pathogens as posited by the biomedical model. Responsibility for health and illness therefore rests on individuals and society rather than on the medical profession alone. Similarly, treatment considers physical, psychological and social contributing factors as opposed to the physical in isolation. A further comparison of the key features of the biomedical and biopsychosocial approaches is given in Table 1.3.

The biopsychosocial approach has implications for research, education, and clinical practice. It should lead to more comprehensive research that examines the multiple levels, systems, and factors involved in health. Moreover, in clinical practice the biopsychosocial approach should result in a more complete understanding of the many factors that can contribute to health or illness. This in turn should lead to a more **holistic approach** – that is, treatment of the whole person. The biopsychosocial approach has already formed the basis for a more person-centred approach to medicine (Borrell-Carrio et al., 2004). It should also lead to better healthcare training, with the inclusion of education about psychological and social factors.

Thus the biopsychosocial approach is an improvement on the biomedical approach and should result in clear clinical benefits if used. It is therefore puzzling that, more than 30 years after it was proposed, the biopsychosocial approach still is not widely used or practised in medicine or psychology. Although the biopsychosocial approach is taught in most training courses for healthcare professionals, it tends to be taught more as a theoretical framework than applied to clinical work.

So we still have a long way to go to properly incorporate the biopsychosocial approach into medicine. There are many reasons why this might be. The biomedical approach has been dominant for centuries and modern medicine and healthcare developed within this framework. Although the biopsychosocial approach may appear simple, in fact the inclusion of all the different elements makes research and medicine more complicated to carry out in practice. In addition, the biopsychosocial approach suggests circular or nonlinear causality. In other words, that physical, psychological, and social factors all influence, and are influenced by, each other. This means there is rarely a simple and linear cause–effect relationship between one factor and illness. This raises difficulties in clinical practice if we need to choose or prioritise one treatment (see Case Study 1.3). To do this, we have to think in terms of a hierarchy of causes (e.g. one cause is more important than others) and linearity of treatment (e.g. removing this cause will remove illness) (Borrell-Carrio et al., 2004).

CASE STUDY 1.3   Applying a biopsychosocial approach

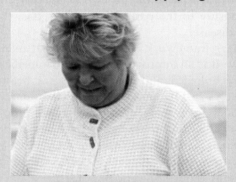

Photo courtesy of Craig Cloutier, taken 28 March 2009

Anne is a 50-year-old woman with hypertension. This hypertension could be due to Anne's high cholesterol, obesity, smoking, demanding job, lack of support at home, or perfectionist tendencies and inflated beliefs about responsibility that mean she works long hours and is stressed. Which of these explanations we adopt will influence the treatment we offer.

If we take the biological cause (high cholesterol), then we would treat Anne with cholesterol-reducing drugs. If we take the behavioural explanations (smoking and obesity), we might offer Anne support to stop smoking or lose weight. If we take the psychological explanation (stress and maladaptive beliefs), we might offer Anne stress-management or psychotherapy sessions. Finally, if we adopt the social explanations (work stress and a lack of support), we might refer her to an occupational health worker, counsellor, or a life coach.

In reality Anne's hypertension will be affected by all these factors and we need to treat her in the most effective way. To decide this, we would need to consider which treatment will provide the best outcome for Anne at the least cost and time for the health service. What do you think would constitute effective treatment in this case?

(Continued)

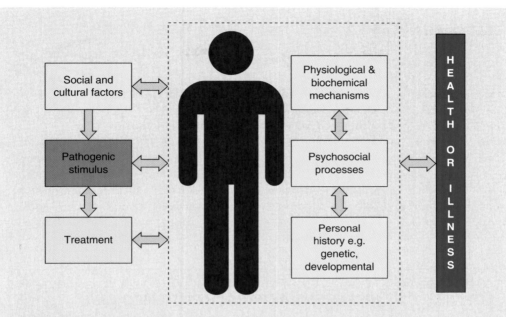

FIGURE 1.3   Biopsychosocial approach to health

TABLE 1.3   Comparison of biomedical and biopsychosocial approaches

	Biomedical	**Biopsychosocial**
Mind–body relationship	Separate; independent (dualism)	Part of dynamic system; influence each other
Cause of disease	Pathogens	Multiple factors at different levels
Causality	Linear	Circular
Psychosocial factors	Irrelevant	Essential
Approach to illness and treatment	Reductionist	Holistic
Responsibility for health	Medical professionals – e.g. to combat disease	Individuals/society – e.g. healthy lifestyle
Focus of treatment	Eradication or containment of pathology	Physical, psychological, and social factors contributing to illness
Focus of health promotion	Avoidance of pathogens	Reduction of physical, psychological, and social risk factors

CLINICAL NOTES 1.2

In clinical practice:

- Promoting healthy lifestyles is an important aspect of medicine and has the potential to save thousands of lives.
- People respond differently to illness so it's important not to assume you know how each person feels.
- Tolerance of ambiguity and the ability to test alternative explanations for symptoms are essential clinical skills.
- The holistic approach means we should consider biomedical factors, lifestyle behaviour, psychological factors (e.g. beliefs, emotions, symptoms), and social factors.

ACTIVITY 1.2   DIFFERENT APPROACHES TO MEDICINE

- Reflect on the last time you saw a doctor.
- To what extent was this doctor working with a biomedical framework or a biopsychosocial one?
- How would their treatment have differed if they'd altered their framework(s)?

We can see that barriers to applying the biopsychosocial approach include the facts that (i) it is not possible to address all the factors that influence illness, and (ii) in order to plan treatment we need to think in terms of linear causality rather than circular causality. However, this does not mean we should abandon it and return to the biomedical approach, which ignores psychosocial and environmental factors completely. There is, after all, a crucial difference between, on the one hand, recognising all potential determinants and then selectively treating an individual and, on the other hand, focusing only on biomedical factors because that's all we look at. Psychologists also need to be reminded of this. Just as medicine and other healthcare professions err toward biological explanations, psychologists err toward psychological explanations. In fact, a search of research published in a leading health psychology journal found that only 26% of studies included biological, psychological, social, and macro-cultural variables (Suls & Rothman, 2004).

Therefore we all need to consciously remind ourselves to explore factors at each level of the biopsychosocial approach when assessing and treating people. This will give us a more complete understanding of the illness, encourage an holistic treatment of the person, include a consideration of potential psychosocial barriers to treatment efficacy, and allow us to change or modify treatments accordingly if our first approach is not as effective as expected.

This tendency to focus on biology or psychology emerges in debates about nature and nurture. Some argue strongly that nature (i.e. genes) is the determinant of behaviour and wellbeing. Others argue just as strongly that nurture (i.e. environment and psychosocial context) is the main determinant. The problem with many **nature–nurture debates** is that health and wellbeing are determined by nature *and* nurture. Furthermore, interactions between nature and nurture are often crucial. As noted in Chapter 16, the likelihood of developing psychological disorders such as schizophrenia may be influenced by a genetic predisposition *and* experiences during pregnancy/birth, early childhood, or later life. Similarly, material presented in Chapter 8 shows how the cognitive potential children inherit in their genes can be optimised or impaired by psychosocial experiences in childhood.

The evolving field of **epigenetics** focuses on how environmental factors – including social contextual factors – regulate the activity and expression of genes (Kundakovic & Champagne, 2015). There is emerging evidence that environmental influences such as a lack of nurturing can lead to physiological changes that can then be passed from parents to children and grandchildren; this is sometimes termed the **intergenerational transmission of vulnerability**. It has led some to suggest that health communication and health education could incorporate epigenetics to explain how parenting practices, lifestyle factors, and social environments affect different people in different ways (McBride & Koehly, 2017). Better knowledge of epigenetic processes could help the planning of public health interventions so that they are delivered at key times when environmental exposures most strongly influence gene expression.

1.6 SOCIAL DIVERSITY AND HEALTH

Within any population, there is wide variation in health behaviours and health outcomes along the lines of age, sex, education, socioeconomic status (SES), ethnicity (sometimes referred to as 'race'), sexual orientation, and other demographic variables.

Health status is more than simply a consequence of biological, physiological, or genetic factors; it is also affected by much broader economic, social, cultural, and environmental elements. The conditions in which people are born, grow up, and live influence their health (WHO, 2008b). Research in different countries has revealed that the general sociopolitical context (social democratic, corporatist, or welfare state) and levels of gender equity affect health outcomes and health-related behaviours such as alcohol use (Bambra et al., 2009; Bosque-Prous et al., 2015). **Socioeconomic status** (**SES**) influences health behaviours and health outcomes, including mortality. Poor health and poverty go hand in hand (Centers for Disease Control and Prevention, 2014; El-Sayed et al., 2011; Wang & Beydoun, 2007). People with lower levels of education and/or income tend to report less healthy patterns of behaviour, report poorer physical and psychological wellbeing, and have shorter life expectancy (Bleich et al., 2012; Braveman & Gottlieb, 2014).

Ethnicity is an important influence on health behaviours and health outcomes, and people from ethnic minorities tend to have poorer health. Some research indicates that our understanding of risk factors may be blind to the important influence of ethnicity.

For example, a 13-year follow-up study of nearly 60,000 Canadians revealed that the risk of diabetes was significantly higher among people of south Asian, black, or Chinese ethnicity than among white adults (Chiu et al., 2011). Furthermore, the risk of diabetes for a white person with a Body Mass Index (BMI) of 30 (the lower boundary of the 'obese' category) was comparable to that of south Asian, black and Chinese people with much lower BMIs at the boundary between 'healthy' and 'overweight'. This highlights a need for ethnicity-specific BMI targets and prevention strategies. In addition to considering how ethnicity interacts with physiological factors to influence disease onset and progression, it is important to consider whether health services and individual health professionals are aware of, and responsive to, cultural diversity (Memon et al., 2016).

Sex and gender also have an influence on health and health outcomes. Statistics reveal some stark differences between women's and men's health. In nearly every country, life expectancy is several years shorter for men than for women. This difference is strongly influenced by patterns of behaviour such as smoking, alcohol use, and poor diets, which are linked to chronic conditions such as cardiovascular disease, diabetes, and some cancers (White et al., 2011; WHO, 2014b, 2014c). In addition, women are more likely than men to engage in screening behaviours or to consult health professionals for psychological or physical concerns (Hing & Albert, 2016; White et al., 2011). Such sex differences should not simply be interpreted as the result of biological differences. The health of men living in different countries can vary greatly, and the health of women within the same country (e.g. women of different ethnicity) can also vary greatly (Bambra et al., 2009; Thümmler et al., 2009; White et al., 2011).

People often use the terms 'sex' and 'gender' interchangeably, but they have quite distinct meanings. Sex and sex differences are biologically based: they refer to comparisons between people who are biologically female and people who are biologically male. Gender refers to the social construction of femininities and masculinities through 'feminine' and 'masculine' behaviours. Of course there are some basic biological characteristics that distinguish all men from all women, but femininity is not a single thing – compare Margaret Thatcher and Marilyn Monroe – and nor is masculinity a single thing – compare Genghis Khan and Freddie Mercury. Some have argued that gender is better conceptualised as a verb than a noun: femininity is not something that women *have*, but something that they *do* (West & Zimmerman, 1987). Many social behaviours – including types of jobs, expressions of emotion, and competitiveness – have clear links to traditional definitions of gender.

Furthermore, many health-related behaviours have clear gender stereotypes: boys and men are encouraged to take risks and not to show weakness, whereas women are often expected to take care of themselves and others (Courtenay, 2000). This helps to explain within-sex differences in health that cannot be explained by biological differences. For example, men who believe more in 'traditional' definitions of masculinity are more likely to engage in unhealthy 'masculine' behaviours, such as excessive alcohol consumption, and less likely to engage in healthy 'feminine' behaviours, such as healthy eating and consulting health professionals about physical or psychological wellbeing (Addis & Mahalik,

2003; de Visser & McDonnell, 2013; Gough & Conner, 2006; Mahalik et al., 2006). Furthermore, health professionals' beliefs about masculinity and femininity can influence how they respond to men's and women's emotional distress (Möller-Leimkuhler, 2002).

Health behaviours and health outcomes also vary along the lines of **sexual identity**. People who identify as Lesbian, Gay, Bisexual, or Transgender – often abbreviated as **LGBT** – tend to have poorer psychological wellbeing and are more likely to attempt or complete suicide (O'Brien et al., 2016). LGBT people are also more likely to report smoking, drinking alcohol excessively, or using illicit drugs, and are also more likely to experience and report barriers to using health services (Conron et al., 2010). Important reasons for poorer wellbeing and less healthy behaviour among LGBT people include minority stress, and responses to stress arising from prejudice, discrimination, and violence (Hughes, 2016). Furthermore, many LGBT people may avoid health services because health professionals do not understand their specific needs or because they feel marginalised by health professionals' heteronormative assumptions (i.e. unquestioningly assuming that heterosexuality is a given and is normal instead of being one of many possibilities).

It is clear that health is shaped by a range of demographic variables. Each of these may be important in its own right and may also intersect with other variables. This concept of **intersectionality** was first introduced in the context of social justice (Crenshaw, 1991), but it has spread to influence social studies of health and illness. Awareness of intersectionality draws attention to the ways in which age-, sex-, gender-, ethnicity-, sexuality- or SES-based inequalities can combine to magnify inequalities in health behaviours and health outcomes (Mereish & Bradford, 2014). When designing and providing health services we must be responsive to diversity and intersectionality.

Summary

- It is difficult to define health. The choice of definition has implications for medical practice and society.
- No single definition of health is adequate and it is perhaps easier to think of health and illness on a continuum from complete wellness to death.
- The separation of psychology and medicine was initially founded on the mind–body divide (dualism).
- Contemporary research challenges dualism by showing that the mind and body are interdependent and influence each other in many ways.
- Medicine was dominated by the biomedical approach for many years but it assumes a mind–body split so cannot account for contemporary research evidence.
- The more recent biopsychosocial approach has the capacity to unify disciplines in theory and practice, and encourage a holistic approach to medicine.

CONCLUSION

In this chapter we have looked at how health is difficult to define and for individuals health is subjective in terms of whether they feel or think they are healthy or ill. It is therefore important to consider psychological and social factors for a number of reasons. First, a substantial proportion of people seen by healthcare professionals have no identifiable physical cause for their symptoms. Second, there is substantial evidence for the importance of psychological and social factors in both the onset, spread, and treatment of diseases, such as Ebola. Third, elements of social diversity and intersectionality are also associated with health and health outcomes.

Historically, the lack of focus on psychosocial factors in healthcare was perpetuated by a widespread belief in mind–body separation (dualism) and the pervasiveness of the biomedical approach. Developments in psychological sciences and neuroscience have shown how the mind and body are integrally linked. Research on embodied cognition and emotion shows how bodily sensations influence our thoughts and feelings, as do the actions of people around us. Epigenetics shows how environmental factors regulate the activity and expression of genes, and there is evidence that psychosocial factors during pregnancy and early childhood influence long-term health and can lead to an intergenerational transmission of vulnerability (see Chapters 8 and 14).

The biopsychosocial approach is consistent with current evidence and shows that we need to consider biological, psychological, social, and macro-cultural factors in health and healthcare. This will lead to a more complete understanding, more accurate and appropriate treatment, and a holistic approach to treating people.

FURTHER READING

Llewellyn, C.D. et al. (eds) (2018) *The Cambridge Handbook of Psychology, Health and Medicine* (3rd edition). Cambridge: Cambridge University Press. Includes short chapters on social, cultural, and ethnic factors and health, health inequalities, socioeconomic status, and medically unexplained symptoms.

Frankel, R.M., Quill, T.E. & McDaniel, S.H. (eds) (2009) *The Biopsychosocial Approach: Past, Present, Future*. Rochester: University of Rochester Press. A comprehensive, edited book on the biopsychosocial approach, clinical applications, patient-centred clinical methods, educational/administrative issues, and the future of this approach.

White, P. (ed.) (2005) *Biopsychosocial Medicine: An Integrated Approach to Understanding Illness*. Oxford: Oxford University Press. Edited book based on experts discussing the application of the biopsychosocial approach in medicine.

REVISION QUESTIONS

1. Describe three specialisms in psychology and outline how they are relevant to healthcare.

2. Outline four different definitions of health.

3. Compare and contrast two definitions of health. What are the implications of each definition for treatment?

4. What is dualism? How has it influenced medicine?

5. Describe the biomedical approach to medicine and outline the strengths and weaknesses of this approach.

6. Describe the biopsychosocial approach to medicine and outline the strengths and weaknesses of this approach.

7. Compare and contrast the biomedical and biopsychosocial approaches to medicine.

8. Explain what is meant by 'intersectionality' and why it is an important influence on health outcomes.

SECTION I

PSYCHOLOGY AND HEALTH

2 MOTIVATION, EMOTION, AND HEALTH

(Continued)

Case studies

Figures

Research box

LEARNING OBJECTIVES

This chapter is designed to enable you to:

- Describe motivation and discuss how it affects health.
- Outline the different components of emotion.
- Appreciate the role of positive and negative emotions in health.
- Consider whether expressing emotion is good or bad for health.

Motivation, emotion, and the way we respond to stress shape our lives in many ways. Emotions are powerful motivators that can even make us risk our lives in extreme cases, such as when parents risk their lives trying to save their children. In medicine and other healthcare professions we are surrounded by stressful and emotional events as people face illnesses and death, either their own or others. How people respond to these situations varies hugely and there are many examples in healthcare of people behaving in ways we might not understand. For example, the woman in Case Study 2.1 was prepared to risk her own and her unborn baby's life rather than have a caesarean section.

The media are full of similar examples: parents refusing life-saving treatment for their child on religious grounds; a man with liver cirrhosis who continues to drink alcohol even though he knows it will kill him; a pregnant woman with cancer who refuses chemotherapy and then dies just after her daughter is born; a teenage girl who cuts her arms with a razor blade. These are real cases that illustrate the importance of beliefs, motivation, and emotion in how people respond to day-to-day stress and extreme situations. They also illustrate the complex interaction between motivation and emotion. In this chapter we shall look at motivation and emotion in turn, examining what these are, and how they are relevant to health.

CASE STUDY 2.1   Refusing life-saving treatment

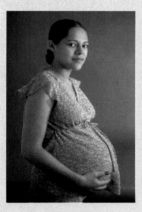

Ms S was a 29-year-old single woman who did not see a doctor for the majority of her pregnancy. When she was 36 weeks pregnant she registered with a doctor, who found she had severe pre-eclampsia – a life-threatening condition marked by high blood pressure, which can develop very quickly and lead to the death of the mother and baby. Women with this condition are usually admitted to hospital immediately, and the baby is delivered by inducing labour or performing a caesarean section. However, Ms S repeatedly refused to be admitted to hospital despite two doctors recommending it. She insisted that she wanted to give birth naturally in a barn in the countryside. When told that she and the baby might die, Ms S responded 'so be it'.

The doctors called in a social worker, who concluded that Ms S had 'little interest in her own survival and certainly none in the survival of her baby'. Ms S talked of punishing her ex-boyfriend and hoping he felt guilty if she died. The social worker and doctors therefore admitted Ms S to a psychiatric hospital against her will. Although a psychiatrist judged her mentally competent, Ms S was then quickly transferred to a nearby hospital and a court application was made to perform an emergency caesarean section. The court granted the injunction and Ms S was forced to have a caesarean section. Her daughter was born healthy.

Ms S took her case to the High Court. Her admission to hospital and caesarean section were deemed unlawful and she was awarded financial compensation. The judge acknowledged that the social worker and doctors appeared to be well-motivated, but concluded that women have the right to refuse operations even if they risk their own life or that of their baby. Ms S argued that she did not want a hospital birth because she did not like medical procedures and was prepared to risk both her own and her daughter's life because she felt very strongly about it.

Photograph © Johanna Goodyear/Fotolia

2.1 MOTIVATION

2.1.1 WHAT IS MOTIVATION?

Motivation is essentially a drive to act. People are motivated to do (or, indeed, not do) things in their life by many different factors. Because of this, theories from various areas of psychology and other disciplines are relevant. These include health behaviour (see Chapter 5) and decision making (see Chapter 17). Some motives are biological – for example, the desire to eat, drink, or reproduce. Others are more psychological and social – for example, the drive for achievement and status. Box 2.1 gives some examples of biological and social motives, although it is worth noting that the distinction between biological and social motives is not clear cut. For example, sexual motives can be both biological (the drive to reproduce) and social (e.g. the need for affiliation and nurturance).

BOX 2.1   Examples of motives

Biological motives

 Hunger
 Thirst
 Sex
 Temperature: need for appropriate temperature
 Excretory: need to eliminate bodily wastes
 Sleep and rest
 Activity: need for optimal stimulation/arousal
 Aggression

Social motives

 Achievement: need to excel
 Affiliation: need for social bonds
 Autonomy: need for independence
 Nurturance: need to nourish and protect others
 Dominance: need to influence or control others
 Exhibition: need to make an impression on others
 Order: need for orderliness, tidiness, organisation
 Play: need for fun, relaxation, amusement

(adapted from Weiten, 2004)

Theories of motivation can be separated into three broad categories, namely drive theories, evolutionary theories, and incentive theories. **Drive theories** use the concept of homeostasis to explain motivation. Homeostasis is a state of physiological equilibrium or stability that organisms strive to maintain. An organism's behavioural and physiological systems operate together to ensure the stability in bodily functions that is necessary to survive. A lack of equilibrium between our current state and our needs creates an internal tension which we are motivated to reduce.

Drive theory is most easily applied to biological drives such as hunger. When we are hungry we are motivated to find food and eat. We are also more likely to think about food and notice food-related stimuli like advertisements for food (Berry et al., 2007). Some studies even suggest that hungry men find heavier women more attractive (Swami & Tovee, 2006) and that this preference for heavier women is driven by the availability of critical resources, such as food and money, in different cultures (Nelson & Morrison, 2005). Drive theory would predict that once we have eaten we are no longer motivated to continue eating. However, although this is usually the case, there are many examples of people continuing to eat when they are no longer hungry and vice versa. Dieting provides a good example of where a drive to eat is not acted on (see Chapter 13). Thus drive theory can account for some biological drives and motivation but is limited in its application to a lot of human behaviour.

Evolutionary theories of motivation argue that social characteristics are shaped by processes of natural selection in the same way as physical characteristics: desirable social characteristics maximise the chances of reproductive success. Thus social motives, such as the need for achievement, affiliation or dominance, are thought to occur because they increase our chances of survival and reproduction. There is some evidence to support this. For example, there is some evidence that when women are at the most fertile point of their menstrual cycle they rate men who are physically masculine and apparently healthy as more attractive (Jones et al., 2008). However, this evidence is inconsistent and it might only be the case if women are asked to rate men as mates in the short term (Little & Jones, 2012). If women are asked to rate men as *long-term* mates this effect disappears completely, indicating that decisions about long-term partners are based on other criteria (Little & Jones, 2012). Evolutionary theories would explain this as long-term mates being chosen on the basis of criteria such as their ability to support and protect a family.

Incentive theories emphasise the role of external factors that trigger and regulate motivation. For example, a man may not be motivated to seek a relationship until he meets a woman he finds particularly desirable. More elaborate incentive theories take into account **expectations** and **values,** which are common in models of health behaviour (see Chapter 5). Expectancies and values allow for the influence of whether people (i) expect to attain their goal, and (ii) how important or valuable that goal is to them. Therefore, when a man meets a woman he finds very desirable he will not act on his desire if he thinks (i) that there is no chance she will be interested in him or (ii) that he does not really value having a relationship at that stage in his life.

These different theories of motivation are not incompatible. Drive theories emphasise internal states as motivating us whereas incentive theories emphasise external stimuli and rewards. The two can be thought of as push and pull theories of motivation: internal states push us to act and external stimuli pull us. However, all these theories are reductionist in one form or another because they concentrate solely on internal, external, or genetic causes. A more comprehensive theory is PRIME theory (West & Brown, 2013), which looks at determinants of addiction and considers a person's motivation, emotions, impulses, evaluations, and plans as important in addictive behaviours. PRIME theory is examined in more detail in Chapter 5.

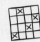

ACTIVITY 2.1 MOTIVATION

- How would different theories explain the motives of Ms S in Case Study 2.1? She refused a caesarean even though it put both her own and her baby's life at risk.

2.2 MOTIVATION AND HEALTH

Clearly, motivation is relevant to health and healthcare professionals. Understanding biological motivations can help us treat abnormal extremes of biological drives, such as obesity, eating disorders, smoking, addiction, risky sexual behaviour, and insomnia. Understanding social motivations can help us comprehend our own behaviour and what motivates us to work as healthcare professionals. It can also help us empathise and deal better with other people's behaviour that we might not understand. Knowing more about another person's motives means we can address situations more constructively. Interventions such as motivational interviewing have been developed to treat disorders with a strong motivational component, such as addiction. Motivational interviewing is defined as 'a collaborative conversation style for strengthening a person's own motivation and commitment to change' (Miller & Rollnick, 2013). It is effective in encouraging and promoting behaviour changes in drug, alcohol, nicotine use, and risky sexual behaviours (Llewellyn, 2017), and is an effective adjunct to standard treatment (Hettema et al., 2005).

Motivation is relevant to many health topics. These include smoking, which is discussed in Chapter 5, and obesity, which we look at in Chapter 13. Here we focus on alcohol use because it is a good example of complex motives preventing people changing their drinking behaviour. Alcohol consumption and alcohol-related problems are high in developed countries. Rates of consumption per capita are shown in Figure 2.1. Alcohol-related diseases account for almost 6% of deaths worldwide, and 5% of the global disease burden (World Health Organisation, 2014b). Harmful use of alcohol is the leading risk factor for death in males aged 15 to 59 worldwide, but alcohol consumption in women is also a concern because it is increasing steadily in countries with economic development where women's gender roles are less traditional (WHO, 2014b). Increased alcohol consumption inevitably affects morbidity and mortality. In the UK there has been a dramatic increase in deaths from liver cirrhosis and alcohol disorders over the last 50 years. However, in most developed countries alcohol consumption now remains stable or is decreasing (WHO, 2014b). There is more information on alcohol use in Chapter 13.

The motivation to drink alcohol involves both biological and social factors. As with many activities that become habitual, drinking alcohol is usually pleasurable. For many people the immediate feeling or reward they get from drinking alcohol outweighs the long-term risks, especially when those risks seem removed or unlikely. The common bias of **health optimism** means that most people will consistently underestimate their own risk of disease compared to others. This is especially the case in young adults (Madey & Gomez, 2003). Therefore the long-term negative consequences are minimised and outweighed by short-term pleasure or

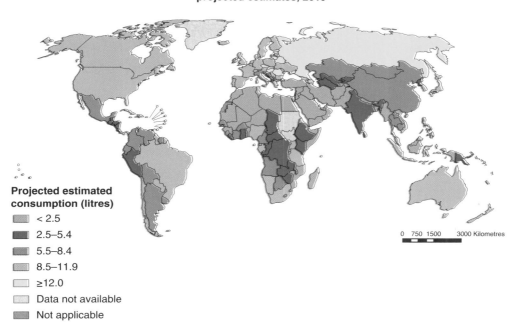

Total alcohol per capita (>15 years of age) consumption, in litres of pure alcohol, projected estimates, 2015

Projected estimated consumption (litres)

- < 2.5
- 2.5–5.4
- 5.5–8.4
- 8.5–11.9
- ≥12.0
- Data not available
- Not applicable

0 750 1500   3000 Kilometres

FIGURE 2.1   Alcohol consumption worldwide

Reprinted from Total alcohol per capita (age 15+ years) consumption, Data sets of FAO and United Nations Statistics Division, 2010 © WHO

gain. Drinking alcohol is also a part of many social rituals and norms. Changing a habitual behaviour such as alcohol consumption is difficult, particularly when it is longstanding and associated with social functions. Case Study 2.2 provides an example of using motivational interviewing with a woman who has an alcohol problem and wants fertility treatment.

CASE STUDY 2.2   Treating alcohol misuse with motivational interviewing

Kate is a 37-year-old senior executive in the music industry. She works 12 hour days and finds it hard to unwind. In the evening she drinks wine to relax. She often has to entertain clients at lunch and will also drink alcohol on these occasions. Her total alcohol consumption is more than three times the recommended maximum. Kate does not think she has an alcohol problem. Many of her friends and colleagues also drink every day.

Kate has been trying to get pregnant for 10 months without success. She knows the chances of getting pregnant decrease with age and wants fertility treatment. Kate's periods

(Continued)

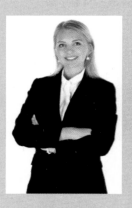

are irregular and she is worried it might be signs of an early menopause. Heavy drinking is associated with disruption to the menstrual cycle and poor fertility, so it is possible this is influencing Kate's situation. She needs to reduce her alcohol intake substantially for it to be within safe levels.

Motivational interviewing

Motivational interviewing rests on the principle of not judging or imposing our own views on Kate but instead trying to understand her situation and helping her harness her own motivation to change.

1   Exploring Kate's reasons for drinking and whether she has any ambivalence brings up the following:

Motives for drinking	Motives against
It helps me relax	I want to get pregnant
I like it – it is my treat	I like it at the time but not afterwards
It switches my brain off	It is not good for me
Entertaining is part of my job	I don't want people to see me as a 'drinker'

2   Making these ambivalent motives explicit leads Kate to re-evaluate her drinking. It also highlights the fact that falling pregnant is the most important motive for her at the moment.
3   Kate sets a goal to stop drinking. Strategies to help her achieve this are explored. For the first week she decides to replace wine with a non-alcoholic alternative and join a yoga class to help her relax. An appointment is made for one week later to review her progress and support her.

CLINICAL NOTES 2.1

Using motivation to encourage behaviour change

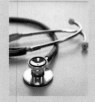

- Understanding motivation can help us treat abnormal extremes of biological drives, such as obesity, eating disorders, smoking, addiction, risky sexual behaviour, and insomnia.

(Continued)

- If you ask people about perceived negative behaviours like smoking or alcohol intake they will often under-report their behaviour.
- Educating people about the negative effects of these behaviours can trigger them to try to change.
- However, imposing our views and making people feel judged will not help them as much as assisting them to harness their own motivation.
- Try to understand why they behave in this way and empathise with their situation. Then support them to change their behaviour.
- Help them believe that they *can* change.

Summary

- Motivation is a drive to act for a range of reasons, including internal and external factors.
- Theories of motivation include drive theories, incentive theories, and evolutionary theories.
- Understanding motivational processes can be used to guide intervention for changing health-related behaviours, such as alcohol misuse.
- Theories of motivation have clinical applications.

2.3 EMOTION

Human life involves a wide range of emotions: indeed, the English language has over 550 words referring to emotion. In psychology the term **affect** is used generally to include **emotions, moods,** and **impulses.** There is cross-cultural evidence of six basic common emotions that have their own distinct physiology. These are happiness, sadness, surprise, anger, fear, and disgust (Ekman, 1992), as shown in Figure 2.2. Additions to this list, including contempt, excitement, embarrassment, love, and jealousy, have also been proposed (Ekman, 1999; Sabini & Silver, 2005).

Our emotions have a huge impact on the quality of our life. When feelings are negative, such as severe depression, this can motivate people to end their life. In healthcare settings where people face stress and personal difficulties, emotion has a huge impact on people's attitude, recovery, and quality of life. For example, one person with terminal cancer may cope with humour and a renewed zest for life, whereas another person with curable cancer may feel devastated, depressed, and convinced they will die.

Emotional disorders such as depression are one of the leading causes of burden of disease in the world and are projected by the World Health Organisation to be the top

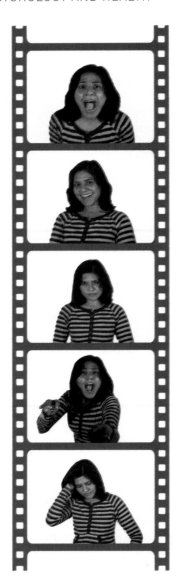
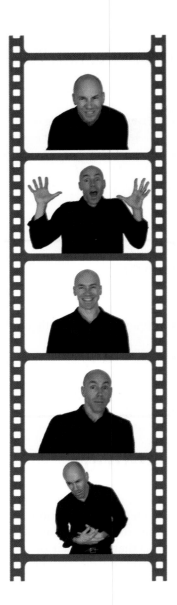

FIGURE 2.2   Facial expressions and emotions

cause of disease burden by 2030 (WHO, 2008c). The costs associated with emotional disorders are therefore huge. For example, in the UK, it was estimated that emotional disorders cost society £12 billion a year through loss of work, incapacity benefits, and absenteeism. Mental illness is also responsible for 40% of physical and mental disability (Layard, 2006). Much research and theory has therefore concentrated on negative

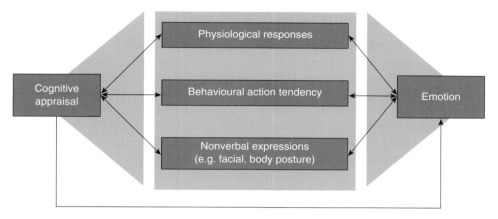

FIGURE 2.3   Components of emotions

emotions, such as anxiety and depression. The development of **positive psychology** over the last 20 years has encouraged the study of positive emotions, such as happiness, and the effect these can have on our wellbeing. There has also been research into normal emotions and their associated physiology: it is thought that they may provide a link between psychosocial factors – such as stress and social relationships – and health. Theories of emotion have therefore emerged from the study of both normal and abnormal emotional processes.

The range and complexity of emotional experiences make it difficult to define. Most theories of emotion start with the premise that emotion has three components: cognitive (thoughts), physiological, and behavioural. The **cognitive component** is the conscious experience of emotion, including the meaning we attach to it. The **physiological component** of emotions is complex and involves the central nervous system, autonomic nervous system, and endocrine system. The **behavioural component** can be further separated into the nonverbal expression of emotions (facial expression, body posture, etc.) and behavioural responses. The interplay between these components is reflected in common phrases such as 'being frozen with fear' or 'blood boiling with anger'. Figure 2.3 shows how these different elements interact to result in emotional experience.

ACTIVITY 2.2   REGULATING EMOTIONS

- Think of the last time you were really upset or angry about something.
- What things did you do to calm yourself down?
- Did this involve cognitive factors, taking action, changing behaviour, or social factors?

2.3.1 COGNITIVE COMPONENTS OF EMOTION

The *meaning* of a situation is critical to how a person responds to it emotionally. For example, if a woman finds a lump in her breast and interprets it as a harmless cyst, she will not be hugely alarmed, whereas if she interprets the lump as cancer, she will be frightened and anxious. Strong negative emotions like this will usually motivate people to take action. A review of 13 qualitative studies of why women delay getting help for breast cancer concluded that how women interpret their symptoms is the most important influence on seeking help (Khakbazan et al., 2014). Table 2.1 illustrates women's emotional responses to discovering a breast lump and how quickly they went to see their doctor (Meechan et al., 2003).

The first cognitive element of emotion is how people **appraise** a situation when it occurs, or what immediate meaning they make of it (e.g. whether it is dangerous, challenging, or harmless). A second element is how people **label** their emotional state when it occurs. The physiological arousal experienced with many emotions is similar. For example, sympathetic nervous system arousal occurs when we are anxious and excited, so how we label our emotional state will influence our emotional experience. On a roller-coaster, some people will label their experience exciting or thrilling, but some (including the authors!) will label it terrifying and aversive. This leads us to a third important cognitive element, which is whether we **evaluate** our response as positive or negative. Those people who evaluate their experience on the roller-coaster as positive will enjoy it and want to do it again.

This process of appraisal, labelling, and evaluation therefore shapes our future emotional responses as well. Panic disorder is a good example of this. Between 3% and 9% of people experience panic at some point in their lives (Grant et al., 2006). Panic is associated with extreme physiological arousal, which is part of the 'fight-flight' response (see Chapter 3). Although panic is very unpleasant, it is not life-threatening or uncommon. Thus long-term panic disorder is most likely to develop in people who interpret their initial experiences of panic in a catastrophic way, such as 'I'm going mad' or 'I'm going to die', and who label and evaluate the panic attack as extremely negative (Goldberg, 2001). Under these circumstances, people will worry about having another panic attack. This

TABLE 2.1   Responses to discovering a breast lump (adapted from Petrie & Pennebaker, 2004)

Visited doctor <4 days after discovering lump	Visited doctor 7-90 days after discovering lump
'I felt sheer panic, I freaked out' (1 day)	'I felt fine' (7 days)
'I was worried – my hands were shaking' (1 day)	'I'm not a worrier – sometimes I'm too relaxed' (90 days)
'Scared stiff' (3 days)	'Just a little bit worried' (14 days)
'Scared – I even cried' (1 day)	'Just "oh, a lump". I was fairly blasé' (7 days)
'I felt bad – panic and worry' (2 days)	'I didn't think anything of it really' (7 days)
'I was scared, nervous and sweaty' (3 days)	'I wasn't really bothered' (21 days)

increases their anxiety levels and physiological arousal, thereby also increasing the likelihood they will experience panic again. In addition, if a person interprets the panic attack as being linked to a particular situation, they will be highly anxious when put in that situation again and may become phobic. For example, if a person has a panic attack in an MRI scanner they are likely to get more anxious when having another MRI, which in turn increases the likelihood they will experience another panic attack.

The meaning that people attach to their experience of panic can therefore result in them becoming anxious about being anxious, which becomes a self-fulfilling cycle. However, although the cognitive component is *necessary* for emotion, it is not *sufficient* on its own. Emotions are rarely consciously initiated – we cannot force ourselves to feel panic, disgust, or anger. As we have seen in Chapter 1, emotions are also embodied and the physical response that accompanies emotion (as well as motorsensory input from movement, posture, and gestures) is an important part of how we feel.

2.3.2 PHYSIOLOGICAL COMPONENTS OF EMOTION

The physiological components of emotion are initiated in the brain from a number of structures that form the **limbic system** (see Chapter 7). Elements of the limbic system control the autonomic nervous system and endocrine responses (see Chapter 3), and are involved in learning and modulating emotion. For example, the amygdala is particularly

---

BOX 2.2   The case of Phineas Gage

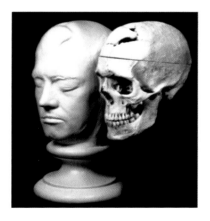

Phineas Gage was working on the railroads in 1848 when a gunpowder explosion drove a large metal rod straight through his head. The rod entered below his left cheek bone and passed through the frontal cortex before exiting and landing many metres behind him. A model of the injury he sustained is shown here. Remarkably he survived his injury and was conscious moments later.

After his injury, Gage is reported to have changed from a hardworking, kind, and likeable man to an impulsive, inconsiderate person who used frequent profanities. Up to this point, the frontal lobes were not considered to affect personality or social interaction. Gage became the first case to indicate the frontal lobes were important. Although there is some controversy over whether the damage was exclusively to the left frontal lobe or involved both lobes, it was apparent that the frontal lobe was involved in the inhibition of inappropriate emotional responses.

Image reproduced courtesy of the Warren Anatomical Museum, Francis A. Countway Library of Medicine.

important in fear. If the amygdala is damaged, animals are unable to learn fear when exposed to a threatening object. In people, imaging studies have shown the amygdala is activated during fear (Lang & Davis, 2006).

Emotion also involves areas of the **frontal cortex**. It is thought that the limbic system provides a fast initial response and the cortex then provides a slower, secondary response that regulates this initial response (Le Doux, 1996). This would explain why we often react or 'feel' before we think. The role of the cortex in inhibiting emotional and behavioural responses was first suspected in the case of Phineas Gage in Box 2.2. Research has since indicated that the orbitofrontal cortex, in particular, plays an important role in inhibiting emotional and behavioural responses. For example, damage to the orbitofrontal cortex is associated with increased anger, anxiety, pride, depression, inappropriate crying or laughing, and the impaired filtering of emotional information (Beer & Lombardo, 2007).

2.3.3 BEHAVIOURAL COMPONENTS OF EMOTION

The behavioural components of emotion can be divided into:

- Action tendencies: the potential or drive to act
- Nonverbal responses: e.g. posture, gestures
- Facial expressions

It is thought that the behavioural components of emotion are part of its purpose. In other words, emotion makes us want to act by intruding on what we are doing and taking priority. This can be clearly seen in Figure 2.4 on the faces of people observing the attack on the Twin Towers on September 11 2001. Thus emotions are early warning signals that there may be something we need to attend to. Research shows that negative emotions lead to people narrowing their focus of attention onto whatever prompted the negative emotion. Conversely, positive emotions lead to a broadening of attention, promoting broader processing of information and events (Fredrickson, 2004).

Emotions therefore direct our attention. The physiological response equips our body for action, and action tendencies provide us with ways to cope with the situation, such as fight or flight if we are under threat. The fight-flight response is certainly observable in extreme situations, but people do not always respond in this way. For example, following the 9/11 attacks, there were reports of people walking in a calm and orderly fashion to get out of the World Trade Center twin towers. Thus, people's responses to threat are more complicated and influenced by social circumstances and norms. Consequently, there has been a substantial amount of research that has examined how people regulate their emotions, and the coping strategies they use to deal with challenging circumstances (Ochsner & Gross, 2005). We shall return to this in section 2.4 on Emotion and Health.

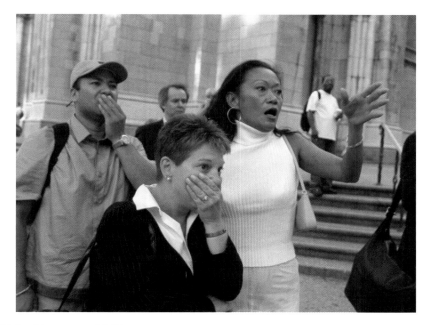

FIGURE 2.4   Observers of 9/11

Photograph reproduced courtesy of Associated Press

The behavioural component of emotion also includes the nonverbal expression of emotion in our posture, movements (e.g. clenched fists), and facial expression. Studies of embodied cognition and emotion show that sensorimotor feedback on our bodily state also affects the way we label our emotions. Research where people have been asked to tense certain facial muscles in ways that resemble a 'smile' has shown that people will report more positive emotion in response to stimuli, such as a film clip or photographs (Arminjon et al., 2015). According to the **embodied cognition hypothesis**, sensorimotor signals are used by the brain to interpret which emotion is being felt (Niedenthal, 2007).

ACTIVITY 2.3   EMBODIED EMOTION AND FACIAL FEEDBACK

- Raise your eyebrows and try to be angry.
- What happens?
- Why do you think this is?

2.3.4 THEORIES OF EMOTION

Early theories of emotion concentrated on the relationship between different components of emotion. In a chicken and egg type of debate, theorists argued about whether physical responses preceded appraisal or not. The current consensus is that appraisal processes initiate our physiological, behavioural, and conscious experience of emotion. These appraisal processes can be preconscious or conscious, which fits with the view that the limbic system is a fast-processing system (preconscious appraisal) that can be moderated later by the frontal cortex (conscious appraisal).

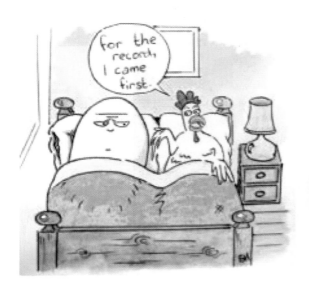

Substantial evidence confirms that preconscious processing occurs and influences our mood and behaviour. For example, Chartrand, Van Baaren and Bargh (2006) flashed positive words (e.g. friends, music), negative words (e.g. war, cancer), and neutral words (e.g. plant, building) very quickly on a screen so people could not consciously 'see' them. They found that even though people could not 'see' the words, they reported a more negative mood after being shown negative words. Other experiments have shown that if we 'see' something preconsciously, we are more likely to prefer it or feel good if it is shown to us so we can consciously see it (Monahan et al., 2000).

Theories of emotion vary in focus. One theory of emotion divides it into positive and negative affect (Watson & Tellegen, 1985). Thus all emotions can be plotted according to whether they are positive (e.g. pleasurable) or negative (e.g. distressing), and on a second dimension according to intensity (high versus low), as shown in Figure 2.5. This has the advantage of simplifying emotions so it is easier to look at relationships between emotions, health, and illness. It also accounts for the *intensity* of emotion, which may be important in the effect emotion can have on health. It is quite reasonable to assume that emotion at a low level of intensity (e.g. irritation) will have a different physiological effect and influence on health than a high-intensity emotion (e.g. extreme anger).

2.4 EMOTION AND HEALTH

A good example of the link between emotions and health is the association of psychological disorders such as clinical depression with an increased risk of morbidity and mortality. For example, there is robust evidence that depression is a risk factor for all-cause mortality and cardiac mortality in people with coronary heart disease (Fiedorowicz, 2014), so much so that depression has been specified as a risk factor for mortality by the American

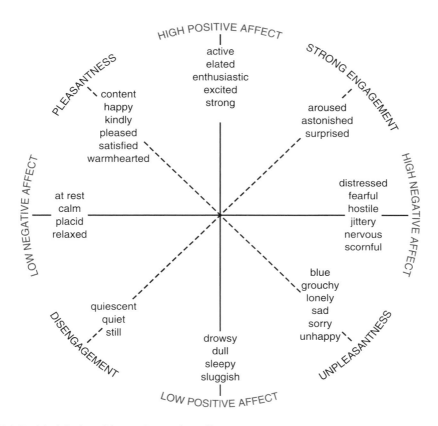

FIGURE 2.5 Model of positive and negative affect

Heart Association (Lichtman et al., 2014). Prospective epidemiology studies have also showed that depression is a risk factor for developing cardiovascular disease and mortality. A study of 5.5 million people in Denmark showed that people who had been admitted to hospital for major depression or bipolar disorder were 60% more likely to die from cardiovascular disease than the general population (Laursen et al., 2007).

In this section the nature of the relationship between emotions and health is considered in three main ways:

1. The association between normal emotions and health.
2. The influence of emotional dispositions on health.
3. The effect of how people regulate and express their emotions on health.

2.4.1 NORMAL EMOTIONS AND HEALTH

Laboratory studies show that any acute, strong, or extreme emotion is associated with increased physiological arousal regardless of whether that emotion is positive or negative.

This arousal has potentially negative effects on health through influencing systems such as the cardiovascular and immune system. However, studies of people's moods in day-to-day settings suggest that positive emotion in natural settings produces less negative physiological responses than negative emotion (Pressman & Cohen, 2005).

Large-scale epidemiological and survey studies of mood and health generally find that positive mood is associated with better health. People with high positive affect report fewer symptoms or pain and have fewer illnesses, such as strokes, colds, and accidents. In people aged 55 and over, positive affect is associated with longer life (Pressman & Cohen, 2005). A review and meta-analysis of 70 prospective studies concluded that positive affect (e.g. emotional wellbeing, positive mood, joy, happiness, vigour, energy) and positive dispositions (e.g. life satisfaction, hopefulness, optimism, sense of humour) are associated with reduced mortality in healthy people (Chida & Steptoe, 2008). Positive wellbeing is also associated with reduced mortality in people with illnesses, such as renal failure or HIV.

However, the association between happiness and health does not mean that one causes the other. Better health may mean people are more likely to be happy: happier people may be more likely to *say* they are healthier, have a stronger support network, be more likely to carry out good health practices, etc. Theories of positive affect and health outline a number of pathways through which positive affect might lead to better health. These include the Broaden and Build model (Fredrickson, 2004), which proposes that positive affect results in: (1) more healthful thought processes by broadening attention which promotes more global information processing, connections across concepts, and more forward thinking; and (2) more resilience by enhancing resources, such as coping and social relationships. Cameron and colleagues (2015) built on this model and other evidence to propose additional pathways, such as increased motivation, more responsiveness to health-related goals, better mood maintenance or repair, physiological arousal, increased self-control and resilience. They conducted a meta-analysis of 39 experimental studies where positive affect was induced in a laboratory through tasks such as watching positive film clips to examine the influence on different aspects of cognition and behaviour. However, this found no reliable effect of positive mood on health cognitions (e.g. intention to drive safely, intention to refrain from alcohol, risk perceptions, perceived control over health behaviours) or behaviour (e.g. food and alcohol consumption, exercise, smoking). The only reliable effect of positive mood was on choosing healthier food (although not reducing food consumption). So it is currently unclear exactly how positive affect results in better health and longevity.

The role of negative emotions in health has been more extensively researched with mixed results depending on which outcomes are examined. There is now substantial evidence that some types of negative emotion are associated with specific illnesses. The main examples of this are associations between anger, hostility and cardiovascular disease (Chida & Steptoe, 2009), and depression and cardiovascular disease (Fiedorowicz, 2014). Depressive disorders are associated with a range of illnesses and with mortality. For example, depressed people are 50–100% more likely to develop cardiovascular disease than healthy people (Lett et al., 2004). The role of hostility and depression in cardiovascular disease is discussed in more detail in Chapter 12.

In summary, there is evidence that positive emotions are associated with good health and that specific negative emotions are associated with certain illnesses, but there are many ways in which one may influence the other. This is often the case with links between psychosocial and biological phenomena and explains why we use terms such as **association** or **relationship**, rather than **cause** or **predict**. For example, the association between emotion and health can in part be explained by biased attention, meaning people focus more on their symptoms or, alternatively, mood influencing the way people interpret these symptoms. Possible pathways between emotion and health are summarised in Figure 2.6. The important point to note is that emotion can influence our health through biological, behavioural, and/or social mechanisms.

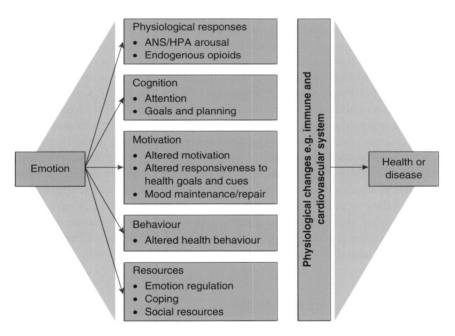

FIGURE 2.6   Pathways between emotion and health (adapted from Pressman & Cohen, 2005, and Cameron et al., 2015)

2.4.2 EMOTIONAL DISPOSITIONS AND HEALTH

Emotional dispositions are personality-like tendencies toward experiencing certain emotions. There are five main personality traits: openness to new experience, conscientiousness, extraversion, agreeableness, and neuroticism (as shown in Table 2.2). Of these, conscientiousness and neuroticism are considered more fully here because they are most consistently linked with health (Heilmayr & Friedman, 2018). **Conscientious** people are defined as having self-discipline and being efficient, organised, reliable, responsible, etc. Evidence suggests conscientious people live longer, although this is probably due to the fact that conscientious people are more likely to practise positive health behaviours, such as exercising, and less likely to practise negative health behaviours, such as smoking. However, conscientiousness is not associated with particular emotions (Heilmayr & Friedman, 2018).

Neuroticism is the personality trait with the most obvious emotional component. People who are high in neuroticism experience a wide range of negative emotions, such as low mood, anxiety, guilt, hostility, and fear. People high in neuroticism report more somatic symptoms and are more at risk of psychological disorders (Contrada & Goyal, 2005). However, it is difficult to know whether this is due to the personality trait of neuroticism or to components of neuroticism such as negative affect, depression, anxiety, and hostility. There is also no consistent link between neuroticism and measures of chronic morbidity such as heart disease, cancer, or mortality (Hielmayr & Friedman, 2018).

Emotional dispositions associated with psychological health are **optimism** and **pessimism**. Optimism is a general disposition toward expecting good things to happen in the future and pessimism is expecting bad things. These are not mutually exclusive and it is possible to be generally optimistic about most things but pessimistic about others. A commonly used measure of optimism and pessimism is shown in Box 2.3.

Optimism is associated with better psychological wellbeing and with some measures of physical wellbeing, such as better recovery from myocardial infarctions and heart surgery (Smith & MacKenzie, 2006). However, as with other dispositions or traits, it is difficult to distinguish the mechanisms involved or to be sure what role, if any, emotions play. As with conscientiousness, evidence shows that optimism is also associated with positive health behaviours, healthier coping strategies, and increased social support, which can in turn affect our responses to illness or stress (Contrada & Goyal, 2005). A review and meta-analysis of 84 studies found optimism is associated with lower premature mortality, fewer physical symptoms, lower risk of cardiovascular disease and better markers of physiological functioning (including immune function) (Rasmussen et al., 2009).

TABLE 2.2   Five main personality traits (OCEAN)

Openness to new experiences	Intellect and interest in culture. Includes characteristics such as being artistic, curious, imaginative, insightful, having wide interests, and being unconventional.
Conscientiousness	Dependable with the will to achieve. Includes characteristics such as being self-disciplined, efficient, organised, reliable, responsible, dutiful, and thorough.
Extroversion	Outgoing. Includes characteristics such as being talkative, gregarious, enthusiastic, seeking excitement, assertive, and active.
Agreeableness	Loving, friendly, and compliant. Includes characteristics such as being sympathetic, appreciative, trusting, kind, forgiving, generous, and altruistic.
Neuroticism	Tendency to experience negative emotions. Includes characteristics such as being anxious, tense, self-pitying, worrying, self-conscious, hostile, and vulnerable.

The mechanism through which optimism affects physical health is unclear. Some immunological studies show that in mild or moderately stressful situations, optimists have a better immune function compared to pessimists. However, in highly challenging or difficult events, optimists show poorer immunological functioning (Segerstrom, 2005). This may be because optimists will engage with stressful situations and try to resolve them. Hence difficult circumstances might lead to greater physiological strain for optimists than for pessimists who disengage.

BOX 2.3 Measuring optimism

The Life Orientation Test (Revised)

Please be as honest and accurate as you can throughout. Try not to let your response to one statement influence your responses to other statements. There are no 'correct' or 'incorrect' answers. Answer according to your own feelings, rather than how you think 'most people' would answer.

4 = I agree a lot
3 = I agree a little
2 = I neither agree nor disagree
1 = I Disagree a little
0 = I Disagree a lot

1	In uncertain times, I usually expect the best.	
2	It's easy for me to relax.	[filler]
3	If something can go wrong for me, it will.	[reverse]
4	I'm always optimistic about my future.	
5	I enjoy my friends a lot.	[filler]
6	It's important for me to keep busy.	[filler]
7	I hardly ever expect things to go my way.	[reverse]
8	I don't get upset too easily.	[filler]
9	I rarely count on good things happening to me.	[reverse]
10	Overall, I expect more good things to happen to me than bad.	

Scoring

To calculate your score, ignore the fillers (items 2, 5, 6, 8). Reverse your score on negatively worded statements (items 3, 7, & 9). Then total your score. Scores range from 0 to 24: high scores indicate optimism, low scores indicate pessimism.

Source: Scheier, M.F., Carver, C.S. & Bridges, M.W. (1994) Distinguishing optimism from neuroticism (and trait anxiety, self-mastery, and self-esteem): A re-evaluation of the Life Orientation Test. *Journal of Personality and Social Psychology*, *67*: 1063–1078. Copyright ©1994 by the American Psychological Association. Reproduced with permission.

2.4.3 EMOTIONAL EXPRESSION, EMOTIONAL REGULATION, AND HEALTH

Research into emotional expression raises a few puzzles. On the one hand, there is a view that not expressing strong emotions is bad for you. Research has found that the suppression of emotion is associated with poorer health, but the evidence is inconsistent (Garssen, 2004). In contrast, we have already seen that anger and hostility, which both involve some expression of these emotions, increase the likelihood of heart disease.

A particularly interesting area of research has looked at the effect of writing about negative or traumatic events on health. This research suggests that writing about negative events can have positive effects on health in some groups of people (Frattaroli, 2006; Mogk et al., 2006). It is not clear why emotional expression in this way might lead to better health. Various explanations have been put forward, including that people find more meaning in the experience, that it helps regulate and decrease negative emotions attached to the event, that people are more likely to talk about it with others, and/or that other people are more supportive when told about the event.

Emotion regulation is critical in how we respond to stress and control our emotions. Regulation may take two forms. There is intrinsic regulation where we attempt to regulate our own emotions through strategies like cognitive reappraisal, talking to others and seeking help from others; and extrinsic regulation where we attempt to regulate someone else's emotion through strategies like providing empathy, comfort, or support (Zaki & Williams, 2013). There is now compelling evidence that other people regulate our emotions. For example, the mere presence of another person can reduce negative responses to stress, particularly if that person is a friend or family member. Research Box 2.1 outlines a study giving an example of this (Coan et al., 2006). Interpersonal factors are therefore a powerful influence in people's experiences of illness and treatment when we frequently have to help individuals face challenging circumstances. An example of how we might use ways to regulate emotions to help people in healthcare is given in Case Study 2.3, which looks at how we might help a person with diabetes manage needle procedures more easily.

CLINICAL NOTES 2.2

Emotions and healthcare

- Emotional disorders cost society billions every year, and mental illness is responsible for 40% of disability.
- How people respond to illness is initially determined by how they appraise it.
- Helping people appraise things more positively can reduce negative emotions and help people cope.
- Positive emotions have the potential to have a positive influence on health.

(Continued)

- Negative emotions, such as anxiety, anger, and depression, are associated with chronic illnesses such as heart disease. Treating people with these dispositions early can prevent later illness.
- Encouraging optimism can help people if they are facing an essentially controllable or modifiable illness.
- Getting people to write about stressful or traumatic events has the potential to improve health in some people.

RESEARCH BOX 2.1   Lending a hand: the social regulation of responses to stress

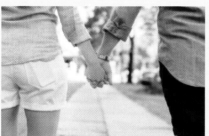

Background

Social support and contact is associated with better health and wellbeing, which might be partly due to the effect of others on regulating emotional responses to stress.

Method and findings

This study used functional magnetic resonance imaging (fMRI) to examine 16 married women's responses to the threat of electric shocks while (1) holding their husband's hand, (2) holding the hand of a male researcher, or (3) not holding anyone's hand. During the experiment, women were shown a series of 'threat cues' or 'safety cues'. Threat cues indicated a 20% likelihood that an electric shock would occur. Ratings were taken of unpleasantness and arousal after each shock. Before the experiment women also rated the quality of their marriage.

When women held their husband's hand there were marked decreases in activation in the neural systems associated with threat, compared to no hand holding. Decreases were also found when holding the hand of a stranger but these were smaller than for the husband. The quality of the marriage also had an effect with larger decreases in neural responses in women who had higher quality marriages. Similar results were found for women's experiences of unpleasantness and arousal after each shock.

Significance

This experiment shows the potential impact that others have on our physiological and emotional responses to stress. It illustrates the importance of other people in regulating emotional responses to negative or challenging events.

Coan, J.A., Schaefer, H.S. & Davidson, R.J. (2006) Lending a hand: social regulation of the neural response to threat. *Psychological Science*, *17*(12): 1032–1039.

CASE STUDY 2.3   Regulating emotional responses to stress in healthcare

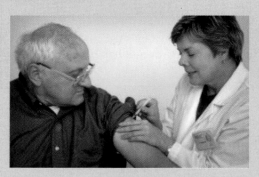

Photograph courtesy of CDC/ Judy Schmidt acquired from Public Health Image Library (Website)

Clive is 62 years old and has Type 2 diabetes, which means he needs regular injections of insulin. Clive is not managing his diabetes well and has been hospitalised twice in the last three months. He does not like needles and cannot face injecting himself. When nurses try to do the injections, he gets very worked up and distressed.

How can Clive regulate his emotional reaction to needles?

Select situations that make things less negative: distraction is useful for dealing with needle anxiety, so it may help for Clive to have his injections in a situation where he can be distracted by something he really enjoys, such as a film, music, or something else he finds interesting.

Modify the situation: the situation can be changed in many ways including (i) finding an alternative mode of delivering insulin; (ii) changing the timing of injections so he has less time to get anxious beforehand; (iii) having a healthcare professional do the injections; (iv) bringing a friend who can support him and help him stay calm.

Focus attention away from the situation or emotion: Clive should be encouraged to concentrate on something else while the injection is being done, by distracting him, asking him to focus on another object, or talking about a happy event. Helping him cope is much more effective than empathy, which often increases distress.

Change the way a situation or emotion is appraised or labelled: Clive's appraisals need to be changed from negative (e.g. the injection will hurt, he won't cope, the nurse will think he's stupid) to positive (e.g. the injection will be over very quickly, he's managed it before, after the injection he will feel better).

Regulate physical, behavioural, and emotional responses: there are many things Clive can adopt to help regulate his responses in injections. For example, he can do physical exercise before the injections to make him more physically relaxed. Before and during the injection he can use relaxation techniques such as focusing on his breathing. He can also use positive self-statements to cope.

(based on Gross & Thompson, 2007)

Summary

- Emotion includes affect, moods, and impulses.
- Emotion has cognitive, physiological, and behavioural components. Behavioural components include action tendencies, nonverbal behaviour, and facial expression.
- Appraisal processes initiate the physiological, behavioural, and conscious experience of emotion.
- Positive emotions are associated with good health and negative emotions, such as anger and depression, are associated with certain illnesses. However, the mechanisms or causes underlying this association are not clear.
- Emotional dispositions of optimism and neuroticism are positively and negatively associated (respectively) with psychological health as well as with some measures of physical health.

CONCLUSION

This chapter has looked at how motivation and emotion are important influences on our behaviour, health, and illnesses such as cardiovascular disease. There is substantial overlap between these different areas and their implications: motivation drives us to act while emotions also include impulses and action tendencies. Appraisal is important in determining how we feel and respond to different situations. In this chapter we have concentrated on the effect of motivation and emotion on health and the possible pathways this works through, including physiological, cognitive, and behavioural changes. A good example of the interplay between appraisal, emotion, cognition, and behaviour, and how this affects our health, is what happens when we are stressed, which we look at in the next chapter.

FURTHER READING

Llewellyn, C.D. et al. (eds) (2018) *The Cambridge Handbook of Psychology, Health and Medicine* (3rd edition). Cambridge: Cambridge University Press. Includes short chapters on emotions and health, personality and health, and social relationships.

Ryff, C.D. & Singer, B. (2001) *Emotion, Social Relationships and Health*. Oxford: Oxford University Press. This is a good book if you want to know more about how social relationships and context affect emotions and health. It includes chapters on immunity, common colds, and breast cancer.

Steptoe, A. (2006) *Depression and Physical Illness*. Oxford: Oxford University Press. A comprehensive text on the effect of depression on physical illness.

REVISION QUESTIONS

1. Describe motivation and give examples of different types of motives.

2. Outline and evaluate three different theories of motivation.

3. Describe the main components of emotion.

4. What are the six basic emotions that are expressed similarly across different cultures?

5. Discuss how the different components of emotion might interact to determine our emotional experience.

6. Outline the effect of positive and negative emotions on health.

7. How might the expression of emotion affect health?

8. Outline the two-factor model of positive and negative affect.

9. Distinguish the various pathways through which emotion may influence health.

10. What emotional dispositions have been associated with health?

3 STRESS AND HEALTH

CHAPTER CONTENTS

(Continued)

LEARNING OBJECTIVES

This chapter is designed to enable you to:

- Define stress and outline aspects of stress, including (a) appraisal and (b) stress responses.
- Describe physical responses to stress and discuss variations, (a) between individuals and (b) between situations, in how we respond physically to stress.
- Discuss the relationship between stress and physical health, and outline the factors that protect us or make us more vulnerable to illness following stress.
- Understand some of the psychological consequences of stress, including burnout.

Most people think that stress is bad for us. In fact, stress is *not* always bad for us – a small amount of stress is necessary for us to rise to challenges such as competitions or exams. However, long-term stress is indeed negative in its effects: there is a lot of evidence linking stress to adverse outcomes like depression, burnout, and cardiovascular disease. Stress is also associated with infections, slower recovery, and a worsening of symptoms in illnesses such as asthma, herpes, and rheumatoid arthritis (Steptoe & Ayers, 2005). In this chapter we look in more detail at stress, our physical responses to it, how it can affect our physical and mental health, and what can protect us against stress.

3.1 WHAT IS STRESS?

The concept of stress originated in physics and mechanical engineering to describe the internal forces in a system caused by external pressures, such as the pressure of water or wind on a bridge. Over time the word **stress** has become widely used to mean many things, including a negative situation, a feeling of pressure, tension, or negative emotion. According to the psychological definition, stress occurs when demands are appraised as exceeding a person's resources to cope.

Like emotion, stress has many components and first it is necessary to distinguish between stressors and stress responses. **Stressors** are external or internal events that may trigger stress responses. If, for example, you feel stressed because you are sitting an exam, we may say that the exam is acting as an external stressor. If, on the other hand, you feel stressed because you are torn between helping a friend who needs you and revising for that exam, the stress is caused by an internal stressor (your conflicting desires). Stressors can be further divided according to their type or duration, such as acute stressors (e.g. the death of a relative), chronic stressors (e.g. caring for a sick relative), daily hassles (e.g. problems getting to work), traumatic stressors (e.g. an assault), and role strain (e.g. balancing home and work roles). Not everyone responds to the same stressors in the same way.

Stress responses are the various ways we respond to a stressor. These can be divided into cognitive, affective, behavioural, and physiological responses. Interestingly, there is not always a strong association between these different responses. In other words, it is possible for a person to have a strong physiological response to a stressor but not report feeling emotionally stressed. This is apparent in people who have a repressive coping style who, when put under stress, will report little or no emotional distress but show strong physiological responses (Myers, 2010). A commonly used questionnaire measure of stress is given in Box 3.1 so you can consider how stressed you are.

BOX 3.1   How stressed are you?

During the last month how often have you...	Never	Almost never	Sometimes	Fairly often	Very often
Been upset because of something that happened unexpectedly?	0	1	2	3	4
Felt that you were unable to control the important things in your life	0	1	2	3	4
Felt nervous and 'stressed'?	0	1	2	3	4
Felt confident about your ability to handle your personal problems?	4	3	2	1	0
Felt that things were going your way?	4	3	2	1	0
Found that you could not cope with all the things that you had to do?	0	1	2	3	4
Been able to control irritations in your life?	4	3	2	1	0
Felt that you were on top of things?	4	3	2	1	0
Felt angered because of things that were outside of your control?	0	1	2	3	4
Felt difficulties were piling up so high that you could not overcome them?	0	1	2	3	4

Scoring: Add your scores together. Scores range from 0–40. The average score for people aged 18–29 is around 14; aged 30–44 is 13; >45 years is approximately 12.

Source: Cohen, S., Kamarack, T. & Mermelstein, R. (1983) A global measure of perceived stress. *Journal of Health and Social Behaviour*, 24: 385–396. Copyright © 1983 American Sociological Association. Reproduced with permission.

3.1.1 PHYSICAL RESPONSES TO STRESSORS

Understanding physical responses to stressors is critical to explaining the link between stress and disease. Our understanding of physical responses to stressors initially comes from research in the 1950s detailing the physiological fight-flight response. The **fight-flight response** involves the sympathetic branch of the **autonomic nervous system** as a fast, first-wave response; and the endocrine pathways of the **hypothalamic-pituitary-adrenal (HPA) axis** as a slower, second-wave response. The sympathetic nervous system (SNS) and HPA responses are illustrated in Figure 3.1. The SNS directly activates body systems to prepare the body for immediate action. The adrenal medulla is stimulated to produce stress hormones such as **adrenaline** (epinephrine) and **noradrenaline** (norepinephrine). This causes stimulation of the heart and lungs and the diversion of energy away from unnecessary functions, such as saliva production, digestion, and reproduction.

At the same time, the HPA axis is activated so the hypothalamus releases corticotrophin releasing factor, which then sets off a cascade of endocrine events culminating in the release of cortisol and other hormones from the adrenal cortex. **Cortisol** is a steroid and is a critical stress hormone. It results in an increase in blood sugar levels and metabolic rate, hence further supporting the body in the need for fight or flight. It also influences the regulation of blood pressure, the immune system, and the inflammatory response. Normally, the HPA axis works as a negative feedback loop so the presence of cortisol in the blood stream triggers the hypothalamus to stop producing corticotrophin releasing factor. Thus cortisol will usually return to normal levels 40 to 60 minutes after a stressful event. However, under prolonged periods of stress the HPA axis can become dysregulated and result in chronically elevated levels of cortisol. In the long term this has negative effects, such as the accumulation of abdominal fat and the wasting of bone and muscle tissue. The effects of excess cortisol are illustrated by Cushing's syndrome – where there is overproduction of cortisol (hypercortisolism). People with Cushing's syndrome have large amounts of fat on their abdomen and face, sweating, thinning of the skin, stretch marks, and facial hair. In some cases it also leads to sleep problems, reduced sexual function, reduced fertility, increased depression, and anxiety.

Understanding of physical responses to stressors has developed substantially since the fight-flight responses were first identified. It is now clear that physiological responses to stressors vary according to the characteristics of a situation. Research with animals shows that stronger physiological stress responses occur in situations that are novel, unpredictable, or uncontrollable. Research examining this in humans is broadly consistent with the findings from animal research. For example, a study of commuters found that those who rated aspects of their journey as unpredictable reported more stress and had higher cortisol levels (Evans et al., 2002). Similarly, research generally indicates that a lack of control is associated with greater stress and a more negative impact on health (Walker, 2001). A study of over 5,000 retired adults in the USA found that the effect of chronic stress on physical frailty was fully mediated by perceived control (Mooney et al., 2016) – i.e. a high sense of control overcame the expected effect of chronic stress on frailty.

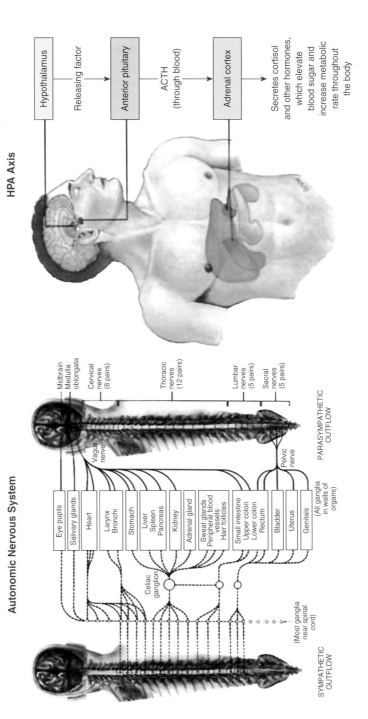

Physical stress response

Autonomic Nervous System

HPA Axis

Hypothalamus

Releasing factor

Anterior pituitary

ACTH
(through blood)

Adrenal cortex

Secretes cortisol
and other hormones,
which elevate
blood sugar and
increase metabolic
rate throughout
the body

Midbrain
Medulla
oblongata

Cervical
nerves
(8 pairs)

Thoracic
nerves
(12 pairs)

Lumbar
nerves
(5 pairs)

Sacral
nerves
(5 pairs)

Vagus
nerve

PARASYMPATHETIC
OUTFLOW

Eye pupils

Salivary glands

Heart

Larynx
Bronchi

Stomach

Liver
Spleen
Pancreas

Kidney

Adrenal gland

Sweat glands
Peripheral blood
vessels
Hair follicles

Small intestine
Upper colon
Lower colon
Rectum

Bladder

Uterus

Genitals

(All ganglia
in walls of
organs)

Pelvic
nerve

Celiac
ganglion

(Most ganglia
near spinal
cord)

SYMPATHETIC
OUTFLOW

FIGURE 3.1   Fight-flight responses to stressors

Source: Kalat, J.W. (1992) *Biological Psychology* (4th edition). Belmont, CA: Wadsworth. © 1992 Wadsworth, a part of Cengage Learning Inc.
Reproduced by permission. (www.cengage.com/permissions)

This has led to the view that it is important to empower people and encourage them to have as much perceived control as possible. Though this is usually true, there is not a simple blanket effect of perceived control on health and it can be moderated by a number of factors. For example, another study of 6,135 adults in the USA found that stronger beliefs of control over one's life were associated with less risk of dying prematurely for people with low levels of education, but not for those with high levels of education (Turiano et al., 2014). It is also worth noting that if a situation is essentially uncontrollable, encouraging someone to strive for control might result in more stress. The evidence for this is not consistent but, if this is the case, it has important implications for uncontrollable situations in healthcare, such as births that involve obstetric complications that women cannot predict or control. In these circumstances, it may be unhelpful to encourage women to strive for control and perhaps more emphasis should be placed on supporting them through such events.

People also vary in *how* they respond physiologically to stress. Some individuals are more responsive than others. This is called stress responsivity. Studies of twins, epigenetic studies, and animal studies indicate that stress responsivity is partly genetically determined but that the early environment is critical in altering and shaping our physical and behavioural responses to stressors. Babies of mothers who had high levels of stress and anxiety during pregnancy are more responsive to stressors, show more anxiety and fearfulness, and are more likely to have cognitive and attentional problems (Talge et al., 2007). This is referred to as fetal programming and makes sense from an evolutionary perspective, because offspring born into a stressful or dangerous environment will need exaggerated stress responses to survive (see also Chapter 14).

The environment is important in shaping infants' stress responses. Animal studies show that offspring of more nurturing mothers have reduced HPA axis responses through less corticotrophin releasing factor (see Figure 3.1) and enhanced negative feedback (Champagne & Meaney, 2001). In addition, the mere presence of the mother alters and reduces their offspring's physiological responses to stressors (Debiec & Sullivan, 2016). Thus, individuals vary in their levels of stress responsivity and this is determined by **nature and nurture**. Classic studies conducted in the 1990s show that young children differ in their level of cardiovascular or immune responsivity to stressors. Children who were less responsive to stressors had a similar risk of respiratory illnesses whether they were raised in high or low adversity settings – nicknamed 'dandelion children' because of their relative resilience under different conditions of adversity. Children who were highly responsive to stressors and lived under high adversity had substantially more illness than all other groups of children. However, unexpectedly, children who were highly responsive but lived in low adversity settings (i.e. supportive family or care settings) had the *lowest* rates of illness (Boyce et al., 1995). These children were nicknamed 'orchid children' to illustrate their sensitivity to their early environment. This finding has since been replicated in many studies: children who are more responsive to their environment have the best or worst outcomes depending on whether they are raised in a positive or negative environment, respectively. This is found for both physical and psychological health outcomes (Del Giudice et al., 2011) (see also Chapter 8).

The fight-flight response provided the initial basis of our understanding of physical responses to stressors. However, the matter is more complex than this. In particular, there is more variation between individuals than the above explanations imply. There is also evidence that fight-flight is only one way of responding to stressors and that an alternative response is a **tend and befriend** response, where animals and humans tend to their off-spring (tend) and seek out others for safety and comfort (befriend) (Taylor, 2012). Tend and befriend responses are more commonly displayed by females so it has been argued that fight-flight responses may be more relevant to males.

The biological basis of affiliative responses to stressors is the hormone oxytocin in conjunction with endogenous opioids. There is substantial evidence from animal studies for the importance of oxytocin and opioids in affiliative behaviours. For example, administering oxytocin and/or opioids leads to an increase in maternal and other prosocial behaviours (Lim & Young, 2006). However, if male animals are injected with oxytocin and then subjected to stressors they are more likely to nurture any young animals present and show tend behaviours (Taylor, 2012).

There is also accumulating evidence from research with humans that oxytocin and opioids are involved in affiliative behaviours and attachment to others. For example, rises in oxytocin and endogenous opioids occur in women during labour, breastfeeding, and in both men and women during sex, which are presumably to increase affiliation and bonding. Increased oxytocin is also observed in people who are socially isolated or those with poor quality relationships – presumably because they need to seek social affiliation (Taylor et al., 2009). The opioid system is involved in reducing physical pain but also in reducing separation distress. Researchers have therefore argued that coping with social pain (as in loss and separation) might be based on similar physiological mechanisms to physical pain (Way & Taylor, 2009).

The tend-befriend response also reduces the negative effects of stressors. Oxytocin is associated with reduced physiological stress responses and psychological distress. Studies administering oxytocin to animals show it reduces fearful behaviour and increases exploration. In humans oxytocin is associated with decreased SNS and HPA activity (Taylor, 2012). It is therefore thought that, although fight-flight responses are good for acute resolution of threatening events, social affiliation and tend-befriend responses can buffer against the long-term negative impact of stressors on health. This is consistent with the extensive literature showing the importance of social support in health (see section 3.2.2). Figure 3.2 summarises how affiliative responses might decrease stress responses.

It can be seen that the fight-flight response to stressors is well established but is not the only biobehavioural response to stressors. Tend-befriend responses and the importance of affiliation and social relationships illustrate the notion that physical responses to stressors will differ according to circumstances, the individual, and the social context.

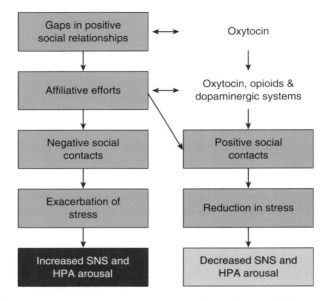

FIGURE 3.2   Affiliative responses to stressors (adapted from Taylor, 2006)

CLINICAL NOTES 3.1

Stress and health

- In uncontrollable circumstances, such as an emergency situation, it may be more helpful to support people through it rather than encourage them to strive for control.
- Severe or chronic stressors are associated with poor health, so helping people manage and reduce their stress has the potential to reduce illness in the long term.
- The physical symptoms of stress will vary between individuals – some may experience cardiovascular symptoms, such as palpitations, whereas others may experience gastro-intestinal symptoms.

3.1.2 STRESS AND THE IMMUNE SYSTEM

Stress has various effects on the immune system, depending on the demands of the situation. Both the SNS and the HPA axis affect the immune system. The SNS increases immune system activity, particularly large granular lymphocyte activity such as natural killer cells. However, the HPA axis suppresses some immune activity through the production of cortisol, which has an anti-inflammatory effect and reduces both the number of white blood cells and the release of cytokines (see Chapter 11).

Different types of stressors make different demands on the body, and the immune response to stress has developed to reflect this. A review and meta-analysis of over 300 studies of stress and immunity showed that immune responses vary according to whether the stressor is acute (lasting a few minutes), a brief naturalistic stressor, a sequence of stressors, or a chronic long-term stressor (Segerstrom & Miller, 2004). Short stressors, such as giving a presentation, lead to an acute increased immune response and redistribution of cells to provide an immediate defence against injuries and the broad risk of infection. This response is very rapid and the immune system quickly returns to baseline levels. Brief stressors that continue for several days, such as studying for exams, have a different effect on the immune system and influence the *function* of the immune system with a switch away from cellular immunity, which protects against injury or damage, to humoral immunity, which protects against infection. This means the body will be more able to coordinate responses against infections: it might explain why students often get sick after exams – because during the stressful revision period they have increased immunity against infections which largely disappears when exams are over. The research on stressful sequences of events has largely looked at bereavement and trauma and these events are associated with different immune responses. Chronic stressors, such as caring for a relative with dementia or unemployment, have a negative impact on almost all aspects of immune functioning, with poorer immune function overall. This makes a person more likely to get ill, particularly if they are already vulnerable (e.g. elderly people) or have pre-existing disease (Segerstrom & Miller, 2004).

ACTIVITY 3.1

- Can you remember how many stressful events you have been through in the last year?
- How accurate do you think you can be? Are there things you might have forgotten?
- What do you think affects whether you remember stressful events or not?

3.1.3 STRESS AS A PERSON–ENVIRONMENT INTERACTION

It is now widely accepted that how we respond to stressors depends on the interaction between a person and their environment. Interactional or transactional explanations of stress provide a more complete account of the different processes involved in stress. This approach argues that stress occurs when a person appraises the demands of a situation as being greater than their ability to cope with these demands (Lazarus & Folkman, 1984). Appraisal processes are central and explain why there is so much variation in how different people respond to stressors.

The interactional approach outlines three processes of appraisal:

1. *Primary appraisal*: the demands of a situation are evaluated as benign or stressful (i.e. challenging, threatening, or potentially involving harm or loss).
2. *Secondary appraisal*: a person evaluates their resources and capacity to cope.
3. *Reappraisal*: after applying a coping strategy (or strategies) a person reconsiders the situation. This may lead to reappraisal of a stressor as less or more stressful than originally thought, depending on the effect of their coping responses.

There is a wealth of evidence for the importance of appraisal in how we respond to stressors. A meta-analysis of 81 studies of people with chronic pain or who had pain induced in laboratory experiments showed that in both these situations appraisals of pain as threatening were associated with greater pain, reduced tolerance of pain, and more passive coping. In people with chronic pain, appraisal of the pain as threatening was also associated with more impairment and psychological distress. In contrast, appraisals of pain as challenging were associated with more pain tolerance and active coping (Jackson et al., 2014). The importance of primary appraisal is illustrated throughout this book (see, for example, the discussion in Chapter 2 of responses to discovering a breast lump). Box 3.2 gives examples of primary and secondary appraisal, and reappraisal. A strength of the interactional approach is the recognition of the appraisal-coping-reappraisal cycle. This constant interplay between appraisal, coping, and reappraisal means stress is conceptualised as a dynamic process.

BOX 3.2   Appraisal and stress

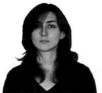

Trigger	Skin rash	Skin rash
Primary	*'It's meningitis'* (threatening)	*'It's probably nothing'* (benign)
Secondary	*'I can't cope with this on my own'*	*'I'll just leave it'*
Feelings	Stressed	Calm
Coping	Visit doctor – find out it's eczema	Keep an eye on it
Reappraisal	*'The cream the doctor gave me should make it better'* (can cope)	*'It doesn't seem to be getting worse so I'll wait a bit longer'*
Feelings	Calm	Calm

The interactional model as originally proposed is not without problems but elements of it are now widely accepted, such as the importance of the interaction between the person and environment, the central role of appraisal, and that coping and other psychosocial factors moderate how we respond to stressors. A biopsychosocial approach to stress incorporates all these elements and is illustrated in Figure 3.3.

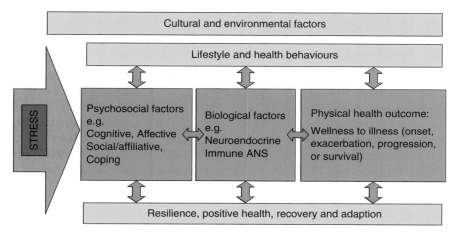

FIGURE 3.3 Biopsychosocial approach to stress (adapted from Turner-Cobb & Katsampouris, 2017)

Summary

- The stress process involves (a) stressors and (b) stress responses.
- Stress responses include physiological, behavioural, emotional, and cognitive changes.
- Stress occurs when the perceived demands of a situation are appraised as exceeding a person's perceived resources and ability to cope (individually or with social support).
- Appraisal is therefore central to whether a person feels stressed or not.
- Physical stress responses involve the sympathetic nervous system, HPA axis, and immunological changes.
- The flight-flight response is not the only biobehavioural response to stressors. The tend-befriend response is an affiliative response to stressors which is more common in females and underpinned by oxytocin and endogenous opioids.
- Physical stress responses vary according to the characteristics of the stressor, for example, novelty, predictability, and control.
- Individuals vary in the strength and nature of their physical responses to stressors (stress responsivity).

3.2 STRESS AND HEALTH

3.2.1 LINKS BETWEEN STRESS AND HEALTH

There is plenty of evidence that stress is associated with morbidity and mortality. For example, studies of bereavement show that older people are more likely to die in the year after their spouse dies than other people of the same age and health (Subramanian et al., 2008). The impact of stress on physical health varies between illnesses. There is good evidence that prolonged stress (whether measured in terms of stressors or subjective experience of stress) results in increased episodes of infectious illnesses like colds (see Research Box 3.1), cardiovascular disease, slower wound healing, and worsens auto-immune conditions such as asthma, rheumatoid arthritis, inflammatory bowel disease, and HIV/AIDS (Steptoe & Ayers, 2005). Examples of research in these areas can be found throughout Section III of this book. Similarly, the association between stress and poor mental health is well recognised. Chronic or severe stress can lead to a number of mental health problems, including anxiety, depression, stress burnout, and post-traumatic stress disorder (PTSD).

However, as with our emotions, it is difficult to establish the definitive pathways between stress and health. There are three main issues. The first is the huge variation in how people respond to stressors. Why is it that if we put two people in the same circumstances, one person becomes stressed and the other does not? Or that one person develops heart disease and another remains healthy? Some of these differences can be accounted for by differences in appraisal and stressor characteristics, as we have already seen, but the effect of stress is also influenced by many other factors, such as an individual's resilience, coping responses, and social support.

The concept of allostasis and **allostatic load** is one way to explain how stress might lead to disease (McEwen, 1998a, 1998b). Allostasis refers to the process of regulating our physiological state to achieve stability, or homeostasis. This is done through physiological systems, such as the autonomic nervous system, HPA axis, neuroendocrine and immune systems, or through changing behaviour. In the short term, these changes are adaptive because they maintain physiological stability while adapting to changing external circumstances. However, frequent or chronic activation of these systems results in a high allostatic load (or strain) on the body. This cumulative allostatic load can lead to an imbalance in allostatic systems and disease. Different types of allostatic load have been proposed. A prolonged response is where physiological systems remain in a continually high state which results in long-term strain on the body. An inadequate response is where one allostatic system does not respond adequately so other systems have to overcompensate. Alternatively, if people are exposed to repeated acute stressors there can be a lack of adaption, with repeatedly high physiological stress responses (McEwen, 1998a, 1998b). Allostatic load is usually measured by a combination of biomarkers from the cardiovascular, metabolic, immune, and neuroendocrine systems.

A review of the evidence for allostatic load shows it is associated with a range of social and environment factors associated with health, and with health disparities between certain groups. Factors associated with allostatic load include ethnicity, socioeconomic status,

RESEARCH BOX 3.1   Stress and the common cold

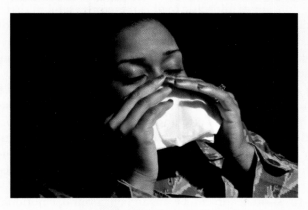

Photo via Senior Airman Tristin English/Scott Air Force Base

Background

Research shows that susceptibility to the common cold is greater when people feel stressed, but also when people have less social support. Other research suggests people with trait-like positive affect are more resilient. This study examined the interactive effects of stress, social support, and dispositional affect on susceptibility to the common cold.

Method and findings

694 healthy adults completed measures of perceived stress, trait positive and negative affect, and social support. They were then given a cold virus, kept in quarantine for five days and monitored for clinical illness (infection and objective symptoms of illness). Overall, 75% of participants became infected with the virus and 30% met criteria for developing a clinical cold.

Results showed that levels of perceived stress or support on their own were not associated with greater risk of catching a cold. However, emotional disposition was an important moderator. People who had negative dispositions were at greater risk of a cold if they felt stressed, regardless of their levels of social support. In contrast, people with positive dispositions were responsive to levels of support: those who felt stressed but who had high levels of support were less likely to develop a cold than those with poor support.

Significance

This study tests the idea that support buffers against the negative effects of perceived stress and shows that this may be moderated by emotional disposition when looking at susceptibility to the common cold (see also Chapter 2 on emotions and health). Part of the significance of this research and previous studies of this kind is in showing that perceived stress, support and emotional disposition can affect whether people catch cold viruses (through an examination of immune antibodies) and also whether they then display the symptoms of a cold (through an examination of coughs, mucus, etc.). These studies illustrate that the effect of stress is strong enough to be clinically relevant.

Janicki Deverts, D., Cohen, S. & Doyle, W.J. (2016) Dispositional affect moderates the stress-buffering effect of social support on risk for developing the common cold. *Journal of Personality*, 28 July.

social relationships, gender, lifestyle factors, exposure to stressors, and genetic factors. High allostatic load is also associated with physical and mental health outcomes, and all-cause mortality (Beckie, 2012). The concept of allostatic load is therefore useful in that it provides a framework through which the interaction between the environment and individuals' biobehavioural responses can lead to poor health outcomes. The use of combined measures from multiple physiological systems has also broadened the focus onto systemic responses to stressors and the impact of this.

However, a second issue is that it is usually not possible to say whether an illness is due (a) entirely to stress or (b) entirely to other factors (i.e. not at all to stress). Illnesses often have multiple causes, ranging from the genetic and biological to the environmental. The role of stress will also vary widely in different illnesses. A traumatic stressor may cause PTSD but only exacerbate the symptoms of asthma. The contribution of stress to illness will therefore vary widely between individuals, circumstances, and illnesses.

A third issue is that the effect of stress on health can be due to behavioural, emotional, or physical responses to stressors. For example, people who are stressed are also more likely to smoke, drink alcohol, and have a poor diet (Wardle et al., 2000). The physical response to stressors is therefore not the only pathway between stress and disease, as illustrated in the biopsychosocial approach in Figure 3.3.

3.2.2 VULNERABILITY AND RESILIENCE

We have already seen how some people are more vulnerable to poor health. Examples of this are 'orchid' children who are more responsive to adverse environments (Boyce et al., 1995), and the health disparities observed between different groups, such as people from lower socioeconomic groups. The vulnerability-stress model (sometimes called the diathesis-stress model) shown in Figure 3.4 summarises how vulnerability factors interact with stressors to influence whether someone develops disease or not.

It is also clear that some people are very resilient in the face of stressors and remain in good health despite adverse circumstances. This is illustrated by the research described earlier where 'dandelion' children had similar health outcomes regardless of whether they were raised in positive or adverse environments (Boyce et al., 1995). It is also clear that even in the face of significant adversity, such as chronic or terminal illness, people can adapt and find happiness and personal growth (see Chapter 6). Resilience has been classified as people showing swift recovery from stressful events, having sustainability of purpose in the face of adversity, and growth or new learning from adversity (Zautra & Reich, 2010).

Research suggests that the majority of people are resilient. For example, trauma and adversity are common and at least 50% of people will experience trauma or adversity

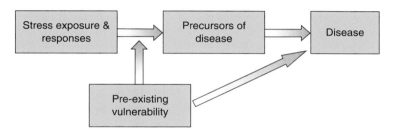

FIGURE 3.4   Pathways between stress and disease (vulnerability-stress model)

in their lifetime. However, the prevalence of PTSD in the general population is approximately 10%, suggesting that most people who experience a traumatic event recover (Horn et al., 2016). A review of factors associated with resilience identified those factors in Box 3.3 as important in developing resilience during childhood and remaining resilient in adulthood (Horn et al., 2016).

BOX 3.3   Psychosocial factors associated with resilience

Childhood	Adulthood
Positive bonds with caregivers	Positive emotions, optimism
Consistent parenting	Active coping
Self-regulation of emotions	Cognitive reappraisal
Intelligence and problem-solving	Altruism
Mastery	Mastery
Positive friendships	Social support
Motivation for achievement	Facing fears
Meaning	Meaning, sense of purpose

(Adapted from Horn et al., 2016)

Here we focus on a few of the factors associated with resilience, namely (1) emotion and emotional disposition, (2) ways of coping, and (3) social relationships and social support.

Emotion and emotional disposition

As we saw in Chapter 2, positive emotions and positive emotional dispositions have a powerful influence on health so are important in resilience. A range of positive emotional states (e.g. emotional wellbeing, positive mood, joy, happiness, vigour, energy) and positive dispositions (e.g. life satisfaction, hopefulness, optimism, sense of humour) are associated with reduced mortality in healthy people and in people with chronic illness (Chida & Steptoe, 2008). Having an optimistic disposition is associated with reduced mortality, increased survival, fewer physical symptoms, lower risk of cardiovascular disease, and improved physiological functioning (including immune function) (Rasmussen et al., 2009).

The role of negative emotions and emotional dispositions as a vulnerability factor is not as straightforward. There is now substantial evidence that some types of negative emotion are associated with specific illnesses. The main examples of this are associations between anger, hostility, depression, and cardiovascular disease (Chida & Steptoe, 2009; Fiedorowicz, 2014). Depression is a clear vulnerability factor and is associated with a wide range of morbidity and mortality. For example, depressed people are between 50% and 100% more likely to develop cardiovascular disease than healthy people (Lett et al., 2004).

The negative emotional disposition of neuroticism has also been implicated as a vulnerability factor. People high in neuroticism experience a wide range of negative emotions, such as low mood, anxiety, guilt, hostility, and fear. People high in neuroticism generally report more pain and somatic symptoms and are at greater risk of psychological disorders (Contrada & Goyal, 2005). For example, a large prospective study of 21,676 adult twins in the USA, who were followed up over 25 years, found that, after controlling for genetic vulnerability in twins, those who were high in neuroticism were significantly more likely to report musculoskeletal pain, headaches, migraine, chronic fatigue, colitis, irritable bowel syndrome, gastroesophageal reflux disease, and cardiovascular disease 25 years later (Turk et al., 2008). However, there is also no consistent link between neuroticism and measures of chronic morbidity such as heart disease, cancer, or mortality (Hielmayr & Friedman, 2017).

ACTIVITY 3.2

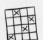

- Do you know anyone who gets stressed very easily?
- Which kind of factors do you think influence why they are like that?
- How much of it is due to circumstances, the person's vulnerability or resilience, and the coping strategies they use?

Coping

As we saw earlier when looking at the interactional model of stress, coping is a vital part of how we respond to stressors. How we cope with stressors partly determines our physical and emotional responses. People who appraise an event as challenging have smaller cortisol responses than people who appraise it as threatening. Research looking at coping defines it as *any* attempt to cope with a stressor, irrespective of whether this is successful or not. This covers a huge range of coping actions and there has been an extensive debate over how to best conceptualise different coping strategies. Categories that are widely used distinguish between emotion-focused and problem-focused coping; or between approach and avoidant coping. **Emotion-focused strategies** are those that concentrate on reducing distress (e.g. not thinking about it, eliciting emotional support) whereas **problem-focused strategies** concentrate on dealing with the problem (e.g. information seeking, problem solving).

For healthcare practice, the distinction between approach coping and avoidant coping may be more useful. **Approach coping** strategies try to deal with the situation proactively, so are predominantly active strategies and share some overlap with problem-focused strategies. **Avoidant coping** strategies try to avoid the problem (e.g. denial, not wanting to talk about it), so are predominantly emotion-focused. The important point for healthcare practice is that a person who is predominantly an avoidant-coper may find it very difficult to discuss their illness, the side effects of treatment, or any potential complications. Conversely, an approach-coper will want to know everything about it and may come to consultations armed with extensive information gleaned from the internet!

In general, coping strategies that enable a person to feel more in control (mastery) increase positive emotions and decrease negative emotions, and are associated with resilience and better health. For example, finding meaning or benefit in adverse events is associated with resilience. A review of the literature on people with cancer showed that those who found some benefit in having cancer had better immune function (Pascoe & Edvardsson, 2013).

However, it is not always as simple as saying one coping style is better than another. Under certain circumstances avoidant or passive coping strategies may be good for reducing anxiety and distress in the short term. Before an operation this can be helpful because it keeps anxiety levels down and once the operation is over the stress or is over. However, for someone with a chronic illness, avoidance can lead to a lack of adherence to treatment regimens and compound illness problems.

ACTIVITY 3.3

- Which kind of coping strategies do you tend to use?
- Can you think of anyone who is clearly an avoidant-coper or an approach-coper?
- How well does this coping approach work for them in different situations?

Social relationships and social support

Interpersonal relationships are vital to our quality of life and health. Negative relationships involving abuse or conflict are some of the most potent stressors. Traumatic events that involve intentional harm from another person, such as rape, assault, or torture, are much more likely to cause PTSD than natural disasters (Charuvastra & Cloitre, 2008).

Social relationships also shape the way we respond to stressors. As we have seen, early mothering influences the way young animals respond physiologically and behaviourally to stressors. In humans, social bonds are very influential in shaping a child's stress responses. Attachment theory (see Chapter 8) proposes that babies are born with an instinct to turn to their parents or significant others when they experience stressors or are in danger. In extreme situations, such as children being abandoned or abused, children are more likely to develop insecure and chaotic responses to stressors. Parents also shape their children's responses to stressors. Studies of parents and children exposed to the same stressor show that their responses are very similar. There is increasing evidence that anxious parents have anxious children, and that having a controlling parenting style is a strong moderator of this (van der Bruggen et al., 2008). It has also been shown that interventions designed to promote positive parenting improve resilience in children (Wolchik et al., 2002)

It is well established that social relationships are associated with improved health outcomes in both healthy people and those with chronic diseases. A review and meta-analysis of over 300,000 people showed that having stronger social relationships is associated with a 50% increase in survival rates (Holt-Lunstad et al., 2010). This is comparable or greater than other well-known risk factors, such as smoking, exercise, and hypertension (Uchino et al., 2017). Conversely, loneliness, social isolation, and living alone are associated with a 26–32% increased risk of premature mortality (Holt-Lunstad et al., 2015).

However, although there is extensive evidence about the importance of social networks and relationships, the impact of an act of support on perceived stress is more complex. Laboratory experiments that induce stress by asking people to undertake social speaking or hard arithmetic tasks show that having someone present can reduce SNS and HPA axis responses, although this is not consistent and varies according to factors such as culture, gender, and the nature of the relationship (Hennessy et al., 2009; see Research Box 3.2). The same effect (and variation in this) has also been observed with pets being present (Schreiner, 2016).

Thus, social relationships are critical to health. Having a strong support network and relationships has a direct positive impact on health and being socially isolated has a direct negative impact on health. Receiving support during a stressful event can buffer against the effects of stress, but this is affected by a number of factors. Individual and cultural differences in how support is interpreted are illustrated in Research Box 3.2. Some have therefore argued that the effect of support on health is due to knowing that other people are close and available to support us should we need it, rather than due to actual support received during stressful events (Taylor, 2010).

RESEARCH BOX 3.2 Interpreting a helping hand: cultural variation in the effectiveness of social support

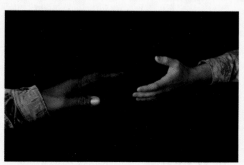

Source: U.S. Department of Defense, June 2016

Background

Support is associated with better health outcomes but there are cultural differences in how people perceive and respond to support.

Method and findings

This study investigated whether the way in which support is offered affects how people respond to stressors. It examined stress responses in adults from an individualistic culture (European Americans) or collectivistic culture (Asian Americans).

An experiment was conducted where people were given a stressful mathematical task to do with another person in the room. They were told that this person was a mathematics major. In one condition, the maths major gave the participant help and support without the participant having to ask for it (unsolicited support). In another condition, the participant had to ask for support (solicited support). 70 people took part in the experiment (38 Asian Americans and 32 European Americans).

Participants from the collectivistic culture (Asian Americans) were less likely to ask for support. They also found the task more stressful when they had to ask for support, as opposed to it being given automatically. In contrast, participants from the individualistic culture (European Americans) did not rate the task as any more or less stressful if they had to ask for support compared to receiving it automatically. Further analysis suggested that this effect of culture might be due to performance self-esteem, which was higher in European Americans.

Significance

This study demonstrates that the way in which support is offered can impact on perceived stress for people from different cultural backgrounds. If people from collectivistic cultures have to ask for help, they may experience this as more stressful. This has implications in healthcare settings where we support people in difficult health circumstances.

Mojaverian, T. & Kim, H.S. (2013) Interpreting a helping hand: cultural variation in the effectiveness of solicited and unsolicited social support. *Personality and Social Psychology Bulletin*, *39*(1): 88–99.

CLINICAL NOTES 3.2

Coping styles and clinical practice

- Consider people's coping styles when giving information in clinical practice.
- People with avoidant coping styles may not want information and may become anxious or distressed if given information.
- Conversely, people with approach coping styles will want information and may become distressed if not given information.
- Social relationships are critical to wellbeing so it is important to identify people who are socially isolated and encourage or help them to increase their support networks.
- Providing support can buffer against the effects of stressors but this varies according to how the individual interprets such support.

Summary

- Severe or chronic stressors are associated with a range of morbidity and mortality.
- Variability in how we respond to stressors makes it difficult to establish causal pathways between stress and disease.
- A vulnerability-stress approach explains how stress may interact with an existing vulnerability to affect health.
- Most people are resilient to stressors.
- Resilience in adulthood is influenced by positive emotions and emotional dispositions, coping, and social relationships and support.
- Interpersonal relationships and social support are critical and shape how we respond to stressors and, in some cases, can buffer against the negative impact of stress.

3.3 STRESS IN MEDICINE AND HEALTHCARE

Working in healthcare and medicine is inherently stressful: it involves dealing with health crises and distressed people, and it may entail making life and death decisions. As we have already seen, stress is associated with negative psychological states, including anxiety, depression, burnout, and PTSD. Stress burnout has three main symptoms:

1. *Emotional exhaustion*: feelings of physical exhaustion, being depleted, worn out.
2. *Depersonalisation*: having an unfeeling, impersonal approach to co-workers or patients, cynicism, and a lack of engagement with the job or people.
3. *Reduced personal accomplishment*: a poor sense of effectiveness, involvement, commitment and engagement, and a poor belief in one's ability to change or improve work patterns or environment.

Burnout can be conceptualised on a continuum from work engagement to burnout. Engagement is characterised by high levels of vigour, dedication, and absorption, and is associated with good performance (Montgomery & Maslach, 2017). Burnout is associated with poor performance, high job dissatisfaction, absenteeism, and staff turnover. In addition symptoms of exhaustion are associated with many other physical symptoms, such as headaches, gastrointestinal disorders, hypertension, colds or flu, and sleep disturbances (Leiter & Maslach, 2000).

Burnout is a particular problem for doctors, nurses, and student healthcare professionals. Rates of burnout among doctors are between 25% and 60% (Goitein et al., 2005), and can even be as high as 75% (Fahrenkopf et al., 2008; Shanafelt et al., 2002). Burnout is also high in nurses with 33–50% being affected (Imai et al., 2004; Poncet et al., 2007). One European survey of family doctors in 12 countries found high levels of burnout were associated with poor job satisfaction, intention to change job, sick leave, younger age, being male, and use of alcohol, tobacco, and psychotropic medication. Burnout also varied according to country and region (Soler et al., 2008). A meta-analysis of burnout in over 28,000 doctors also found differences between countries, with doctors in the USA having lower levels of emotional exhaustion than those in Europe. In the USA, burnout was associated with work–life conflict and poor coping strategies, whereas in Europe burnout was associated with negative attitudes to work (Lee et al., 2013). Lifestyle and health behaviours are also affected: a study of burnout in seven European countries found that burnout led to more fast-food consumption, less exercise, and greater use of alcohol and painkiller use. These associations remained even after controlling for individual differences and country of residence (Alexandrova-Karamanova et al., 2016).

Risk of burnout operates at three levels: individual (healthy lifestyle/behaviours, adequate coping), the individual and the environment (social support structures, relationships, improving person–organisation fit), and at the organisational level (adequate working conditions, organisation of work, design). Interventions to prevent burnout should therefore be aimed at all three levels. However, although there is evidence for individual risk factors for burnout, there is more substantial evidence for the importance of organisational risk factors (Montgomery & Maslach, 2017). The six main organisational factors associated with burnout are shown in Box 3.4. Ways to change these to engender a positive organisational culture and staff engagement have also been proposed. There is some evidence that interventions such as Civility, Respect and Engagement in the Workplace

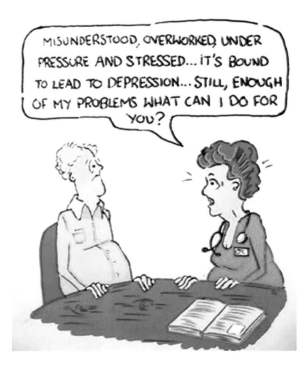

(CREW) promote change and a work culture that is more empowering for staff (Spence Laschinger et al., 2012).

BOX 3.4   Workplace and burnout

Evidence suggests that burnout is more likely in jobs that involve:

- A high workload.
- A lack of control.
- Insufficient rewards.
- An absence of fairness.
- Value conflicts.
- A poor sense of community.

(*Source*: Leiter & Maslach, 2004)

Students training in medicine and other healthcare professions also face many stressors. These include keeping up with coursework and exams; dealing with death, suffering, and difficult ethical issues; performing intimate examinations of others at a young age; and demanding work hours. Longitudinal studies that have followed medical students over a number of years have identified some characteristics that are associated with stress and burnout later in life. Medical students who are disorganised, have poor time management, feel overwhelmed, and who are unsure of the demands of different tasks are more likely to report stress and burnout in their 30s (McManus et al., 2004). Students who are self-critical, neurotic, perfectionists, report feeling like an 'imposter', and if they are female are also more likely to suffer from stress and burnout later in their career (Firth-Cozens, 2001). Learning positive ways to manage stress is therefore extremely important for healthcare professionals. These include using appropriate support and learning positive stress management techniques. Case Study 3.1 shows how the interactional model of stress can be used to help a student cope with exam stress.

3.4 MANAGING STRESS

Understanding the processes of stress provides a basis for helping people manage stress more effectively.

Most stress management interventions aim to reduce arousal and build coping skills so the person is able to manage stress better. There are many different approaches to stress management which can broadly be divided into two main categories: (1) those that focus on physical and mental relaxation, such as relaxation exercises, meditation, mindfulness, and yoga; and (2) those that focus on cognition and behaviour, such as psychoeducation,

CASE STUDY 3.1   Managing stress in medicine and healthcare

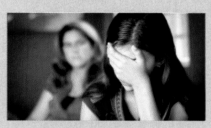

Source: Kamira's portfolio, obtained via Shutterstock

Isha is a medical student approaching the end of her first year. Before medical school Isha was a straight-A student. At medical school her results have varied. She has passed everything but has lost confidence. She is particularly worried about the Clinical Examinations where she has to demonstrate clinical skills with a patient in front of an examiner. Isha is very anxious and not coping well. She is convinced she is going to freeze up, look stupid in front of the examiner, and fail the exam.

Isha finds the constant examinations and evaluation of medical school really hard. She feels tired, tense, and is finding it difficult to concentrate on her studies. She is beginning to doubt whether medicine is the right career for her.

Stress management

Stress management involves education about stress and coping, exploring each person's unique way of dealing with stressors, and facilitating more adaptive coping. When based on the interactional model, stress management looks at demands, appraisal, resources, and coping as follows:

Demands

The demands of medical school on Isha may be explored in order to make them explicit. For example:

- *What are the triggers to this situation?* e.g. clinical examinations.
- *What demands does it place on Isha?* The exams make Isha feel evaluated, not good enough, and she has lost confidence.
- *How real are these demands?* Are they based on fact or Isha's fears?

Appraisal

This stage would look at her appraisals and how they are affecting her feelings and coping, such as:

- When she is feeling unable to cope, what thoughts are going through her head? This would emphasise the role of appraisal in how Isha feels. Current appraisals include: 'I am going to fail', 'I will freeze up and look stupid', 'Maybe medicine isn't right for me'.
- How could she think differently to help her feel and cope better? This would highlight appraisals and coping strategies that might be more adaptive: 'Exams are hard but I

(Continued)

have got through them before', 'It's not only me that finds exams hard', 'If I freeze up it's not the end of the world', etc.

Resources to cope

This stage would involve exploring with Isha which resources she can use to cope. This includes helping her to learn new coping strategies and to draw on existing ones. For example:

- *What support is available?* Including other students, teachers, friends, family, and healthcare professionals. *How can she use this now?*
- *How has she coped with difficult situations in the past?* This would raise awareness of which coping strategies are available to her.
- *What worked and what didn't work?* This would help Isha realise what are adaptive and maladaptive coping strategies in different situations.
- *How can she use these strategies to cope now?* This could help Isha realise she has resources to cope and should reduce her feelings of helplessness, increase her confidence, and encourage her to use strategies that will help her feel better.
- *What new coping strategies might help her now?* This encourages Isha to learn and use new ways of coping.

Managing stress

Drawing on the previous stages, you can explore practical steps and strategies to help Isha manage her exam preparation now and in the future. To some extent this is very individual. For example, Isha might realise that talking to other students really helps because it normalises a certain amount of anxiety and worry. She might find that working with a group of students to revise and practise together boosts her confidence. Or she might realise that in a previous stressful situation she was able to think about it differently and 'talk' herself out of her fears.

cognitive restructuring, assertiveness training, and stress inoculation. More information about relaxation, mindfulness, and cognitive behaviour therapy (CBT) is given in Chapter 19. Interventions such as stress inoculation are based on exposing people to potential stressors and training them in skills (e.g. skills drills) so they become 'inoculated' against these stressors and are able to work effectively under potentially stressful conditions. For example, paramedic training will often include rehearsals or 'mock ups' of major road traffic accidents in order that when paramedics are in a real accident situation they are equipped with the right knowledge and actions to deal with it effectively.

Building resilience is frequently suggested as a preventative strategy against burnout among doctors and healthcare professionals. This is a broad approach that can draw on many of the techniques above to help an individual cope better with stress and recover quicker. A qualitative study of physicians in Canada found resilience was a dynamic, evolving process of positive attitudes and effective coping strategies. Four main aspects of resilience in these physicians were: (1) attitudes and perspectives, which included valuing the physician role, maintaining interest, developing self-awareness, and accepting personal limitations; (2) balance and prioritisation, which included setting limits, taking effective approaches to continuing professional development, and honouring the self; (3) practice management style, which included sound business management, having good staff, and using effective practice arrangements; and (4) supportive relations, which included positive personal relationships, effective professional relationships, and good communication (Jensen et al., 2008).

Cognitive-behavioural stress management programmes focus on appraisals and coping responses to help people manage stressors and perceived stress better. These can be useful to assist people who are coping with illness. Stress management techniques have therefore been widely implemented and evaluated for people with cardiovascular disease, cancer, and chronic headaches – but with mixed results. The evidence suggests that stress management has positive effects on psychological outcomes, such as reducing depression and increasing self-esteem, but the impact on physical morbidity or mortality is mixed. Early studies showed stress management programmes led to decreased mortality from heart disease (Friedman et al., 1986) and cancer (Spiegel et al., 1989). However, research since then has failed to replicate this effect. For example, a Cochrane review of 148 studies of cardiac rehabilitation found that psychological and educational interventions have little or no impact on morbidity or mortality but can improve quality of life (Anderson & Taylor, 2014).

One particular type of stress management programme, called critical incident debriefing, has proved controversial. Debriefing was initially developed to help people deal with very stressful or traumatic events and prevent the development of PTSD. Debriefing programmes vary but they usually involve one session within four weeks of the event, during which a person is encouraged to talk about their thoughts and feelings during the event and their symptoms since the event. The therapist will then educate the person about responses to traumatic events, in an attempt to normalise these experiences. A number of studies have shown that debriefing has little effect on symptoms of PTSD or depression, and one study of using debriefing with people with burns found it made them worse (Bisson et al., 1997). Some clinical guidelines therefore explicitly recommend *against* using debriefing interventions as a treatment after traumatic events (National Institute for Clinical Excellence (NICE), 2005).

Interventions to prevent work stressors and perceived stress in healthcare professionals have mixed results. Some interventions have good results in particular settings. For example, an intensive training programme for oncology nurses to help improve attitudes, communication skills, and reduce perceived stress led to nurses having better communication skills with patients, reporting less stress, and patients being more satisfied with their care (Delvaux et al., 2004). Another review of mindfulness interventions to help nurses cope with stressors and perceived stress found it led to improved wellbeing, reduced anxiety and depression, and improved performance at work (Guillaumie et al., 2016). However, reviews that look at multiple interventions across multiple settings generally find more moderate effects. A Cochrane review of interventions aimed at preventing stress in healthcare workers concluded there is moderate evidence that physical and mental relaxation exercises and CBT reduce work stress compared to no intervention, but that relaxation and CBT interventions are similar in their efficacy (Ruotsalainen et al., 2015).

CLINICAL NOTES 3.3

Looking after yourself

- Studying and working in healthcare can be very stressful. It is therefore really important that you are aware of your own stress levels and take steps to look after yourself.
- Recognise the signs and symptoms of stress in yourself and take steps to manage your stress.
- Avoid trying to 'go it alone'. Use formal and informal support available to you, such as student counsellors (at university) and colleagues (in practice). Some areas have groups where healthcare professionals can talk through stressful or difficult issues in healthcare practice (e.g. www.balint.co.uk).
- If you have symptoms of burnout or other psychological problems, then get help as soon as possible, before the problem becomes chronic or severe.
- Skills in organisation, time management, and finding positive ways of dealing with stressors are worth developing early on in your career.
- Perfectionism and self-criticism will increase the stress you put on yourself.

CONCLUSION

It is clear that we need to take a more sophisticated approach than thinking there is a simple dose–response relationship between stress and illness. As we saw in Chapter 2 on emotion, some negative emotions, such as depression and anger, are associated with illnesses such as heart disease. However, as this chapter on stress has shown, we need to account for individual differences in many factors, including a pre-existing vulnerability and resilience, exposure, health behaviour, and social and environmental factors in determining whether a person will become ill and the type of illness they may suffer.

In the last two chapters we have concentrated on the effects of motivation, emotion, and stress on health. In trying to explain the mechanisms underlying the association between emotion, stress, and health we have primarily concentrated on physical and behavioural pathways. However, emotion and stress will also influence symptom perception, help-seeking, and illness behaviour. In the next chapter we examine the role of symptom perception and illness beliefs in more detail.

Summary

- Severe or chronic stress is associated with psychological problems such as anxiety, depression, stress burnout, and PTSD.
- Burnout occurs when people feel exhausted, depersonalised, and have a poor sense of personal accomplishment.
- Health professionals are at increased risk of burnout and stress-related psychological problems, particularly in demanding specialties such as intensive and palliative care.
- Understanding stress processes is important to develop interventions that help people manage stressors more effectively.
- Stress management interventions are generally associated with increased psychological wellbeing, but evidence of their effect on physical health is mixed.

FURTHER READING

Llewellyn, C.D. et al. (eds) (2018) *The Cambridge Handbook of Psychology, Health and Medicine* (3rd edition). Cambridge: Cambridge University Press. Includes short chapters on stress, coping, personality, emotions, physical activity, social factors, social relationships, psychoneuroimmunology, and burnout in health professionals.

Cooper, C.L. & Campbell Quick, J. (2017) *The Handbook of Stress and Health*. Malden, MA: Wiley Blackwell. This is a comprehensive book covering all aspects of stress and health.

Folkman, S. (ed.) (2010) *The Oxford Handbook of Stress, Health, and Coping*. Oxford: Oxford University Press. This is a comprehensive book covering all aspects of stress and health.

REVISION QUESTIONS

1. How is stress defined in psychology?
2. Outline the different elements of the interactional model of stress.
3. Describe the physiological responses to stress.
4. What factors are important in the variation in how we respond physiologically to stress?
5. Outline the vulnerability-stress explanation of how stress influences health.

6. Discuss four factors that moderate the effect of stress on health.

7. Define 'coping' and describe two different ways in which coping strategies have been classified.

8. Outline the evidence that social support affects health.

9. What is stress burnout and how does it affect healthcare professionals?

10. Describe two types of stress management interventions and briefly discuss the evidence that they are effective.

4 SYMPTOMS AND ILLNESS

(Continued)

LEARNING OBJECTIVES

This chapter is designed to enable you to:

- Discuss the role of different psychological factors in physical symptoms.
- Describe the multidimensional nature of pain and the role of psychological factors in the perception of pain.
- Outline the placebo and nocebo effects and how they affect illness and recovery.
- Describe different representations of illness and understand how these impact on the psychological and physical outcomes of illness.
- Understand how these principles can be used in clinical interventions to improve health outcomes.

Understanding symptoms is fundamental to providing good healthcare. Symptoms are a sign that something might be wrong, they motivate people to seek help from healthcare services, help doctors and other healthcare professionals to diagnose the problem, and give an indication of whether a treatment is working and people are getting better. All of this would be fairly straightforward if there were a simple relationship between having symptoms and having a disease, or the severity of a symptom and disease. In reality, however, the relationship is not simple or straightforward.

First, symptoms are remarkably common – indeed, a population survey carried out in New Zealand found that, on average, people reported having experienced five symptoms of illness in the previous week (Petrie et al., 2014). The most common symptoms were back pain, fatigue, headache, runny or stuffy nose, and joint pain, which had been experienced by between 34% and 38% of people in the previous week. In this survey, only 11% of people reported having no symptoms at all (Petrie et al., 2014), which is consistent with other population studies. For example, a study of almost 50,000 people in Denmark found only 10% of people did not report any symptoms in the previous four weeks (Elnegaard et al., 2015). A second complication is that most people with symptoms do not consult doctors, preferring to ignore the symptoms, treat themselves, or rely on a natural recovery. Research suggests that only a third of people see their doctor for symptoms that they experience (Elnegaard et al., 2015).

Thus symptoms are remarkably common. They are often also ambiguous: they are strongly influenced by psychological factors, such as the degree of attention paid to symptoms, how they are interpreted, and beliefs about illness and healthcare. The previous chapters have described how the perception of symptoms is influenced by emotion and stress, and how motivation determines whether people will act and in what way. In this chapter, we examine more specifically how people perceive symptoms and illness, including pain, which is a primary symptom of many disorders. Placebo and nocebo effects demonstrate the importance of beliefs in the perception of symptoms and illness. These show that in some cases people recover because they believe they will recover, or feel ill because they believe they will get ill.

Symptoms are not only a sign of the *onset* of illness but also indicate the *progression* of illness. Chronic illnesses, such as rheumatoid arthritis or multiple sclerosis, involve remitting or slowly worsening symptoms and disability. Perhaps unsurprisingly, beliefs about symptoms play an important role in how people adjust to chronic illness and predict further symptoms, distress, and disability. For example, a person who believes that their illness is uncontrollable, incurable, and disrupts every area of their life will be highly distressed and focused on their symptoms, worrying about whether the disease is getting worse. In contrast, a person who that believes their illness is controllable and requires adjustment but does not disrupt every area of their life will be less distressed and less focused on their symptoms. As we have seen in previous chapters, distress such as anxiety or depression is in turn associated with poorer health and slower recovery. Thus negative beliefs, distress, and negative interpretation of symptoms can become a vicious downward cycle. This is often seen in people with chronic pain. This chapter therefore examines the perception of symptoms, pain, placebo and nocebo effects, and finally looks at how beliefs about symptoms and illness influence the experience and progression of chronic illness.

4.1 SYMPTOM PERCEPTION

A **symptom** can be thought of as any variation in a physiological or emotional state that is interpreted as unusual and labelled as potentially harmful. Therefore, as with emotion and stress, appraisal and interpretation are central. For example, a racing heartbeat just before giving a presentation could be interpreted as nerves (unusual, transient, not harmful) or a possible heart problem (unusual, potentially chronic, harmful). Symptoms of a myocardial infarction (MI) are also experienced and interpreted differently by men and women (Lefler & Bondy, 2004). This affects how women respond to these symptoms – which may cost them their life if medical treatment is delayed. Evidence shows women suffering a heart attack can take up to twice as long to get to hospital as men (Walsh et al., 2004). The main reasons that women delay getting treatment include: experiencing different symptoms than those typically associated with a heart attack; not perceiving symptoms as severe; having other illnesses; incorrectly attributing or labelling symptoms as due to something else; and women believing they are less likely than men to have a heart attack (Lefler & Bondy, 2004).

How people appraise and interpret symptoms is therefore critical. Unfortunately, people are generally not very good at interpreting their physical state accurately. This has huge implications for treatment. For example, people with asthma are expected to monitor their symptoms and use inhaler medication when they need it. However, up to 60% of people with asthma are unable to detect changes in their lung function reliably (Kendrick et al., 1993). Similarly, people with hypertension are not able to detect consistently when their blood pressure goes up, although 90% of them believe they can (Meyer et al., 1985). There are a few exceptions to this. Some individuals are more accurate at detecting symptoms than others, and most people can accurately perceive extreme symptoms or physical changes that need immediate action, such as a bad injury or strong pain.

4.1.1 PSYCHOLOGICAL FACTORS AND SYMPTOMS

Psychological factors can affect the perception and interpretation of symptoms in a number of ways, including (a) the role of *attention* in whether people notice their symptoms, (b) the effect of the *environment* on symptom perception and interpretation, (c) *individual differences in the interpretation* of symptoms, and (d) the *influence of emotions* on symptom perception and interpretation.

Attention and the environment

The degree of attention we pay to our internal physical state has a strong influence on the perception of symptoms. Most theories of attention assume we have a limited capacity to pay attention to different stimuli at the same time. Therefore, changes in our internal states have to compete with what is going on around us for attention. There are many examples of injured soldiers fighting on and not feeling the injury, or of athletes continuing to play with serious injuries (see Case Study 4.1). This can be explained on different levels. Physiologically, the release of endogenous opioids like endorphin reduces the level of pain we feel. Psychologically and socially, the demands of an immediate situation mean people are less likely to attend to their physical symptoms.

Research evidence confirms the importance of attention in the perception of symptoms. People are more likely to report symptoms if they are in boring environments. More symptoms are reported by people who are unemployed, living alone, or who are put in boring situations in laboratory research (Broadbent & Petrie, 2018). People also report more symptoms if they are instructed to attend to their internal physical stimuli rather than to external stimuli. For example, one study asked overweight and obese women to exercise with or without listening to music. Listening to music resulted in women paying less attention to the exercise and bodily cues, and rating the exercise as less demanding (Silva et al., 2016). The implications of this for healthcare are that taking a person's attention away from internal stimuli by using strategies such as distraction can lower the perception of symptoms. Attention is covered in more detail in Chapter 10.

CASE STUDY 4.1   Claire Markwardt: running through the pain

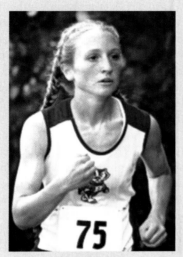

Claire Markwardt was competing in the Ohio State high school cross country championships when she broke her leg in two places. Two miles around the course she was running at her personal best. About 400 metres from the finish line she heard her left leg crack. Claire thought she'd pulled or torn a muscle so continued to run for the finish:

> 'There was a runner from one of our rival schools right in front of me – I kept staring at the back of her jersey and pushing myself to catch her.'

200 metres further on her leg cracked again and gave out. She fell to the ground but a team mate encouraged her to get up and continue. She tried, using her right leg. But as soon as she shifted weight to the left, her leg cracked again loudly and gave out again:

> 'At that point, I knew that my leg was hurt. I had a suspicion it was broken, but I also thought it might be a muscle. It was such a short time I wasn't overly analyzing it, but I knew I couldn't get up again so I started crawling.'

She said she didn't think of her coach, her parents, or team mates, but just of the many stories she had heard about runners who collapsed before the end of a race and somehow found the courage to cross that last line. She managed to crawl to the finish line and was only 18 seconds under her personal best time.

Reproduced courtesy of Claire Markwardt; image reproduced courtesy of Carl Chrzan

Individual differences in the interpretation of symptoms

People differ in the amount of attention they pay to internal states and also in which types of symptoms they are more likely to attend to. Most people have sets of beliefs, or **schemas,** about which illnesses they are vulnerable to, which symptoms indicate potential illness, and which illnesses comprise a threat to their overall health. Schemas are mostly developed during childhood and are not always rational. Events in adulthood may lead to schemas changing or being modified. Schemas people have about their health and illness will therefore be influenced by their past experience of illness and others' attitudes to illness – particularly those of their parents.

Schemas usually operate unconsciously to influence what symptoms people attend to and how they interpret them. For example, in one study, healthy volunteers were shown either a neutral TV programme or a programme on the negative effects on health of being exposed to Wi-fi. Afterwards, volunteers were exposed to sham Wi-fi and asked to rate various physical sensations. Volunteers who had watched the programme on the negative effects of Wi-fi on health rated their physical sensations as more intense and were more anxious about being exposed to Wi-fi (Bräscher et al., 2017). A similar phenomenon is apparent in the finding that up to a third of medical students worry they have an illness they have just studied. This is probably because they scan their symptoms for any that fit with the illness they are learning about (Broadbent & Petrie, 2018).

Thus the perceived cause of symptoms is important. In the example above, medical students were more likely to think their symptoms were due to a serious disease they had just learned about. This process of interpreting the cause of something is called **attribution**. At a very simple level, people can attribute the cause of their symptoms to somatic causes, psychological causes, or environmental causes. If a middle-aged woman feels hot and faint she could attribute this to the menopause (somatic), being upset or embarrassed (psychological), or the room being too hot (environment). Within each category there are potentially many explanations. Which attribution a person makes will affect the action they then take. For example, an aching muscle could be attributed to exercise (somatic but benign) or to the start of flu (somatic, threatening) and this will influence whether someone seeks help for a symptom.

Research into attribution indicates that people have different **attributional styles**. Individuals might be more or less likely to attribute events internally (to themselves) or externally (to the environment or others). In relation to symptoms, it is possible that some individuals who have an internal/somatic attribution style may also have increased health-care use in response to symptoms.

Influence of emotion

Emotion is strongly associated with the perception and reporting of symptoms, which was covered in Chapter 2. Strong emotion is accompanied by physiological changes that can be misinterpreted as symptoms. There is a large amount of evidence that negative emotions or emotional dispositions are related to increased reports of symptoms, pain, disability, and psychological distress. In part this is due to negative emotions making people more likely to notice symptoms and interpret them as threatening. Research into anxiety shows it leads to a narrowing of attentional focus and a bias toward the perception of threat. Anxiety will therefore make people hypervigilant, in which case they will scan themselves and the environment for any potential threat (Bar-Haim et al., 2007). In addition some people are very sensitive to the physiological symptoms of anxiety and do not tolerate them well. High anxiety sensitivity is associated with more fearful appraisal of pain, reduced tolerance of pain, and more pain-related disability (Ocañez et al., 2010).

Research that induces negative moods in people finds similar associations. Negative moods are usually induced by showing upsetting films or asking people to recall difficult episodes from their past. Such research finds people report more symptoms and think they are more vulnerable to illness when they are in a negative mood. People are also more likely to attribute the cause of symptoms to illness. For example, one study looked at people a week after a vaccination and found that those with high negative affect reported more symptoms from the vaccination than people who were low in negative affect (Petrie et al., 2004). Our emotional state and dispositions therefore influence attention to symptoms, appraisal, and interpretation of symptoms.

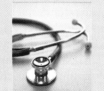

CLINICAL NOTES 4.1

Symptoms

- There is no straightforward relationship between the extent of reported symptoms and disease.
- Most people are bad at detecting physical changes so do not rely on self-reported measures of physical processes such as lung function or blood pressure.
- Getting people to focus on external stimuli (e.g. distraction) is a useful technique for reducing symptoms such as pain. It is particularly useful for brief painful procedures such as injections or venepuncture.

4.1.2 EFFECTS OF SYMPTOM PERCEPTION ON HEALTH

The misperception of symptoms potentially compromises the effectiveness of healthcare services through:

- Delay in seeking help if symptoms are interpreted as non-threatening.
- Overuse or underuse of healthcare services if symptoms are interpreted wrongly.
- Compromised treatment if people self-treat or do not adhere to a treatment because they misattribute the cause of symptoms.

For example, someone might stop taking medication, such as antibiotics, because they feel a bit better but are not 'cured'. This is an obvious waste of resources and undermines effective treatment (adherence is discussed in Chapter 17).

Understanding the processes that affect symptom perception can therefore help us to design more effective interventions, particularly for chronic illnesses where people have to adhere to intensive treatment regimes. For example, interventions have been developed to increase awareness of blood glucose in people with diabetes. This includes education about symptom recognition, biases, and management, and leads to better metabolic control of diabetes than standard educational interventions (Kim & Lee, 2016; Tan et al., 2015).

4.1.3 MEDICALLY UNEXPLAINED SYMPTOMS

Many people have persistent symptoms that do not have an identifiable physical cause. Medically unexplained symptoms (MUS) are common and in the UK account for a fifth of all consultations in primary care and a larger proportion of consultations in specialties such as gynaecology, neurology, and gastroenterology (Nimnuan et al., 2001). MUS are defined as persistent bodily symptoms with functional disability but no explanatory structural or other pathology (Chalder & Willis, 2017). Diagnostically, MUS have been classified as somatoform disorders or somatic symptom disorders (American Psychiatric Association, 1994, 2013). These disorders include conditions where the cause is poorly understood, such as irritable bowel syndrome, fibromyalgia, chronic fatigue syndrome, non-cardiac chest pain, and chronic pain, as well as those with a clear psychological component such as hypochondriasis.

MUS are strongly associated with psychological disorders such as anxiety or depression, illustrating the close relationship between negative emotions and physical symptoms discussed in the previous section. In fact, the presence of physical symptoms, whether explained or unexplained, is highly associated with psychological morbidity. A study of 4,864 people in the USA found that experiencing more physical symptoms was associated with anxiety, depression, psychological distress, substance use disorders, and increased use of healthcare services, regardless of whether these symptoms had an identifiable physical cause (Escobar et al., 2010). MUS are also more common in women, lower socioeconomic groups, and people with a history of child abuse. Symptoms might also run in families – there is some evidence that children of parents with MUS are more likely to report symptoms themselves (Shraim et al., 2013).

Evidence shows that symptoms and disability are perpetuated by both cognitive and behavioural factors, such as increased attention to symptoms, fear and avoidant coping, and attribution of symptoms to physical causes (Chalder & Willis, 2017). There is also considerable overlap of symptoms between different conditions, such as chronic fatigue and irritable bowel syndrome, despite different aetiological pathways. Chalder and Willis (2017) outline a model of MUS that shows how predisposing vulnerability (e.g. childhood abuse, neuroticism), precipitating factors (e.g. life events, stress, viral infections), and perpetuating factors (focus on symptoms, attribution, catastrophic misappraisal, rumination) might interact to perpetuate the disorder. They use this model to propose an individualised treatment based on cognitive behavioural therapy (CBT). Given the close association between medically unexplained symptoms and psychological factors, it is perhaps unsurprising that psychotherapy – particularly cognitive behaviour therapy (CBT) – is associated with a reduction in symptoms and disability (Chalder & Willis, 2017; van Dessel et al., 2014). Self-help programmes are also associated with reduced symptoms and better quality of life compared to usual care (van Gils et al., 2016).

MUS are a challenge for doctors and other healthcare professionals because of the uncertainty about cause and, therefore, treatment. A review of 13 studies of doctors' experiences with MUS found a key difficulty for doctors was the lack of congruence between the dominant biomedical model of disease and the reality of trying to help people suffering from chronic symptoms with no known biomedical cause. Doctors reported feeling stuck, inadequate, frustrated, and powerless to help, which could lead to a difficult relationship with the patient. Doctors had to work flexibly and use a more psychosocial approach through establishing a good relationship, alliance, and partnership with the patient. This led to positive experiences of mutual trust and validation. Part of this process was doctors learning to balance the 'ideal versus real', where the ideal is biomedicine as a learnt discipline and the real is experience-based knowledge (Johansen & Risor, 2017).

MUS therefore highlight the limitations of a biomedical approach to disease (Lipsitt et al., 2015; Rosendal et al., 2017). The classification systems used in healthcare services are diagnostic so require some certainty about physical cause. This has led to proposals for new classification systems that, instead of focusing on physical disease, focus on a range of prognostic factors (Rosendal et al., 2017), such as symptom characteristics (e.g. number, multi-system, frequency, severity), concurrent psychological disorders, and sociodemographic characteristics (e.g. female, low socioeconomic status). These characteristics can be used to group symptoms according to whether they are likely to be self-limiting, recurrent, persistent symptoms, or symptom disorders (Rosendal et al., 2017).

In the next section we look at symptoms of pain and how psychological knowledge and research can help provide effective treatments for chronic pain, which in many cases is a type of medically unexplained symptom.

Summary

- Understanding symptoms is fundamental to good healthcare.
- Symptoms are any variation in our physiological state that are interpreted as unusual and labelled as potentially harmful.
- Symptoms can be a sign of the onset and progression of a disease. However, there is not a straightforward relationship between symptoms and disease.
- How people appraise and interpret their symptoms is critical to whether they act and receive appropriate treatment.
- Psychological factors affect the perception and interpretation of symptoms though variables such as attention, beliefs, or schemas about illnesses and individual vulnerability.
- Negative mood is associated with increased symptom perception.
- Medically unexplained symptoms are common. They illustrate the importance of psychosocial factors in the onset, perpetuation, and treatment of such symptoms.

4.2 PAIN

Pain is a common symptom and often an important signal that the body has been damaged or something is wrong. In rare cases of congenital insensitivity to pain, children have a reduced ability to feel pain and are unable to recognise physical damage or danger. These children are at risk of a range of problems, including biting off parts of their tongue, being prone to eye infections following damage by foreign objects, and suffering bone fractures or burns.

Pain has been defined as a distressing experience that is associated with actual or potential tissue damage and which has sensory, emotional, cognitive and social elements (Williams & Craig, 2016). A number of distinctions are important in understanding pain. First, it is important to distinguish between nociception, sensation, and suffering. **Nociception** is the stimulation of peripheral pain receptors, which send pain messages to the central nervous system. The **sensation** of pain is how this is interpreted and this will be influenced by many factors, including attention, schemas, emotion, etc. **Suffering** refers to the perceived pain, distress, and disability that can arise from pain and other related factors.

Second, it is important to distinguish between pain threshold and pain tolerance. The **pain threshold** is the point at which a stimulus becomes painful and is similar for most people, regardless of their gender, race, or culture. **Pain tolerance** is the degree to which a painful stimulus can be tolerated and this varies widely between individuals, cultures, and contexts. For example, music and humour can increase people's tolerance of pain. Research shows that simply listening to music or watching a funny film increases pain tolerance (Lee, 2016; Zweyer et al., 2004). Indeed, music is increasingly used to help people undergoing difficult procedures or with severe illnesses. For example, a Cochrane review of music therapy for people with cancer found it reduces pain and anxiety, increases mood and quality of life, and has positive effects on heart rate, respiratory rate, and blood pressure (Bradt et al., 2011).

Acute pain is necessary to protect us from damage or infection. **Chronic pain** is somewhat different. In the general population, chronic pain is common and thought to affect around 20% of adults. An Australian survey of over 17,000 people found that 17% of men and 20% of women reported experiencing pain every day for at least three months (Blyth et al., 2001). In the USA, chronic pain affects nearly one in three people and is estimated to cost over $560 billion per year through treatment costs and lost work days (Institute of Medicine, 2011). Prolonged aches or pains are usually a signal that a part of our body is damaged or healing. However, if pain continues for three months or longer it is possible that the original physical damage has healed but that pain pathways have become over-sensitised or dysregulated so that pain is still felt in the absence of physical injury. Research has shown that after three months of stimulation to a pain pathway, molecular changes occur in the ribonucleic acid (RNA) in the neurons of the spinal cord. Thus pain neurons adapt and change in the face of constant stimulation. Similarly, imaging research has shown extensive cortical reorganisation in response to chronic pain and that some maladaptive coping strategies, such as thinking the worst (catastrophising), can affect this (Friebel et al., 2011; Gracely et al., 2004). This has implications for the treatment of chronic pain. Rather than taking a 'wait and see' approach, early intervention is important to prevent changes to the neural pathways.

How we view pain has implications for understanding and treatment. Biological explanations of pain assume that pain results from physical damage. Treatment will therefore comprise analgesia to numb the pain and, if possible, surgery to repair the damage. However, as we have seen above, there can be many instances where pain occurs in response to threat of injury or even the absence of physical injury. Pain is increased by negative emotion, cognitive processes, and behaviour, such as inactivity.

Overall, it is clear that pain is highly subjective and influenced by many factors, including biological, psychological, and social factors. The range of factors that can affect pain perception is illustrated in Figure 4.1. The point at which a person complains of pain will vary according to the immediate context, their background and characteristics, and what they have learned from others about pain expression. The implication for healthcare is that each person's pain should be treated *as needed*, without referring to stereotypes about how much pain they 'should' be in.

4.2.1 THEORIES OF PAIN

Historically, pain was viewed from a biomedical perspective, where pain was a direct result of injury and the severity of the pain would be proportionate to the severity of injury. Recent literature emphasises the importance of a biopsychosocial understanding of pain such as that shown in Figure 4.1. A biopsychosocial approach acknowledges that pain occurs within a social context and that there are different aspects to it: biological factors, such as injury, genetics, immune and central nervous system responses; psychological factors, such as emotional, cognitive, and behavioural responses; and social factors, such as support from others, reactions of others, and cultural norms for expressing pain. In many ways, this is similar to the models of emotion in Chapter 2 that also highlight the interdependence between physical sensations, thoughts, and emotion.

Theory has made a significant contribution to our understanding of how psychological and physical factors interact in the perception of pain. The **Gate Theory of pain** (Melzack & Wall, 1965) was influential in our understanding and is based on the notion of a synaptic gate between peripheral nerves and neurons in the spinal cord, as illustrated in Figure 4.2. Pain signals from peripheral nerves compete with other neural signals to get through the gate. The gate can be open or closed by physical factors (e.g. counter-stimulation of other peripheral nerves, endogenous opioids) or by psychological factors (e.g. attention, downward stimulation from the brain, moods). This theory therefore provides a basis on which to understand the interplay between physical and psychological factors in pain. It also accounts for the phenomenon of pain being reduced through touch, such as when a child is hurt and someone 'rubs it better' (see Research Box 4.1). This theory was later expanded

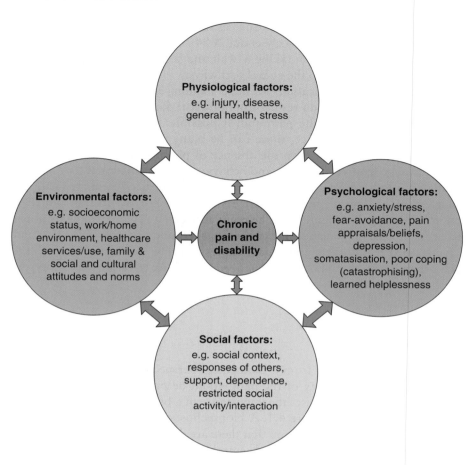

FIGURE 4.1 Biopsychosocial model of pain (adapted from Stinson et al., 2016)

by Melzack into the *neuromatrix* model, where pain is due to interacting neural networks with somatosensory, limbic, and cognitive components (Melzack, 1999).

The advantage of Gate Theory is that it provides a physiological explanation for how psychological factors affect pain perception. It also makes it clear that pain is not simply physical or psychological, but a combination of both. However, evidence for this theory is mixed. There is a large amount of supporting evidence showing that psychological factors influence pain but the physiological evidence for Gate Theory is less consistent (Mendell, 2014). Nonetheless, Gate Theory is an important and useful part of pain management programmes because it helps people with chronic pain understand that their mental attitude and behaviour can influence their pain. This can help them feel less helpless and more in control. It provides them with knowledge about the things they can do that can open or close the gate, such as those shown in Box 4.1, so they can actively work to reduce their pain by increasing those things in their life that will close the gate.

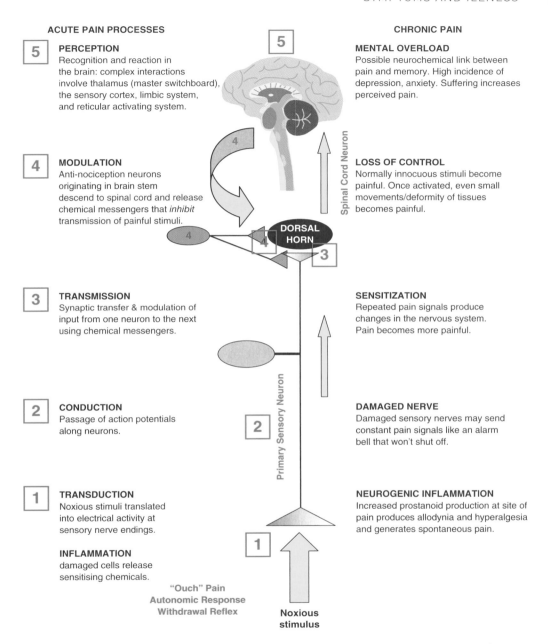

ACUTE PAIN PROCESSES

5 PERCEPTION
Recognition and reaction in the brain: complex interactions involve thalamus (master switchboard), the sensory cortex, limbic system, and reticular activating system.

4 MODULATION
Anti-nociception neurons originating in brain stem descend to spinal cord and release chemical messengers that *inhibit* transmission of painful stimuli.

3 TRANSMISSION
Synaptic transfer & modulation of input from one neuron to the next using chemical messengers.

2 CONDUCTION
Passage of action potentials along neurons.

1 TRANSDUCTION
Noxious stimuli translated into electrical activity at sensory nerve endings.

INFLAMMATION
damaged cells release sensitising chemicals.

"Ouch" Pain
Autonomic Response
Withdrawal Reflex

CHRONIC PAIN

MENTAL OVERLOAD
Possible neurochemical link between pain and memory. High incidence of depression, anxiety. Suffering increases perceived pain.

LOSS OF CONTROL
Normally innocuous stimuli become painful. Once activated, even small movements/deformity of tissues becomes painful.

SENSITIZATION
Repeated pain signals produce changes in the nervous system. Pain becomes more painful.

DAMAGED NERVE
Damaged sensory nerves may send constant pain signals like an alarm bell that won't shut off.

NEUROGENIC INFLAMMATION
Increased prostanoid production at site of pain produces allodynia and hyperalgesia and generates spontaneous pain.

DORSAL HORN

Spinal Cord Neuron

Primary Sensory Neuron

Noxious stimulus

FIGURE 4.2 The psychophysiology of pain reproduced courtesy of Christine Whitten MD (Whitten et al., 2005)

RESEARCH BOX 4.1   Counter-stimulation, attention, and pain

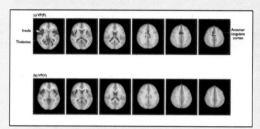

fMRI showing brain activation when participants focused on the pain (i) VP(P) or on the vibratory stimulus (ii) VP(V).

Background

Gate Theory of pain suggests that stimulating another part of the body during pain can reduce perceived pain. This experiment looked at people's subjective pain responses and their central nervous system responses using fMRI.

Method and findings

Five healthy people took part in a series of experiments where pain was induced using a rapid heat stimulus. In one condition people just had the painful heat applied. In other conditions the painful task was coupled with an unpainful vibratory stimulus. Participants were asked to pay attention to the pain, the vibratory stimulus, or a neutral image.

In keeping with the Gate Theory, counter-stimulation with the vibratory stimulus led to participants reporting less pain. Attention was also important. Participants reported less pain when they focused on the vibratory stimulus compared to when they focused on the pain. Brain regions involved in processing pain were also less active when participants focused on the vibratory stimulus as shown above.

Significance

This study confirms that counter-stimulation reduces pain and also highlights the importance of attention in the perception of pain and central nervous system processing of pain.

Longe, S.E., Wise, R., Bantick, S., Lloyd, D., Johansen-Berg, H., McGlone, F. & Tracey, I. (2001) Counter-stimulatory effects on pain perception and processing are significantly altered by attention: an fMRI study. *Neuroreport*, *12*(9): 2021–2025.

Since Gate Theory was proposed, more has become known about psychological processes and pain. Theories within the psychology aspect of a biopsychosocial approach include the role of conditioning, cognitive-behavioural models, and functional-contextual approaches in chronic pain. **Conditioning** approaches to chronic pain focus on the role of operant conditioning in behavioural responses to pain (Fordyce et al., 1973). Although the initial behavioural response may be triggered by injury, this approach focuses on how long-term pain behaviours are shaped by how others respond to these behaviours. If behaviours are reinforced, then they are more likely to continue, whereas behaviours that are not reinforced or are punished are likely to stop. Thus long-term behavioural responses to pain are contingent on

BOX 4.1 Factors that open or close the pain 'gate'

	Factors that tend to open the gate	Factors that tend to close the gate
Physical	Further injury	Appropriate use of medication
	Inactivity/poor physical fitness	Heat/cold
	Long-term drug and alcohol use	Massage
Behavioural	Poor or too little pacing of activity, i.e. doing too much	Exercise
		Relaxation training
	Poor sleep	Meditation
Emotional	Anxiety, depression	Laughter/humour
	Stress, distress	Love
	Hopelessness/helplessness	Pleasure/happiness
Cognitive	Focusing on the pain	Focusing on other things, e.g. hobbies
	Worrying about the pain	
	Catastrophising (thinking the worst)	Distraction
	Focusing on the negative consequences of pain	Positive coping strategies
	Wishing it would go away	

reinforcement from others (Chapter 10 gives more information on conditioning). There is evidence to support this. For example, a study of children with chronic pain showed that when parents responded maladaptively to the child's pain, their children reported increased symptoms and disability. This occurred regardless of whether parents' responses were positively reinforcing (e.g. paying more attention to the pain, granting special privileges) or negatively reinforcing (e.g. criticism, discounting the pain) (Claar et al., 2008). Behavioural interventions for chronic pain therefore aim to reduce symptoms and disability through training healthcare professionals and family members to reinforce 'well' behaviours, such as increased functioning, and to ignore pain behaviours, such as verbal or nonverbal expressions of pain or disability (Scott & McCracken, 2018). However, behavioural interventions alone are not effective treatments for chronic pain (Williams et al., 2012).

Cognitive-behavioural approaches to chronic pain incorporate behavioural factors, such as operant conditioning, as well as individual factors, such as perceived pain, pain-related beliefs, cognitions, and emotions. There are many approaches within this, one of which is the **fear-avoidance model**. This model suggests that if people catastrophise about their pain (e.g. focus on how awful it is, feel helpless and out of control), this leads to greater fear of pain, greater focus on pain, and restricted functioning such that people actively avoid any activity that might increase their pain. This avoidance leads to disuse, disability, and depression, as shown in Figure 4.3 (Crombez et al., 2012).

Cognitive behaviour therapy (CBT) for chronic pain draws on these and other approaches to identify and change maladaptive thinking, emotional and behavioural responses, and coping styles. CBT for pain management might involve education about the role of psychological factors in pain, examination of current appraisals, beliefs and responses to pain, and looking at more adaptive ways of thinking and coping. People are taught coping strategies such as relaxation, distraction, or stress management. Functioning is increased through setting goals and gradually increasing activity. CBT is an effective treatment for chronic pain. A review of 42 randomised controlled trials with 4,788 participants showed CBT led to small to moderate improvements in pain, disability, and mood immediately after treatment (Williams et al., 2012).

The **functional-contextual approach** to chronic pain (McCracken & Morley, 2014) was developed in line with third-wave CBT, particularly **acceptance and commitment therapy (ACT)**. The functional-contextual approach focuses on the *processes* and *function* of thoughts and behaviours, rather than the *content* of thoughts (e.g. pain-beliefs) which is the focus of standard CBT. The contextual aspect of this model is a focus on psychological flexibility, i.e. the function and workability of responses to pain and whether people's responses to pain are consistent with their values and goals in life (Scott & McCracken, 2018). The focus of treatment is therefore to improve functioning and quality of life, rather than specifically targeting pain. This is done through a range of techniques, such as acceptance of chronic pain, identifying life values, and using mindfulness and cognitive defusion to help people manage their pain and live according to their values and goals. More information on ACT, mindfulness and other techniques is given in Chapter 19. Meta-analyses suggest that ACT is an effective treatment for chronic pain. It is comparable to traditional CBT in terms of improvements in pain, disability, and emotional functioning and appears to be superior to mindfulness-based interventions (Hann & McCracken, 2014; Veehof et al., 2016).

The **communal coping model (CCM)** is also a social-contextual approach. The CCM looks at the relationship between pain and catastrophising thoughts and behaviour. It suggests that some people may be predisposed to dealing with distress by catastrophising in order to communicate their distress and attempt to increase social proximity and support from others. In this way, it is similar to operant conditioning approaches, because the behaviour of others is important. However, like the functional-contextual approach, it looks at the social function of catastrophising behaviour to the person in chronic pain. The CCM distinguishes between pain severity, the emotional components of pain, catastrophising thoughts, catastrophising behaviour, and reinforcing or solicitous behaviours of others (Thorn et al., 2003).

4.2.2 BIOPSYCHOSOCIAL APPROACH TO PAIN MANAGEMENT

The section on theories of pain showed how different theories have led to the development of various treatments for chronic pain. Because pain is multidimensional, interventions for chronic pain need to tackle the physiological, psychological, and social factors involved in pain. Chronic pain management programmes should therefore involve physicians, physiotherapists, psychologists, and specialist nurses, who work together to use pharmacological, behavioural, and psychological techniques to help people with chronic pain. The aim of these programmes is to assist people in effectively *managing* their pain so that they can lead a functional and positive life. These programmes are usually effective, particularly if they involve a psychological component such as CBT or ACT. Psychological components include educating people about the different dimensions of pain and how vicious cycles can arise, such as the fear-avoidance cycle shown in Figure 4.3. People are encouraged to take control of their life and through a process of empowerment to become more active. This can then lead to a positive cycle of less fear, less focus on the pain, and therefore less pain.

Pain management programmes are usually effective and reduce pain, depression or other negative emotion, and abnormal pain behaviours. They can also lead to more successful coping, increased activity, and improved social functioning (Morley, 2007). Programmes vary widely in their specific approach. Case Study 4.2 illustrates a broad approach.

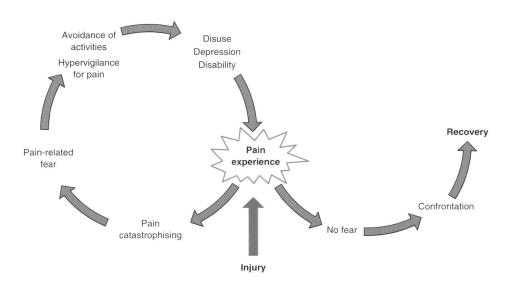

FIGURE 4.3 *Fear-avoidance model of pain (Crombez et al., 2012)*

CASE STUDY 4.2   Treating chronic back pain

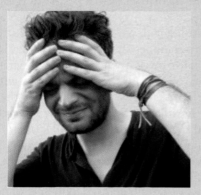

Robert is a 40-year-old man who works as a laboratory technician and has chronic lower back pain. The pain started following a work-related accident three years ago. In the last six months the pain has become constant and seems to get much worse when Robert is driving or sitting. Robert's back occasionally 'goes into spasm'. When this happens he feels semi-paralysed and has to lie down on the floor until the attack passes. This has only happened twice but Robert is very worried and frightened of the possibility of another attack.

Robert is on long-term sick leave. He does not go out much because he is worried he will have another attack and collapse. Robert is depressed and says the pain has taken over his life. He uses a number of pain relief medications every day but says it doesn't help. He is physically inactive.

Treatment

In a typical pain management programme Robert would be seen by a doctor to rule out any physical cause for his pain and agree an effective approach to analgesia. A physiotherapist would work with Robert to do exercises that strengthen his back. The physiotherapist might also help Robert gradually increase his activity levels each week.

Psychological treatment might involve education about psychological aspects of pain to help Robert understand how his actions and thoughts affect his pain. He would be encouraged to manage his pain, rather than allowing it to control him. A traditional CBT approach might involve deconstructing the pain through monitoring of pain-related thoughts and behaviour, and increasing Robert's awareness of pain processes. Robert might complete a pain diary to identify any pattern to his symptoms, the effect it is having on his life, and how his pain is linked to triggers like stress, thoughts, emotions, and general activity levels. Maladaptive thought processes or behaviours would be identified and Robert would be encouraged to change these. Robert would be taught coping strategies such as relaxation techniques, mindfulness, positive self-talk, and setting and achieving personal goals.

This should help Robert exercise and go out more often, which in turn should reduce his fear and avoidance of activity, and help him feel more in control of his pain. Providing Robert with positive coping strategies may consolidate his feelings of control and empowerment and help him have a better quality of life.

Summary

- Pain is a common symptom: up to 20% of the adult population is estimated to suffer from chronic pain.
- Pain is multidimensional: it involves nociception, pain sensations, thoughts, emotions, pain behaviours, and suffering.
- Attention, anxiety, and distress are associated with increased pain.
- The Gate Theory of pain provides a physiological explanation for the influence of psychological factors on pain.
- Pain management programmes help people cope better with chronic pain. They are often effective at reducing pain, depression, negative emotion, negative coping, and maladaptive pain behaviour; and increasing activity, positive coping, and social functioning.

4.3 PLACEBO AND NOCEBO EFFECTS

Placebo and nocebo effects provide clear examples of the effect of beliefs on symptoms. The term 'placebo' is Latin for *I shall please*. A **placebo effect** is when people are given a fake treatment that has no active ingredient yet report an improvement. Placebo effects are not limited to fake drugs but can also occur in response to fake surgery. For example, a study comparing arthroscopic procedures (debridement or lavage) for osteoarthritis of the knee with sham surgery (where incisions were made but no debridement or lavage done) show that people who have sham surgery have less pain and better functioning after the surgery than those who had real surgery (Evidence Development and Standards, 2014). Similarly, a placebo effect can occur with an active drug, where part of the drug effect is due to the active ingredients and part due to a placebo effect. For example, studies have been conducted where people consent to having medication administered intravenously without their knowledge so they do not know when, or if, they are being given medication. Comparing their responses to medication with people who know when they receive medication shows that a substantial proportion of the effects of morphine on pain, beta-blockers on heart rate, and diazepam on anxiety are due to the placebo effect (Benedetti et al., 2003; Colloca et al., 2004). An example of research showing a placebo effect is given in Research Box 4.2.

Some people respond to placebo more strongly than others, and some illnesses are more amenable to placebos. Evidence suggests that placebo effects are most powerful for conditions with psychological components such as pain, depression, asthma, and insomnia. Placebos are not effective for disorders with a clear simple biological basis, such as anaemia and infections (Wampold et al., 2005). Characteristics of placebos affect how well they work. For example, injections have a larger effect than pills; fake morphine has a larger effect than fake aspirin; and placebo effects are larger if the doctor or healthcare professional expresses a belief it will work (Kirsch, 2018).

RESEARCH BOX 4.2   Listening to prozac and hearing placebo

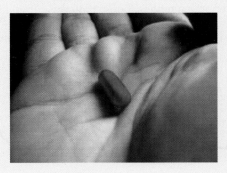

Background

Meta-analysis is a technique used to synthesise the results of several studies to give a statistical summary of the findings. However, to produce the most accurate information, meta-analysis should be based on published and unpublished research.

Method and findings

Information from published and unpublished randomised controlled trials of the most widely used antidepressant medications (SSRIs) was collected. Thirty-five trials were found involving 5,133 people with major depressive disorder. All trials compared the effect of SSRIs with a placebo drug.

For most people, the effect of SSRIs was so small it was not clinically significant. A placebo could duplicate 80% of the effect of antidepressants. In people with extremely severe depression, antidepressants had a small effect on recovery, but this seemed to be mainly due to these people being less responsive to placebos rather than being more responsive to antidepressants.

Significance

Previous meta-analyses of published research had found more positive results, with small effects of some SSRIs on depression. This meta-analysis was the first to include unpublished evidence and clearly shows that SSRIs are no better than a placebo for treating mild or moderate depression. SSRIs are therefore only clinically useful for the treatment of very severe depression.

Photograph reproduced courtesy of Clix (stock.xchng)

Kirsch, I., Deacon, B.J., Huedo-Medina, T.B., Scoboria, A., Moore, T.J. & Johnson, B.T. (2008) Initial severity and antidepressant benefits: A meta-analysis of data submitted to the Food and Drug Administration. *PLoS Medicine*, 5(2): 260–268.

The **nocebo effect** is less well known than the placebo effect. The term 'nocebo' is Latin for *I shall harm*. The nocebo effect occurs when people develop symptoms that fit their beliefs even when they have not been exposed to a pathogen. For example,

Lorber et al. (2007) asked students to inhale an inert substance, which they said was a toxin that could result in particular symptoms. In addition, half the students watched another person, who was secretly a research confederate, inhale the substance first and show these symptoms. All students who inhaled the placebo reported the symptoms they were told they might have. Women were particularly influenced if they saw the confederate display symptoms. Nocebo effects with demonstrable physical changes have also been observed. For example, giving people with asthma a sham inhaler which they are told is an allergen leads to bronchoconstriction, even when they are given nebulised saline (Colloca & Miller, 2011).

There is substantial evidence for placebo and nocebo effects (Kirsch, 2018). What is less clear is the mechanisms through which these effects are produced. Explanations include conditioning (including modelling) and the effect of expectations. **Classical conditioning** occurs when a stimulus (in this case an active drug or treatment) is paired with a response (an improvement in health) and over time becomes associated with a neutral stimulus that also occurs in this context (pills, injections, the actions of healthcare professionals). The neutral stimulus then becomes a conditioned stimulus, which results in some of the changes observed to the initial active stimulus. **Modelling** occurs when one observes the effect in someone else and learns it. These types of learning are covered in more detail in Chapter 10.

Another key explanation is that placebos work through a person's **expectations** – they expect to get better or worse, so they do. There is evidence that both classical conditioning and expectations can contribute to the placebo effect, and that these are not incompatible (Kirsch, 2018). More recently, an integrated framework has been proposed where the placebo response is thought to be a learned response, where a variety of cues trigger expectations that generate placebo or nocebo effects via the central nervous system. These cues can be verbal, conditioned, or social, such as being influenced by what healthcare professionals say about the placebo, as well as by observation of others' responses. Evidence from neurological studies supports the role of the central nervous system in the placebo effect. A review of fMRI studies of responses to placebo analgesia found reduced activity in brain areas associated with pain, such as the insula, dorsal anterior cingulate cortex, thalamus, amygdala, and right lateral prefrontal cortex (Atlas & Wager, 2014). Genetic research into possible determinants of why people are more or less responsive to placebos suggests genetic variation in the dopamine, opioid, serotonin, endocannabinoid, and oxytocin systems may be involved (Colagiuri et al., 2015; Fabbro & Crescentini, 2014).

4.3.1 USING THE PLACEBO EFFECT IN CLINICAL PRACTICE

The placebo effect has many clinical implications. The first is that the effect of many active drugs can be increased by the way they are presented – both in form (e.g. pill or injection) and in manner (e.g. with enthusiasm and conviction). A healthcare professional

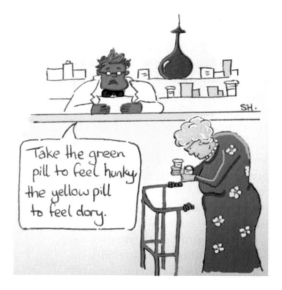

who encourages people to believe treatments will work can harness the placebo effect in addition to the drug. The second implication is that placebos can result in a positive change without any negative side effects, so are useful treatments for those conditions that are amenable to placebos, such as depression. In fact, surveys of healthcare professionals in different countries show that up to 80% of doctors and even more nurses have used placebos such as saline injections (Fässler et al., 2010). However, if we use these strategies we must be mindful of the ethical and legal issues. People should be encouraged to have positive expectations, but within realistic limits. The dilemma when using placebos is how to do so without employing deception, although recent research suggests placebos can be effective even when people know they are placebos (Carvalho et al., 2016). Kirsch (2018) recommends using treatments that do not have active components where there is some evidence they might be effective, such as some complementary therapies or physical exercise.

CLINICAL NOTES 4.2

Pain and placebo

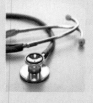

- Pain is subjective so each person's pain should be treated *as needed*, without reference to stereotypes about how much pain they 'should' have.
- Chronic pain results in extensive neural changes that may be difficult to reverse so we should intervene as early as possible to avoid these.
- Placebo effects can duplicate 80% of the effect of antidepressants in people with mild or moderate depression.
- Use the placebo effect to increase the effect of treatment: express confidence that treatments will work to increase people's positive expectations.
- Conversely, if you tell people to expect side effects or negative symptoms they will be more likely to experience them (the nocebo effect).

Summary

- A placebo effect occurs when someone's health improves in the absence of any active substance or treatment.
- A nocebo effect occurs when someone reports symptoms in the absence of any active pathogen.
- These effects can account for a substantial proportion of recovery, particularly in illnesses with strong psychological components, such as asthma and depression.
- The extent of the placebo effect varies between individuals.
- Placebos are thought to work through a combination of expectations, classical conditioning, and modelling.
- The placebo effect can be used in clinical practice to aid recovery.

4.4 ILLNESS BELIEFS AND REPRESENTATIONS

Earlier in this chapter we looked at the effect of unconscious schema on the perception of symptoms. In addition to this, people hold conscious beliefs about illness which will shape their behaviour in response to symptoms. Beliefs about illness will determine the action a person chooses to take, which information they give to a healthcare professional, the kind of treatment they want, whether they adhere to that treatment, and their emotional, behavioural, and cognitive responses to the illness. Illness beliefs are not necessarily accurate or coherent. **Illness representations** are people's organised sets of beliefs about the experience, impact, effect, and outcome of an illness. They are unique to each individual and are shaped by many factors, including their personal history, experience of different illnesses, and social and cultural learning.

Five main dimensions of illness representations have been identified: identity, timeline, cause, control, and consequences (Leventhal et al., 1984; Leventhal et al., 2003). Here we will outline each of these in more detail. The concept of **illness identity** refers to the way a person labels the illness and symptoms, such as what multiple sclerosis is and what it involves. People will have mental models of which symptoms go with different illnesses. The more various symptoms match a person's model of a particular illness the more likely it is they will diagnose themselves as having that illness. For example, a headache could be due to many things, such as a hangover, tension, migraine, a brain tumour, or meningitis. A self-diagnosis of meningitis is more likely if a person experiences a headache, stiff neck, and a rash. Making a self-diagnosis is important in seeking help. Research shows that people are more likely to attend a doctor if they have self-diagnosed a specific illness (Cameron et al., 1993; Simons et al., 2015).

The **timeline** is the length of time that a person believes the illness will last and the pattern it will take, for example chronic, acute, remitting, or cyclical. This affects their adjustment to the illness and adherence to treatment. For example, people who believe their illnesses are chronic will report more disability and distress compared to other people with the same illness who believe it is acute or cyclical (Millar et al., 2005).

The **cause** is what a person thinks caused their symptoms or illness. This overlaps with the attributions and interpretation of symptoms discussed earlier. However, they may not be medically accurate. For example, stress is commonly believed to cause a range of illnesses including cancer, diabetes, multiple sclerosis, and arthritis (Cameron & Moss-Morris, 2004).

Beliefs about **control** concern whether the person believes their illness can be prevented, controlled, or cured. People who think their illness is controllable are more likely to take an active part in their treatment and rehabilitation. Conversely, thinking an illness is uncontrollable is associated with using passive coping strategies (e.g. avoidance) and poorer mental health outcomes (Dempster et al., 2015; Hudson et al., 2014; Richardson et al., 2016). In a chronic or terminal illness, we should therefore encourage people to focus on those aspects of their illness they can control, such as their symptoms, disability, and the timeline.

Beliefs about **consequences** are concerned with the effect of the illness, for example physical, psychological, social, and economic effects. Perceived consequences are usually closely linked to the severity of someone's symptoms. Therefore asymptomatic illnesses, such as hypertension, are often viewed as having no consequences.

The diagram in Figure 4.4 shows how illness representations can affect the way a person copes with their symptoms, illness, and treatment (Leventhal et al., 1984; Leventhal et al., 2003). This is known as the **self-regulation model of illness behaviour** because it accounts for how people will self-manage their illness as a result of their personal beliefs. The strengths of this model are that it recognises the importance of appraisal, emotion, and coping in managing illness. Case Study 4.3 illustrates how illness beliefs can affect perceptions of chest pain. A difficulty with the illness representations model is that severe

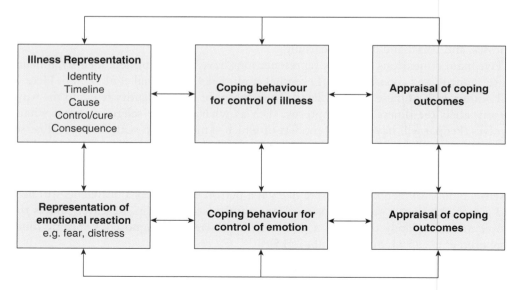

FIGURE 4.4   Self-regulation model of illness cognition and behaviour (Leventhal et al., 1984)

illnesses like cancer are more likely to result in negative illness representations, for example being chronic, uncontrollable, and having severe consequences. A key question is therefore whether illness representations can affect a person's adjustment over and above the severity of the illness itself. Many studies have shown that this is the case. Beliefs about the consequences of chronic diseases such as rheumatoid arthritis and multiple sclerosis are associated with poorer psychological outcomes, reports of more symptoms, and an increased use of health services (e.g. Dempster et al., 2015; Hudson et al., 2014; Jopson & Moss-Morris, 2003; Richardson et al., 2016).

CASE STUDY 4.3   The self-regulation model and chest pain

The self-regulation model illustrates how symptoms, such as chest pain, will be perceived and interpreted by a person on the basis of their illness representations, which in turn will influence their coping behaviour. The symptom will also evoke an emotional reaction that will lead to coping strategies to control that emotion. Both the emotional and cognitive strands will influence each other. Coping and reappraisal can then lead to an adjustment of beliefs, emotions, and coping responses and so on, as illustrated below.

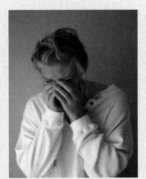

Source: Kennedy, Wikipedia Commons, August 2009, CC-by-2.0

Tanya is 48 years old and has a pain in her chest one evening after she has eaten a large dinner and had a heated argument with her husband. Tanya's uncle died of a heart attack a few years ago, aged 65. Tanya thinks that men are particularly vulnerable to heart attacks but women are not (identity). Tanya knows that indigestion or heartburn can also cause pain in the chest (cause). She also knows that arguments and stress can lead to an upset stomach (cause). She therefore interprets this pain as indigestion, which will pass if she relaxes (consequences). She makes herself a calming cup of tea and goes to lie down (coping response).

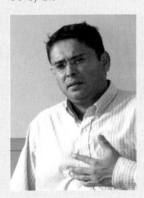

Photo courtesy of Ronald Sumners, obtained via Shutterstock

Vinay is 48 years old and has a pain in his chest one evening after he has eaten a large dinner and had a heated argument with his wife. Vinay's uncle died of a heart attack a few years ago, aged 65. Vinay knows that men in their 40s are particularly vulnerable to heart attacks (identity) and that they can be caused by stress (cause). He therefore immediately interprets this pain as a possible heart attack and potentially fatal (consequences). He becomes very anxious and upset and feels his heart pounding. He calls an ambulance to take him to hospital immediately (coping response).

RESEARCH BOX 4.3   Self-management after a myocardial infarction

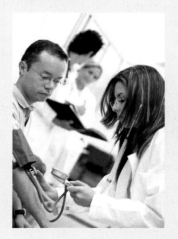

Photo courtesy of ESB Professional, obtained via Shutterstock

Background

Self-management interventions focus on people's illness representations and coping skills in order to promote effective self-management for a range of illnesses. This study compared a self-management intervention to standard care for people who had a myocardial infarction (MI).

Method and findings

Sixty-five people who had had an MI were randomly allocated to receive a self-management intervention or standard care while in hospital. People were assessed before and after the intervention and followed up three months later. The self-management intervention involved three sessions of half-an-hour each:

- Session 1: educating about MI and exploring people's beliefs about the cause of their MI; challenging the common perception that an MI is largely caused by stress; educating people about the importance of lifestyle (e.g. exercise and diet).
- Session 2: exploring people's perceptions of the timeline and consequences; encouraging people to develop beliefs of control; developing an individualised written illness management plan to minimise future risks and encourage returning to normal levels of activity.
- Session 3: reviewing the action plan from session 2 and educating about distinguishing normal symptoms of recovery from symptoms that might indicate another MI.

People who had the self-management intervention did much better. They felt more prepared for leaving hospital, had a better understanding of MI, were less distressed at discharge, were more likely to attend cardiac rehabilitation, viewed their MI more positively, and had more positive beliefs about control, consequences, and the timeline of MI. Three months later, people in the self-management group had returned to work quicker and reported fewer symptoms of angina.

Significance

This study shows how a brief intervention in hospital based on the principles of illness representations helped people understand and manage their MI better, return to work quicker, and have fewer symptoms in the long term.

Photograph © Andres Rodriguez/Fotolia

Petrie, K.J., Cameron, L.D., Ellis, C.J., Buick, D. & Weinman, J. (2002) Changing illness perceptions after myocardial infarction: An early intervention randomized controlled trial. *Psychosomatic Medicine*, 64: 580–586.

ACTIVITY 4.1 ILLNESS REPRESENTATIONS

- Think of a person you have seen who was particularly upset by their illness.
- What sort of beliefs did they have about their illness identity, timeline, cause, control, and consequences?

4.4.1 APPLICATIONS TO CLINICAL PRACTICE

Illness representations have many implications for clinical practice. Managing an illness which seems abstract is harder than managing an illness when a person has concrete experience of it. In other words, people are less likely to adhere to treatment for an illness where there are no concrete symptoms. This can be the case in asymptomatic illnesses like hypertension, or illnesses that do not have regular symptoms such as diabetes or HIV. This links to the issue of motivation: if people do not have symptoms, they may be more likely to favour an immediate reward (such as sugary food for diabetics) over the long-term consequences.

People can also have beliefs and representations about treatment procedures that will affect how likely they are to adhere to particular treatments. For example, the use of corticosteroids will not be effective if a person associates it with the steroids used by body builders and is put off by this. Some people may also worry about the addictive properties of certain drugs and will therefore not take them. For example, a survey in Germany found that 80% of people believed antidepressants were addictive (Althaus et al., 2002). For this and other reasons, 30–60% of people on antidepressants do not take them as prescribed (Demyttenaere, 2001).

The self-regulation model of illness beliefs can therefore be useful when treating people. By exploring and changing a person's illness beliefs we can maximise the chances of them managing their illness appropriately, both through changing their lifestyle and adhering to treatment. These types of intervention are broadly referred to as **self-management interventions** because they target people's beliefs and coping in order to help them manage their illness and treatment effectively. Research has shown that self-management interventions are usually effective at promoting the positive self-management of diabetes, asthma, HIV, and cancer (Petrie et al., 2003). Research Box 4.3

gives one example of a study that used a self-management intervention with people following MI. This was found to be very effective at reducing people's distress, symptoms, and increasing their return to work.

Summary

- Beliefs about illnesses will affect how people appraise symptoms, interpret symptoms, whether they seek help, and their adherence to treatment.
- Illness representations include illness identity, timeline, cause, control, and consequences.
- Illness representations are associated with both the psychological and physical outcomes of illness.
- The self-regulation model explains how illness representations can interact with coping to determine health outcomes.
- Illness representations can be used to develop effective self-management interventions for chronic illnesses that will help people cope with and manage their illness and treatment more effectively.

CLINICAL NOTES 4.3

Illness representations

- How a person thinks about their illness will affect their distress, symptom perception, and disability.
- Self-management interventions can educate people and help them think about their illness in more adaptive ways.
- To help people manage their illness better we need to help them:
  o Correct any misperceptions about the cause of their illness (and therefore future risk).
  o Focus on an aspect of their illness that they can control – such as treatment adherence or symptom management.
  o Reduce their perceptions of severe consequences through education and joint treatment plans. In cases of terminal illness this may involve tackling worries about pain relief and dying.

CONCLUSION

In this chapter we have seen how the perception of symptoms is strongly influenced by psychological factors, including attention, emotions, beliefs, and environmental factors. The importance of psychological factors in the outcome of illnesses has been illustrated by placebo and nocebo effects, which can be substantial. Research and theory in this area are therefore highly relevant to clinical practice and have been used to develop effective treatments such as pain management programmes and self-management programmes in order to help people manage their symptoms and illness more effectively.

FURTHER READING

Llewellyn, C.D. et al. (eds) (2018) *The Cambridge Handbook of Psychology, Health and Medicine* (3rd edition). Cambridge: Cambridge University Press. Includes short chapters on pain, pain management, placebo and nocebos, and illness representations.

Cameron, L.D. & Leventhal, H. (2003) *The Self-Regulation of Health and Illness Behaviour*. London: Routledge. This book has more in-depth information on illness beliefs and self-regulation, with chapters on the theory of self-regulation, illness representations, social and cultural influences, and interventions.

Friedman, H.S. (ed.) (2011) *The Oxford Handbook of Health Psychology*. Oxford: Oxford University Press. This book has chapters on health and illness perceptions, and chronic pain.

REVISION QUESTIONS

1. What is a symptom? How accurate are people at detecting changes in physiological states (e.g. blood pressure)?

2. Discuss the role of two psychological factors in the perception of physical symptoms.

3. What is the difference between a person's pain threshold and pain tolerance? Briefly outline the role of psychological factors in both.

4. Outline the Gate Theory of pain and discuss how it has extended our understanding of the interplay between psychological and physical factors.

5. What is the communal coping model of pain? What implications does it have for treatment?

6. What is a placebo effect? What factors affect how strong it is?

7. What is a nocebo effect? What is the evidence it affects symptom perception?

8. Outline three different explanations for why placebo and nocebo effects might occur.

9. Describe the five main dimensions of illness representations.

10. Describe a self-management intervention based on the self-regulation model.

5 HEALTH AND BEHAVIOUR

(Continued)

LEARNING OBJECTIVES

This chapter is designed to enable you to:

- Discuss the importance of health behaviour and of health behaviour change.
- Outline the different models of health behaviour.
- Understand how to apply these models in clinical practice to help people change.

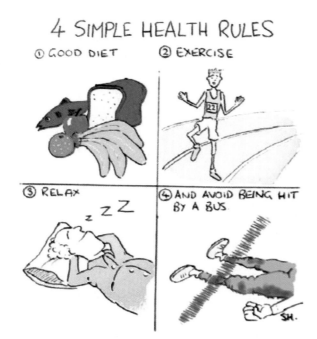

4 SIMPLE HEALTH RULES
① GOOD DIET   ② EXERCISE
③ RELAX   ④ AND AVOID BEING HIT BY A BUS

Understanding and changing health behaviour effectively would do more than anything else to reduce morbidity and mortality in our society. The leading global risks for mortality – in high, middle, and low income countries – are high blood pressure, tobacco use, high blood glucose, physical inactivity, and being over-weight (World Health Organisation, 2009b). These raise the risk of chronic diseases such as heart disease, diabetes, and cancers. Globally, over three quarters of premature deaths are caused by cardiovascular diseases, cancer, diabetes, and chronic respiratory diseases, including lung cancer (World Health Organisation, 2016a). Most people know cigarette smoking is bad for their health, yet around one in five people smoke. Even when they are in hospital some people will continue to smoke, despite often having to stand outside to do so.

5.1 PREDICTING AND CHANGING HEALTH BEHAVIOUR

5.1.1 WHAT ARE HEALTH BEHAVIOURS?

It is not only risky behaviours like smoking that affect our health. In a famous longitudinal study of almost 7,000 people living in Alameda County (USA), it was found that seven key behaviours were associated with a longer life: not smoking; being physically active; moderate weight; moderate alcohol intake; getting 7–8 hours sleep a night; eating breakfast regularly; not snacking (Belloc, 1973; Kaplan et al., 1987). Table 5.1 shows key health behaviours at the global level.

TABLE 5.1 Top five global risks for mortality and burden of disease (World Health Organisation, 2009b)

Mortality	Burden of disease (disability-adjusted life years: DALYs)
high blood pressure	underweight
tobacco use	unsafe sex
high blood glucose	alcohol use
physical inactivity	unsafe water
overweight and obesity	sanitation and hygiene

Thus our health is affected by a range of behaviours, which can be categorised as (a) health protective behaviours and (b) health risk behaviours. Health protective behaviours consist of things like exercise, a good diet, sleep, and dental care. They also include **screening behaviours** such as attending regular screening checks for chlamydia, cervical

CLINICAL NOTES 5.1

Smoking and health

- Smoking is the number one cause of preventable illness and death.
- Every person you help to give up smoking reduces a lot of morbidity and mortality – not only for them, but also potentially for their children too.
- Advice from a health professional is one of the most effective triggers for people to give up smoking.
- Even *brief* advice from a health professional makes it more likely a person will give up smoking and remain non-smoking a year later.

cancer, hypertension, and dental checks. Health risk behaviours include things such as smoking, substance misuse, unsafe sex, and risky driving. Behaviours particularly pertinent to morbidity and mortality include smoking, diet, physical activity, alcohol consumption, screening behaviour (particularly for cancer), sexual behaviour, and driving behaviour.

We need to understand why people choose to behave in ways that will harm their health in order to help them change. This is not simple: behaviour is determined by many factors, including individual differences, social surroundings and influences, and cultural aspects. In order to have effective health promotion programmes we need to know the main causes of specific behaviours in different groups of people. For example, young people might be more motivated to eat a low-fat diet and regularly brush their teeth to improve their appearance rather than to improve their health, so emphasising the health benefits of these behaviours would not result in significant change in this group. The range of factors that influence health behaviour is shown in Table 5.2. Research and theories of health behaviour try to identify the strongest or proximal causes of behaviour so intervention can target those factors which are most likely to result in change.

TABLE 5.2   Factors that influence health behaviour

Biological factors	Heredity (i.e. genetic factors)
	Sex
	Age
Psychological factors	Conditioning
	Modelling
	Emotional state
	Cognitive factors
Social factors	Demographic factors
	Social factors
	Financial/employment status
Cultural factors	Legislation
	Economics
	Healthcare provision
	Systems of provision

5.1.2 THEORIES OF HEALTH BEHAVIOUR

Many theories of health behaviour have been proposed. In recent years, social-cognition models have been most successful at explaining health behaviour. These models account for the interplay between social and cognitive factors, such as social pressures, social norms, beliefs, and attitudes. These models are based on an *expectancy-value* principle. This assumes that a behaviour is most likely to be maintained or changed if (a) a person expects it to result in certain outcomes and (b) the person values these outcomes as important or positive. These models account for up to a third of the variance in people's behaviour. Other theories integrate aspects of social-cognition models with other factors, such as an individual's readiness or motivation to change.

This chapter discusses four models of health behaviour: two social-cognition models and two integrative models. We examine the evidence for these models and explore how we can use them in clinical practice to help people change their behaviour. This is illustrated by a case study that shows how each model can be adopted to help a young woman stop smoking.

Predicting and changing health behaviour

The social-cognition models that have been most widely used in the study of health behaviour are the Health Belief Model and the Theory of Planned Behaviour. Examples of integrative approaches are the Transtheoretical Model and PRIME Theory. These models are not necessarily in competition. Although one model may be more successful at predicting a particular type of behaviour, aspects of all of these models can be used in clinical practice.

5.2 THE HEALTH BELIEF MODEL

→ transtheoretical model   OR PRIME THEORY

The Health Belief Model (HBM) (Rosenstock, 1974; Strecher et al., 1997) is shown in Figure 5.1. It suggests that the likelihood of someone changing their behaviour is primarily determined by the perceived threat of their current situation, coupled with an evaluation of the outcome if they change. Perceived threat is thought to be influenced mainly by the perceived susceptibility to negative consequences and the perceived severity of these consequences for the person. For example, if a person thinks they are not susceptible to tuberculosis (TB) then obviously TB will not be a threat to them so they are unlikely to attend screening. Another person might think they are susceptible to TB but that TB is not severe enough to do anything about. Perceived susceptibility and severity then combine to produce a level of perceived threat that motivates people to take action or change their behaviour.

However, even when the perceived threat is high, people might still not change their behaviour. There is another factor here that influences behaviour, namely how a person evaluates the outcome. This evaluation is affected by perceived benefits and perceived barriers. Perceived benefits are what a person thinks they will gain from the behaviour or behaviour change. This can be the removal of negative factors as well as positive gains. For example, attending TB screening can mean the threat of the illness is removed or the illness is treated in its early stages before it causes a disability. Perceived barriers are things that make it difficult for a person to carry out the behaviour. For TB screening this might include not being able to take time off work, the screening clinic being a long distance away, difficulty in finding childcare, a lack of transport, etc.

The HBM is the only model that explicitly recognises the importance of cues to action that will prompt people to change. These cues can be internal (such as perceived symptoms),

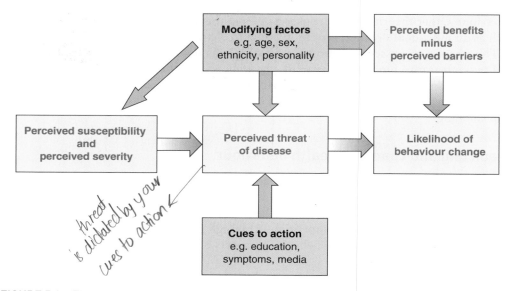

FIGURE 5.1   The Health Belief Model

or external (such as health promotion, the advice of a doctor or nurse, the warning labels of products, or the illness or death of a known person). The illness or death of a public figure can provide strong cues to act that may be wide-reaching through extensive media coverage. For example, media coverage of the deaths of British celebrities Linda McCartney (from breast cancer) and Jade Goody (from cervical cancer) was followed by marked increases in the number of women being screened.

Cues to action can take many forms. Smoking research has indicated that one of the most effective triggers in persuading someone to quit smoking is for a health professional to tell a person that they should give up. Even brief simple advice from a physician can make it more likely a smoker will quit and remain a non-smoker 12 months later (Stead et al., 2013). However, cues to action are not always necessary for change. If an individual has a sufficient perceived threat and positive evaluation of the outcome of change, then they will often change without needing a cue. In other cases, cues can be the final trigger that will tip the balance between a perceived threat and barriers and will prompt someone to act.

Later versions of the HBM have included health motivation as a factor. This relates to how much a person is concerned about their health and prepared to consider behaviour change. Surprisingly, research has given less attention to health motivation and cues to action than other model components. However, it seems that health motivation might have a small but significant effect on behaviour (Abraham & Sheeran, 2007).

The HBM is one of the longest-standing models of health behaviour. It has been researched in relation to many health behaviours, including breast self-examination, flu vaccinations, diabetes management, medication for hypertension, and cancer screening (Janz & Becker, 1984). Reviews of the evidence for the HBM have been generally positive and find that perceived barriers and benefits are often the most important factor in

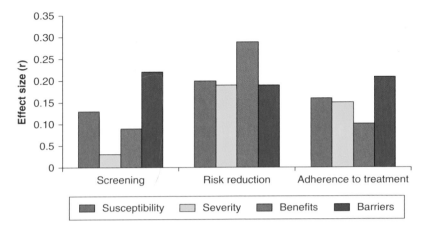

FIGURE 5.2 The Health Belief Model and different types of behaviour (adapted from Harrison et al., 1992)

determining change (Carpeneter, 2010; Janz & Becker, 1984). The importance of the HBM for different categories of health behaviour is shown in Figure 5.2. It can be seen that screening behaviours are most influenced by perceived barriers and susceptibility. When changing risky behaviours it is the perceived benefits that are most important. Adherence to medical treatment is most affected by perceived barriers to the treatment.

Interventions using the Health Belief Model

To use the HBM in clinical practice we would explore people's perceived susceptibility, severity, benefits and barriers, as well as any cues. People's perceptions of threat and benefits can be improved through education. Problem solving and action plans can be used to reduce perceived barriers. Using the HBM to design interventions has proved very effective. For example, a meta-analysis of medication adherence revealed that interventions based on the HBM were more likely to be effective than those based on other theories (Conn et al., 2016).

ACTIVITY 5.1   YOUR OWN HEALTH BEHAVIOUR

- Think back to the last time you:

    o Went to the doctor.
    o Checked yourself for breast or testicular lumps.

- How much (if at all) was your behaviour affected by the perceived severity, susceptibility, benefits, and barriers in these different situations?

Case Study 5.1 shows how we might use the HBM to help a young woman give up smoking. This illustrates how the model may be implemented as a guide if we wish to help people change a risky health behaviour.

CASE STUDY 5.1   Smoking cessation using the Health Belief Model

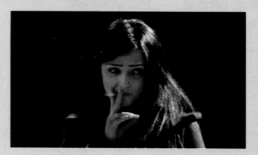

Divya is a 22-year-old woman who has smoked 20 cigarettes a day since she was 15 years old. She coughs every morning and gets breathless easily. Although she has a family history of asthma, she has never been checked for asthma herself.

Cues to action
Explore whether anything has triggered her to consider giving up smoking:
- Has anything made you think about giving up smoking?

If so, capitalise on this by reinforcing it. Give her positive feedback if she has thought about giving up smoking.

Health motivation
Explore how motivated or concerned she is about her health:
- How concerned are you about your health? (abstract health concern)
- How important is it to you to stay healthy/not to get ill? (concrete health concern)

Susceptibility and severity
Explore the perceived susceptibility and severity:
- How do you think smoking is affecting your health? (current susceptibility)
- How might it affect your health in 10 years' time? (future susceptibility)
- What would it be like if that happened to you/you got [illness]? (severity)

Educate about the negative effects of smoking to increase the perceived susceptibility and severity:

(Continued)

- If you smoke you are more likely to have heart disease, a stroke, circulation problems, lung cancer, and many other cancers.
- Every cigarette you smoke contains over 4,000 chemicals.
- The toxins in cigarettes put huge strain on your body.
- Other effects of smoking are that your skin ages quicker, teeth become discoloured, gum disease, poor sense of smell, reduced fertility, and blindness.
- Smoking is therefore the single most preventable cause of illness and death.

Perceived benefits and barriers

Explore the perceived benefits and barriers:

- What are the pros and cons of smoking for you? (current benefits and costs)
- Is there anything stopping you from giving up? (current barriers)

Problem solving to reduce barriers:

- How can you/we change this? What steps can you/we take to help you give up? (reducing current barriers and focusing on taking action)

Educate about the positive benefits if they give up smoking now, to increase the perceived benefits:

- If you give up smoking you will improve your health and live longer.
- Your risk of heart disease drops dramatically in the first year after quitting.
- You will feel healthier and, as smoking damages the skin, you might look better too.
- You will save a huge amount of money! Someone who smokes 20-a day will spend over £3000 a year on cigarettes.

5.3 THE THEORY OF PLANNED BEHAVIOUR

The Theory of Planned Behaviour (TPB) (Ajzen, 1988) originated from social psychology and was first proposed to explain all kinds of behaviour, not just health behaviour. This theory is shown in Figure 5.3. It starts from the assumption that a person's **intention** will be the strongest determinant of how they will actually behave.

Intentions are thought to be determined by two factors. The first is a person's attitudes toward the behaviour (see Chapter 9). This is influenced by their *beliefs about the outcomes of the behaviour* (e.g. the pros and cons) and their *evaluation of these outcomes* (e.g. whether these are positive or negative). Consider our case study. If Divya believes smoking will keep her slim and reduce stress (pros), and that these outcomes

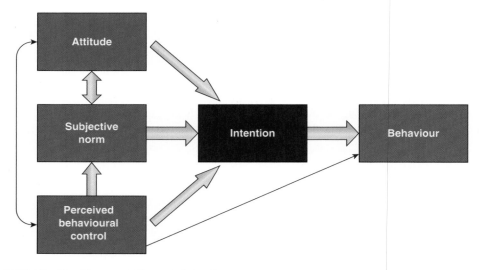

FIGURE 5.3 The Theory of Planned Behaviour

are the most important to her (her evaluation of outcome), then she will not be motivated to quit.

The second factor that determines intentions is the subjective norm. This is the perceived social norm about the behaviour in a person's environment. This is influenced by the *perceived beliefs of others* about the behaviour and the person's *motivation to comply* with these beliefs. For example, young people are often most motivated to comply with the norms of their friends. Family-based interventions for young people are therefore less likely to be successful than interventions targeted at peer groups.

ACTIVITY 5.2   SOCIAL NORMS VERSUS ATTITUDES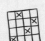

- Has there ever been a time when you have been persuaded to do something against your better judgement because everyone else was doing it? For example:

  o Drinking and driving.
  o Drinking too much.
  o Smoking or other drug use.

- What do you think is more powerful: your own attitudes or social pressure/group norms? Why is this?

A strength of the TPB is that it takes account of the importance of social pressures and norms as well as how much control a person believes they have over their behaviour. Research has shown that control is indeed important in behaviour change (Wallston, 2007). The TPB accounts for control quite broadly in the form of **perceived behavioural control**. The link between perceived behavioural control and intentions is via the amount of overall control people believe they have over their behaviour and changing this behaviour. If a person believes they do not have any control over their smoking, then they will not intend to quit. The direct link between control and behaviour is thought to be due to an *actual* lack of control over the factors needed to support or change a behaviour, rather than a *perceived* lack of control. An actual lack of control might involve not having suitable transport to attend a smoking cessation clinic, not being able to afford nicotine replacement therapy, or living in an environment where many other people also smoke.

There are numerous ways in which we can look at control. For example, we can distinguish between an internal **locus of control**, where people believe they can control their behaviour or the outcome of events, or an external locus of control, where people believe that other people or fate are controlling the outcome of events (see Chapter 9). This will vary between different situations but is very relevant to medicine. For example, a person with an external locus of control is more likely to expect medical professionals to control or sort out their illness. A person with an internal locus of control will be more proactive and likely to make lifestyle changes or adhere to treatment because they believe they have control over the outcome of their illness. This is a useful characteristic to look out for in clinical work because it can help to develop a more effective treatment plan for each individual. For example, a person with diabetes who has an external locus of control might be more effectively treated with regular outpatient appointments to monitor their progress and adjust their medication.

The TPB therefore proposes that attitudes, subjective norms, and perceived behavioural control are the major determinants of intentions. The relative importance of these three factors will vary according to different behaviours and individuals. There is evidence that the TPB predicts around half of the variance in intentions for a wide range of health behaviours, including smoking, testicular self-examination, exercise, abortion, condom use, diet, and oral hygiene (McEachan et al., 2011). The TPB is therefore very good at explaining people's intentions to act in certain ways. However, although many of us intend to live healthier lifestyles – especially at New Year – this does not always mean we will do so! The TPB is slightly less successful at predicting actual behaviour. TPB components explain around 20% of variance in physical activity and diet, but slightly less variance in risk behaviour, safer sex, and drug use (McEachan et al., 2011). Researchers therefore endeavour to improve the theory by adding such factors as **anticipated regret** about changing a behaviour, **moral norms**, and **implementation intentions** (i.e. how a person plans to take to change). These additions have appeared to be useful, particularly the implementation intentions. However, they have not added greatly to the predictive power of the model.

CLINICAL NOTES 5.2

Changing a health behaviour

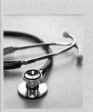

- Information (education) from a healthcare professional is a strong trigger for a behaviour change.
- Models of health behaviours are useful guides for clinical practice when helping someone change their behaviour (see case studies).
- It is important to identify barriers to change: even when people are motivated to change, perceived and actual barriers can prevent it happening.
- Explore how a person's social environment and norms may facilitate or prevent a behaviour change.
- If a person thinks they have no control over a behaviour, they will not attempt to change. Re-education and support can help increase a person's perceived control.
- Helping someone develop a plan for how they will change their behaviour makes it more likely they will succeed.

Interventions using the Theory of Planned Behaviour

Reviews of the evidence indicate that interventions based on the TPB can lead to significant behaviour change (Steinmetz et al., 2016). It appears to be better for predicting physical activity and dietary behaviours than risk behaviours or detection behaviours (Stead et al., 2013). One well-designed study used the TPB to develop a structured intervention to increase exercise and improve dietary behaviour in older people with diabetes. Different sessions emphasised different elements of the TPB, and participants were helped to apply techniques for setting goals and making plans to meet them. Compared to people who were in a control group, those who participated in the intervention had significantly greater levels of physical activity at the six-week follow-up. The study design and results are shown in Research Box 5.1.

Case Study 5.2 illustrates how the TPB might be used as a guide for intervention in clinical practice. Next we look at a completely different model, which focuses on the *processes* of change rather than on the factors that determine behaviour.

RESEARCH BOX 5.1 A Theory of Planned Behaviour intervention to improve diet and physical activity

Background

The Theory of Planned Behaviour (TPB) suggests that healthy behaviour can be promoted by changing attitudes, normative beliefs, and feelings of control over behaviour. This study looked at whether an intervention based on an extended TPB could improve

(Continued)

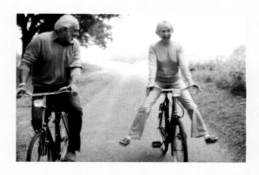

healthy eating and increase physical activity in older people with cardiovascular disease and/or Type 2 Diabetes (NIDD).

Method and findings

183 older adults recruited from seven community health centres were allocated to a control group or to an intervention group. The intervention group took part in four weekly group sessions. Sessions lasted two hours and were run by trained health professionals. Session content was as follows:

- Session 1: exploration of attitudes and beliefs about healthy eating and physical activity to help participants consider the advantages (e.g. feeling healthy, losing weight) and disadvantages (e.g. reducing the taste of food, feeling tired) of healthy eating and physical activity.
- Session 2: consideration of the barriers (e.g. cost, time) that prevented participants from making healthy eating choices and being physically active, common triggers to unhealthy behaviours, and how unhealthy habits develop. Discussion of social interactions that influence unhealthy behaviour and sources of social support for healthy behaviour.
- Session 3: learning and practising techniques for setting goals and making plans for achievable behaviour change.
- Session 4: consideration of their sense of control over behaviour change, and generating strategies for dealing with barriers preventing them from meeting their diet- and activity-related goals.

At six-week follow-up, data were available from 111 people. The intervention led to significant improvements in levels of physical activity, intentions, planning, perceived behavioural control, and subjective norms. The intervention did not produce significant changes in dietary behaviour.

Significance

The results of this study indicate that interventions based on the TPB can encourage physical activity among older people with diabetes and cardiovascular disease. The results suggested that key components of the original model – subjective norms, perceived behavioural control, and intentions – were significant influences on behaviour change. The study also found that a key component of the intervention's impact was the inclusion of planning strategies for dealing with barriers to intended behaviour change.

White, K.M. et al. (2012) An extended theory of planned behaviour intervention for older adults with Type 2 diabetes and cardiovascular disease. *Journal of Aging and Physical Activity*, *20*: 281–299.

CASE STUDY 5.2   Smoking cessation using the Theory of Planned Behaviour

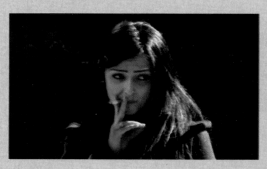

Divya is a 22-year-old woman who has smoked 20 cigarettes a day since she was 15 years old.

Attitudes

Explore her attitudes toward smoking:

- What do you think about smoking? (general attitude)
- Is smoking a good or bad thing for you? In what way? (evaluation of attitude/behaviour)

Educate about the negative effects of smoking to try to change the attitude from positive to negative.

Social norms

Explore the norms of important people around her:

- What do your friends/family/partner think about smoking? (general norm)
- What do your friends/family/partner think about *you* smoking? (specific norm)
- Whose opinion is most important to you? (who she is motivated to comply with)
- Would you like to give up smoking for [person]? (motivation to comply with norms)

Discuss the pros and cons for her if she were to comply with the person or group norms she values most.

Intentions

Explore whether she intends to quit smoking:

- Have you ever thought about giving up smoking? (previous intention)
- Do you intend to give up smoking in the next few months? (current intention)

Perceived behavioural control

Explore how much control she thinks she has over quitting smoking.

- Do you think you can give up smoking? (perceived control over quitting)

If she indicates low control, explore the reasons for this, for example:

- What makes you think you can't give up?

Normalise the difficulty in quitting:

- Many people find it hard to give up.

(Continued)

Increase the perceived control:
- Most people are successful if they keep trying.

Explore the actual control:
- Is there anything in particular that stops you from trying to quit?

Action implementations

If she is ready to try quitting, discuss the steps she can take to give up smoking:
- What steps are you going to take to give up smoking? (concrete plans)

Discuss how these can be changed or added to in order to increase chances of success, for example:
- Nicotine replacement, smoking cessation groups.
- Setting personal goals about quitting, and setting rewards for not smoking.

5.4 THE TRANSTHEORETICAL MODEL

The Transtheoretical Model (Prochaska & DiClemente, 1983) was an early attempt to integrate models of health behaviour and psychotherapy to produce an effective model for smoking intervention. This model is often referred to as the 'Stages of Change' model. The stages that characterise this model are illustrated in Figure 5.4. It includes four components: (1) the stages of change, (2) decisional balance, (3) confidence and temptation, and (4) processes of change.

The **stages of change** are a series of stages that people are thought to go through when changing their behaviour. In *precontemplation* a person is not even considering changing their behaviour. In *contemplation* they begin to consider changing. If they want to change, then this leads into *preparation*, where the individual plans how to change. The final two stages are *action*, where the person makes the initial change in behaviour, and *maintenance* if this behaviour change is consolidated and maintained in the long term. An important aspect of this model is the inclusion of relapse, based on the recognition that people can relapse back to previous behaviour at any point, and that they may have to go through the cycle a few times before the new behaviour becomes permanent. The advantage of this is that it normalises relapse and encourages people not to see this as a failure, but to keep trying to change their behaviour. In clinical practice a healthcare professional can emphasise this and explore what a person has learned from the relapse, and how this can be used to increase chances of success next time.

Decisional balance involves the relative pros and cons of changing the behaviour. People are asked to write down the pros and cons of changing their behaviour in a decisional balance task (note the parallels to identifying barriers and benefits in the HBM).

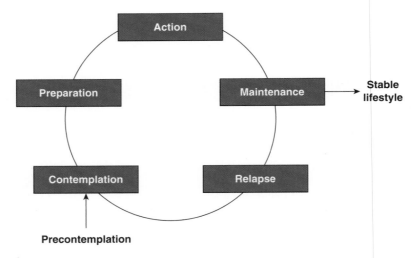

FIGURE 5.4 The Transtheoretical or 'Stages of Change' Model

This helps them to clarify whether there are more pros than cons (or vice versa) and might prompt a person to consider changing thei r behaviour (i.e. move from precontemplation into contemplation).

Confidence refers to the confidence a person has in their ability to change. This over-laps with perceived behavioural control from previous models. **Temptation** is which factors will tempt a person to continue with an unhealthy behaviour in particular circum-stances. For example, in our case study, Divya may want to give up smoking but finds it difficult to resist smoking when out with friends.

The fourth aspect of the model is that it specifies ten **processes of change** which can be used to help people change their behaviour. These include consciousness raising, replacing smoking with other behavioural responses (counter-conditioning), helping a person to plan rewards (reinforcement), and using social support (helping relationships).

ACTIVITY 5.3   CHANGING YOUR OWN BEHAVIOUR

- Do you have a bad habit or behaviour you would like to change?
- If so, what stage do you think you are at?
- How could you use the Transtheoretical Model to help yourself change that behaviour?

The strengths of the Transtheoretical Model are that it recognises people may be at dif-ferent stages of readiness for change and that interventions should be tailored to their particular stage. For example, if in our case study Divya had never thought of giving up smoking (precontemplation), there is little point in trying to develop an action plan with her. It might make more sense to educate her about the dangers of smoking and encourage her to think about quitting (contemplation). Another strength is the inclusion of relapse. This is particularly important in addictive behaviours where relapse is common. However, the model has been criticised on the grounds that people do not necessarily move through the various stages consecutively. People might move backwards and forwards through the stages or miss out other stages completely.

CLINICAL NOTES 5.3

Working with resistance and relapse

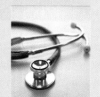

- Whether a person is ready to change will affect the type of approach you should take.
- If a person has not considered changing, educate them about the negative impact of their current behaviour and encourage a change.
- Looking at the pros and cons of the current behaviour can also get people thinking about changing.
- Help them plan how they are going to change and build in rewards to reinforce the new behaviour.
- Relapse is a common part of behaviour change and not a failure. Explore why this happened and work out how to avoid it happening again the next time.

Interventions using the Transtheoretical Model

There is a surprising lack of strong evidence for the Transtheoretical Model, and there is a need for well-designed intervention studies to provide a stronger evidence base (Mastellos et al., 2014). There is, at best, weak evidence and, at worst, no evidence that interventions targeting people in particular stages are more effective than interventions that do not target such stages (Sutton, 2007). This is not to say that interventions based on the model have been completely unsuccessful, but rather that targeting stages does not significantly *improve* on interventions developed from other models, such as the Theory of Planned Behaviour. The Transtheoretical Model at least provides a way to think about how the other models of behaviour may operate at different stages. In other words, this is not an alternative to other models but a framework in which to place them. Case Study 5.3 illustrates how we might use the Transtheoretical Model in clinical practice.

CASE STUDY 5.3 Smoking cessation using the Transtheoretical Model

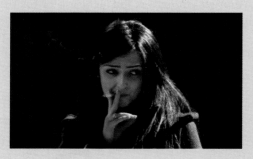

Divya is a 22-year-old woman who has smoked 20 cigarettes a day since she was 15 years old.

Stage of change
Identify which stage she may be at:
- Have you ever thought about giving up? (contemplation)
- Have you ever planned to give up or tried to give up? (preparation and action)

Decisional balance
Explore her perceived pros and cons of smoking. This is best done by writing them down and then looking at the list together:
- What are the positive things for you about smoking? (pros)
- What are the negative things for you about smoking? (cons)
- Looking at this list, what does it make you think about your smoking?

Confidence
Explore how confident she is that she can control her smoking:
- How much do you think your smoking is under your control?
- How confident are you that you can reduce or quit smoking?

Temptation
Explore which situations are particularly tempting for her to smoke and how this might affect a relapse:
- Are there certain times or situations when you find it difficult not to smoke?
- How can you prevent this from happening if you give up smoking?

Processes of change
Use any of the processes to plan with her how she can quit smoking. For example:
- Is there someone who can help you quit, or give up with you? (helping relationships)
- Can you do something instead of smoking that distracts you and makes you feel better, e.g. something relaxing, or exercise? (counter-conditioning)
- It's important to reward yourself to continue not smoking – especially in the beginning. What would be a good reward for you? (reinforcement)

5.5 PRIME THEORY

A difficulty with many theories of health behaviour is that they tend to assume people will think rationally about their behaviour. Very few theories consider the role of emotions, or why people behave without thinking or in ways that they do not intend. **PRIME Theory** (West, 2006) is an attempt to incorporate motivation, emotions, impulses, and cognitive factors into one model.

The structural elements of PRIME Theory are shown in Figure 5.5. These consist of five factors thought to determine health behaviour:

1. *Plans*: conscious representations of future actions, including a commitment to act.
2. *Responses* that start, stop, or modify any action.
3. *Impulses* or inhibitory forces that are experienced as urges.
4. *Motives* that are experienced as desires.
5. *Evaluations* or evaluative beliefs.

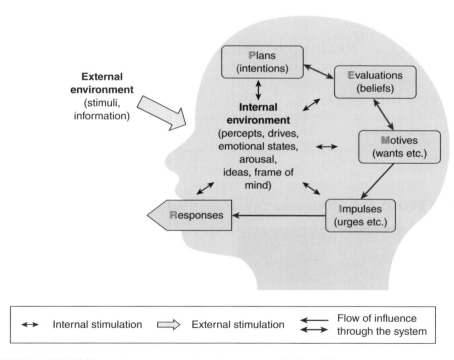

FIGURE 5.5 PRIME Theory Image reproduced courtesy of Robert West

As illustrated in Figure 5.5, momentary responses are influenced by external stimuli such as triggers, and internal states such as arousal and emotion, and then directly moderated by impulses and inhibitions. Impulses and inhibitions are in turn influenced by motives and evaluations. Motives and evaluations can be consciously experienced but not necessarily so. PRIME theory suggests that it is only at this level that beliefs and higher thought processes come in. Finally, plans are cognitive intentions for future action that moderate motives and evaluations.

PRIME Theory is based on four assumptions about motivation and health behaviour: (1) we need to understand the moment-to-moment control of health behaviour before we can understand the long-term influences on behaviour; (2) the system has plasticity – that is, it can be modified by experience; (3) self-identity is highly important to our motives, plans, and behaviour (see Chapter 9); (4) a system can appear complex but still be determined by relatively simple processes.

One strength of PRIME Theory is that it integrates motivation (e.g. arousal, drives, motives) and emotion (emotional states, impulses) with cognitions (e.g. plans, evaluations) in a theory of health behaviour. Also, the model includes self-identity, something which is rarely considered in other models. A difficulty with PRIME Theory is that there is little evidence available on whether it is effective at explaining health behaviours. However, PRIME Theory can still be used in clinical practice to help people change their behaviour, as is illustrated in Case Study 5.4.

ACTIVITY 5.4   HELPING OTHERS CHANGE

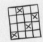

- If you wanted to help a friend to become more physically active, how would you use these models?
- What four things do you think would be most appropriate and useful for this person?
- How would you incorporate this into a behaviour change programme?

CASE STUDY 5.4   Smoking cessation using PRIME Theory

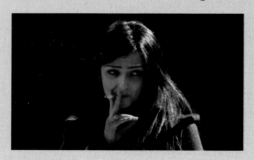

Divya is a 22-year-old woman who has smoked 20 cigarettes a day since she was 15 years old.

Plans
Explore whether she plans or intends to give up smoking:

(Continued)

- Have you ever thought about giving up smoking? (previous intention)
- Do you intend to give up smoking? If so, when? (intention and timeframe)

Evaluations/beliefs

Explore her beliefs about smoking and evaluation of it:
- What do you think about smoking? (beliefs)
- Is smoking a good or bad thing? In what way? (evaluation of smoking)

Educate about the negative effects of smoking to try to change her attitude from positive to negative.

Motives

Explore her motives and motivation to quit:
- Do you want to quit? If so, how much do you want to do this?
- What motivates you to give up?
- How important is that to you?

Impulses

Explore the positive and negative impulses:
- Are there times when you have strong impulses to quit? (positive impulses)
- What triggers this, or when do you feel this? (triggers to positive impulses)
- How can you make the most of this to help you quit? (harnessing these impulses)
- Are there times when you have strong impulses to smoke? (negative impulses)
- What triggers this, or when do you feel this? (triggers to negative impulses)
- How can you avoid this or change it? (harnessing these impulses)

Responses

Explore her responses in these situations:
- How do you usually respond to these (positive) impulses/circumstances?
- How do you usually respond to these (negative) impulses/circumstances?

Self-identity

Examine her self-identity and how this is affected by smoking:
- How does smoking affect how you feel about yourself? (self-identity)
- Do you think being a smoker affects how other people see you? (perceptions of others)
- How would you feel about yourself if you quit smoking? (develop new positive self-identity)
- How do you think other people would see you if you were a non-smoker? (develop the reinforcing views of others)

CONCLUSION

There is good evidence that the Theory of Planned Behaviour and Health Belief Model can explain some of the factors that determine health behaviour, and that interventions based on these models are effective at changing behaviour. There is limited evidence to support the effectiveness of interventions based on the Transtheoretical Model. PRIME Theory has not yet been tested empirically, so it is not clear how effective it actually is at predicting behaviour and behaviour change.

From this chapter it should be clear that all of these models have various strengths and weaknesses. It should also be apparent that, although the models possess different concepts and underpinnings, many of the questions in the different case studies are similar and overlap. Thus, in clinical practice aspects of all these models can be mixed and used effectively to encourage people to change unhealthy behaviours. To aid choices of strategies, a taxonomy of behaviour change strategies has been developed (Abraham & Michie, 2008). It can be used to synthesise evidence, implement effective interventions, and test theory (Michie et al., 2015).

It is probable that different aspects of the models described above and different behaviour change strategies will work better for different health professionals and different people, and may be more effective for some conditions or situations than others. Despite differences between models, a common implication is that we need to explore each person's beliefs and reasons for behaving in the way they do in order to be most effective in helping them to change and develop an appropriate plan of change.

Summary

- Social-cognition models of health behaviour take an expectancy-value approach and include the Health Belief Model and the Theory of Planned Behaviour.
- The Health Belief Model states that health behaviour change is determined by the threat of illness (perceived susceptibility and perceived severity) balanced by the perceived benefits and barriers to change. Triggers or cues to action can also be important in some cases.
- According to the Theory of Planned Behaviour, health behaviour is determined by intentions, which in turn are determined by attitudes toward the behaviour, social norms, and perceived behavioural control.
- The Transtheoretical Model of behaviour change is an integrative theory that focuses on the stages and processes of change, rather than the determinants of health behaviour.

(Continued)

- PRIME Theory attempts to integrate motivational and health behaviour theories to explain moment-to-moment behaviour. This theory focuses on plans, responses, impulses and inhibitions, motives, and evaluations as determining behaviour.
- There is evidence that the Theory of Planned Behaviour and Health Belief Model explain some health behaviours, and that interventions based on these models are effective at changing behaviour.
- There is limited evidence to support the effectiveness of interventions based on the Transtheoretical Model. PRIME Theory has not yet been tested empirically so it is not yet clear how effective it is.
- Each model results in slightly different approaches to intervention, but aspects of all these models can be combined in clinical practice to encourage behaviour change.

FURTHER READING

Llewellyn, C.D. et al. (eds) (2018) *Cambridge Handbook of Psychology, Health and Medicine* (3rd edition). Cambridge: Cambridge University Press. This book has short chapters on models of health behaviour, health behaviour change interventions, health promotion, motivational interviewing (often used to change addictive behaviours), physical activity interventions, and implementing changes in practice.

Anisman, H. (2016) *Health Psychology*. London: Sage. This is a new textbook designed to introduce undergraduate students to the broad field of health psychology. It includes chapters on lifestyle factors and behaviour change.

Ogden, J. (2012) *Health Psychology* (5th edition). Buckingham: Open University Press. Now in its fifth edition, this book provides a wide-ranging introduction to health psychology. It covers factors that influence susceptibility to disease and illness, as well as the psychological experience of being unwell.

REVISION QUESTIONS

1. What are health behaviours and how can they been categorised?

2. What biological, psychological, social, and societal factors influence health behaviours?

3. What is the expectancy-value principle? How is this relevant to health behaviour change?

4. Outline the Health Belief Model. How effective is it for behaviour change?

5. Outline the Theory of Planned Behaviour. How effective is it for behaviour change?

6. What is locus of control? How might it be relevant to clinical practice?

7. Outline the Transtheoretical Model. How effective is it for behaviour change?

8. Outline PRIME Theory. How might it be used to promote health behaviour change?

9. Compare and contrast two models of health behaviour change.

10. Describe how you might use one model of health behaviour to help someone give up smoking.

6 CHRONIC ILLNESS, DEATH, AND DYING

(Continued)

Figures

Research box

LEARNING OBJECTIVES

This chapter is designed to enable you to:

- Learn more about the experience of chronic or terminal illnesses.
- Outline some of the psychosocial interventions to help people adjust and cope with chronic illness.
- Understand the difficulties of palliative care, in particular the tension between helping a person have a good death and euthanasia.
- Describe the processes of normal bereavement and pathological grief.

As we become more successful at treating disease and delaying death, the proportion of people living with long-term illnesses increases. Chronic illnesses or long-term conditions are illnesses that cannot be cured, and so need to be managed with drugs and other treatments. In developed countries approximately one in three people have a chronic illness at any given time. Many of us will have a chronic illness at some point in our lives.

Treatment of chronic illness presents healthcare professionals with a particular challenge: it requires a change from focusing purely on a cure to focusing on helping people manage their symptoms. The implications of this are examined later when considering quality of life for people with chronic and terminal illnesses. Chronic illnesses raise some of the most difficult ethical issues in medicine. For example, how do we decide who gets a transplant and who does not, when should we stop resuscitation or turn off a life support machine, and what is the doctor's role in cases of assisted suicide?

Chronic diseases vary hugely. They include disorders such as epilepsy, arthritis, cancer, diabetes, chronic fatigue syndrome, asthma, hypertension, liver disease, and dementia. Chronic diseases account for approximately 80% of deaths in developed countries. Figure 6.1 shows the top 10 causes of death worldwide in 2015 (World Health Organisation, 2017b). Ischaemic heart disease and stroke are the largest killers, accounting for 15 million deaths in 2015. The order of other diseases then varies between regions.

It can be seen that in Europe fewer communicable diseases and more cancers are in the top 10 causes of death. Interestingly, deaths that receive a lot of media attention, such as those from HIV or homicide, are much less likely. For example, in the UK, homicide accounts for the deaths of seven men and two women in every one million people.

Given the wide range of chronic illnesses, it is difficult to generalise about the role of psychosocial factors. In previous chapters (Chapters 2, 3, and 5) we have seen how psychosocial factors such as social support, lifestyle, stress, and negative emotion can affect the onset and prognosis of illness. We have also seen the importance of beliefs, attention, and behaviour in how we interpret symptoms and what we do about them (Chapters 2 and 4). The role of psychosocial factors in specific illnesses is covered in the chapters on different body systems in Section III. In this chapter we shall focus on the experience of chronic illness: the impact of chronic illness, how people adapt and cope, and whether psychosocial interventions can help. In the second half of the chapter we will look at the impact of terminal illness, coping with dying, the effect of death on others, bereavement, and dealing with death in medical practice.

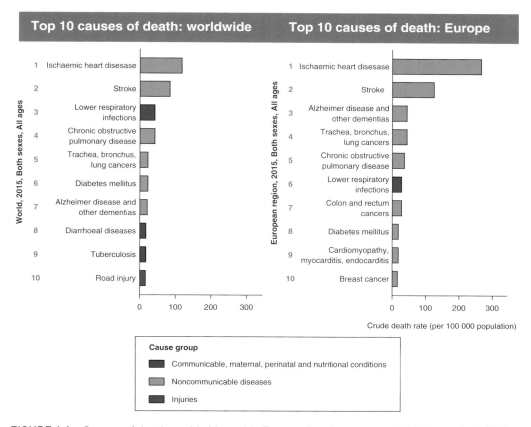

FIGURE 6.1 Causes of death worldwide and in Europe. Death rates per 100,000 people in 2015 (World Health Organisation, 2017b)

6.1 CHRONIC ILLNESS

The onset and diagnosis of a chronic illness brings with it profound changes in a person's life that can lead to a reduced quality of life and wellbeing. The onset and diagnosis of chronic illness raise significant challenges, including:

- Adjusting to symptoms and disability.
- Maintaining a reasonable emotional balance.
- Preserving a satisfactory self-image and sense of competence.
- Learning about symptoms, treatment procedures, and self-management.
- Sustaining relationships with family and friends.
- Forming and maintaining relationships with healthcare providers.
- Preparing for an uncertain future.

The enormity of these tasks, coupled with the emotional distress brought on by chronic illness, mean that people are at high risk of depression. For example, studies of people with multiple sclerosis show that 35% are severely depressed and 34% have severe anxiety (Boeschoten et al., 2017).

The crisis theory of chronic illness (Moos & Schaefer, 1984) assumes that we need a social and psychological equilibrium similar to physiological homeostasis. This is similar to the concept of **allostatic load** in stress and how we respond to stress (see Chapter 3). The diagnosis of an illness can put someone in an extreme state of disequilibrium, which is accompanied by negative emotions such as fear, anxiety, and depression. Because people cannot remain in a state of disequilibrium, some resolution must be found. People in disequilibrium are more susceptible to outside influence, such as the actions of healthcare professionals. In chronic illness, people's equilibrium may be very fragile and can be destroyed at any moment by even small setbacks or other stressful events. This explains why people may overreact to seemingly minor setbacks or difficulties.

Crisis theory is a useful analogy for the challenges of chronic illness. Theories of stress and coping (Chapter 3) are also useful in understanding people's responses. For example, the demands of illness are more likely to overwhelm a person if they have existing psychological problems, make negative or catastrophic appraisals, and have poor coping skills and resources. Case studies illustrating how our understanding of stress can be used to help people cope with difficult events are given in Chapters 3 and 11.

6.1.1 IMPACT OF CHRONIC ILLNESS

Common emotional responses to illness are denial, anxiety, and depression. **Denial** is a psychological defence that allows people to avoid thinking about the illness and its consequences. People may refuse to accept that they have an illness, play down the severity of it, or insist they will recover and the illness will be cured. Denial is not helpful in the long term because it interferes with adherence to treatment and self-management. However, denial can be helpful in the short term – particularly if people are physically weak and not able to cope with the full psychological consequences of the illness. In these circumstances, denial can help to keep fear and anxiety lowered until they have recovered and feel more able to cope with the emotional consequences of the illness. For example, denial is associated with faster initial recovery from a heart attack and fewer treatment side effects (Sirois, 1992).

Anxiety and depression are common in people with chronic illness. The substantial overlap between chronic illness and mental health is illustrated in Figure 6.2 which shows that 30% of people with chronic illness have a mental health problem. Similarly, if looked at the other way, 46% of people with a mental health problem have another chronic illness (Naylor et al., 2012). A review of heart disease, stroke, diabetes mellitus, asthma, cancer, arthritis, and osteoporosis found that depression is more common in people with these illnesses than in the general population (Clarke & Currie, 2009). Anxiety is more common in people with heart disease, stroke, and cancer than in the

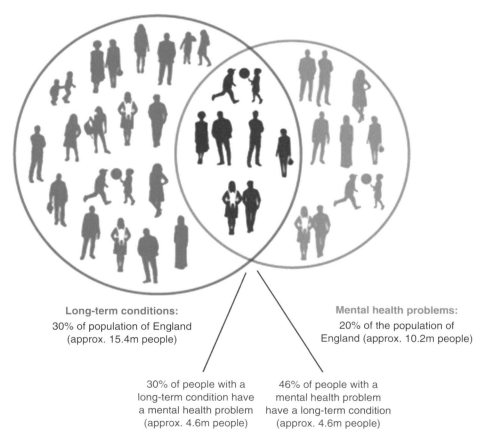

Long-term conditions:
30% of population of England
(approx. 15.4m people)

Mental health problems:
20% of the population of
England (approx. 10.2m people)

30% of people with a
long-term condition have
a mental health problem
(approx. 4.6m people)

46% of people with a
mental health problem
have a long-term condition
(approx. 4.6m people)

FIGURE 6.2   The overlap between long-term conditions and mental health problems (Khan, 2015)

general population (Clarke & Currie, 2009). Depression and anxiety can be a response to illness, present before illness, or both. As we saw in Chapter 2, there is strong evidence that positive and negative emotions are associated with health outcomes. Both anxiety and depression have been associated with physiological states that might affect the course of chronic illness. Anxiety is associated with sympathetic nervous system and HPA axis arousal, and depression is associated with neuroendocrine changes that can affect inflammatory and immune pathways (see Chapters 3 and 11). For example, depression is associated with an increased risk of cardiovascular disease (Steptoe, 2006) and mortality from a wide range of other illnesses (Everson-Rose et al., 2004). Anxiety is associated with more frequent or severe symptoms in disorders such as asthma or irritable bowel syndrome (see Chapters 12 and 13).

Though anxiety and depression are often comorbid (occurring together), they stem from different types of appraisal. Anxiety is a response to threat. In chronic illness this is likely to be a threat to a person's wellbeing, work, self-image, etc. Anxiety can increase in medical settings because of potentially threatening events such as getting test results, having painful procedures, dependence on healthcare professionals, and uncertainty about the disease course. For example, a review of anxiety related to dental procedures found it was associated with the severity of the procedure and expectations and experience of pain, among other things (Astramskaite et al., 2016). Depression, on the other hand, is usually a response to loss, failure, or helplessness. In chronic illness this will include a loss of health or physical capacity, a loss of social status, a failure to conform to healthy standards, and helplessness in the face of illness.

Learned helplessness occurs when people believe they have no control over events, become hopeless, helpless, and subsequently depressed (Seligman, 1975). This is particularly relevant to chronic illness. If people believe they have no control over their illness or outcome, it can lead to detachment, withdrawal, and depression (see illness representations, Chapter 4). Self-management programmes and cognitive behaviour therapy (CBT) deal with this by encouraging people to identify and challenge maladaptive beliefs, educating them about the importance of psychosocial factors and empowering them to manage their illness.

In chronic illnesses the emphasis of treatment is on improving **quality of life** rather than curing the illness. However, there are tensions between improving quality of life on the one hand, and side effects of medical treatments that may decrease quality of life on the other. There is also the controversy of deciding the point at which gains in quality of life are worth expensive treatments, such as those for advanced cancer. Finding treatments that maximise physical wellbeing and quality of life can therefore be difficult. For example, NICE guidelines for dementia care aimed to combine best practice in social and physical care for dementia, but formulating these guidelines was so complex that the panel published information on how to do it (Gould & Kendall, 2007).

The measurement of quality of life in chronic illnesses is therefore critical to inform healthcare guidelines. However, it is also fraught with problems. Self-report measures typically ask people about pain, disability, restricted functioning or roles, mental health, energy, and overall ratings of health. Unsurprisingly, research using these measures has found that people with chronic illnesses report a poorer quality of life. Measures of quality of life are often not specific to the illness being studied and do not take into account changes in people's goals and priorities during illness. For example, standardised measures of pain may be interpreted differently by people with chronic illness. Similarly, some domains of life may be more or less important to someone with a chronic illness.

Specialised measures of quality of life in chronic illness have therefore been developed, such as patient-generated indexes, where people list the five domains of life that are important to them and then rate how much each domain has been affected by their illness (e.g. the Patient-Generated Index, Ruta et al., 1994). Research using these measures shows that people generate a wide range of domains, including some not encompassed in traditional quality of life measures. Such domains include memory, writing, and sexual function. Domains may also change over time as people adjust to continuing disease and incapacity. This type of measure is moderately related to global measures of quality of life, life satisfaction, and mental health, but only weakly associated with health and functional status (Wettergren et al., 2009). General quality of life is usually best predicted by psychological functioning (Arnold et al., 2004).

6.1.2 FINDING MEANING AND BENEFIT

So far, we have focused on negative aspects of chronic illness. However, many people with chronic illnesses adapt and some even report positive changes to their lives. Figure 6.3 summarises the interplay between crisis, resilience, and growth that can occur in response to a crisis such as the onset and diagnosis of a critical illness. Factors associated with resilience include emotional disposition, coping, and social support (see Chapter 3).

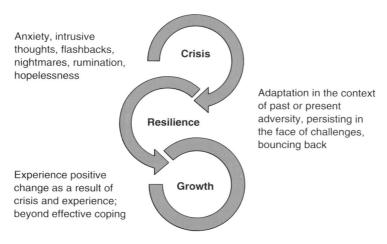

FIGURE 6.3   Crisis, resilience, and growth

Positive responses to illness are referred to as stress-related growth, post-traumatic growth, or benefit-finding (Tedeshi & Calhoun, 2004). Three main types of positive changes can occur:

1. *Enhanced relationships* – people need support from others and positive interpersonal experiences may strengthen their appreciation of relationships.
2. *A changed view of themselves* – people may develop a greater sense of personal resilience and strength, an acceptance of their vulnerabilities and limitations, or a heightened awareness of the fragility of life.
3. *Changed life philosophy* – the concern that illness might result in incapacity and a shorter life can lead to changes in priorities and values, a different approach to life, and a greater appreciation of living.

These positive changes can lead to a whole new approach to life. Reviews have shown that 60–90% of people with HIV or cancer report positive growth. Growth is associated with less distress in the short term and better physical and mental health overall (Barskova & Oesterreich, 2009; Sawyer et al., 2010; Shand et al., 2015).

6.1.3 ILLNESS AS A STORY – NARRATIVES IN MEDICINE

The events of chronic illness, positive and negative changes, become part of people's story about themselves (Case Study 6.1). Books, internet sites, and blogs provide millions of examples of people writing about their experiences of illness. Stories or narratives have a number of functions (Greenhalgh, 2016; Hydén, 1997). Illness narratives:

- Transform events and construct meaning from the illness.
- Help people reconstruct their history to incorporate the illness and reconstruct their identity to retain a sense of self-worth in the face of illness.
- Help people explain and understand their illness.
- Relate the illness to their values and life priorities.
- Make illness a collective experience.

The importance of illness narratives is reflected in **narrative-based medicine** (Greenhalgh & Hurwitz, 1998), in which the emphasis is on listening to people's narratives and using these to improve clinical care. In diagnosis, narratives are useful because they provide an insight into someone's experience of ill-health and encourage empathy and understanding between doctor and patient. Narratives encourage a holistic approach to treatment. Talking through illness narratives can prove therapeutic or palliative for people. In addition, it may suggest other treatment options. In patient education, narratives are memorable, grounded in experience, and encourage reflection. The use of narratives can therefore be helpful both for patients and doctors at many stages of illness (see Chapter 18).

CASE STUDY 6.1   Narratives of illness

Fighter in the face of adversity

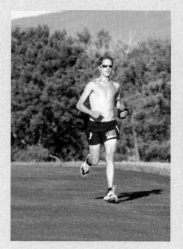

Brooks Williams was diagnosed with cystic fibrosis at 5½ months old. He says, 'when I was 21 I had a serious bout of pneumonia: my lung function was down to 40% and I was coughing up lots of blood. After I was released I was told that due to scarring in my lungs I might never make a full recovery. It made me realise how quickly my health could take an irreparable turn and this fear is what made me start running seriously. I started running to live and I attribute my improved health to running. My doctor told me not many people with cystic fibrosis try running marathons so I'm a guinea pig.

I have been running for six years now and have completed ten marathons and seven ultramarathons. I just completed a 100 mile ultramarathon in Texas in 17.5 hours and finished 12th overall. I think only half of finishing is down to your physical conditioning – the rest is down to mental fortitude.'

(Reproduced with the kind permission of Brooks Williams; photograph reproduced courtesy of Thomas Dewane)

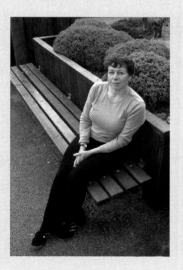

Reactions, struggles and changing priorities

Ten years ago I was diagnosed with multiple sclerosis – I was going blind and was scared to death. I had young kids and more than anything I was scared I would never see them again. All I knew about MS was the worst so I was convinced I'd become totally handicapped and have a terrible life. However, the treatment worked well and my sight came back, although I have other side effects to deal with. My hands and feet are numb and I am allergic to some drugs so can't take them – so it is an ongoing process of trying different drugs and finding out what works.

I try to look on the bright side – I have a great husband, good friends, and God. On good days I can see how wonderful life is. On bad days I try not to take anything for

(Continued)

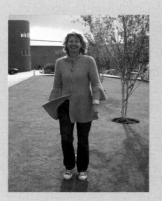

granted and concentrate on what I can do, rather than what I can't. I am excited by the new drugs they are working on and pray for a cure. I take each day at a time and am thankful for what I have. (Anonymous)

Acceptance of death – strength in existential issues

My dad died of cancer when I was young so I was really scared of cancer. When the doctor told me I had cancer I was shocked and frightened. I was so scared of dying – I had young children so was really worried about what would happen to them. It took a while to get my head around it but eventually I realised that we all have to die sometime. I can't run away from it – none of us can. I feel connected to all the people who died before me and those who will die after me. I am just a small part of a big circle of life.

I am doing everything I can to get rid of the cancer because I don't want to die, but I am not worried anymore. I enjoy my time with family and friends. I know my children will be okay because other people will be there for them. My experience of cancer has been a revelation and I have a very different perspective now. I'm not afraid of dying. I think nature has its own way of making it alright because who wants to live in pain? I see that my life has been good – it has been a privilege. (Anonymous)

ACTIVITY 6.1   USING NARRATIVES IN MEDICINE

- Think about a person you saw recently. How much do you remember about:
  - The clinical details?
  - The person and their story?

Summary

- Chronic illnesses affect approximately one in three people in developed countries and account for approximately 80% of deaths.
- The onset and diagnosis of a chronic illness brings with it profound changes in a person's life which can lead to a reduced quality of life and wellbeing.
- Common emotional responses are denial, anxiety, and depression. Depression and anxiety may be a response to the illness, present before the illness, or both.

(Continued)

- The relationship between quality of life and physical health is not straightforward, which is partly due to variations between illnesses and how quality of life is measured.
- Many people with chronic illness are resilient and report positive life changes, such as enhanced relationships and a changed view of themselves and their philosophy of life.
- Illness narratives are important in how people make sense of their illness. Narrative-based medicine uses narratives to improve diagnosis, treatment, and the education of patients.

6.2 PSYCHOLOGICAL INTERVENTION

The previous section highlighted the importance of psychological factors in chronic illness. Psychological interventions for chronic illness are usually associated with improvements in psychological wellbeing, quality of life, coping, the self-management of illness, and general functioning (Sansom-Daly et al., 2012). However, there is little evidence that they affect morbidity or mortality. Information is given elsewhere on specialist interventions (CBT, stress management, and support – see Chapter 19; self-management – see Chapter 4). The interventions we look at here are relaxation training and expressive writing, which are both easy to learn and use.

Relaxation training can take many forms, including physical relaxation techniques such as progressive muscle relaxation, mental relaxation techniques such as meditation, or a combination of both (see Box 6.1). Relaxation is useful for coping with pain (Kwekkeboom & Gretarsdottir, 2006), reducing anxiety and depression, and coping with nausea and the side effects from treatment (Luebbert et al., 2001; van Dixhoorn & White, 2005). However, relaxation training is not effective for all illnesses. For example, there is little reliable evidence that relaxation can have an effect on asthma (Huntley et al., 2002).

The internet can also be a significant resource for people with chronic illness. It provides easy access to information, blogs, and online support. This raises the possibility that many interventions can be accessed via the internet. Computerised cognitive therapy treatments for anxiety and depression are already widely used, with evidence showing these are effective (Foroushani et al., 2011; Newby et al., 2016; Pennant et al., 2015). Online support groups for illnesses are also widely available (e.g. www.dailystrength.org, www.bigwhitewall.com).

Expressive writing offers a simple intervention for chronic and terminal illness. People are asked to write for 15 minutes every day for three or four days about things they find (or have found) stressful or very upsetting. It is important that people write about their thoughts and feelings and do not just describe factual events. Evidence suggests that this intervention can have small but significant effects on psychological wellbeing, physical health, general functioning, and health service use in some people (Frattaroli, 2006; Meads

& Nouwen 2005; Mogk et al., 2006). Meta-analyses examining expressive writing find that in healthy people expressive writing can have a positive effect on physical and psychological functioning (Frattaroli, 2006) and reduced healthcare use (Harris, 2006). In clinical populations, expressive writing is associated with improved physical health (but not psychological health) (Frisina et al., 2004), and is effective for reducing post-traumatic stress and comorbid symptoms of depression (van Emmerik et al., 2013). However, it does not appear to be effective for some groups, such as people with cancer (Zachariae & O'Toole, 2015), although the authors of this review conclude that it is possible expressive writing can be helpful for a subgroup of people with cancer. Writing interventions are easy to use in clinical practice with the instructions given above and some encouragement.

BOX 6.1   Three-minute relaxation exercise

1   Make sure you are sitting comfortably and are as relaxed as possible.
2   Ask yourself, **what am I experiencing right now?** What body sensations do you have? What thoughts are going through your mind? What sounds can you hear? Just observe all these experiences without trying to change them. (*1 minute*)
3   **Focus on your breathing.** Breathe slowly and deeply: count to 4 as you inhale, then count to 4 as you exhale. Focus on the physical sensations of breathing, such as the movement of your stomach as your breath goes in and out. Let all thoughts go. (*1 minute*)
4   **Expand your awareness** to the sensations throughout your body. If you have strong feelings it's OK, just allow yourself to feel them – breathe with the feelings. If you have worries try saying to yourself '*let it go*' when you breathe out. (*1 minute*)

(Adapted from www.cci.health.wa.gov.au)

Summary

- Psychological interventions for chronic illnesses include expressive writing, relaxation, stress management, self-management, and support interventions.
- Psychological interventions are associated with better psychological wellbeing, quality of life, the self-management of illness, less pain, reduced symptoms, improved general functioning, and reduced pain and healthcare use.
- There is no consistent evidence that psychological interventions have an effect on morbidity or mortality.
- The internet has become a significant resource for people with chronic illness providing access to information, blogs, and online support.

CLINICAL NOTES 6.1

Treating chronic illness

- Be especially alert to depression or anxiety in people with chronic illness and treat it appropriately.
- When adjusting to illness, people may have a fragile psychological equilibrium and react strongly to minor setbacks or difficulties.
- Reactions and adjustment to illness vary hugely, so do not assume you know how a person thinks and feels about their illness.
- When diagnosed, people may use denial to avoid being emotionally overwhelmed. Do not challenge denial too much at this stage – it is only a problem if it continues in the long term and interferes with treatment.
- Helping people consider any positive life changes since an illness can reduce distress.
- Listening to people's narratives will help us know them and treat them better.

6.3 DEATH AND DYING

The way we die has changed substantially. At the beginning of the twentieth century the majority of people died at home and their bodies were laid out for friends and family to see, touch, and mourn. By the 1960s the majority of deaths in developed countries occurred in hospitals. For example, in England 57% of deaths between 2001 and 2010 happened in hospitals, 19% at home, 17% in care homes, and the rest in hospices or elsewhere (Gao et al., 2014). Although most people would prefer to die at home, the majority will die in an institution (Murray et al., 2009). Death is therefore much less on display in our society, which means it is perceived as less 'normal' or acceptable.

The fact that the majority of deaths in our society occur in hospitals raises a number of tensions and ethical issues. Healthcare staff are trained to save life rather than support death. Medical technology is rapidly advancing to help people live with severe disease. People have increasing expectations about their ability to survive, which can make it harder to come to terms with dying. As healthcare professionals, it is often difficult to decide the point at which we stop prolonging life and let someone die. Which criteria should we base these decisions on, and how much autonomy does the person have in decisions about dying? In this part of the chapter we shall look at death and bereavement from the perspective of the individual and family. We will then consider death in medical practice, including palliative care, assisted suicide, and decisions to end life.

6.3.1 DYING AND THE END OF LIFE

For most of us who are healthy, when and how we will die remains unknown. Deaths in modern society can be divided according to three main patterns: a gradual death typified by a slow decline in ability and health; a catastrophic death through sudden and unexpected events; and premature deaths through accidents or illness (Clark & Seymour, 1999). With most terminal illnesses, people will be aware that they are going to die for some time before their actual death.

ACTIVITY 6.2   HOW LONG WILL YOU LIVE?

- Life expectancy counters or 'death clocks' use a combination of questions about lifestyle to estimate your lifespan. These are just for entertainment as they are the technological equivalent of a crystal ball! See www.livingto100.com, www.myabaris.com/tools/life-expectancy-calculator-how-long-will-i-live/

As illustrated in the case studies earlier, responses to illness are very individual. Table 6.1 summarises some of the main challenges of terminal illness for the individual. It is also common for honest and open communication between terminally ill people, family, friends, and health professionals to break down because of taboos about death, worries that others do not want to talk about it, or finding it difficult to talk about. This combination of the impact of terminal illness and difficulties in communicating can result in reduced social interaction. Dying has subsequently been referred to as a 'falling from culture' as terminally ill people become increasingly isolated (Seale, 2008).

TABLE 6.1   Challenges of terminal illness

Illness-related	Self-concept	Social
• Illness symptoms and disability • Continuous treatment and side effects • Possible invasive surgery • Decisions whether to continue treatment • Threat of death	• View of self as patient • View of self as terminally ill • Changes in physical function due to illness or treatment, e.g. tremors, pain • Changes in appearance • Changes in mental function, e.g. cognitive ability	• Depression or anxiety leading to withdrawal • Preparing for loss and withdrawing from others • Mental or physical decline leading to shame, embarrassment, or concern about the impact on others • Worries about being a burden on others • Feeling bitter, angry, or resentful of healthy people

RESEARCH BOX 6.1   Doctor–patient collusion about dying

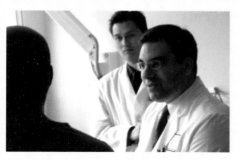

Source: National Cancer Institute, August 2005

Background

This study stemmed from the clinical observation that many people with terminal lung cancer had unrealistic optimism about their prognosis. The researchers wanted to discover why this was.

Method and findings

A qualitative study of 35 people with small-cell lung cancer were followed from diagnosis to death over four years in the Netherlands.

False optimism was put down to a 'collusion' between doctors and patients, where doctors focused on the benefits of treatment and this fed into people's need to believe they could recover. In keeping with this, false optimism was highest during chemotherapy treatment but disappeared when the tumour recurred. People became more realistic about prognosis as the disease progressed and by having contact with people at a more advanced stage. Below is the view of one of the consultants.

> 'This is one of the most difficult things in my work. Just before the therapy I told him that his life expectancy was short and that this was the last thing I could do. He and his wife were crying all the time. Because they were very upset, I could not continue my explanation. That's why I wanted to talk to them again today. You saw what happened. They asked me again whether other therapies are available. Must I ruin their life by being honest? By telling things again that I have already told them? Or just leave it? That's a huge problem. I tell them once or twice what the situation is. If people want to know more, they must ask for it. I leave it to them.'

> 'Do you find it difficult to break bad news?' the researcher asks.

> 'I think people must know what their situation is, but I find it difficult. What are the effects of what I say? That's my problem.'

Significance

This study highlights the difficulty that doctors face when discussing prognosis with people and why it might be easier to collude with the patient. More research is needed to explore whether false optimism is helpful or unhelpful to the patient and their family.

The, A.M., Hak, T., Koeter, G. & van der Wal, G. (2000) Collusion in doctor–patient communication about imminent death: an ethnographic study. *British Medical Journal, 321*: 1376–1381.

Doctors and other healthcare professionals may also find it difficult to 'diagnose' death and discuss prognosis in terminal illness (see the Research Box 6.1) and people may have a false optimism about their prognosis which helps them in the short term but makes it harder to accept death if it comes quickly. Barriers that make it hard for healthcare professionals to diagnose dying include:

- A hope that the person will get better.
- The lack of a definitive diagnosis.
- Pursuing unrealistic or futile treatments.
- Disagreements about the person's condition.
- A failure to recognise the severity of an illness.
- A lack of knowledge about specific care.
- Poor communication skills.
- Concerns about withholding treatment.
- A fear of foreshortening a person's life.
- Concerns about resuscitation.
- Cultural and spiritual barriers.
- Medico-legal issues.

ACTIVITY 6.3   DIAGNOSING DYING

- What do you think people should be told about their illness?
- Should people always be given a complete and honest prognosis?
- Are there reasons why we should withhold information?

6.3.2 RESPONSES TO TERMINAL ILLNESS

Death is the ultimate existential crisis when we are forced to confront our very existence. Existentialism assumes that most personal crises are prompted by realising our mortality. Therefore people will tend to question their purpose in life, the meaning of their life, the values they have held, the foundations of their life, their relationships with others, and their religious beliefs. This realisation of mortality may make people feel alone and isolated.

One of the most influential views of dying was put forward by the psychiatrist Kübler-Ross (1969), who proposed that people go through five stages:

1. *Denial*, where the person uses denial to adjust to the fact they are dying without being emotionally overwhelmed.
2. *Anger*, which stems from a frustration at dying and is often directed at those closest to the person. Questions like 'why me?' are common. Understanding that the person is angry at dying (not at people around them) can help carers to cope with angry outbursts.

3. *Bargaining*, where people try to make a deal with God or the medical professionals so they live, promising good behaviour in return for their life.
4. *Depression*, which occurs when the person realises there is nothing that can be done. This is seen as 'anticipatory grief' where people prepare for, and mourn, their own death.
5. *Acceptance*, where the person accepts their death with calmness and peace.

We now know that people with terminal illness do not go through discreet or consecutive stages of tasks or emotions. People may experience any of these feelings concurrently or move between them. Many people never reach the stage of acceptance, and anxiety and a fear of death are common. Many people fear death, pain and suffering, loneliness, and the unknown. Fear of death is higher in people with poor physical health, low life satisfaction or purpose in life, and those who have anxiety or depression (Neimeyer et al., 2004).

6.3.3 BEREAVEMENT

Dying does not occur in isolation but affects family, friends, and the community. In this section we shall consider the process of bereavement, the impact of bereavement on health, and normal and pathological grief processes.

Process of bereavement

Bereavement involves loss, grief, and mourning. **Loss** occurs when a person or object we are emotionally attached to becomes permanently unavailable. Loss is an integral part of terminal illness – people lose the ability to function physically, occupationally, and at home. **Grief** is a normal reaction to loss. It involves emotional reactions (e.g. anger, guilt, anxiety, sadness, despair), physical reactions (e.g. changes in appetite, sleep, somatic complaints), and social reactions (e.g. changes in social functioning, inability to work). Mourning is the process through which people adapt to loss.

How we grieve and mourn is strongly influenced by cultural customs and rules. What happens after death is prescribed by society. For example, work regulations affect the process and length of mourning. In the UK, health service workers are allowed three days' paid leave following a bereavement. Compare this with specific cultural and religious values, such as Hindu funeral rituals, which can last for up to 13 days.

The symptoms that people can experience during bereavement are given in Table 6.2. Although there are individual differences in how people grieve, 85% of people will usually adjust by the second year of bereavement (Figure 6.4). The duration and severity of a person's grief depends on:

- How attached they were to the deceased person.
- The circumstances of the death and situation of loss.
- How much time they had to work through anticipatory mourning.

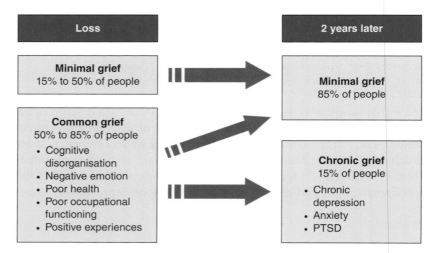

FIGURE 6.4   Responses to bereavement (adapted from Bonanno & Kaltman, 2001)

Bereavement is associated with an increased risk of illness and mortality, particularly in older adults who lose their spouse. This is probably due to a range of factors, such as stress (see Chapter 3), depression (see Chapter 2), and lifestyle (Chapter 5).

What we classify as 'normal' during bereavement will depend on the theoretical view we take. Traditional views focus on the *work* of grieving. Bereavement is seen as a time during which people work through unresolved conflict or issues to do with the deceased, accept the reality of their loss, adjust to life without them, and emotionally detach from them to continue living (Worden, 2009). Stage theories emphasise the different stages a person will go through, such as numbness, yearning, despair, and recovery (Buglass, 2010). Stress theories emphasise stress and coping with bereavement as a dynamic process involving changes in orientation toward loss or restoration (Stroebe et al., 2007). When people are orientated toward loss they will be preoccupied with their loss, think about and yearn for the deceased, and carry out behaviours such as seeking out common places or searching for the deceased. When orientated toward restoration people will adjust their lifestyle, cope with day-to-day life, build a new identity, distract themselves from painful thoughts, and take over the tasks and roles that the deceased used to do.

In pathological or chronic grief, people are severely affected and can develop mental health problems such as depression or anxiety disorders. Pathological grief is more likely if the death was sudden or unexpected, if the deceased was a child, and/or there was a high level of dependency in the relationship. Risk is also increased if the bereaved person has a history of psychological problems, poor support, and additional stressors, such as financial difficulties. Psychological interventions for bereavement appear to have little effect on depression, grief, or physical symptoms except in high risk people (Jordan & Neimeyer, 2003). Support appears to help bereaved people generally but does not buffer them against the grief (Stroebe et al., 2007). This suggests that for most people bereavement is a process they have to go through and, although support or intervention may be a comfort to them, it will not 'solve' their grief.

TABLE 6.2 Responses to loss (adapted from Bonanno & Kaltman, 2001; Payne et al., 1999)

Physical	Behavioural	Emotional	Cognitive
• Fatigue • Sleep pattern changes • Aches and pains • Appetite changes • Digestive problems • Shortness of breath • Palpitations • Restlessness • Increased vulnerability to illness	• Irritability • Restlessness • Searching • Crying • Social withdrawal • Inability to fulfil normal roles	• Depression • Anxiety • Hypervigilance • Anger/hostility • Guilt • Pining/yearning • Emotional loneliness • Social loneliness • Feeling detached or distant	• Lack of concentration • Shorter attention span • Memory loss • Confusion • Preoccupation • Helplessness/hopelessness • Sense of disrupted future • Search for meaning • Disturbances of identity

Summary

- Death is the ultimate crisis when people are forced to confront and question their existence.
- Fear of death is common in terminal illness, especially in people who are younger, have worse physical health, low life satisfaction, anxiety or depression.
- Honest communication between terminally ill people, family, friends, and health professionals may break down, and health professionals may collude with patients to promote false optimism.
- The severity of grief and mourning will depend on how attached a person was to the deceased, the circumstances of death and situation of loss, and the extent of anticipatory mourning.
- Bereavement is associated with an increased risk of illness and mortality, particularly in older adults who lose their spouse.
- 15% of people develop chronic grief. This is more likely if the death was sudden, unexpected or a child, if there was high dependency in the relationship, or if the person has a history of psychological problems, poor support, and additional stressors.

6.4 DEATH AND HEALTHCARE PRACTICE

In the 1960s people with terminal illnesses were usually not told they were dying but were instead heavily sedated and kept separate from other patients (Glaser & Strauss, 1966). Hospices today are founded on the idea that terminally ill people should have compassionate care that addresses the medical, psychological, social, and spiritual aspects of dying (see Box 6.2). Palliative care focuses on relieving symptoms such as pain rather than curing disease. Painful or invasive treatments are usually discontinued. A greater emphasis is placed on the person's psychological wellbeing. The person is given as much control and choice as possible. Honest communication is emphasised and family are encouraged to be involved. Palliative care is increasingly provided to people in their own homes by specialist nurses or multidisciplinary teams. Dying at home or in a hospice is associated with better control of pain and symptoms and greater satisfaction on the part of the main carer (e.g. spouse). However, the evidence is inconsistent over whether hospice care does result in a better quality of life (Finlay et al., 2002).

BOX 6.2   Aims of palliative care

1   To promote quality of life.
2   To manage emotional and physical symptoms.
3   To support people to live productively.
4   To empower people to take control of life.

Working in palliative care puts considerable strain on staff, and burnout rates are high (see Chapter 3). A review of people working in oncology found that around 30% had symptoms of burnout (Trufelli et al., 2008). The inability to cure people and the fact that every patient dies can be unrewarding and frustrating. Healthcare professionals may detach or withdraw from patients to protect themselves emotionally. Others may focus their attention on people who will benefit from medical intervention. Palliative care implicitly supports the idea of a 'good death', that is one where the person is psychologically prepared, physically comfortable, and able to die in the best way possible. There has been extensive debate over the notion of a 'good death' and how far we should go to help people achieve this.

CLINICAL NOTES 6.2

Working with terminally ill people

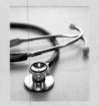

- Talk to people about their illness and treatment.
- Involve them in decisions wherever possible.
- Try to address their fears and reduce anxiety.
- Be calm and mindful when with a terminally ill person – even if you don't feel like this.
- Empathise (e.g. 'that sounds…', 'I can imagine …') but do not say you 'know' or 'understand'.

(Continued)

- If they are angry do not take it personally – it is usually anger and frustration at their illness.
- Help them make the most of the time they have left in the best way for them.
- Help them and their family work through anticipatory loss and grief.
- Help them die with dignity. If possible this should be where and how they wish.

Euthanasia and assisted suicide

Euthanasia comes from the Greek words for 'good death'. Voluntary euthanasia is when death is hastened at the dying person's request and with their consent. Involuntary euthanasia is killing a person who has not specifically requested assistance in dying. This occurs in situations such as brain-death or coma where family and/or doctors withdraw life support. The way in which euthanasia is done can be active or passive. Active euthanasia involves an active acceleration of death through the use of drugs or by other means. Passive euthanasia involves the withdrawal of treatment so that the person dies. This is relatively common in critical care settings as it involves any situation where life support is removed. Passive euthanasia is therefore already practised in countries where active euthanasia is illegal. Assisted suicide is a form of active voluntary euthanasia where someone assists a terminally ill person to commit suicide in as painless and dignified a way as possible.

Some of the ethical arguments for and against euthanasia are given in Table 6.3. Euthanasia and assisted suicide are currently illegal in the UK, Australia, and most of the USA. Other countries have decriminalised euthanasia, for example the Netherlands, Belgium, and Switzerland. Attitudes and laws on euthanasia are increasingly challenged

TABLE 6.3   Arguments for and against euthanasia (adapted from www.dignityindying.org.uk)

For	Against
<ul><li>People should have the right to decide when and how to die</li><li>Euthanasia happens anyway</li><li>It allows people to have a good quality of life when they are alive</li><li>People will die in less pain and with dignity</li><li>Passive euthanasia already occurs so is there any difference between passive and active euthanasia?</li><li>Most lay people (82%) are in favour of euthanasia</li><li>The alternative is a protracted death with poor quality of life</li></ul>	<ul><li>Sanctity of life</li><li>Intentional killing is not allowed</li><li>A cure may be found</li><li>Voluntary euthanasia will lead to the involuntary euthanasia of people who do not want it but cannot express this</li><li>People who chose euthanasia are depressed and/or not given adequate care</li><li>Legalising killing leads to reduced respect for human life, and this is potentially damaging for society</li><li>Good palliative care means euthanasia is unnecessary</li></ul>

by pressure groups such as Dignity in Dying, and terminally ill people who fight for the right to take their own life. Medical opinion is also slowly changing, with many professional organisations changing their stance from explicitly opposing assisted suicide to being neutral.

ACTIVITY 6.4   INVOLUNTARY EUTHANASIA

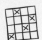

Consider the scenarios below and think about what you would do:

- In intensive care you have a 78-year-old woman on life support with no hope of recovery. The family are unsure what to do. There is a 21-year-old car accident victim who has just arrived and needs intensive care but you have no bed available. He will probably not survive the journey if you send him to the nearest alternative hospital.
- A terminally ill 67-year-old man is in the advanced stages of cancer. He looks uncomfortable and is having trouble breathing. His relatives are very distressed. Should he be given a drug that will settle his breathing but will also mean he dies quicker?
- A 60-year-old woman collapses in the Accident and Emergency department and is being actively resuscitated when the medical team find out she has advanced bowel cancer and has refused chemotherapy. Should they stop resuscitation?

Research on healthcare professionals' experience of euthanasia is remarkably limited. One study in the USA carried out confidential interviews with 10 nurses working

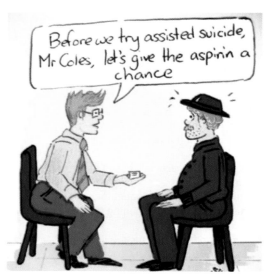

in palliative or critical care settings (Schwarz, 2004). All of the nurses had been asked by patients to help them die. When patients asked for help the nurses reported (a) refusing assistance; (b) administering palliative drugs that might secondarily hasten dying; (c) ignoring and not interfering with the patient's or family's plans to hasten death; or (d) actively assisting the patient in dying. How nurses responded was influenced by the context and circumstances of each request. It was rare for nurses to consult with colleagues or the professional guidelines. Very few nurses immediately agreed or refused to help people die; most struggled to find morally and legally acceptable ways to help them. Regardless of how they responded, nurses who had hastened death described feelings of guilt and distress.

This study illustrates a number of very important issues. First, it shows that medical professionals in critical and palliative care are sometimes asked by people for assistance to die. Second, the current legislation means staff will not be professionally supported when faced with these difficult ethical and moral decisions. Third, acting alone in these circumstances may have negative repercussions for emotional wellbeing. Consequently, some doctors and healthcare professionals are active campaigners for legal euthanasia (see Case Study 6.2).

CASE STUDY 6.2 Helping people to die

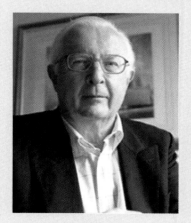

Retired doctor Michael Irwin is working to highlight the plight of people who are terminally ill and wish to commit suicide. His actions have increased the pressure on the UK government to legalise assisted suicide.

At present, British people with chronic or terminal illnesses have to travel to a clinic in Switzerland if they wish to commit suicide. So far, approximately 140 people have done this and most friends or relatives that accompany them have not been prosecuted. However, a few people have been investigated or arrested.

One such case is the arrest of the partner of a man who killed himself at a Swiss clinic in 2007 with Dr Irwin's help. Dr Irwin helped pay for the trip and was there at the assisted suicide. Dr Irwin was also arrested and they were both held on bail for more than five months. Dr Irwin has been completely open about his involvement. He provided police with a diary of his trip that detailed how the suicide was carried out.

Dr Irwin has been investigated before for his involvement in assisted suicide. He spent two years under investigation after accompanying a woman with a severe degenerative disease to Switzerland to commit suicide. However, police did not have enough evidence to press charges. In 2003, he was held on bail for three months because he admitted helping a cancer sufferer die because the patient was too ill to swallow the pills that Dr Irwin provided him with.

Dr Irwin has publicly stated that he intends to help other terminally ill people to end their lives.

> I've done this before and I would do it again if someone is terminally ill. It's so wrong that people have to travel abroad to die when they could die here at home with dignity. I say to the police 'arrest me'.

Reproduced courtesy of Dr Michael Irwin. All rights reserved.

In countries where euthanasia is not illegal, most guidelines insist that physicians are involved. For example, the guidelines in the Netherlands state that a doctor must ensure the request for terminating life is made voluntarily by the person. They must also establish that the person's situation means they are in unbearable suffering with no prospect of improvement. The procedure of euthanasia must include the consultation and agreement of two doctors; euthanasia can only be carried out on request and must be assisted by a doctor; and the death must be reported to the authorities as euthanasia or physician-assisted suicide.

CLINICAL NOTES 6.3

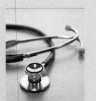

Dealing with death

- When people are grief stricken the best thing you can do is calmly support them, e.g. through touch or gentle words.
- If they are very distressed, a useful technique is to get them to talk about something specific (but relevant). This will focus their mind and should reduce their immediate distress.
- Working with people who are dying is emotionally draining. It is OK to cry and feel upset.
- Make sure you look after yourself: use available support whether informal (e.g. peers, family) or formal (e.g. colleagues). Maintain activities that nourish you (e.g. exercise, music, being with friends).
- Be self-aware. If you start to feel overwhelmed or burnt out then get help straight away.

Summary

- Palliative care is founded on providing terminally ill people with compassionate care that addresses the medical, psychological, social, and spiritual aspects of dying.
- Palliative care implicitly supports the notion of a 'good death' but there is often tension between this and the ethical, moral, or legal opposition to euthanasia.
- Euthanasia can be voluntary (death hastened at the person's request) and involuntary (killing a person who has not requested it).
- Methods of euthanasia can be active (e.g. accelerated by drugs), or passive (e.g. the withdrawal of life-sustaining treatment).
- Assisted suicide is a form of active voluntary euthanasia which is legal in only a few countries.

(Continued)

- Research suggests that medical professionals in palliative care are asked by patients to assist death. Staff therefore face difficult ethical and moral decisions while being professionally unsupported.
- In countries where euthanasia is legal, most guidelines state that physicians must be involved in (a) establishing that assisted suicide is appropriate and (b) assisting death.

CONCLUSION

This chapter has addressed the challenges of chronic and terminal illness, including the significant impact these illnesses can have on the lives of people and their family. In the final section we have also seen that these illnesses are a challenge for healthcare professionals – confronting us with difficult ethical and moral decisions as we watch people die. In a medical system founded on saving life, it can be hard to accept that sometimes there is nothing to do except support a person's death. Yet it is this support they often most appreciate. As one doctor observed:

> In my office adjacent to the medical intensive care unit, I have a growing file of letters from relatives of patients we have treated, thanking us for our care. But the majority of these letters are not from families of patients who survived. Rather, most come from people who have lost a loved one, from the bereaved survivors of patients who died in our intensive care unit. Yet they are deeply grateful for what we did. At first, I found these letters ironic and odd. I expected and basked in appreciation for lives saved. But the ones about lives we could not save – those I had trouble understanding. And I feel guilty. I read the letters over and over, wondering what the writers meant to me ... Saving deaths, I have come to realize, is as important and rewarding as saving lives. (Nelson, 1999: pp. 776–77)

FURTHER READING

Llewellyn, C.D. et al. (eds) (2018) *Cambridge Handbook of Psychology, Health and Medicine* (3rd edition). Cambridge: Cambridge University Press. This handbook contains brief chapters on many topics in this chapter, including chronic illness, health status and quality of life, stress and crisis management, and peer support interventions.

Fallon, M. & Hanks, G. (eds) (2006) *ABC of Palliative Care*. Oxford: Blackwell. This book covers both the medical and psychological aspects of palliative care and includes chapters on managing physical symptoms, communication, carers, and bereavement.

Martz, E. & Livneh, H. (eds) (2007) *Coping with Chronic Illness and Disability: Theoretical, Empirical, and Clinical Aspects*. New York: Springer. This is a comprehensive account of our psychological understanding of chronic illness. It also includes chapters on specific disorders, such as AIDS, arthritis, burns, cancer, diabetes, heart disease, and MS.

REVISION QUESTIONS

1. Outline the common emotional responses to chronic illness and discuss how these may affect health.

2. Describe one psychological intervention for people with chronic illness and discuss the evidence for its effectiveness.

3. What is narrative-based medicine and how can it improve clinical care?

4. What challenges does terminal illness raise for individuals?

5. What are the reasons why healthcare professionals can find it difficult to 'diagnose' death and discuss this prognosis with terminally ill people?

6. Outline Kübler-Ross's stages of dying. Discuss how accurate and how useful these are in clinical practice.

7. Describe the processes of normal bereavement and pathological grief.

8. What are the common symptoms of bereavement?

9. What are the different types of euthanasia and what type of euthanasia is assisted suicide?

10. Describe some of the main ethical arguments for and against euthanasia.

SECTION II

BASIC FOUNDATIONS OF PSYCHOLOGY

7 BRAIN AND BEHAVIOUR

(Continued)

LEARNING OBJECTIVES

This chapter is designed to enable you to:

- Describe the functional organisation of the brain and nervous system.
- Describe how messages are communicated within neurons and from neurons to other cells.
- Describe how the nervous system controls involuntary and voluntary muscle movement.
- Outline explanations of the mechanisms of sleep, dreaming, and consciousness.

Medical and healthcare professionals need to understand the normal functioning of the brain and nervous system. This chapter introduces the structure and function of the nervous system, the control of movement, as well as sleep, consciousness, and biological clocks. Medical and healthcare professionals also need to be able to recognise the physical and psychological aspects of normal and abnormal brain functioning. Abnormal functioning is covered in Chapter 16.

7.1 COMPONENTS AND ORGANISATION OF THE NERVOUS SYSTEM

7.1.1 ORGANISATION OF THE NERVOUS SYSTEM

There are two major divisions of the nervous system: the central nervous system and the peripheral nervous system (see Figure 7.1). The central nervous system (CNS) consists of

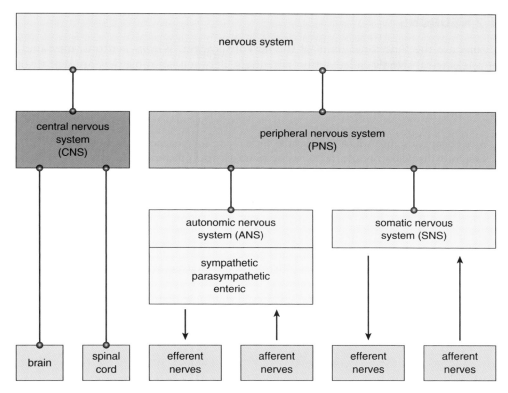

FIGURE 7.1 Organisation of the nervous system

nerves in the brain, brainstem, and spinal cord. Afferent nerves carry nerve impulses toward the CNS; efferent nerves carry impulses away from the CNS. The structure and function of the CNS are described more fully later in this chapter.

The second major division is the peripheral nervous system (PNS). It consists of nerves that lie outside the CNS. It also consists of two components: the automatic nervous system and the somatic nervous system. The **autonomic nervous system** (ANS) consists of nerves that innervate internal and glandular organs and regulate processes that are not normally under voluntary control. The ANS comprises *sympathetic* and *parasympathetic nervous systems*. In general, the sympathetic nervous system prepares the body for action – e.g. opening airways, increasing the heart rate, inhibiting digestion, and stimulating the release of hormones from the adrenal glands. The parasympathetic nervous system tends to work in the opposite way to produce relaxation – e.g., slowing the heart rate, promoting digestion. The *enteric nervous system* controls the gastrointestinal system, and is often considered as part of the ANS.

The somatic nervous system (SNS) receives sensory information (what we see, hear, smell, touch, and taste) and relays this to the CNS via afferent nerves. The CNS acts on this sensory information and sends motor signals (e.g. signals to pick and sniff a flower or to catch a ball thrown to us) via efferent nerves to the skeletal muscles.

7.1.2 NEURONS

Neurons are the functional units of the nervous system. Within neurons, messages are sent as electrical signals called action potentials. Between neurons, they are sent through the release of neurotransmitters into synapses, which are the small gaps between neurons. Neurons process and transmit information within the nervous system. Each neuron consists of:

- A cell body (or soma), which contains the nucleus and components vital for cell life.
- Dendrites that allow one neuron to receive messages from other cells.
- An axon, which carries messages from the cell body to the terminal buttons.
- Terminal buttons, which are important for passing messages from a neuron to other cells.

Neurons have a very high rate of metabolism. They cannot store their fuel and cannot extract energy in the absence of oxygen (unlike some other cells, such as muscle cells). They therefore rely on a supply of glucose and oxygen from supporting cells. If blood flow to the brain is interrupted for as little as a few minutes, then permanent brain damage can occur.

Until quite recently, it was generally believed that new neurons could not be produced in developed adult brains. However, research conducted over the past two decades has identified that generation of new neurons (neurogenesis) does occur in some regions of the adult brain (e.g. Bischofberger, 2007; Jessberger & Gage, 2014). Similarly, it was previously believed that the CNS was unable to repair itself. However, there is now evidence that there is the potential for some degree of neural regeneration and reorganisation within an adult CNS (e.g. Okano & Sawamoto, 2008; Williams, 2014). These advances in understanding have raised hope for effective treatments for conditions such as Parkinson's disease, Alzheimer's disease, and stroke.

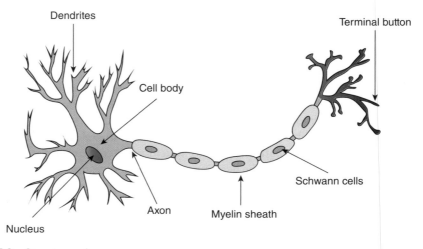

FIGURE 7.2   Structure of a neuron

In the PNS, destruction of cell bodies leads to a permanent and irreversible loss of axons in the peripheral nerve. Severe damage to peripheral axons causes permanent impairment such as a loss of sensation and muscle bulk. If the damage is not severe, the nerve may be able to repair itself (Navarro et al., 2007). Some brain systems are able to be re-modelled in response to changes in input resulting from nerve damage (Sharma et al., 2013). The ability of neural circuits to undergo changes in organisation or function as a result of previous activity or damage is called neural plasticity.

Summary

- The two major divisions of the nervous system are the central nervous system (CNS) – the brain, brainstem, and spinal cord – and the peripheral nervous system (PNS) – nerves that carry information to and from the CNS.
- The PNS consists of three components: (i) the autonomic nervous system, which regulates bodily processes not normally under voluntary control; (ii) the enteric nervous system, which controls the gastrointestinal system; and (iii) the somatic nervous system, which processes sensory information.
- Neurons are the nervous system's functional units. Their dendrites receive information from outside the cell. Their axons transfer signals to other cells.

7.2 COMMUNICATION WITHIN AND BETWEEN NEURONS

7.2.1 ACTION POTENTIALS WITHIN NEURONS

An action potential is an electrical pulse used to send signals from a neuron to another cell. An action potential is a burst of electrical activity that is of a fixed size and is an all-or-nothing response. A sequence of changes to the action of ion channels in the neural membrane results in an action potential travelling along the axon toward the axon terminals.

7.2.2 SYNAPSES

When an action potential reaches the end of an axon it triggers the release of neurotransmitters from the terminal buttons into the synapse. Neurotransmitters are chemical messengers that bind to specialised receptors on the postsynaptic membrane of the target cell (which may be another neuron, a muscle cell, or a gland cell). The response may be the generation of an action potential in a neuron, the inhibition of neurotransmitter release, the contraction of a muscle, or the release of a hormone. Once a neurotransmitter has bound to its target cell receptor, it is broken down to prevent any further excitation or inhibition of the target cell. Many neurotransmitters are taken up and recycled by the pre-synaptic neuron to produce more of the neurotransmitter.

Whereas neurotransmitters within the central nervous system are involved in direct one-to-one neuron-to-neuron communication, neuromodulators secreted by some neurons diffuse through large areas of the nervous system and affect multiple neurons. Neuromodulators are not metabolised or re-absorbed by the pre-synaptic neuron. As a result, they influence the brain's overall levels of activity.

A number of different neurotransmitters and neuromodulators have been identified, some of which are briefly described in the remainder of this section.

Acetylcholine is released by neurons that stimulate the contraction of voluntary muscles. It also serves as a neurotransmitter in many regions of the brain and appears to be involved in the regulation of normal attention, memory, and sleep. Acetylcholine-releasing neurons die in people with Alzheimer's disease.

Monoamine neurotransmitters are divided into catecholamines and indolamines. The *Catecholamines* dopamine and noradrenaline (norepinephrine) are widely distributed in the brain and PNS. Within the brain, dopamine is present in three principal circuits:

- One circuit controls movement. Dopamine deficits in Parkinson's disease produce muscle tremors, rigidity, and difficulty in moving, but the dopamine precursor levodopa (L-Dopa) is an effective treatment.
- A second circuit is important for cognition and emotion and may be involved in psychosis.
- A third circuit regulates the endocrine system. In response to dopamine, the hypothalamus is stimulated to store or release hormones within the pituitary.

Noradrenaline (norepinephrine) appears to be involved in learning and memory. Deficiencies in noradrenaline occur in people with Alzheimer's disease, Parkinson's disease and Korsakoff's syndrome – a cognitive disorder associated with chronic alcoholism. Depression is also often associated with low levels of noradrenaline.

The *indolamine* serotonin is implicated in sleep, mood, depression, and anxiety. Because serotonin appears to control various emotional states, much research has been directed toward developing serotonin analogues – chemicals with molecular structures similar to that of serotonin. Drugs that supplement or alter the action of serotonin can relieve the symptoms of depression and anxiety disorders.

Amino acids can act as neurotransmitters in the brain. Some inhibit the firing of other neurons, such as glycine and gamma-aminobutyric acid (GABA), whereas other proteins have excitatory functions, such as glutamate and aspartate.

Peptides are chains of amino acids linked together that are smaller than proteins. Opioid peptides have been the focus of much research. For example, endorphins act like opium or morphine to reduce pain and cause sleepiness.

Hormones are able to affect neural activity because hormone receptors are present on many neurons. In the brain, hormones can alter the structure and function of neurons. For example, stress hormones such as cortisol can affect learning. Severe and prolonged stress can cause permanent changes to the brain.

Thus far, the discussion of communication between neurons has focused on neurotransmitters acting at axon–dendrite synapses. However, the brain does contain axon–axon synapses in which the terminal buttons of one axon connect to a second axon and modulate the release of neurotransmitters from the second axon. In addition, direct electrical transmission between neurons occurs at some sites in the brain. These fast-conducting gap junctions promote the rapid and widespread propagation of action potentials between neurons and may be important for synchronising complex brain activity.

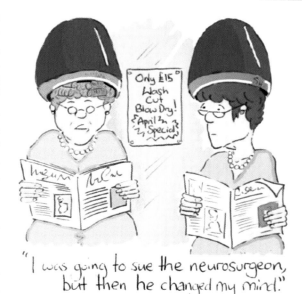

"I was going to sue the neurosurgeon, but then he changed my mind."

Clearly, numerous events or processes can interfere with the transmission of action potentials within neurons and between neurons. Damage to the myelin sheath impairs the coordination of neuronal activity (see multiple sclerosis, Chapter 16). Disruptions or modifications to neurotransmitter or neuromodulator activity may impair memory and cognition and have been implicated in a range of psychiatric disorders (see Chapter 16). The normal effects of neurotransmitters on neurons become disrupted by addiction to alcohol or other drugs. The specific effects of different drugs vary, as do the neurotransmitters involved. Neurotransmitters involved in addiction include GABA, glutamate, opioid peptides, serotonin, and dopamine (Koob & Volkow, 2016). Note that although the physiological aspects of drug dependence are important, the biopsychosocial explanation of addiction highlights the importance of psychological and social aspects of addiction. The psychosocial aspects of addiction and its treatment are illustrated at various points in this book (see the Case Studies on smoking cessation in Chapter 5, and Case Study 2.2 on alcohol use in Chapter 2).

Summary

- Communication between a neuron and another cell (a neuron, or muscle, or gland cell) occurs across a synapse.
- When an action potential reaches the presynaptic neural membrane, it triggers the release of a neurotransmitter which crosses the synapse and binds to the target cell's postsynaptic membrane.
- The effect of a neurotransmitter on its target cell may be the excitation or inhibition of its function.
- Different neurotransmitters have specific roles within different regions of the CNS.

7.3 STRUCTURE OF THE BRAIN AND CENTRAL NERVOUS SYSTEM

7.3.1 SUPPORTING CELLS

Neurons rely on supporting cells to supply nutrients and oxygen and provide the optimal environment for neural functioning. The most important supporting cells are glia. There are several different kinds of glia – each with different functions. For example, oligodendrocytes provide physical support to CNS neurons and produce the myelin sheath. This appears as a string of beads along the axon and helps to insulate the axon and speed up the transmission of action potentials (see Figure 7.2). In the PNS, Schwann cells perform the same functions as oligodendrocytes: they support axons and produce myelin.

The myelin sheaths of neural axons are vital for the efficient conduct of action potentials. Multiple sclerosis is characterised by inflammation in the CNS and the destruction of the myelin sheaths of CNS axons (see Chapter 16). As a result, the myelin is completely or partially stripped from the nerves. There may also be damage to the underlying neurons. Damage to the myelin disrupts the passage of action potentials. Virtually all functions controlled by CNS innervation can be affected. The myelin produced by Schwann cells in the PNS has a different composition from the myelin produced by the oligodendrocytes in the CNS and it is not affected in multiple sclerosis.

7.3.2 MENINGES, CEREBROSPINAL FLUID, AND VENTRICLES

The whole of the nervous system – the brain, spinal cord, and nerves – is covered by tough connective tissue. The connective tissue that surrounds the brain and spinal cord is called the meninges and is arranged in three layers:

- The dura mater – the tough outer layer.
- The arachnoid membrane – the spongy web-like middle layer.
- The pia mater – the inner layer, which is closely attached to the brain.

The subarachnoid space between the arachnoid membrane and pia mater is filled with cerebrospinal fluid (CSF). Because the brain is completely immersed in liquid, pressure on the base of the brain is reduced. In the PNS there is no arachnoid matter or CSF and the dura and pia mater are fused to form a protective sheath.

The brain contains a number of CSF-filled spaces called ventricles. In addition to providing physical support for the brain, the CSF protects against acute changes in blood pressure; is involved in intra-cerebral transport; helps maintain the ionic homeostasis of the CNS; and is a route for waste excretion.

7.3.3 BRAIN REGIONS

The brain has three major divisions: the forebrain, midbrain, and hindbrain (see Figures 7.3 and 7.4). The term 'brain stem' is often used to refer to the midbrain, pons, and medulla.

The cerebral cortex is the largest part of the human brain and is involved in 'higher' brain functions. It distinguishes mammals from other vertebrates and is thought to be responsible for the evolution of intelligence. The cortex is the outer surface of the forebrain. It is highly wrinkled in order to increase the surface area of the brain and the number of neurons within it. The outer region of the cortex contains neural cell bodies. Below this 'grey matter' is the 'white matter': this consists of axons which carry signals between cerebral neurons and other parts of the brain and body.

The cerebrum is divided into the left and right hemispheres. Although the two hemispheres look mostly symmetrical, each side has slightly different functions. In each hemisphere, the cerebral cortex is divided into four sections, or 'lobes' – the frontal, parietal, occipital, and temporal. Each lobe has different functions, as described below. A bundle of millions of axons called the corpus callosum connects the right and left frontal lobe, right and left parietal lobe, right and left occipital lobe, and right and left temporal lobe.

The frontal lobe is involved in reasoning, planning, problem solving, aspects of speech, movement, and emotions. It contains the primary somatosensory cortex, which

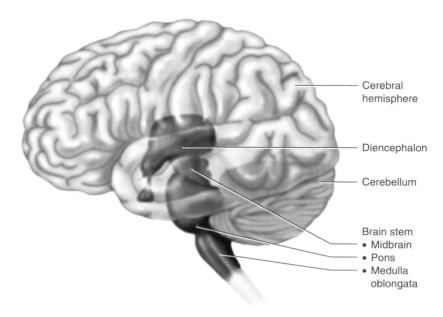

FIGURE 7.3   Anatomy of the brain

major division	subdivision	principle structures	
Forebrain	Telencephalon	Cerebral cortex	
		Basal ganglia	
		Limbic system	
	Diencephalon	Thalamus	
		Hypothalamus	
Midbrain	Mesencephalon	Tectum	
		Tegmentum	
Hindbrain	Metencephalon	Cerebellum	
		Pons	
	Myelencephalon	Medulla oblongata	

FIGURE 7.4   Divisions of the brain (adapted from Carlson, 2007)

receives sensory input, and the primary motor cortex, which controls movement. The frontal lobe contains most of the dopamine-sensitive neurons in the cerebral cortex (recall that dopamine systems are involved in cognition and emotion). The frontal lobe is involved in more complicated or 'higher' mental functions. These include our capacity to: choose between different options; imagine the future consequences of our behaviour; and suppress socially unacceptable behaviour. The frontal lobe also plays an important part in our long-term memory of experiences by processing messages from the limbic system (see below).

The parietal lobe is important for integrating sensory information from various parts of the body and is also important for movement, orientation, recognition, perception of stimuli, and manipulation of objects.

The most important functional aspect of the occipital lobe is that it contains the primary visual cortex. Damage to specific areas of the occipital lobe leads to specific losses of visual capacity located in those areas.

The temporal lobe is the location of the primary auditory cortex. It is important for processing the meaning of both speech and vision. The temporal lobe also contains the hippocampus, which plays a key role in the formation of our long-term memory. Wernicke's area – in the left temporal lobe – is particularly specialised for language comprehension. It is believed to have special connections to Broca's area in the left frontal lobe. Although it has long been held that language comprehension and speech production are localised in Wernicke's and Broca's areas respectively, more recent research now suggests that these capacities may not be so clearly demarcated (see Research Box 7.1).

RESEARCH BOX 7.1   Localisation of speech capacity

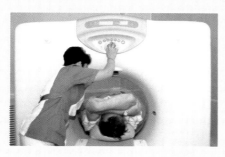

Background

Historically, understanding of the brain's functional anatomy derived from post-mortem studies of people with brain damage. Later advances in neural imaging have led to dramatic changes in understanding how the brain works. It was traditionally thought that Broca's area was responsible for speech production, with speech comprehension localised in Wernicke's area.

Method and findings

The day after a surgical procedure, a 67-year-old man referred to as MJE suddenly became unable to speak. He soon regained some speech capacity, but was only able to produce short phrases or say single words. Functional Magnetic Resonance Imaging (fMRI) revealed an infarction and a severe restriction of the blood supply in Broca's area. In addition to the expected impairments to language production, MJE also had impairments in some aspect of language comprehension. Restoration of normal blood flow to the affected area resulted in an immediate recovery of these functions.

Significance

Advances in imaging have improved our understanding of the brain's functional anatomy. This study shows that language comprehension and language generation may not be as separate as was originally thought. It is important, however, to note the limitations of this study. First, there was only a short time for observations before blood flow was restored to the affected area. Second, it may be difficult to generalise from case studies (this is a limitation common to many studies of brain abnormalities).

Photograph © Mikhail Malyshev/Fotolia

Davis, C., Kleinman, J.T., Newhart, M., Gingis, L., Pawlak, M. & Hillis, A.E. (2008) Speech and language functions that require a functioning Broca's area. *Brain & Language, 105*: 50–58.

The basal ganglia consist of a cluster of neural nuclei connected with the cerebral cortex, thalamus, and brainstem. They are involved in motor control, cognition, emotions, and learning. Disorders linked to the basal ganglia include cerebral palsy, Huntington's disease and Parkinson's disease.

The limbic system lies buried within the cerebrum, forming the inner border of the cortex. In evolutionary terms, this is an old structure. It contains the thalamus, hypothalamus, amygdala, and hippocampus. It is often referred to as the 'emotional brain' and is important for the formation of memories. The limbic system operates by influencing the endocrine system and the ANS, and is highly interconnected with the nucleus accumbens, which is the brain's pleasure centre.

The thalamus is a large mass of grey matter deep in the forebrain. Axons from every sensory system (except olfaction/smell) synapse here as the last relay site before the cerebral cortex. However, it is not just a relay system. The thalamus also processes sensory information. It also plays an important part in regulating sleep, wakefulness, and consciousness (see section 7.5).

The hypothalamus is located just below the thalamus. It is mainly involved with homeostasis, including the regulation of thirst and hunger. It is also involved in the regulation of emotions and the control of the ANS and circadian rhythms (see section 7.5). Consequently, it receives input from a number of regions of the body and the brain. The hypothalamus sends messages to the rest of the body in two ways: via the ANS and via instructions sent to the pituitary gland (the 'master gland' of the endocrine system).

The amygdala are two almond-shaped masses of neurons located in each temporal lobe on either side of the thalamus. These are involved in memory and emotion (especially aggression and fear). Damage to this area of the brain makes people indifferent to things that would normally invoke fear.

The hippocampus consists of two 'horns' of neurons projecting back from the amygdala. It is important for converting short-term memory into long-term memory, so it is important for learning (see Chapter 10). Damage to this region means that people may keep their old memories but will be unable to form new ones.

The term 'brain stem' is often used to refer to the midbrain, pons, and medulla. Collectively, these structures are responsible for basic vital functions such as breathing, heartbeat, and blood pressure. In evolutionary terms, these are old structures present in the ancestors of mammals and modern reptiles (indeed, the entire brains of some reptiles resemble the human brain stem). The midbrain lies at the 'top' of the brain stem. The anterior part of the midbrain contains the cerebral peduncle, which is a large bundle of axons involved in voluntary motor function.

Like the cerebrum, the cerebellum (literally the 'little brain') has a highly folded surface and is divided into two hemispheres. Although it makes up only 10% of brain mass, it contains more than half of its neurons. Its functions include the regulation and coordination of movement, posture, and balance. In evolutionary terms, the cerebellum is an old structure.

The **pons** is involved in the regulation of consciousness, sleep, and sensory processing. Some structures within the pons are linked to the cerebellum and are therefore involved in movement and posture. The myelencephalon consists mainly of tracts carrying signals between the brain and the rest of the body. The medulla oblongata is responsible for maintaining vital body functions, such as breathing and heart rate.

Luria's functional model provides a useful summary: the brainstem regulates the arousal of the brain and muscle tone; the posterior areas of the cortex are involved in processing sensory information from the internal and external environments; and the frontal lobes and prefrontal lobes are involved in planning, executing, and monitoring behaviour (Zillmer et al., 2008).

Summary

- The brain is organised into different regions, each of which has different activities and functions. Major divisions of the brain are the forebrain, midbrain, and hindbrain. The forebrain is divided into two linked hemispheres.
- The frontal lobes are involved in reasoning, planning, problem solving, speech, movement, and emotions. They process sensory input and control voluntary movement. They also process information from other brain regions.
- The temporal, parietal, and occipital lobes all have specialised capacities for processing and integrating sensory information.
- The limbic system is the 'emotional brain', and is also important for memory.
- The brain stem and the cerebellum are involved in regulating basic functions such as posture, movement, breathing, and heart rate.

Disruptions to normal functioning in different brain regions are related to different disorders and diseases. Disorders with primarily psychological symptoms are covered in Chapter 16. Other chapters discuss the regulation of emotions (see Chapter 2) and pain (see Chapter 4). The following sections will focus on control of movement and movement disorders, and sleep and consciousness.

7.4 CONTROL OF MOVEMENT

All muscular activity is influenced by the nervous system. Although smooth muscle cells may contract spontaneously, their rate of contraction is influenced by motor neurons of the ANS. Although the contraction of the cardiac muscle is triggered by an internal pacemaker, the motor neurons of the ANS modulate the intrinsic rate and strength of the heartbeat. Reflexive action in skeletal muscle is coordinated via the spinal cord without the involvement of the brain. Voluntary skeletal muscle activity is controlled by the CNS.

Motor neurons control muscle movement. Skeletal muscles are innervated at the neuromuscular junction (NMJ) and convert electrical action potentials from motor neurons into mechanical force by means of contraction. The presynaptic neuron membrane releases acetylcholine at the NMJ. The binding of acetylcholine to specific receptors on the muscle cell membrane causes muscle contraction. A single impulse from a neuron produces a single twitch in a muscle fibre. However, because muscle has a certain degree of elasticity, the duration of a muscle twitch is longer than the duration of the action potential. A rapid series of action potentials causes a muscle to produce a sustained contraction (rather than twitches). The overall strength of a muscle contraction depends on how many motor units fire and how rapidly they do so.

7.4.1 REFLEXES

If you touch something that is too hot, you will automatically move your hand away from it. This is not a conscious process: you do not think 'Oh, that pan is too hot, I should let go of it'. This type of movement is a reflex – an involuntary almost instantaneous movement in response to an external stimulus. Reflex actions can be made quickly because most sensory neurons do not pass directly into the brain. Instead they form synapses with other motor neurons in the spinal cord. The stimulus could come in any sensory form (e.g. heat or pain). This stimulus input is sent to the spinal column where it may directly synapse with a motor neuron, or an interneuron may relay the signal to an efferent motor neuron. The motor neuron then fires an action potential which causes the appropriate muscle movement (e.g. a withdrawal from heat). This arrangement of afferent and efferent neurons is referred to as a reflex arc. Although reflex arcs mean that the brain does not have to process sensory information before producing the appropriate response, the brain does receive sensory input while the reflex action occurs so that we can become aware of reflexive movements.

Spinal reflexes do not occur in isolation: rather, they involve control from the brain. In some cases the brain can inhibit the reflexive muscle action. The brain contains circuits which recognise that in some situations the reflex action may do more harm than good. For example, imagine you take a hot casserole out of the oven using a thin oven glove and begin to walk toward the kitchen table. After a few moments the heat will trigger a withdrawal reflex. However, your brain will recognise that dropping the casserole on the floor would be disastrous, so it overrides the reflex, allowing you to hold on until you get to the table.

7.4.2 VOLUNTARY CONTROL OF MOVEMENT

The nerves involved in generating the impulses for voluntary movement are located in the primary motor cortex. This is a band of neurons in the posterior frontal lobes which is organised like a map of the body. This 'motor homunculus' (see Figure 7.5) is not a scale model of the body. Instead, the size of each region indicates the level of innervation and reflects the degree of control of fine movements: the hands and fingers occupy more space than the rest of the arm, and more space than the feet and toes. The image on the right of Figure 7.5 shows what we would look like if we were a scale model of the motor homunculus.

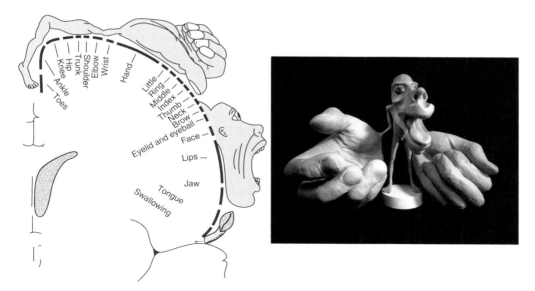

FIGURE 7.5   The motor homunculus. Photograph reproduced courtesy of the Natural History Museum

Each area of the primary motor cortex controls the movements of particular groups of muscles. It receives feedback from these muscles and the joints that they influence, via the somatosensory cortex. The term 'descending pathway' is used to refer to nerve pathways that go from the brain toward the spinal cord and allow the brain to control movement of the body below the head. In contrast, ascending pathways go upwards from the spinal cord toward the brain. They carry sensory information from the body to the brain.

Electrical stimulation to the various areas of the motor homunculus produces muscle action in the relevant area of the body (but not other areas). Extensive damage to areas of the primary motor cortex may impair people's ability to move the corresponding body part independent of others (e.g. moving only one finger). However, voluntary movement is still possible because of the existence of pathways that descend directly from the secondary motor cortex without passing via the primary motor cortex.

The secondary motor cortices perform several functions. They are responsible for:

- Transforming visual information into motor commands (posterior parietal cortex).
- Guiding movement and controlling the proximal and trunk muscles (premotor cortex).
- Planning and coordinating complex actions such as those requiring two hands (supplementary motor area).

The secondary motor cortices may be involved in programming specific patterns of movement according to instructions received from the prefrontal cortex (which is involved in forming plans and strategies) and sending their output to the primary motor cortex.

In addition to these cortical areas, other brain regions are important for controlling motor function. Although skilled rapid movements are initiated in the frontal cortex, the control and timing of such movements require the involvement of the cerebellum. Extensive damage to the cerebellum results in a loss of ability to control movements, impairments in capacities to modify movements in changing conditions, and difficulty in maintaining posture. The basal ganglia also modulate movement. They do this via neural loops that receive input from a wide array of cortical areas and feed this back

CASE STUDY 7.1 Parkinson's disease

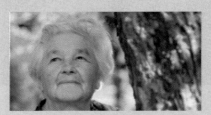

You can't think straight... it's a horrible feeling, you feel as if, er, you you're not connecting, you know, that's all I can explain it, you're brain isn't telling your body what to do.

Beth is 62 years old and married with four adult children. When she was in her late 30s, she began to experience tremors in her arm, which were attributed to her response to the recent death of her son. However, the symptoms persisted and she was diagnosed with Parkinson's disease at the age of 44. Since then it has been treated with L-Dopa. Before she takes her medication and sometimes between doses, Beth often feels 'dull' and is often barely able to move and communicate properly.

Overcoming her reduced capacity to control her movements requires purposeful effort: she talks herself through sequences of actions, such as walking or eating. Whereas she used to enjoy being active and 'never felt tired', Beth now feels fatigued and has difficulty doing things that used to be easy. Parkinson's disease has led to profound changes in how she sees herself and how others see her:

They think that you're senile because you're moving like this and... finding things hard to do like take a top off a bottle.

These changes to daily activities and quality of life are soul-destroying: Beth feels 'young at heart' but appears to others to be an 'old lady' who cannot manage. However, her efforts to conceal her muscle tremors so as to avoid negative evaluations from others usually only make the situation worse:

I try and stop myself from moving. So I hold my arm or I put my arms to the back and clasp my fist... but I look worse when I disguise it because I'm doing contortions.

To minimise such experiences, Beth adheres to her medication regimen. This lets her achieve daily activities at the right times, but it also limits her capacity to be spontaneous. She therefore feels empowered, but also disempowered by her medication.

(Adapted from Bramley & Eatough, 2005)

via the thalamus to the primary motor cortex, premotor cortex, and supplementary motor area. They also send outputs to the motor nuclei of the brain stem. Damage to the basal ganglia causes severe motor deficits such as Parkinson's and Huntington's disease (see Chapter 16).

Summary

- All muscular activity is influenced by the nervous system.
- Spinal reflexes are muscular contractions made in response to sensory information that do not have to be processed by the CNS. However, the brain can override reflexive muscle actions.
- Voluntary muscle movement is initiated in the primary motor cortex, a band of neurons in the posterior frontal lobe arranged as a motor homunculus. It also involves the secondary motor cortices, basal ganglia, and cerebellum.
- Damage to neurons in any of the areas involved in the control of movement can lead to severe motor impairments.

7.5 SLEEP, CONSCIOUSNESS, AND BIOLOGICAL CLOCKS

Sleep is an important topic: many people experience sleep difficulties (Grandner et al., 2015; Stranges et al., 2012), and quality of sleep affects our wellbeing (see below). Given the high levels of neural and muscular activity described in the last section, one might think that sleep involves an absence of such activity. However, when we are asleep our brains are not simply at rest: important activities are going on.

Sleep research uses a range of devices to monitor the body's activity during sleep: electroencephalograms (EEG) record electrical activity in the brain; electromyograms (EMG) record muscle activity; and electrooculograms (EOG) record eye movement. Researchers may also monitor markers of arousal such as heart rate, breathing, and galvanic skin response (i.e. changes in the electrical resistance of the skin). The information gathered shows that rather than there being a single entity called 'sleep' there are various phases of sleep, each with specific patterns of bodily activity.

Sleep can be divided into five stages: REM sleep (so named because it is characterised by Rapid Eye Movement), and four stages of increasingly deep **non-REM sleep**. Typically, people will progress through Stages 1–3 of non-REM sleep before entering REM sleep, which is when dreaming occurs. This progression usually takes around 90 minutes. Normally, REM sleep must be preceded by slow-wave sleep (SWS: Stage 3), and there is a refractory period after each bout of REM sleep when REM sleep does not occur (Figure 7.6).

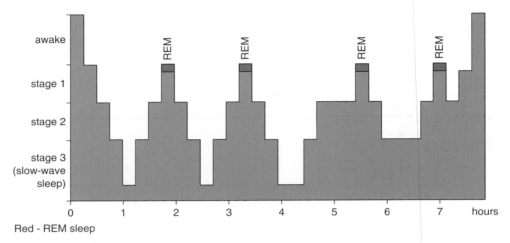

FIGURE 7.6   Stages of sleep

The progression from Stages 1 to 3 leads to 'deeper' sleep. People are easiest to wake during Stage 1 and hardest to wake during Stage 3 sleep. If people do wake from Stage 3 they are often groggy and confused. In Stage 3, EEGs show slow synchronised waves of neural activity. In contrast, EEGs during REM sleep show high frequency desynchronised activity more similar to those that can be seen when awake. During REM sleep the brain becomes activated: levels of neural firing, blood flow, and oxygen consumption increase to waking levels. REM sleep also differs from non-REM sleep stages because of the eponymous rapid eye movements that are observable through closed eye lids and via EOG. The EMG shows a marked loss of skeletal muscle tone compared to the moderate muscle tone in Stage 3, so movement is restricted.

EEG and fMRI studies indicate that neural activity during REM sleep corresponds to the content of dreams (Hobson, 2009). For example, talking and listening during dreams is associated with the increased neural activity in brain regions involved in talking and listening (Hong et al., 1996). However, physical movements made during sleep do not occur during dreams in REM sleep because of the loss of skeletal muscle tone. Sleepwalking and night terrors occur during slow-wave sleep.

7.5.1 WHY DO WE DREAM?

There is no definitive explanation of why we dream. That there are specific patterns of brain activity during REM sleep that are absent from other stages of sleep suggests that it may have a distinct function. Studies of REM sleep deprivation show that the body tries to ensure a certain amount of REM sleep. In such studies, people will be allowed to sleep

CASE STUDY 7.2   Insomnia

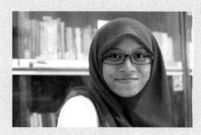

Aisha is 27 years old and is part of the one-third of the population who experience insomnia. She has always been healthy otherwise, and has tried to cope with her disrupted and unsatisfying sleep for a few months. However, now she feels that she needs help. Her performance at work is slipping and she has noticed that she is snappy and less pleasant company than she used to be.

My insomnia seems to be getting worse every day. I am worried that the sleep part of my brain has been destroyed. There is nothing worse than being awake and knowing that other people are sleeping... and knowing how exhausted I will feel the next day. I get really frustrated and I try to relax, but it seems that the more I think about it, the harder it is to sleep.

Aisha discussed her insomnia with her doctor, but she was not satisfied with the treatment options. Her doctor was reluctant to prescribe medication (hypnotics), and instead suggested focusing on 'sleep hygiene'. This refers to behavioural strategies, such as avoiding stimulants like caffeine close to bedtime, limiting alcohol intake, avoiding rich, fatty foods, exercising to promote good quality sleep, and ensuring adequate exposure to natural daylight. It also entails having a regular, relaxing bedtime routine which should include the avoidance of bright lights in the bedroom or smartphone/computer screens in bed.

Aisha understands that some of her sleep hygiene behaviours could be better, but she also wants a rapid solution to her predicament:

My friends and family try to understand, but I don't think they get just how serious it is and the impact it has on my life. I don't think my GP does either. I don't want to have to rely on drugs to get to sleep – or stay asleep, but I need something that will work now! Maybe with a little help from the medication I will be able to sort out my sleeping in general.

Health professionals in primary care who are working with people with insomnia may advise short-term medication, improved sleep hygiene, and cognitive behavioural therapy. However, they should be aware that it is unlikely that there will be a quick-fix solution.

as much as they want, but will be woken each time they enter REM sleep. In response to REM deprivation, the body appears to enter REM sleep more rapidly than normal and on subsequent nights there is evidence of the body catching up on REM sleep.

Some research has indicated that REM sleep is important for consolidating learning and memory (Stickgold et al., 2001). However, there is also some evidence that deficits in total sleep or REM sleep do not affect learning and memory. For example, although REM sleep is significantly reduced by the three major classes of antidepressant drugs, there are no corresponding disruptions to learning and memory (Vertes & Eastman, 2000). Recent reviews suggest that REM sleep and non-REM slow-wave sleep may be important for different elements of memory consolidation (Ackerman & Rasch, 2014).

Just as there is disagreement about why we dream, there is also disagreement about what dreams mean. As you will probably know from your own experience, dreams will often relate to things you are preoccupied about. The content of dreams may have a literal interpretation. For example, if we are dehydrated we may dream about drinking water. However, objects and events within dreams may also have symbolic meanings. For instance, feeling thirsty but not being allowed to drink may symbolise some other frustration in our lives. When interpreting dreams, it is important to consider the individual items or events in dreams, their links to other objects/events in the dream, and the context of the dreamer's waking life.

Freud (1999 [1990]) believed that dreams are the 'royal road' to understanding our unconscious mental processes. In his psychoanalytic theory, he argued that subconscious urges and emotions appear in a disguised form during dreams. An alternative to the psychoanalytic model is the activation-synthesis model, which proposes that dreams are simply the result of the brain trying to make sense of the activation of neural circuits in the brain stem and parts of the limbic system during REM sleep (Hobson & McCarley, 1977).

7.5.2 WHY DO WE SLEEP?

Sleep deprivation appears to be a risk to human health because it is related to lapses of attention, deficits in cognition and memory, and involuntary sleep onset (Goel et al., 2013). A meta-analysis of neuroimaging studies revealed that sleep deprivation results in decreased activation in the fronto-parietal attention network and in the salience network (Ma et al., 2015). As noted earlier, poor quality and/or quantity of sleep may impair the consolidation of memories and performance in learning tasks.

Sleep affects our physical health. People with a shorter average sleep duration tend to have poorer immune function, are at greater risk of neurological disorders, diabetes, and cardiovascular disease, and have higher premature mortality rates (Gallicchio & Kalesan, 2009; Knutson, 2012; Palma et al., 2013). For example, sleep deprivation leads to changes in blood pressure, inflammation, and autonomic tone and hormone activity that increase the risk of cardiovascular disease (Mullington et al., 2009).

Sleep seems to serve a restorative or recuperative function, allowing the body to repair and replenish itself following our daily activities. The primary function of slow-wave sleep in Stage 3 appears to be to allow the brain to rest. Sleep loss causes impairments in cognitive performance, particularly in relation to creative tasks (Killgore, 2010; Reynolds & Banks, 2010), heightens pain perception (Schrimpf et al., 2015), and can also impair mood (Finan et al., 2015). Research Box 7.2 highlights the consequences of sleep deprivation for surgeons. Other studies have shown how sleep deprivation due to working long on-call shifts significantly impairs junior physicians' mood and alertness (Wali et al., 2013). Not all studies have found such links in real-world contexts (Chu et al., 2011), possibly because surgical outcomes are the result of teamwork, rather than one individual. However, studies such as that described in Research Box 7.2 have strengthened calls for legislation to limit doctors' working hours.

RESEARCH BOX 7.2   Sleep deprivation and surgical skill

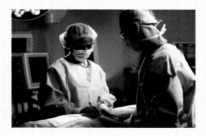

Photo courtesy of U.S. Army

Background

Although it is known that sleep deprivation can lead to lapses in attention and impaired problem-solving capacities, less is known about how sleep deprivation affects the performance of resident physicians when spending 24 hours 'on call'.

Method and findings

The skills of 35 surgical residents were assessed using a laparoscopic surgery simulator. Participants were assessed at three time points – the morning of the day before going 'on call' (well-rested), the morning of the 'on call' period (well-rested), and the morning after being 'on call' (sleep-deprived). Compared to the two 'rested' assessments, performance in the sleep-deprived state was poorer: residents took significantly longer to complete the task and made significantly more errors.

Significance

It is well known that 'on call' schedules lead to acute sleep deprivation and fatigue. This study shows that such sleep deprivation and fatigue led to significant reductions in surgical performance. This may cause poorer clinical performance and patient outcomes.

Eastridge, B.J. et al. (2003) Effect of sleep deprivation on the performance of simulated laparoscopic surgical skill. *American Journal of Surgery, 186*: 169–174.

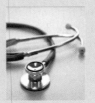

CLINICAL NOTES 7.1

Sleep deprivation in medicine

- For your own sake, and for the safety of your patients, ensure that you get enough good quality sleep.
- Shift work can impair physical and psychological health, particularly if you are over 40 years of age.
- Be aware of how sleep deprivation impairs learning and memory.
- Be aware of the effects of sleep deprivation on your own performance.
- Shift patterns are better if they are forward rotating (i.e. move the biological clock forward with each shift) rather than backward rotating.
- These issues are important while you are a student, and will remain important throughout your working life.

7.5.3 WHY DO WE SLEEP WHEN WE DO?

Although sleep may have a restorative function, it is not simply the case that we sleep more when we have been more active, or sleep less when we have been inactive (e.g. Driver & Taylor, 2000; Ryback & Lewis, 1971). Rather than being responsive to activity levels, sleep patterns appear to be determined internally and to follow a circadian (literally 'about a day') rhythm. The body also has circadian rhythms for body temperature and hormone secretion. These rhythms are determined by the body's internal pacemaker, the **suprachiasmatic nucleus (SCN)** in the hypothalamus. In the case of sleep, the SCN produces a circadian rhythm via the output of melatonin from the pineal gland. Increased melatonin output occurs during darkness and causes drowsiness.

The intrinsic rhythms provided by the SCN are around 24 hours long. They are kept in this pattern by the daily cycle of daylight and darkness. Jet lag occurs when there is a rapid desynchronisation of the endogenous rhythms of the SCN and external patterns of light and darkness. A similar desynchronisation happens among shift workers. In this case, the external patterns of light and darkness stay the same, but workers must adjust their sleep–wake cycles. Both people with jet lag and those working shifts tend to have disrupted sleep, feel more tired, and show impairments in cognitive function. Exposure to bright light at key times can make it easier for people to adjust to shift work or recover from jet lag (Emens & Burgess, 2015). Melatonin-analogue drugs can also be used to treat the range of symptoms associated with shift work and jet lag (Rajaratnam et al., 2009). A simple explanation is that they move the hands of the circadian clock.

Whereas the SCN regulates the periodicity of sleep, other brain regions are involved in the changes between stages of sleep. The reticular formation lies at the core of the brainstem and runs through the midbrain, pons, and medulla. Stimulation of this region ends sleep and may act as a 'wake up call' to the basal ganglia, thalamus, and forebrain.

Serotonin activity within this region appears to be involved in sleep regulation. Activity in the pons appears to regulate REM sleep. Acetylcholine activity in the pons is involved in eye activity during REM sleep, whereas the inhibition of acetylcholine release in the forebrain causes slow-wave sleep. Increased norepinephrine release in the pons is linked to the change from sleep to wakefulness. Sleep–wake cycles can be disrupted in many disorders (including depression and seasonal affective disorder) and following brain injury. For example, 10–40% of people with affective disorders report excessive sleep at night and napping during the day (Kaplan & Harvey, 2009).

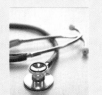

CLINICAL NOTES 7.2

Self-treating insomnia

- Only go to bed when you are sleepy.
- Set your alarm for a normal waking hour and get up at the same time every day – regardless of how much you have slept.
- Do not sleep more than 10 hours a night and do not nap during the day.
- Paradoxically, if you wake up in the night it can sometimes help you get back to sleep if you try to force yourself to stay awake.
- Avoid alcohol, caffeine, or nicotine after 6 pm and do not eat a large meal late at night.
- Keep your bedroom for sleeping and sex – do not work in your bedroom.
- If you wake in the middle of the night for more than 20 minutes, get up and do something else. Only go back to bed when you feel sleepy.
- Do not worry about how much sleep you are getting or watch the clock – this may make it worse.

ACTIVITY 7.1   CONSCIOUSNESS

- Take a few seconds to write down everything that you are currently aware of – what you can see, hear, smell, feel, and taste.
- How much of your body's activities do you think you are consciously aware of?

7.5.4 WAKEFULNESS AND CONSCIOUSNESS

Sleep is not a single state and neither is wakefulness. Consciousness consists of the things that we are aware of – information, memories, or the rumblings in our stomach. Consciousness is the 'tip of the iceberg' of mental processes. There are other levels of mental activity which may or may not enter our conscious awareness. **Non-conscious** brain processes are those that we are never conscious of, such as the control of our heart-beat or digestion. The **pre-conscious** consists of information that is readily available to us should we need it, but of which we are not actively aware. For example, we may be able to tell someone what we ate for breakfast this morning, or where we were born, but that is not to say that we walk around all day consciously aware of this information just in case someone asks. The term **unconscious** is used to refer to information that we process but are never aware of knowing. In psychoanalytic thinking the unconscious contains primitive urges and repressed memories that are never available to consciousness. This psychoanalytic concept of the unconscious mind is controversial and less widely accepted than the concept of unconscious mental processes.

Levels of wakefulness and alertness are influenced by various neurotransmitters acting at different sites in the brain. Neurotransmitters with important influences on arousal are:

- Acetylcholine – released from neurons in the pons and the basal forebrain.
- Norepinephrine – released from neurons in the pons.
- Serotonin – released from neurons in the reticular formation.
- Histamine and hypocretin (or orexin) – both released from neurons in the hypothalamus.

The axons of these neurons branch to many important areas of the brain; some have direct effects on cortical arousal and others have indirect effects via the thalamus and hypothalamus.

7.5.5 DISORDERS OF CONSCIOUSNESS

Disorders of consciousness allow us insights into the physiology of consciousness. Narcolepsy is a neurological disorder characterised by brief bouts of sleep at inappropriate times. It affects around one in 2,000 people, and it appears to be caused by hypocretin/orexin ligand deficiencies – neurotransmitters involved in arousal and alertness (Nishino, 2007). Narcoleptic sleep attacks can occur at any time, but are most common in boring, monotonous situations. People with narcolepsy may also experience cataplexy – a sudden muscular weakness caused by the inhibition of motor neurons in the spinal cord. This often leads to a collapse, followed by a period of immobility during which the person will remain fully conscious. Whereas narcoleptic sleep attacks are often preceded by boredom, cataplexy is usually precipitated by very strong emotions.

Epilepsy is a serious neurological disorder, with a population prevalence of around 0.5%. It is characterised by recurrent seizures – bursts of excess electrical activity in the brain which cause a temporary disruption to normal neural functioning. For around 70% of people with epilepsy there is no known cause, but 30% of cases can be linked to diseases or abnormalities such as imbalances in GABA-inhibition and the glutamate-excitation of neural activity. Partial seizures are localised and affect specific sites in one hemisphere (e.g. one temporal lobe). Simple partial seizures involve no impairment of consciousness, whereas complex partial seizures do. Partial seizures may be precursors to generalised seizures, which affect several areas of the brain and impair consciousness. These are also called tonic-clonic seizures: in the tonic phase the person briefly loses consciousness and their muscles tense up; in the clonic phase rapid contraction and relaxation of the muscles cause convulsions. Such seizures are usually followed by a period of sleep. Upon waking people are often confused and may not remember events just prior to the seizure. Around two-thirds of people with epilepsy cease having seizures within five years, usually as a result of anticonvulsant drug treatment. If such seizures have a localised origin and anti-convulsant medication proves ineffective, surgical solutions may be considered.

Summary

- Sleep is not a period of complete rest for the brain: it consists of several phases, each characterised by specific patterns of neural activity.
- Dreaming occurs during Rapid Eye Movement (REM) sleep. The body tries to ensure a certain amount of REM sleep. This suggests that dreaming has important functions (e.g. the consolidation of memory). However, the functions of dreaming are not fully understood.
- Similarly, the functions of sleep are not fully understood. However, sleep does appear to have restorative functions, and sleep deprivation leads to impaired performance on cognitive tasks, and can lead to impaired health.
- The timing of sleep is determined by circadian rhythms in physiological systems controlled by the suprachiasmatic nucleus. These rhythms usually match natural patterns of daylight and darkness.
- Fluctuations in neurotransmitter levels affect levels of consciousness, and are involved in disorders of consciousness such as narcolepsy.

FURTHER READING

Carlson, N.R. & Birkett, M.A. (2017) *Physiology of Behavior* (12th edition). Boston, MA: Allyn & Bacon. A standard textbook for neuropsychology and biological psychology. It contains detailed descriptions and illustrations of brain structures and functions.

Pinel, J.P.J. (2014) *Biopsychology* (9th edition). Boston, MA: Pearson. Another standard textbook for neuropsychology and biological psychology. It also contains detailed descriptions and illustrations of brain structures and functions, along with descriptions of practical applications of concepts.

REVISION QUESTIONS

1. Describe the organisation of the nervous system (i.e. central, peripheral, autonomic, somatosensory) and the functions of each division.

2. How are action potentials conducted within and between neurons?

3. Outline the functions of the four lobes of the cerebral cortex.

4. Describe the action of the brain regions involved in the control of voluntary movement.

5. Discuss the accuracy of this statement: 'When a person is asleep her/his body and brain are at rest'.

6. Why do we sleep? Why do we sleep when we do?

7. Describe the effects of sleep deprivation and dream deprivation.

8. Describe how sleep deprivation may affect healthcare professionals' competence.

9. Outline the key features of epilepsy and narcolepsy. Describe how neurotransmitters are involved in these disorders of consciousness.

8 PSYCHOSOCIAL DEVELOPMENT ACROSS THE LIFESPAN

CHAPTER CONTENTS

Tables

Case study

(Continued)

Figures

8.1   Still face study
8.2   Nim Chimpsky using sign language
8.3   Piaget's stage model of intellectual development

Research boxes

8.1   Developmental delay and catch-up following severe deprivation
8.2   Child-friendly interventions enhance understanding of illness

LEARNING OBJECTIVES

This chapter is designed to enable you to:

- Describe the major psychosocial developmental changes that occur in childhood.
- Outline how language and thinking develop through childhood and adolescence.
- Describe the physical and psychological changes and challenges of adolescence.
- Discuss stability and change in physical and cognitive capacity during older adulthood.
- Appreciate how changes across the lifespan affect practitioner–patient communication.

Psychosocial development occurs across the lifespan. At different ages, we acquire different cognitive and social skills and enact different social roles (see Chapter 9). One way of thinking about these changes is by using Erikson's (1950) division of the lifespan into eight stages, each characterised by a particular developmental challenge that must be resolved for optimal psychosocial functioning (see Table 8.1).

Although these challenges are psychological in nature, health and illness can influence the extent to which people are able to resolve them. For example, physical disabilities may affect the development of autonomy in childhood. Similarly, people's health may be affected by their experience of each developmental conflict, such as adolescents engaging in risky behaviours as part of identity explorations. This model indicates that although childhood is important, development and change occur across the lifespan.

This chapter, therefore, outlines a lifespan approach to development. Medical professionals must be able to identify abnormal patterns of development and treat these appropriately to minimise disturbances to physical and psychological growth. We also need to be aware of people's capabilities at different ages to allow optimal practitioner–patient communication.

TABLE 8.1   Erikson's model of lifespan development

Age	Conflict	Outcomes
Infancy	Trust vs. Mistrust	Children develop a sense of trust in other people when their carers provide reliable care and affection.
Early childhood	Autonomy vs. Shame/Doubt	Children develop a sense of autonomy and independence derived from acquiring physical skills. Failure leads to shame and doubt.
Preschool	Initiative vs. Guilt	Children begin to assert control over their environment and develop a sense of purpose. Efforts to exert too much power result in disapproval and guilt.
School age	Industry vs. Inferiority	Children need to cope with new social and intellectual demands and develop feelings of competence.
Adolescence	Identity vs. Role Confusion	Adolescents need to develop a strong personal identity. Failure leads to role confusion and a weak sense of self.
Young adulthood	Intimacy vs. Isolation	Adults need to form strong intimate relationships. Failure leads to loneliness.
Middle adulthood	Generativity vs. Stagnation	Adults need to create and nurture things that will outlast them (e.g. children or social changes) to provide feelings of accomplishment and usefulness.
Maturity	Ego Integrity vs. Despair	Older adults need to feel fulfilled when they reflect on their lives. Failure leads to regret and despair.

8.1 CHILDHOOD

8.1.1 ATTACHMENT AND DEVELOPMENT

Attachment is a strong affectional tie felt for another. Children feel pleasure and joy when interacting with caregivers with whom they have a secure attachment, and comfort from being near them in times of stress. Unless infants have secure trusting attachments to their adult caregivers, normal cognitive, social, and emotional development may not occur.

Quality of attachment

Four different types of attachment have been identified by using a research technique known as the 'strange situation' (Ainsworth et al., 1978). This is a situation in which a mother brings her child to a room with toys in it, leaves the child for a short while, and then returns. By observing how much exploration and play the child engages in, and how they respond to their mother's departure and return, children's attachments may be categorised as shown in Table 8.2. The most common type of attachment is the most adaptive one: around 70% of children display secure attachment. Although there is some variation in the proportions found in each group, these general patterns have been observed in different cultures (van Ijzendoorn & Kroonenberg, 1988).

The importance of secure attachment

Secure attachments to carers are important because they develop feelings in children that they are worthy of love and care and that others will be available to them in times of need. They establish children's 'internal working models' for all subsequent close relationships (Bowlby, 1973). The internal working models of children with less secure attachments do not include an expectation that they are worthy of love and care.

TABLE 8.2 Attachment styles in the 'strange situation'

Attachment style	Child's behaviour when mother leaves	Mother's parenting style
Secure attachment	Child gets upset when mother leaves but calms down quickly when she returns, and explores the environment when she is there.	Mother is quick to respond to physical and emotional needs of the child. Helps the child to cope with their stress.
Avoidant attachment	Child explores the environment and does not respond when mother leaves or returns.	Mother does not respond when child is upset: tries to stop child crying and encourages independence and exploration.
Ambivalent attachment	Child gets upset when mother leaves but can be comforted by a stranger. When mother returns the child will act ambivalently and may resist contact or appear angry.	Mother is inconsistent – varies between responding quickly and appropriately on some occasions and not responding on other occasions. Child is therefore preoccupied with whether mother is available before they can use her as a secure base.
Disorganised attachment	Can be secure, ambivalent, or avoidant but also shows some difficulty coping when the mother returns with behaviour such as rocking themselves or freezing.	Mother's behaviour can be negative, withdrawn, inappropriate, roles not clearly defined, sometimes child maltreatment.

Secure attachment during childhood has broad and lasting influences on development. It promotes optimal development of the brain – especially the limbic system, which is crucially involved in emotional regulation (see Chapter 7). Insecure attachment resulting from neglect and a lack of stimulation can lead to serious underdevelopment in these brain regions (Gerhardt, 2004). Secure attachment also results in better social competence and peer relations, better emotional competence and self-reliance, better cognitive function, and better physical and psychological health (Brumariu & Kerns, 2010; Ranson & Urichuk, 2008).

The importance of the interaction between genes and environment for neurological and cognitive developmental is an archetypal example of why 'nature versus nurture' debates are beginning to be replaced by an understanding of the interaction between genes and environment. The evolving field of **epigenetics** focuses on how environmental factors – including social contextual factors – regulate the activity and expression of genes (Kundakovic & Champagne, 2015). There is emerging evidence that environmental influences such as a lack of nurturing can lead to neurological and endocrine changes that can then be passed to the next generation.

Given the importance of attachment, one might wonder whether all is lost if a secure attachment to parents does not develop or is not possible. Research has indicated that adopted children can develop secure attachments with their adoptive parents – especially those adopted at an earlier age (van den Dries et al., 2009). Most children also have a degree of resilience which will allow them to recover to some extent from earlier neglect or abuse (see Research Box 8.1). Others have also questioned the emphasis on secure attachment (Ein-Dor & Hirschberger, 2016).

How does attachment develop?

Several different accounts for the development of secure attachments have been offered. Freud's **psychoanalytic theory** proposed that the mother becomes the primary love object in the baby's life because she satisfies the infant's need for food and oral pleasure. **Learning theory** argues that a positive perception of the mother is formed because the baby learns that breastfeeding satisfies hunger (and the mother learns that breastfeeding calms the baby).

Ethological theory argues that although breastfeeding is important for building the mother–baby relationship, attachment does not depend solely on the satisfaction of hunger and the provision of oral pleasure. Otherwise, how could we explain strong attachments between infants and their fathers? Bowlby (1969) argued that Freud's psychoanalytic perspective fails to acknowledge attachment as a psychological bond in its own right rather than an instinct derived from feeding or sexuality. Bowlby's view was supported by Harlow's (1958) research with monkeys separated from their mothers, which showed that attachment is formed on the basis of comfort rather than nourishment. In that research, baby monkeys separated from their mother were found to prefer a fake surrogate 'mother' covered in soft fabric to a wire 'mother' – even when the wire 'mother' provided milk.

RESEARCH BOX 8.1   Developmental delay and catch-up following severe deprivation

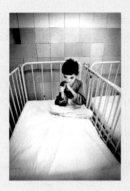

Background

In the 1960s President Ceausescu tried to boost Romania's population by banning birth control and taxing childless adults. As a result, many couples had more children than they wanted and children were left in state orphanages. Conditions in the orphanages were appalling: hygiene and nutrition were poor; children spent much of their time confined to cots with few toys and little interaction with adults or other children. Following the overthrow of Ceausescu in 1989 many of these children were adopted by families in other countries.

Method and findings

Longitudinal follow-up was conducted with 111 Romanian infants adopted by UK families and a comparison group of British adopted children. When they arrived in the UK the orphans had severely impaired physical and cognitive development.

This study showed there was some 'catch-up' to normal levels of physical and cognitive development. This catch-up was nearly complete for children adopted in the UK before they were six months old. However, significant delays remained among those who were older when they were adopted.

Significance

For ethical reasons, it would never be possible to design an experiment in which children were subject to severe deprivation: the researchers took advantage of an unfortunate social experiment. Although all children displayed some resilience in being able to overcome early deprivation, severe prolonged deprivation produced significant deficits in physical and psychological development that were difficult to overcome fully.

Photograph © Forca/www.photoxpress.com

O'Connor, T.G. et al. (2000) The effects of global severe privation on cognitive competence. *Child Development*, 71: 376–390.

Bowlby argued that humans have a set of in-built attachment behaviours designed to maintain close contact with a particular person perceived to be better able to cope with the world. In babies, these include clinging to caregivers, crying for their attention, and smiling at their return. Even in the first week after their birth, babies prefer to look at faces that engage them in a mutual gaze, and assessment of neural activity in four-month-old infants shows that they have enhanced neural processing of direct gaze (Farroni et al., 2002). Older infants become distressed if adults do not respond to their attempts at interaction (Figure 8.1) (Meman et al., 2009).

Attachment develops in stages as infants develop greater skills for directing their attention and actions – the kinds of following and clinging behaviours assessed in the 'strange situation' with children aged 12 to 18 months.

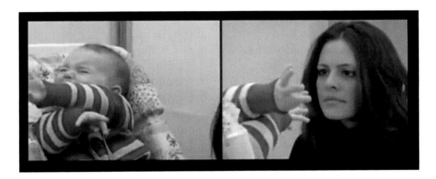

FIGURE 8.1   Still face study – very young infants become distressed if carers do not respond to them. [Watch a video here: www.youtube.com/watch?v=apzXGEbZht0]

Parent–infant bonding

For an attachment to parents to occur, infants must know who their parents are. The process of **bonding** to carers begins before birth. In the first few days of life, babies use various senses to learn who their carers are. It is important, therefore, for parents to engage in behaviours which maximise this multisensory input for their children as follows:

- Physical contact: mothers should be encouraged to keep babies in contact with them as much as possible to provide sensory input in the form of touch, warmth, smell, sound, and sight.
- Smell: babies quickly learn to associate their mother's smell with comfort, pleasure, and nourishment.
- Sound: from an early age, babies can distinguish between their mother's voice and the voices of other people, and will prefer their mother's voice to other similarly pitched female voices.
- Sight: even though their focal distance is only around 25 cm, three-day old babies can visually distinguish between their mothers and others.

Although most of the research has focused on mothers, bonding with fathers is important and the principles described above also apply. Parent–infant bonding in the first days sets an important foundation for subsequent parent–child interaction. However, all is not lost if there is less contact during the early period. Strong parent–child bonds can be formed with premature or sick babies who must spend time in incubators, and between parents and adopted children.

8.1.2 BREASTFEEDING AND DEVELOPMENT

Breastfeeding is an important mother–infant interaction. On the basis of solid empirical evidence, the World Health Organisation advocates that infants be exclusively breastfed for the first six months of life (Kramer & Kakuma, 2012). However, in developed countries most children are not exclusively breastfed for six months. For example, in the UK around 20% of infants receive no breastfeeding and around 45% are breastfed until six months (McAndrew et al., 2012).

Studies that follow children from infancy into middle childhood or adulthood have found that those who were breastfed perform better on tests of intelligence (Horta et al., 2015). The optimal duration for breastfeeding appears to be around 6–9 months, with lower test scores found for those not breastfed at all, breast fed for less than six months, or exclusively breastfed for more than nine months. Exclusive breastfeeding beyond nine months may produce nutritional deficiencies.

Several different factors may explain the links between breastfeeding and intelligence. First, nutrients in breast milk – especially long-chain fatty acids – may contribute to better neural development. Second, physical and psychological attention during breastfeeding may foster greater intelligence. Third, factors related to both breastfeeding *and* children's intelligence may be important. Chief among these are characteristics of mothers who breastfeed, because better educated and more intelligent mothers are more likely to commence and continue breastfeeding (Horta et al., 2015).

Meta-analyses of studies designed to follow children over time show that greater breastfeeding during infancy is associated with lower rates of childhood asthma, and may also protect against eczema and allergic rhinitis (Lodge et al., 2015). Some of the positive effects of breastfeeding may be due to immunomodulatory qualities of breast milk and/or the avoidance of allergens. Longer breastfeeding also appears to reduce the risk of subsequent overweight/obesity, high blood pressure, and Type 2 diabetes (World Health Organisation, 2013).

A recent review revealed that rates of early initiation of breastfeeding, exclusive breastfeeding, and continued breastfeeding can be improved when counselling and education are provided concurrently in home, community, and health systems settings (Sinha et al., 2015).

8.1.3 LANGUAGE DEVELOPMENT

Learning to talk is one of the most important intellectual capacities a child will ever develop. As well as being essential for communication in its own right, language is important for many other learning skills: imagine what school would have been like if you were not able to understand your teacher or ask questions! Various theories have been developed and applied to explain how children progress from nonsensical babbling at six months of age to grammatically sophisticated speech just a few years later.

Some researchers have emphasised the importance of **operant conditioning** and **observational learning** (Skinner, 1957; Chapter 10). Such perspectives argue that children develop their capacity for language in response to encouragement and correction from parents and other people. They also argue that children's imitation of adult speech is important. Although children may learn the meanings of words in these ways, they cannot explain how children learn the complex rules of grammar – that is, rules about how words must be put together so as to make sense.

In contrast to behaviourism and social learning theories, **nativism** argues that children have an innate predisposition for language, that is, they have in-built capacities for making sense of language. Chomsky (1965) argued that humans are unique in having an innate biologically-based language acquisition device (LAD) which allows children who know a few words to generate grammatically correct utterances and understand what others say. The argument that the LAD is a *unique* human feature has received support from studies of language learning in primates. Such research indicates that although primates can learn to use sign language or symbols to communicate, they possess no understanding of grammar (Figure 8.2). Although Chomsky's ideas have been influential, they have some limitations. In particular, although there are specialised language areas in

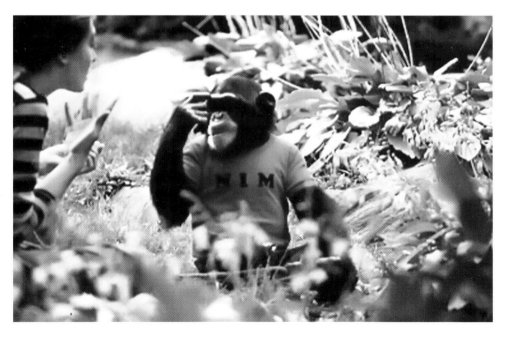

FIGURE 8.2 Nim Chimpsky using sign language. Photograph reproduced courtesy of Susan Kuklin

TABLE 8.3 Comparison of 'motherese' and adult–adult speech

	Adult–child	Adult–adult
Utterance length	4 words	8 words
Utterances with conjunctions (e.g. because)	20%	70%
Utterances with a pause at the end	75%	51%
Speed (words/min)	70/min	132/min

the human brain (see Chapter 7), there is no evidence that the LAD is located in a specific brain region.

Interactionism appears to offer a bridge between the opposing perspectives of Skinner (1957) and Chomsky (1965). Interactionism argues that language learning is a combination of nature *and* nurture. Children learn language via the combination of an innate linguistic capacity, a strong desire to connect with others, a rich linguistic and social environment, and the reinforcement of their efforts.

Evidence for the interactionist perspective comes from the observation that adult–child communication is quite different from adult–adult communication. It involves closer physical proximity, more prolonged eye contact, exaggerated facial expressions and gestures, and the use of **motherese**. Motherese is an alternative name for adult–child speech, which is a simplified version of adult–adult speech. Table 8.3 shows that compared to adult–adult speech, motherese is shorter, less complicated, and much slower.

These differences are significant changes, not slight adjustments. Other features of motherese are that it is more likely to be in present tense; is more likely to use proper names rather than pronouns (e.g. 'Daddy's nose is bleeding' rather than 'My nose is bleeding'); has more repetition; and features exaggerated intonation. Young children appear to have a preference for motherese – the intonation and rhythm can attract and hold their attention. These features mean that children's natural predisposition for language learning is nurtured through interactions with others.

Stages of language development

Babies babble long before they speak their first real words. This is not a simple imitation of adult speech: it includes sounds that may not even be used in the language(s) spoken in a child's home. Babbling is a generalised system of vocalisations – nature provides infants with the sounds they may need, and nurture gradually moulds the use of sounds that are appropriate for their language. It is important that parents show interest in babbling because this indicates to the child that they are part of the social system. Parents' communication with babies at this stage can also help them to learn that vocal sounds have meanings (e.g. people's names).

The mean age of babies saying their first word is 12 months (but the range is 8–18 months). By this age, infants begin to use sounds to convey meaning. However, the meaning of these single word utterances is not always clear: when an infant says 'ear', this may mean 'This is my ear', or 'My ear hurts', or something else entirely. Parents can help their children learn words by giving a 'running commentary' of what they are doing and using expressions and gestures to provide clues to meaning.

From around the age of two, children begin to use 'telegraph speech' which contains mainly nouns and verbs. The sentences are similar to the sentences made by Nim Chimpsky (Figure 8.2). Words are used to express desires (e.g. 'Feel tired'). From age three there is a rapid progression to complete sentences. In addition to using more words per sentence, children begin to use possessive pronouns ('mine', 'Daddy's'), negatives (e.g. 'can't' rather than 'no'), and modifiers (adjectives like 'big' and adverbs like 'quickly'). Language begins to be used to express thoughts and emotions. Some of these changes can be linked to developments in cognitive capacity. By age five, children have vocabularies of thousands of words and can understand quite complex sentences.

Implications for practitioner–child communication

As in all contexts, communication will be best when there is a match between the demands of the situation and the capacities of the people involved. Medical consultations with children are affected by:

- Children's language capacity: very young children may not possess the precise vocabulary used by medical professionals (e.g. what does 'I have a tummy ache' really mean?).
- Practitioners' communication skills: healthcare professionals should be sensitive to how a child's age may affect their ability to understand and should make appropriate adjustments to their manner of speech.
- Interaction between practitioner and child: it is important to consider whether parents can be used as 'translators' for their children.

Healthcare professionals need to be aware of how language capacity develops with age and adjust their communication style as appropriate.

Summary

- All children have an innate capacity to learn language – the language acquisition device (LAD).
- The interactionist perspective argues that in addition to LAD, experience is important, e.g. 'motherese' helps children to learn to use their innate capacity for language.
- Adults can help children develop their language capacity by encouraging them and providing feedback.
- Healthcare professionals should match their language to the capacities of children – e.g. use elements of 'motherese' in consultations with young children.

8.1.4 INTELLECTUAL DEVELOPMENT

How does a child's mind grow? When and how do children begin to think symbolically, reason logically, and see things from another person's perspective? The following section attempts to provide answers to these questions and discuss the implications for medicine and healthcare. It will commence with the influential theory of Piaget, followed by a discussion of some criticisms of Piaget's theory and the insights offered by Vygotsky.

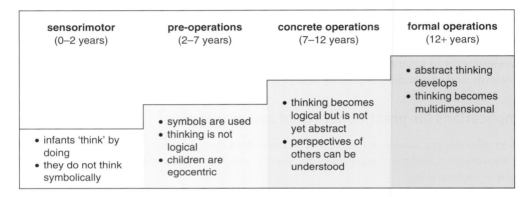

FIGURE 8.3   Piaget's stage model of intellectual development

Piaget's stage theory

Central to Piaget's (1954) influential theory was the idea that a child's mind is not a miniature version of an adult's mind waiting to be filled with information: the child's mind develops into an adult mind through four discrete stages (see Figure 8.3). Although each stage can be broken into sub-stages, development always proceeds in the same order and the order of stages is universal. In this theory, the term 'operations' refers to the ways in which children work out problems. The stages in Piaget's theory are:

- **Sensorimotor stage** – Babies experience the world through their senses. They cannot 'think' because they live in the moment with no abstract concepts. However, they can exhibit intelligent behaviour (e.g. pulling a blanket to get a toy that is out of reach but resting on it). Before eight months, infants do not understand object permanence – the awareness that things which are out of sight still exist.
- **Pre-operations** – Language acquisition brings a fundamental change to intellectual development because language is symbolic: words are symbols that refer to real things. Linked to this capacity for symbolic thought, a major change from the sensorimotor stage is the capacity to imagine things. This is reflected in play, where a stick can become a sword or a magic wand. In this stage, children are **egocentric**. They are unable to see things from another person's perspective or consider the point of view of others. For example, in hide-and-seek children may think that if they cannot see you, then you cannot see them. In medical and healthcare contexts, children may not be aware that other people do not know what symptom they are experiencing.

- **Concrete operations** – Children begin to learn to use logical processes. They can manipulate real (concrete) objects to solve problems, such as using their fingers or blocks to do addition and subtraction. In addition children can learn the principle of conservation, i.e. that moving, spreading out, or rearranging objects does not change them. In this stage, children develop the capacity to see things from another person's perspective.
- **Formal operations** – Children become able to reason not just on the basis of real physical objects, but also on the basis of hypotheses or propositions: e.g. '$x^2 + 4 = 13$, what is the value of x?' During this stage, thinking becomes multidimensional: children become able to consider various possibilities rather than just the most obvious solution to a problem. Other important developments include metacognition (the capacity to think about thinking) and introspection (the capacity to think about emotions).

Numerous studies have shown that development tends to follow Piaget's order. However, Piaget's ideas have been criticised (e.g. Amsel & Reninger, 1997). Development of intelligence is smoother and more gradual than Piaget's argument for step-like jumps between stages. Piaget also seems to have underestimated children's capacities and overestimated adults' capacities. For example, many adults fail to always use formal operational reasoning. It has also been suggested that younger children's difficulty with reasoning tasks is strongly influenced by their inability to understand complex adult language. Furthermore, pre-operational children do have some capacity to consider others' perspectives.

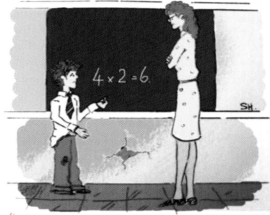

"It's a guess, I never said it was an educated guess."

Vygotsky's theory of social development

A fundamental principle of Vygotsky's theory of social development is that full cognitive development requires social interaction (Daniels, 1996). Vygotsky emphasised the importance of culture for learning. At a broad level, culture teaches children both *what* to think and *how* to think. At the individual level, children learn through problem solving that is shared with someone else (e.g. adult, peer). Compared with Piaget, Vygotsky gave greater emphasis to the importance of language in learning. Vygotsky argued that language is crucial for collaborative problem solving and that such collaborative problem solving is important for children's cognitive development.

Vygotsky argued that learning occurs in the 'zone of proximal development', which is the gap between what a child can do without help and what they could do with appropriate guidance or collaboration. With such help from adults or peers, children can perform tasks they would be incapable of completing on their own. Furthermore, teaching and learning will be more effective if there is a continual adjustment of the level of help given so that children become more independent at solving problems.

Understanding others' perspectives

As noted earlier, young children are egocentric: they cannot take on the perspective of others. Young children also lack a '**theory of mind**': they do not understand that other people have different thoughts, emotions, and perceptions. Children aged two or three use words like 'want' which reflect the development of knowledge of an inner self. Over time, this understanding is applied to other people and children come to understand that they can infer the mental states of other people. Thus, we may say that they possess a naïve theory of mind. Having a theory of mind allows us to empathise with others. However, it also allows us to deceive. For example, children who possess a theory of mind can understand what they need to do to feign illness to avoid school. Similarly, when poker players bluff they are applying their theory of mind.

Healthcare consultations with young children clearly need to take into account the issues of egocentrism and an absence of a theory of mind. Young children may assume others know what they are feeling and experiencing. Healthcare professionals therefore need to encourage young children to explain all of their symptoms and concerns, even if these appear obvious to the child.

Children's understanding of illness

Children's understanding of illness varies with age (see Research Box 8.2). An understanding of illness progresses from concrete, egocentric explanations to abstract, multidimensional explanations.

Although Table 8.4 suggests a stage-like development of an understanding of illness, this is not strictly true: understanding illness is influenced by experience. Thus young children with leukaemia may understand the disorder much more than other children of the same age. Such findings support Vygotsky's argument that children's understanding develops best if they receive appropriate help from considerate adults. These findings also

TABLE 8.4   Children's explanation of illness (Bibace & Walsh, 1980)

Age	Explanation of illness
2–4	Phenomenism – particular objects are believed to cause illness but there is no sense of the mechanisms involved
4–7	Contagion – illness is caused by proximity to ill people or to particular objects
7–9	Contamination – illness is caused by physical contact with an ill person and may be viewed as punishment for misbehaviour
9–11	Internalisation – illness is located within the body but may be caused by external factors, e.g. people get colds from being cold
11–16	Physiological – illness is caused by malfunctions in organs or systems which may be due to infections
16+	Psychophysiological – psychological factors like stress and fatigue can affect physiological processes, rather than only being an outcome

suggest that explanations of illness and disease should build on prior experience and not be based simply on chronological age.

Children's understanding of illness can be enhanced by the use of developmentally appropriate interventions that break complex information into more easily digested pieces and present them in child-friendly ways (see Research Box 8.2). Medical communication with young children – whether it is verbal consultations or information leaflets – should therefore avoid using abstract concepts. With all children, it is important to focus on their 'here and now' experiences and concerns.

RESEARCH BOX 8.2   Child-friendly interventions enhance understanding of illness

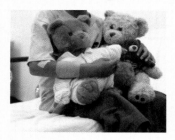

Source: U.S. Department of Defense, November 2006

Background

The 'Teddy Bear Hospital' is a worldwide concept designed to reduce children's fear of hospitalisation and medical procedures and to enhance their medical knowledge. Children bring their teddy bears to be treated by medical students playing the part of 'teddy docs'. Based on theories of child development and previous research, it was expected that taking part in a role-play situation suitable for children's developmental stage should enhance their knowledge of the body, health, and illness.

Method and findings

The participants were 139 children aged 4–5 years attending kindergartens in Germany. Eight kindergartens were randomised to be intervention schools where the Teddy Bear Hospital was run, and eight kindergartens served as a control group. Children's understanding was assessed at the beginning and of a two-week period. Children in the intervention group were assessed before and after visiting the Teddy Bear Hospital.

Results showed that children were able to learn effectively through role-play in the Teddy Bear Hospital. Children who visited the Teddy Bear Hospital had enhanced knowledge of the body, health, and disease at the second assessment. This was particularly clear in relation to their knowledge of internal organs.

Significance

Children's understanding of illness can be enhanced by providing age-appropriate information in an appropriate format and context.

Leonhardt, C., Margraf-Stiksrud, J., Badners, L., Szerencsi, A. & Maier, R.F. (2014) Does the 'Teddy Bear Hospital' enhance preschool children's knowledge? A pilot study with a pre/post-case control design in Germany. *Journal of Health Psychology*, 19: 1250–1260.

Summary

- Young children's thought processes are fundamentally different from those of adults.
- Initial thought processes are based on real-world objects and an egocentric perspective.
- Before developing a 'theory of mind' children will not know that others do not share their thoughts/feelings and may not disclose pain/symptoms.
- Young children cannot understand abstract or unobservable concepts such as infection.
- Experience interacts with the developmental stage to produce an understanding of illness.
- Age-appropriate information increases children's understanding of illness and recovery.

CLINICAL NOTES 8.1

Communicating with children

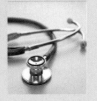

- Adjust your consultation style to the capacities of children: pay attention to the language you use and the complexity of the ideas you are trying to convey.
- Younger children will not understand abstract concepts or internal bodily processes. However, be aware that some children can have very advanced knowledge of illnesses they have been exposed to.
- Explain things to children in age-appropriate ways, e.g. use dolls or action figures to get their attention and help them to understand.
- Age-appropriate information booklets can increase children's understanding of illness, treatment, and recovery.
- If necessary, use parents or other adults to help you communicate with children.

8.2 ADOLESCENCE

Although adolescence is often equated with the physical changes of **puberty**, it is a biopsychosocial phenomenon that involves physical, cognitive, and social changes. The major psychological challenges of adolescence include adjusting to a changing body size and shape, coming to terms with sexuality, adjusting to new ways of thinking, and striving for emotional maturity and economic independence.

The average age of the onset of puberty is around 13 years, but there is a range of a few years around this average. Puberty begins one to two years earlier for girls than boys. It is the most rapid growth period after prenatal development and early infancy. During a period of around four years, adolescents grow an average of 25 cm/10 inches in height and gain 18 kg/40 lb in weight. There are also marked changes in hormone levels, especially testosterone and oestradiol (estradiol). The end point is sexual maturation and an adult physique.

In developed countries, the age of onset of puberty has fallen by three to four years over the last few hundred years due to improved standards of living, including better health and better nutrition. These factors are important because puberty's onset is associated with girls reaching a critical body mass (~48 kg/7.5 stone) and body fat proportion (~17%). These changes mean that it is now common to reach biological maturity at an age when cognitive and social maturity have not been reached.

8.2.1 PSYCHOLOGICAL ASPECTS OF PUBERTY

Responses to puberty are different for boys and girls and are tied to different body shape ideals. In terms of body shape, girls tend to be less satisfied than boys (Brooks-Gunn & Paikoff, 1992). This is influenced by the fact that in high-income countries, the socially ideal body shape for women is often seen to be similar to that of pre- or early-adolescent girls (i.e. very thin), whereas the socially ideal body shape for men is adult (i.e. tall and muscular). However, it is important to note that during puberty both boys and girls feel worse about their bodies than before or after. There are also observed changes in mood. Boys tend to express more anger and irritability; girls tend to express more anger and depression. These alterations could be due to hormonal changes or responses to new life events and developmental challenges.

Puberty onset is earlier for girls than boys, and girls who mature early tend to dislike the experience. Boys tend to like maturing early because they are the first of their male peers to gain height and musculature. Many boys and girls express dissatisfaction with their body image during adolescence. For example, research indicates that although girls express more dissatisfaction with their bodies, the majority of adolescent boys and girls express a desire to change their body shape (Lawler & Nixon, 2010). Such studies also show that many girls and boys feel under pressure to conform to the ideal body shapes of modern consumer culture and that peer criticism of appearance is an unavoidable part of adolescent life for both boys and girls. Concerns about appearance do not only apply to body shape; they are also influenced by cultural ideals of clear, blemish-free skin (Revol et al., 2015).

Relationships with parents and other adults

There are many explanations for the changes that occur in the parent–child relationship during adolescence. One explanation proposes that these occur because adolescents separate their identity (individuate) from their parents, becoming more emotionally and behaviourally independent (Steinberg & Silverberg, 1986). An alternative view suggests changes in parent–child relationships can lead to psychological independence with continued connectedness. Although older adolescents spend diminishing amounts of time in family interactions, the time they spend with parents one-to-one does not change and the quality of such interactions often improves (Larson et al., 1996). The decline in time spent with family members appears to be due to pulls from external factors such as friends and work rather than pushes away from bad interactions with parents.

One important domain of adolescent–adult interaction is medical consultations. Research indicates that many adolescents are dissatisfied with their interactions with healthcare professionals. Some of this dissatisfaction stems from concerns about privacy and confidentiality; some arises from embarrassment arising from talking about sensitive issues such as body image, sexual behaviour, or illegal behaviours such as alcohol or drug use. It is therefore important to be sensitive to these concerns and to remind adolescents that information exchanged in consultations will be private and confidential. Such reassurance can make it more likely that adolescents will disclose sensitive health information (Berlan & Bravender, 2009; Revol et al., 2015). It is also important to encourage adolescents to develop their capacity to discuss their health concerns during medical consultations (Towle et al., 2006).

We often think of practitioner–patient communication as a two-way interaction. However, it must be acknowledged that parents may have legal rights and responsibilities relating to medical consultations involving children below the age of consent. Older adolescents may feel uncomfortable or dissatisfied with three-way communications involving themselves, health professionals, and their parents. This may be more likely if they feel that they are being spoken about rather than spoken to. If parents insist on being involved in medical consultations involving their adolescent children, it may be helpful to ensure that at least part of the consultation involves seeing the adolescent without their parents in a confidential context (Duncan et al., 2011).

CLINICAL NOTES 8.2

Working with adolescents

- Adjust your consultation style to the capacities and experiences of adolescents: pay attention to the complexity of your explanation and check that they understand the terminology used.
- Be aware of adolescents' concerns about their appearance and body image.
- Be aware of people's embarrassment when talking about their health concerns. Respond in a non-judgemental way and reassure them that information will be treated confidentially.
- You may need to be tactful when negotiating with adolescents and their parents about the role of parents in consultations and decision making.

8.2.2 COGNITION, RISK TAKING, AND IDENTITY

Piaget's (1954) stage theory argued that formal operational thought develops during adolescence. In this stage, adolescents become able to understand abstract principles and use propositional logic. Thinking also become multidimensional: a range of possible situations can be imagined.

The improved decision-making capacity of adolescents is supposed to make them better able to: identify alternative courses of action; identify the consequences of each alternative; evaluate the desirability of each consequence; assess the likelihood of each consequence; and logically combine all of this information to make the best decisions about their behaviour. This should reduce the likelihood that they will make bad decisions. However, adolescents seem to be good at making bad decisions! This is reflected in the fact that accidents are the leading cause of death among young people (WHO, 2016), and in the high rates of unintended pregnancies (Sedgh et al., 2015), and unhealthy behaviours (e.g. de Visser et al., 2006) among young people.

Although the development of metacognition (the capacity to think about thinking) and introspection (the capacity to think about emotions) should facilitate a better understanding of others, much of adolescents' thinking is directed toward themselves. Thus, adolescents may become self-absorbed and **egocentric**. However, this is different from the egocentrism characteristic of the pre-operational stage: pre-operational children cannot help their egocentrism whereas adolescents can. The combination of metacognition, introspection, and egocentrism can lead to feelings of there being an imaginary audience observing our actions. Adolescents tend to have a heightened sense of self-consciousness and may feel that their behaviour and appearance are the focus of everyone else's concern and attention. In this stage they may develop a 'personal fable' (Elkind, 1967). This is a belief that all of their experiences are novel and unique (e.g. 'nobody has ever felt love this strong'). The personal fable may be dangerous when it is applied to health risk behaviour (e.g. 'I won't get pregnant' or 'I won't have a car crash'). Although young people may express unrealistic optimism about health risks, unrealistic optimism is not necessarily more common among adolescents than adults (Cohn et al., 1995).

The term 'subjective expected utility' is used to explain the value people give to a particular outcome. Higher rates of risky or unhealthy behaviour may, however, reflect differences in beliefs about the subjective expected utility of different behaviours (Savage, 1954). Put another way, adolescents may not think the 'bad' outcomes of their risky behaviour are as likely or as bad as adults think they are.

A certain amount of risk taking is appropriate during adolescence. For example, Erikson's developmental theory highlights the importance of 'trying out' different identities and related behaviours during adolescence (Erikson, 1968). Adolescents have increased access to a range of potentially risky behaviours – such as alcohol consumption, motor vehicle use, and sexual activity – and some of these behaviours are important aspects of their socialisation into adulthood. Furthermore, many health risk behaviours are gendered and adolescents may engage in risky behaviours as part of the development of their gender identities. Thus, many young men seek to test or display their masculinity by engaging in risky or unhealthy behaviours (de Visser & McDonnell, 2013).

Risky behaviour is also influenced by social contextual factors. For example, adolescents are more likely to take risks when they are with same-age peers but less likely to do so when alongside or with older adults (Gardner & Steinberg, 2005), whereas brain scanning studies suggest that the presence of an adolescent's mother results in greater neural rewards for less risky behaviour (Moreira & Telzer, 2016).

Summary

- Puberty onset is earlier today than 100 years ago. This has been influenced by improved standards of living and better diet.
- Responses to the process and outcomes of puberty are different for boys and girls.
- Major developmental tasks include: adjusting to a new body size and shape, coming to terms with sexuality, using new cognitive capacities, developing maturity and independence.
- Adolescents begin to disengage from family activities but one-on-one quality interactions with parents often stay the same.
- Adolescents' interactions with healthcare professionals can be affected by embarrassment when talking about sensitive issues, concerns about confidentiality, and the presence of parents during consultations. It is important to be aware of, and responsive to, these concerns.
- Although adolescents have an improved decision-making capacity, their egocentrism may distort risk perception.

8.3 ADULTHOOD

There is no clear line separating adolescence and adulthood. The differences between adolescence and adulthood have been blurred by the fact that in developed countries young people now take longer than previous generations to complete their education, gain their financial independence, establish their own households, form long-term relationships, and have children. It has therefore been suggested that the period from the late teens to the early twenties should be conceived of as 'emerging adulthood' (Arnett, 2004).

After rapid and profound changes in cognitive and psychological functioning during childhood and adolescence, adulthood is a time of relative calm. However, it is during adulthood that patterns of behaviour and psychological states linked to the major causes of morbidity and mortality become established. There are many examples of these throughout this book, but particularly in the chapters on body systems (see Chapters 11 to 16).

Although adulthood is often thought of as a period of stability, there can be important changes. Many of these relate to changes in social roles and adjustment to major life events, such as having children, moving house, changing jobs, and experiencing the death of loved ones. As noted elsewhere, gaining, losing, or changing social roles can be stressful and may lead to depression (see Chapter 9). Furthermore, prolonged stress can have serious negative consequences for immune and endocrine function (see Chapters 3 and 14). Although stressful life events and negative role changes tend to be linked to poorer physical and psychological wellbeing, the impact of such events will vary according to coping responses and social support. It is therefore important that adults develop and maintain effective individual coping skills and supportive social networks.

8.4 OLD AGE

Current life expectancy in Europe and the Americas is 80 years for women and 73 years for men (World Health Organisation, 2017d). Life expectancy today is around 30 years longer than it was at the beginning of the twentieth century. Although life expectancy has increased, birth rates have fallen (WHO, 2017d). As a result, the proportion of the population who are elderly is increasing, and will be around 25% by the year 2050. Unless you work in paediatrics or obstetrics, you are likely to encounter increasing numbers of older people.

Control of infectious diseases means that there is a lower burden of disease among young people and a concentration of illness and death among the elderly. This **compression of morbidity** has occurred over the last century because the age of onset of chronic disease increased more rapidly than life expectancy – i.e. people stay well for longer, but illness is compressed into the final phase of life (e.g. Fries et al., 1989). This, combined with changes in population composition, means a greater proportion of medical consultations and expenditure will be concentrated on older people.

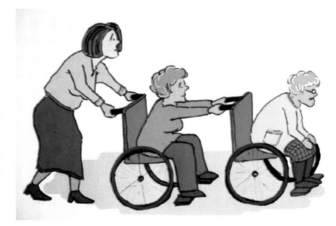

8.4.1 HEALTH PROMOTION AMONG THE ELDERLY

It is generally accepted that ageing involves reduced physical capacity. So should older people resign themselves to physical decline? The answer to this is a definite 'no'. Physical decline can be significantly reduced by encouraging older people to maintain or initiate healthy lifestyles. Research suggests that regular moderate physical activity among older men can lead to significant improvements in immune function (Smith et al., 2004). In addition, lung cancer and cardiovascular risk among smokers falls rapidly within a few years of quitting smoking (Department of Health & Human Services, 1990). Furthermore, even among people aged 65+ the likelihood of an earlier death is influenced by whether they continue or change unhealthy behaviours (Morey et al., 2002). However, behaviour change may be more difficult among older people than among younger people because their patterns of behaviour may have become more habitual.

ACTIVITY 8.1   BELIEFS ABOUT AGEING

- Stop for a moment and note the images that come to mind when you think about elderly people.
- Are the images that come to mind mostly positive or negative? Is there a mixture?

8.4.2 AGEING AND PSYCHOLOGICAL WELLBEING

Stereotypes of elderly people are often contradictory. On the one hand, elderly people are seen as 'sages' with a lifetime's knowledge and experience. On the other hand, they are seen as 'senile' or 'demented'. In general, our society has a negative view of ageing, which is seen as the loss of youth and a decline in physical, cognitive, and social functioning.

Dementia is present in around 3% of European adults aged 70–74 and 25% of European adults aged 85+ (Ferri et al., 2005; WHO, 2012). However, it is a myth that *all* old people suffer from fundamental intellectual decline (see Case Study 8.1). When discussing the intellectual capacities of the elderly, we must distinguish between 'crystalline intelligence', which reflects experience and long-term memory, and 'fluid intelligence', which reflects processing speed and short-term memory. Tests of fluid intelligence (e.g. IQ tests) suggest many older people are 'mentally disadvantaged'. However, their behaviour does not match this description. One reason for this is that crystalline intelligence may compensate for declines in fluid intelligence. In addition, IQ tests may not assess real-world skills. Age-related declines in fluid intelligence may be associated with physical health and organic change in the central nervous system. Some early trials suggested that enhancing older adults' physical fitness could improve cognitive function in older adults without cognitive impairment, but recent reviews have not found significant effects (Young et al., 2015).

CASE STUDY 8.1   Successful ageing

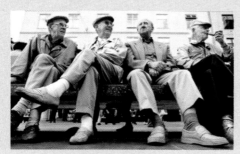

It is a myth that all old people suffer from a fundamental intellectual decline and restriction of their lifestyle.

When Fred Hale Senior died in November 2004 at the age of 113 he was documented as the world's oldest man. Although few people achieve such old age, his experiences show that many elderly people maintain fully active lives:

- At 95 he tried boogie-boarding while visiting Hawaii.
- He participated in his last deer hunt at age 100.
- At 103 he was still living independently – shoveling the snow off his rooftop.
- His driving licence was renewed at age 104, but he gave up driving at 108, because slow drivers annoyed him.
- He maintained an active interest in sport and bee-keeping.

Although his longevity may have been influenced by genetic factors, his lifestyle was also important. He attributed it to eating three full meals at the same time each day, never smoking, rarely drinking alcohol, and eating at least a teaspoonful of honey and bee pollen every day.

Photograph © Nordic Co-operation website

Depression in older age

The prevalence of depression tends to increase with age. Depression tends to be associated with declines or losses in other areas, including functional disability, cognitive impairment, and social deprivation (Aziz & Steffens, 2013; Luppa et al., 2012; Panza et al., 2010). As in earlier phases of life, depression is more common among elderly women than men. Psychosocial influences on increased rates of depression include role loss (see Chapter 9) – particularly among men for whom work was an important component of identity – and negative life events. Bereavement has an important impact on rates of depression. Older people are more likely than younger people to experience the death of their spouse and friends. Given that average life expectancy is longer for women, in each age band there is a greater proportion of widows than widowers. This may help to explain higher rates of depression among older women than men.

CLINICAL NOTES 8.3

Working with elderly people

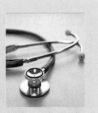

- Be aware of your own stereotypes and prejudices related to ageing and the elderly. Do not let these lead to poorer care for older people.
- Adjust your consultation style to the capacities of older people.
- Do not assume elderly people are frail or senile – difficulty with hearing or talking does not mean they are stupid!

8.4.3 HEALTHCARE OF OLDER PEOPLE

As older people are an increasing proportion of the population, there are concerns that increased demands for health and social care will have to be met by a smaller proportion of tax payers of working age or an increased reliance on informal or voluntary care (Robine et al., 2007).

Negative stereotypes about ageing can lead to the stigmatisation of older people and a neglect of issues concerning them. It is often assumed that older people are physically frail, cognitively impaired, and have diminished social engagement. These stereotypes and prejudices then affect the quality of service provision: many elderly people are not treated with the respect and dignity to which all people are entitled. Mistreatment of older people in hospitals is not purely due to a lack of resources, but also reflects negative attitudes (Care Quality Commission, 2013; Healthcare Commission, 2007).

Although some elderly people experience substantial declines in cognitive function with age, most do not. It is therefore important for healthcare professionals to check their patients' cognitive function and adjust their consultation skills accordingly. During consultations with older people who have clear declines in fluid memory, allow more time for information to be considered before asking further questions. It is important not to fill silences with more questions, as this can lead to a communication breakdown.

It is also important to consider people's expectations of consultations. Although younger people may expect and appreciate a more patient-centred approach to consultations, older people may be more comfortable with a patriarchal approach wherein the practitioner is the expert who is expected to provide solutions and make decisions. At any age, it is important to tailor consultation styles to people's capacities and preferences.

Summary

- Compression of morbidity means that people stay healthier for longer, but have a concentration of illness and/or disability at the end of their lives.
- Even in old age, changes in health-related behaviour are beneficial to physical and psychological wellbeing.
- Ageing is linked to declines in fluid intelligence (i.e. cognitive processing speed), but not crystalline intelligence.
- Depression is common in old age, particularly in women.

FURTHER READING

The three textbooks below have been prepared for psychology students. They give a lot of detail, but little attention is given to medical applications.

Bee, H. & Boyd, D. (2012) *The Developing Child* (13th edition). Boston, MA: Allyn & Bacon. A standard text for development during childhood and adolescence, which is very reader-friendly and has a range of illustrations of the major points.

Berk, L. (2008) *Child Development* (8th edition). Boston, MA: Allyn & Bacon. Also a standard text for child and adolescent development. It has reader-friendly images and text boxes to help with the understanding of key points.

Santrock, J. (2013) *Life-span Development* (14th edition). Columbus, OH: McGraw-Hill Education. This text covers the whole lifespan, and although much of it covers childhood, it has a broader focus than the first two books. It does still give information on childhood development.

REVISION QUESTIONS

1. Why is infant–adult attachment important for children's development?

2. Describe the link between breastfeeding and intelligence.

3. How does the interactionist approach to language learning differ from the nativist (LAD) approach?

4. What should practitioners do to promote effective practitioner–child communication?

5. Describe the central features of Piaget's theory of cognitive development.

6. How is 'theory of mind' important for medical consultations with young children?

7. Adolescents are supposed to have adult-like capacities for risk assessment, so why are they more likely to take risks?

8. What is meant by the compression of morbidity? How does this affect the number of medical consultations with older people?

9. Summarise the major changes in cognitive capacity observed in old age.

10. What factors need to be considered during consultations with older people?

9 SOCIAL PSYCHOLOGY

CHAPTER CONTENTS

(Continued)

Case study

9.1   Self-image and body building

Figure

9.1   Group behaviour and dress

Research boxes

9.1   Nurse–physician relationships
9.2   Doctors' attitudes to mental illness

LEARNING OBJECTIVES

This chapter is designed to enable you to:

- Discuss the links between attitudes and behaviour and the importance of attitude change in encouraging healthy behaviour.
- Describe how self-perceptions influence a range of health-related behaviours.
- Discuss the importance of group membership to individuals and how group membership can influence individual behaviour.
- Outline the different explanations of aggressive behaviour.
- Identify the factors that can increase the likelihood of prosocial behaviour.

Social psychology helps us to consider such issues as how we present ourselves to others, our health behaviour, how a group makes decisions – and even whether we are able to challenge senior doctors if we believe they are wrong. For example, in 2003 one junior doctor was ordered by a senior doctor to administer a combination of two drugs to a man with leukaemia. The combination was lethal. The junior doctor asked the senior doctor twice if this was correct but was told to go ahead, with devastating consequences (Ferner & McDowell, 2006). Social psychology examines why we carry out such actions and which social forces contribute to them. In this chapter we shall consider how people's attitudes and beliefs about themselves can influence their behaviour, including health-related behaviour, and then the issues of conformity and aggression, and how individuals behave as members or leaders of groups.

9.1 ATTITUDES

In social psychology and health promotion a great deal of attention is given to attitudes. **Attitudes** can be defined as a measure of people's like or dislike of an object. The 'object' may be a real object, a person, or a behaviour such as 'healthy eating'.

The expectancy-value model suggests that attitudes are the product of expectancy about an object, and the value given to that object (see Chapter 5). For example, attitudes toward condom use will be shaped by expectancies (e.g. condoms reduce sexual pleasure) and the value of the expectancies (e.g. sexual pleasure is important). Thus, two people with the same expectancy may have different attitudes because they give different values to this expectancy.

Attitudes reflect what we think and feel about something and how we plan to behave (Eagley & Chaiken, 1993). Ideally, the thinking, feeling, and behaving components of attitudes will be consistent with each other. When we hold inconsistent beliefs or when our behaviour does not match our beliefs it leads to unpleasant cognitive dissonance, which we will be motivated to reduce (Festinger, 1957). People may seek to reduce cognitive dissonance by changing either their attitudes or their behaviour. Thus, an overweight person who knows this is unhealthy may either decide to lose weight or change their beliefs about their weight.

9.1.1 MEASUREMENT OF ATTITUDES

Attitudes cannot be observed. However, there are different ways to measure expressions of attitudes. Indirect measures of attitudes may use physiological measures (e.g. heart rate or galvanic skin response) or observations of behaviour (e.g. stopping to help a stranger) to infer people's attitudes. Direct measures of attitudes using questionnaires are more common.

A direct assessment of attitudes can be made in various ways. Likert scales are commonly used to collect people's responses to various statements of attitude (Table 9.1). Ideally, assessments of attitudes using Likert scales will include a mixture of positively and negatively phrased statements which are then combined to give an overall assessment of attitudes. Likert scales are useful because they measure the direction of a person's attitude (i.e. positive or negative) and the intensity of the attitude (see Table 9.1).

An alternative to Likert scales are semantic differential scales (Table 9.2). These also measure the direction and intensity of attitudes. However, rather than being based on participants' agreement with statements, semantic differential scales assess individuals' position in relation to pairs of opposites. Each response is converted into a number, with higher summary scores indicating more positive attitudes toward the behaviours.

TABLE 9.1 Measuring attitudes: Likert scale

	strongly disagree	disagree	neither	agree	strongly agree
People should have the right to die if they are terminally ill and suffering	☐	☐	☐	☐	☐
No one should be allowed to decide to end a suffering person's life	☐	☐	☐	☐	☐

TABLE 9.2   Measuring attitudes: semantic differential scale

		−2	−1	0	+1	+2	
Euthanasia is:	bad	☐	☐	☐	☐	☐	good
	cruel	☐	☐	☐	☐	☐	kind
	unacceptable	☐	☐	☐	☐	☐	acceptable

9.1.2 ATTITUDES AND BEHAVIOUR

Attitudes measured at one time can often be used to predict behaviour at a later time. Attitudes are therefore central to many models of health behaviour (see Chapter 5). However, it is important to note that other beliefs (e.g. normative beliefs) and social factors will influence whether attitudes are acted upon.

Changing attitudes and changing behaviour

Because attitudes predict subsequent behaviour, it is generally accepted that attitude change should be a productive way to change behaviour. The enormous sums of money spent on advertisements for cars, soft drinks, cosmetics, and so on reflect the belief that people's purchasing behaviour will change if their attitudes toward products are changed. For example, in the last decade fast-food chains have changed their advertising to counter concerns that their meals are unhealthy in an effort to retain their market share. Mass media health promotion campaigns also try to encourage behaviour changes by changing peoples' attitudes toward healthy and unhealthy behaviours.

These efforts are based on the hypothesis that there is generally agreement between people's behaviour and the affective, cognitive, and behavioural components of attitudes (Eagley & Chaiken, 1993). According to the theory of cognitive dissonance, if we change people's attitudes toward their current unhealthy behaviours, this will set up a dissonance between their new attitude and their established behaviours: they should then change their behaviour to reduce the dissonance between their attitudes and behaviour.

'Foot-in-the-door' techniques are an interesting illustration of how our desire to behave consistently with our attitudes can be manipulated (Burger, 1999). These techniques involve asking people to agree to a simple request which they are likely to comply with. Later the same person is asked to agree to a substantially more demanding request, which is the actual target behaviour. For example, one study of French university students found that smokers who had previously agreed to a request to stop smoking for two hours were significantly more likely than other smokers to agree to a request to stop smoking for 24 hours (Guéguen et al., 2016). 'Foot-in-the-door' techniques produce better responses to requests for the target behaviour because once a person has agreed to the small initial request they have demonstrated to themselves and others that their attitudes toward the cause are favourable and that they are committed to the behaviour. Other techniques for encouraging behaviour change through attitude change are addressed below.

Persuasive messages

If we wish to change health-related behaviour by changing attitudes, then we must be sure about the most effective ways to do so. A message is most likely to change people's attitudes if it:

- Gets to its recipient – different approaches can be used, including discussion during consultations, leaflets, or the mass media.
- Is attention-grabbing.
- Is understood by the recipient – it must be couched in the appropriate language and 'pitched' at the appropriate level of complexity.
- Is seen by the recipient as relevant and important.
- Is remembered by the recipient, translated into an intention to change behaviour, and acted upon.

The characteristics of the sender of the message – be they individual healthcare professionals or organisations such as the Department of Health – will influence whether the message will be persuasive. We are more likely to be persuaded if the sender of the message is:

- Credible – the qualifications and occupational status of healthcare professionals may increase their persuasive power.
- Trustworthy – the perceived objectivity of healthcare professionals may increase their ability to encourage an attitude and behaviour change.
- Appealing – healthcare professionals must ensure that their personal presentation is attractive.

Inducing a certain amount of fear may motivate people to change their behaviour, but fear campaigns can be counterproductive. If fear-based campaigns do not also include sufficient information about what people can do to avoid a feared outcome, and do not boost self-efficacy for self-protective responses to the feared outcome, then people may simply avoid the issue rather than focusing on the issue and their behaviour (Ruiter et al., 2014).

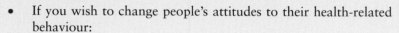

CLINICAL NOTES 9.1

Persuading people to change their behaviour

- If you wish to change people's attitudes to their health-related behaviour:
    - Make sure the message is clear, relevant to them, and easy to remember.
    - Think of whether it is better to emphasise the gains or losses associated with current and desired behaviour.
    - Pay attention to your own persuasive power based on your qualifications, occupational status, and credibility.
    - Be aware that how you present yourself can influence people's perceptions of your status and credibility.

Framing effects can also be important (Rothman & Salovey, 1997). They refer to whether a message emphasises the benefits of a certain behaviour or the losses associated with that behaviour. For example, a gain-framed message may be something like 'A regular saving plan will let you have your dream vacation' whereas a loss-framed message would be 'If you do not save regularly you will not be able to afford a vacation'. When we want people to take up behaviours aimed at detecting health problems or illness (e.g. breast self-examination or HIV testing), loss-framed messages may be more effective. When we want people to take up behaviours aimed at promoting prevention behaviours (e.g. using sunscreen or using condoms), gain-framed messages may be more effective. It is also important to consider the types of gains (or losses) that may be most motivating for people: for example, messages designed to promote sunscreen use to prevent skin cancer may be more effective if they emphasise the impact of sun exposure on people's appearance, not just their health (Thomas et al., 2011).

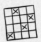

ACTIVITY 9.1   FRAMING MESSAGES

Which of the two statements below will be most effective for breast self-examination?

1. If you do not undertake breast self-examination you may be more likely to die from cancer.
2. If you undertake breast self-examination you may decrease the risk of dying from cancer.

Which of the two statements below will be most effective for promoting sunscreen use?

3. If you do not use SPF15 sunscreen, your skin will be damaged and you may die younger.
4. If you use SPF15 sunscreen, your skin will stay healthier and you may prolong your life.

*Statements 1 and 4 will be the most effective

Ambivalence

For many attitudinal objects we do not have simple positive or negative attitudes. Instead, our feelings are often mixed. For example, we may have positive attitudes toward certain aspects of living in the countryside (fresh air, open space, less traffic, etc.) but negative attitudes toward other aspects of country life (social isolation, having to travel to town for movies and shopping, etc.). People are also ambivalent toward many health behaviours, such as alcohol use, smoking, and condom use (Miller & Rollnick, 2002). This ambivalence can influence efforts to change health behaviours because ambivalent attitudes tend to be worse predictors of behaviour than homogeneous attitudes (Conner et al., 2003). The results of one study of adolescents suggested that interventions to reduce initiation or continuation of marijuana use may be better able to counter peer influences by addressing young people's ambivalence toward marijuana use (Hohman et al., 2014).

Summary

- People are motivated to keep their attitudes consistent with their behaviour. Thus, efforts to change health behaviour will often focus on changing attitudes.
- Attitude change messages should be tailored to maximise their persuasiveness. This means paying attention to the content of the message, the style of delivery, and the characteristics of the person delivering the message.

9.2 SELF PSYCHOLOGY

One important focus of our attitudes is ourselves. Here we shall examine why a person's self-image is important for their health and wellbeing. We naïvely tend to assume that our selves are singular, continuous, and consistent: I think that when I woke up this morning I was more or less exactly the same person I was yesterday and will be when I wake up tomorrow. People with some psychiatric conditions may not always have this sense of unity (see Chapter 16).

Despite feeling that we have a singular self, it is possible to think of different definitions or different components of our selves. One important distinction is the difference between a personal self (how I perceive myself) and a social self (how others perceive me). These two selves may not always be in agreement. For example, someone may be perceived as calm and confident when talking in public but will actually be a bundle of nerves. An important distinction can also be made between personal identity, which consists of everything that makes someone a unique person, and social identity, which consists of the things someone shares with members of groups that are important to them (e.g. family resemblance, national identity, occupation). Processes of group affiliation and conformity will be addressed later in this chapter. For now we will focus on ideas of the self.

9.2.1 SELF-ESTEEM AND SELF-IMAGE

Self-esteem has important links to behaviour and health. Self-esteem consists of feelings and evaluations about ourselves. It is often thought that low self-esteem is unhealthy, but research suggests that this assumption is simplistic (Baumeister et al., 2003). For example, children and adolescents with high self-esteem may be more likely to experiment with smoking and using alcohol or sex rather than avoiding such behaviours. One area in which there are clear links between low self-esteem and ill-health is in relation to eating disorders. One study of over 95,000 adolescents found that low self-esteem was a significant predictor of binge and purge eating practices and other weight loss behaviours (French et al., 2001). Self-esteem can also be lowered in certain illnesses, such as depression (see Chapter 16). Positive self-esteem is reflected in the promotion of a positive self-image to oneself and other people.

Most of us put a lot of effort into developing and promoting a favourable self-image. An important part of self-image is our appearance. Goffman (1959) used the analogy of acting in a play to explain how and why we modify our appearance and behaviour depending on where we are (the scene) and who we are with (our audience). For example, the clothes we wear and the amount of time we spend on our appearance will probably vary depending on whether we are at home studying, going to a party, or attending a formal meeting (see Activity 9.2). Appearance can also be an important marker of group membership (Figure 9.1).

ACTIVITY 9.2   SELF-PRESENTATION AND CLOTHING

Compare the following three settings:

1. The last time you were studying.
2. The last time you went out on a first date with someone.
3. The last time you had a formal interview.

In each of these situations:

*   How much time did you spend planning what you would wear and getting ready?
*   Did you do your hair and use cosmetics/shave?
*   How did the clothes you chose reflect the self-image you were trying to project?

People also use appearance as a shorthand way of evaluating others. However, looks can be deceiving. In some cases this can have implications for health. For example, we often assume that if a person looks healthy they are healthy. This assumption can prove costly in the case of serious illnesses such as HIV/AIDS and cancer where there may be no visible signs of illness.

Hippocrates stated that physicians should be 'clean in person, well-dressed, and anointed with sweet-smelling unguents'. Research suggests that how physicians present themselves via clothing and accessories influences people's trust and confidence in them (Petrilli et al., 2015). In general, people feel less positive about medical professionals wearing casual clothes or jeans. However, preferences do vary between cultures and contexts: formal attire and white coats are generally preferred by older people; and preferences for attire are less obvious in intensive care or emergency settings.

How we behave in social situations is an important component of maintaining a positive self-image. Most of us will try to obey social conventions about appropriate and inappropriate behaviour in order to be perceived favourably. It is also important for our self-esteem to affirm positive aspects of ourselves when we are criticised. This can be done in various ways. The example in Box 9.1 shows that when we are criticised we often try to publicly affirm positive aspects of our selves and/or denigrate the person who has criticised us.

One way to boost our self-image is to make downward social comparisons with people whose problems or situation are worse than our own. For example, a person who has had a leg amputated following a car accident may feel better off than someone who has been made quadriplegic in a car accident. Another example is the responses of some drug addicts to criticism of their behaviour: 'functional' heroin addicts may compare themselves favourably to 'junkies' who engage in crime or prostitution to support their drug use. In contrast, upward comparison occurs when people highlight the similarities between themselves and others who are deemed socially superior so as to make their self-images more positive (Suls et al., 2002). People's upward and/or downward comparisons to other people can lead to changes in anxiety and mood (Petersen et al., 2012).

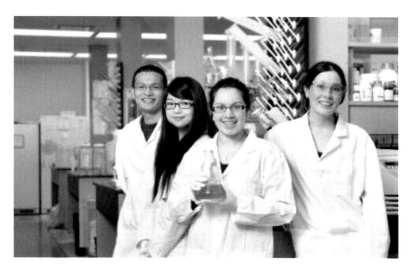

FIGURE 9.1   Group behaviour and dress

Photo courtesy of Selin Jessica, Simon Fraser University, April 2013, Public Domain

BOX 9.1   Self-affirmation

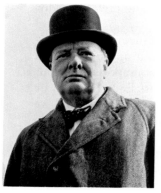

The following exchange is reputed to have occurred between Labour MP Bessie Braddock and Conservative Prime Minister Winston Churchill:

Braddock: Mr. Churchill, you are drunk.
Churchill: And you, madam, are ugly. But in the morning, I shall be sober.

Churchill's response protected his self-image and self-esteem by highlighting the fact that his undesirable behaviour was temporary (and therefore not a fundamental part of him), whereas his critic's undesirable appearance was permanent.

Quote copyright © Winston S. Churchill

9.2.2 ATTRIBUTIONS

Our efforts to create and maintain a positive self-image are also influenced by the attributions we assign to our own and others' behaviour. Internal attributions are based on the belief that a person's behaviour is internally motivated – that it is voluntary and reflects the person's attitudes. In contrast, external attributions are the belief that a person's behaviour is due to external factors such as luck, chance, or someone else demanding it.

In terms of our own behaviour, we tend to prefer internal attributions for our successes (e.g. 'I got an A for the exam because I studied really hard') and external attributions for our failures (e.g. 'I failed the exam because the lecturers set difficult questions'). In contrast, we tend to attribute others' behaviour to internal or dispositional causes rather than external or situational causes. This is known as the fundamental attribution error (Ross, 1977). This error means we are more likely to attribute negative facts about other people (e.g. being unwell, anxious, or depressed) to their own behaviour or characteristics rather than to the broader social context. Examples of internal and external attributions for health are given in Table 9.3.

TABLE 9.3   Attribution errors and illness

	Internal attribution	External attribution
Obesity	They are lazy, ignorant, greedy	There are not the right facilities or incentives to encourage activity and healthy eating
Depression	They are weak and unable to cope	They have experienced severely stressful life events

From this, it should be clear that attribution errors can have wide-ranging repercussions on clinical care through their impact on the doctor–patient relationship and understanding of the person's illness, and therefore treatment. In healthcare practice, we must be aware of making this error and ensure we consider external and situational factors such as life circumstances and competing demands.

One application of attribution concepts within healthcare settings is the health locus of control (Wallston et al., 1978). An individual's locus of control reflects the extent to which they believe that they have control over their health. This can be divided into three components:

- Internal – the belief that what they do will affect their health. These people are more likely to seek information and to initiate and persist with changes in health behaviour.
- Powerful others – the belief that the most important influence on their health is other people, such as medical and healthcare professionals who possess important knowledge and skills. These people may be more likely to seek and follow professional advice but they are less likely to initiate changes in health behaviours.
- External – the belief that the maintenance of health and the onset of illness are due to fate, chance, or luck. These people are unlikely to take action to protect or promote their health.

One example of the importance of attributions of control over health and illness comes from a longitudinal study which showed that children with a higher internal locus of control had a reduced risk of obesity, hypertension, and poor physical or psychological wellbeing during adulthood (Gale et al., 2008). Furthermore, a review of published research showed that a lower internal locus of control and a greater powerful other or external locus of control are associated with more symptoms of depression (Presson & Benassi, 1996).

9.2.3 IDEAL SELF AND ACTUAL SELF

To varying degrees most of us have biased appraisals of ourselves. Most of us probably think that we are more generous, helpful, and caring than others think we are. Often, this discrepancy between our own self-image and how others see us is inconsequential. There may also be a discrepancy between our *actual* self (how we currently are) and our *ideal* self (how we would like to be) (Higgins, 1987). Perceived gaps between our ideal and actual selves can motivate a behaviour change. For example, a man may be motivated to take up regular exercise because when he looks in a mirror he does not see the ideal athletic physique he desires.

Sometimes, the discrepancy between the ideal self and actual self can be distorted, with important consequences for our physical and psychological wellbeing. This is often observed among people with eating disorders such as anorexia and bulimia (Fitzsimmons-Craft, 2011; Peat et al., 2008). Influenced by cultural preferences and media images, many young women (and increasingly men) with eating disorders desire an ideal body image which is unrealistically thin and unhealthy (see Case Study 13.1). Men may also be affected and strive to attain an ideal physique which is unrealistically muscular (see Case Study 9.1).

CASE STUDY 9.1   Self-image and body building

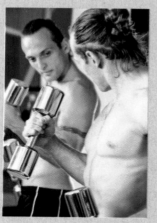

Sometimes the discrepancy between the ideal self and actual self can be distorted, with important consequences for physical and psychological wellbeing. Muscle dysmorphia is a form of body dysmorphic disorder in which men who are already more muscular than most men become preoccupied with the desire to be more muscular than they are.

Tony initially became interested in weight training when he was in high school. He had always felt small and was impressed by a friend's change in physique after he started weight training. Tony quickly became 'hooked' on training. He began spending increasing amounts of time at the gym and less time with friends. He found himself constantly thinking about his body and comparing it to those of other men at the gym. Although he had developed an extremely muscular physique according to any objective standard, he felt ashamed of his lack of musculature, and when he was not at the gym he would wear baggy trousers and loose t-shirts to hide his body.

> No matter how big I got, or how much bigger I was than other guys, it didn't matter – I had to be even bigger. I started using supplements, but I wasn't getting bigger fast enough... so last year I started using steroids.

The steroids have produced some benefits, but they also have unwanted side effects. For someone so concerned about his appearance, the development of acne has been hard to bear. Tony's desire to be bigger has also led him to suffer in other ways:

> I started pushing myself too hard and was getting all these injuries... but that only made me want to train harder when I recovered to make up for the lost time. My shoulders and knees are shot from pushing weights that are too heavy.

Photograph © Sokolovsky/Fotolia

Summary

- Our beliefs about who we are and who we want to be can exert important influences on our behaviour.
- We tend to attribute our successes to our efforts and our failures to external factors.

(Continued)

- The fundamental attribution error is our tendency to attribute other people's poor health or lack of success to their disposition or character rather than to the broader social context.
- Our beliefs about what influences our health (our efforts, other people, or fate) can influence the likelihood of initiating and maintaining healthy behaviours.

9.3 INDIVIDUALS AND GROUPS

Humans have a basic need for the company of others to avoid loneliness, gain attention from other people, bolster our self-image, and reduce anxiety. Some people do prefer to live in isolation, but they are exceptions to a very strong social norm. For most people, group membership and group identity are important components of individual identity. Having a strong positive group identity can benefit our psychological and social well-being. However, group membership may restrict our individual freedom due to pressures to conform to group norms, and membership of some groups may expose individuals to prejudice, stigmatisation, and victimisation.

When you start working as a healthcare professional you will acquire various identities from the broad group of 'healthcare professionals' down to the specific group forming the discipline or team in which you work. Social identity theory (Tajfel & Turner, 1986) proposes that a sense of belonging to valued groups is an important component of maintaining a positive self-image. Our membership of groups may be based on things we cannot change, including obvious physical characteristics such as ethnicity, sex, and age. However, our membership of other groups reflects the choices we make, such as our occupation, sporting team, or subcultural group (e.g. punks, Goths, hipsters). Important markers of group identity include styles of dress and the kind of language use (vocabulary, accent, slang, etc.).

9.3.1 SOCIAL ROLES

Most everyday interactions run smoothly because of shared beliefs and assumptions about how people should behave. Many social interactions are quite complex, and most of us behave in ways that indicate our awareness of what is appropriate and inappropriate behaviour. It is usually only when someone 'breaks the rules' that we will become conscious of them.

Goffman's (1959) dramaturgical theory suggests that social interactions can be thought of as being like a play in which interactions between people inhabiting different **social roles** are guided by shared assumptions about normal or appropriate behaviour. Social roles can be ascribed or acquired. Ascribed roles are those given to us independent of what we do (e.g. daughter/son). Acquired roles are those we attain through experience and social recognition (e.g. doctor). Each social role entails certain rights and responsibilities.

Different social roles also allow us to behave in certain ways. To be recognised as socially competent we must behave in ways that are appropriate to our social roles.

Changes in social roles can be stressful because of the links between social roles, identity, and social recognition. Gaining new roles can also be stressful because we need to learn new patterns of behaviour and prove that we are competent (e.g. getting a job promotion, becoming a parent). Feelings of failure or incapacity in social roles can lead to depression. Role loss can also be stressful (e.g. someone who has retired after 45 years working for the same employer). Role conflict can also be stressful (e.g. people trying to balance the new role of 'parent' with the established role of 'professional').

The concept of social roles is important in medicine and healthcare (Parsons, 1975). A person inhabiting the sick role has the right to relinquish other obligations – they can take time off work/school and avoid having to do daily activities such as washing the dishes or take out the rubbish. However, the sick role also entails obligations, such as the obligation to strive to get better, follow medical advice, and not engage in activities that may hinder recovery. This may be difficult for people who possess other important or valued social roles. Another important aspect of the sick role (as an ascribed role) is that it must be formally acknowledged. Because medical professionals usually have to certify sick leave they can be thought of as gatekeepers of the sick role. The social role of doctor bestows certain rights on them, such as the right to ask personal questions and conduct physical examinations. However, it also entails responsibilities such as upholding professional standards and maintaining patient confidentiality.

9.3.2 CONFORMITY

People generally have strong tendencies for conformity to the expectations of the groups to which they belong. The more we want to belong to a group, the more important it is for us to conform. Research has shown that people tend to go along with what others think – sometimes going against their own better judgement (Asch, 1956). When other group members have expressed a unanimous opinion, many people may find it hard to speak out against this.

ACTIVITY 9.3   CONFORMITY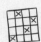

- Imagine you are a junior doctor on your first day. On ward rounds a senior consultant suggests a treatment you believe to be wrong. Several of the other group members seem to agree with the senior consultant.
- How easy would it be to say what you think rather than conforming to the group?
- What would you do?

An important reason to conform to group norms is to maintain distinctions between groups. One way to protect or improve our self-image is to make favourable comparisons between the groups to which we belong (the ingroup) and other groups (outgroups). For example, if the team I support wins an important match, I will feel good about myself and happy to be part of my ingroup rather than the outgroup (i.e. not part of a losing team). However, making favourable comparisons often means relying on and reinforcing prejudices and stereotypes about outgroups.

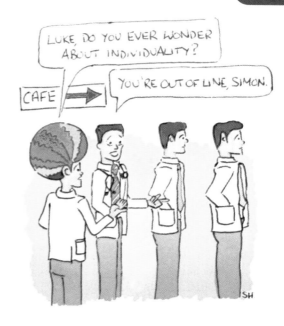

Groups can also have powerful effects on decision making. With group decision making it is not always the case that 'the whole is greater than the sum of its parts' (Mesmer-Magnus & DeChurch, 2009). This seems to be because the urge to conform can sometimes stifle creative thinking. This may be particularly so for new members of groups. For example, junior doctors or medical students may have fresh insights but find it difficult to question the professional opinions of other members of the team.

Group decisions are often more narrow than the decisions of individual group members. The phenomenon of polarisation means that through group discussion, agreement within a group tends to intensify so that each individual's attitude becomes stronger. For example, imagine we have six individuals who have moderately positive attitudes toward euthanasia. Following a group discussion there will tend to be a concentration and polarisation of attitudes: the group will become more positive toward euthanasia. If individuals were moderately opposed to euthanasia before the group discussion, the group attitude would be more extremely opposed following group discussion. Three explanations have been given for why this polarisation occurs (Hogg & Vaughan, 2008):

- Persuasive arguments: people in groups of like-minded people will hear arguments that they already agree with as well new arguments supporting their original beliefs. These will galvanise the initial attitude. In addition, making public commitments to our own beliefs via statements to other people may strengthen our initial attitudes.
- Social comparison: to prove they really belong to the group and seek approval, individuals will make more intense statements of their initial belief.
- Self-categorisation: people will develop stereotypes of group members and be aware of what distinguishes the ingroup prototype from stereotypical outgroup members. Therefore for individual and group identity reasons, people's opinions will move toward the ingroup prototype.

Another example of how group decision making may be worse than individual deci-sion making is called **groupthink** (Janis & Mann, 1977). Groupthink occurs when the desire for group unanimity overrides rational decisions. It is more likely to happen when a group is already homogeneous and cohesive. However, groupthink also depends on the characteristics of the situation, such as if a decision has to be made in stressful or rushed situations or when the group is isolated from external sources of informa-tion. Thus, groupthink may be most likely to occur when cohesive groups are placed in stressful situations. Given the urgency of many medical situations, it is vitally impor-tant that health teams are aware of how groupthink can lead to erroneous or poor decision making.

9.3.3 OBEDIENCE, POWER, AND LEADERSHIP

The processes of conformity just described refer to situations in which people think or behave in certain ways because of a perceived pressure to do so. Of course, there are many situations in which we behave in certain ways because of a need to be obedient to people who have power or authority.

Obedience

The powerful effects of obedience to authority have been observed in many settings, including those directly relevant to medicine and healthcare practice. The study described in Research Box 9.1 shows how an unquestioning obedience to authority may have disas-trous consequences.

In a classic study of obedience, study participants were told by a researcher in a white coat to give increasingly strong electric shocks to 'learners' who made mistakes in a word memory task (Milgram, 1974). No shocks were actually given, but the 'voltage generator' included descriptions of increasing voltage levels – 375v was labelled 'Danger: Severe Shock', and 435v was labelled 'XXX'. At different levels of shock, the 'learner' (actually a co-researcher) gave standard responses: after 150v they asked to leave the study; after 250v they screamed in agony; after 300v they lapsed into silence. If partici-pants hesitated or asked to stop, the researcher urged them to go on, informing them to treat silence or non-responses as errors and to administer another shock. Although it was predicted that fewer than 10% of participants would administer shocks greater than 195v (labelled 'Very Strong Shock'), all of the participants went beyond this. In fact, 63% went all the way to 450v. Subsequent analyses have indicated that key influ-ences on obedience in this study included how legitimate the researcher was perceived to be, and how directive and consistent he was, as well as the proximity of the participant and the 'learner' (Haslam et al., 2014).

RESEARCH BOX 9.1   Nurse–physician relationships

Background

The professional status of nurses is sometimes challenged by doctors' behaviour. One example of this is when nurses are directed by doctors to behave in ways that go against their professional standards or established procedures.

Method and findings

Twenty-two nurses were observed in their normal work environments. The researchers placed a bottle of a fictional drug 'Astroten' in the ward drug cabinet. The label on the bottle clearly stated 'Maximum daily dose 10mg'. A researcher posing as 'Dr Smith' – someone unknown to the nurse – telephoned each nurse and asked her to administer 20mg of Astroten to a patient, stating that he would sign for it when he arrived at the hospital.

Nurses had four good reasons not to administer the drug:

1. The requested dosage was double the safe daily dose stated on the bottle.
2. Hospital procedures stated that they should only take instructions from doctors they know.
3. Hospital procedures also stated that nurses should not take telephone instructions.
4. Astroten was not on the approved medication list and had not been signed for.

Nevertheless, 21 of the 22 nurses complied with the request to give an overdose of the drug. They were intercepted by the researchers after they prepared the dose.

Significance

Power differentials in the status of doctors and nurses can affect nurses' behaviour. No nurses involved in this study expressed concern about the excessive dose – indeed, many repeated and clarified the dosage without questioning it. Such conformity has consequences for the professional and personal esteem of healthcare professionals and the health of patients.

Hofling, C.K., Brotzman, E., Dalrymple, S., Graves, N. & Pierce, C.M. (1966) An experimental study of nurse–physician relationships. *Journal of Nervous and Mental Disease*, *143*: 171–180.

Leadership and influence

Effective leadership involves the appropriate use of authority and influence to ensure the efficient management of people and resources to achieve group aims. Good leadership involves more than simply 'getting the job done'. Good leaders will aim to develop and maintain good team relationships and provide appropriate opportunities for individual input.

Leadership styles can be grouped into three broad categories. Autocratic leaders assume total responsibility for making all decisions and managing team members. This style characterises dictators who do not tolerate the views and decisions of ingroup or outgroup members. Democratic leaders are consultative, allowing group members to be involved in decision making, planning, and the monitoring of performance if they possess the appropriate knowledge and skills. Laissez-faire leaders do not impose their leadership, but allow group members to decide on goals and strategies. In most professional settings it is rare to find purely autocratic or laissez-faire leaders. However, democratic leaders may tend more toward autocratic or laissez-faire styles: the context may determine the extent to which they do so.

Leaders often vary in terms of how they try to encourage or enforce compliance with their decisions (Raven, 1965). One common strategy is to apply the principles of operant conditioning (see Chapter 10). According to this approach, good performance may be recognised via bonuses or other material rewards. One example is performance-related pay. In contrast, coercive leadership is based on a leader threatening to remove privileges if their instructions are not obeyed.

It is also possible to identify different sources of authority or reasons for leadership. One basis for power is recognised hierarchies of power. These are often based on the leader possessing superior knowledge, experience, or expertise. Thus a consultant is in a superior position relative to a junior doctor. However, this is not always the case. For example, in the military a newly commissioned officer has a higher leadership position than a senior non-commissioned officer with 40 years of experience. It is also important to note that people sometimes become leaders not because of their expertise or experience but because of their charisma, charm, or connections to powerful people.

CLINICAL NOTES 9.2

Hierarchy and leadership in medicine

- Being a doctor entails certain rights and responsibilities. Your reputation will be damaged if you disregard these responsibilities or abuse these rights.
- Pay attention to the different leadership skills people use. Use good leaders as role models and avoid following the examples set by bad leaders.
- Be aware of your own tendency to conform to authority. Ask yourself whether it is always in patients' best interests to do what your superiors suggest.
- Be brave enough to challenge your superiors if you think they have made a decision that will not result in the best care for patients.

9.3.4 STEREOTYPES AND PREJUDICE

An important aspect of the study of individuals and groups is stereotypes and prejudice. **Stereotypes** are generalisations that we make about specific social groups and members of those groups. They are 'rules of thumb' which are broadly correct, but may sometimes be erroneous (Tversky & Kahneman, 1974). The social groups for which people have stereotypes are various and include nationality, occupation, and religion. However, they can be more specific.

Stereotypes form the basis of many jokes in which a dominant ingroup denigrates an outgroup that is perceived as being inferior. For example, Australians make jokes about New Zealanders. You may also be aware of jokes based on stereotypes of different medical specialisations (e.g. orthopaedic surgeons, anaesthetists, psychiatrists). Although many of these jokes may appear harmless, it is important to note that incorrect or inaccurate stereotypes can lead to undesirable social behaviour.

Prejudice toward particular social groups is commonly based on inaccurate stereotypes. Taken literally, prejudice means to judge prior to having relevant facts. History is replete with clashes between groups based on erroneous assumptions about differences due to sex, sexuality, nationality, ethnicity, or religion.

ACTIVITY 9.4 STEREOTYPES OF PATIENTS

- Take two minutes to write down quickly words that describe people with AIDS, people with chronic fatigue syndrome, and people with cancer.
- How did you acquire these beliefs?
- How were your interactions with people with these conditions shaped by your initial beliefs?
- How have your initial beliefs been changed by your interactions with people with these conditions?

Stereotypes and prejudice can also affect medical care. Stereotypes and prejudices about people with certain health conditions, ethnic minorities, or the elderly (see Case Study 8.1) are important because of the known links between attitudes and behaviour noted earlier. Indeed, research has highlighted how prejudice and stereotyping can lead to increased ethnic disparities in health (Hall et al., 2015). The example in Research Box 9.2 shows that prejudices about mental illness can result in poorer care for some people (Lawrie et al., 1998). It is notable that many medical students also express prejudices about people with mental illnesses (Dixon et al., 2008). There is some evidence that doctors working in primary care who receive training in community mental health have less stigmatising attitudes toward people with mental illnesses (Lam et al., 2015). However, public attitudes toward mental illness are generally negative despite improved mental health literacy (Schomerus et al., 2012).

Stereotyping in healthcare is not restricted to medical professionals. People's stereotyped beliefs about medical professionals are also important. One study found that people who expressed more negative stereotypes about doctors were less likely to seek medical care when they became ill, were less satisfied with the medical care that they did obtain, and were less likely to adhere to the treatment prescribed by their doctor (Bogart et al., 2004). Identifying the reasons for people's negative stereotypes in an attempt to change these may help to improve the health of the population. It may also be important for doctors to try to change their behaviour so that they do not reinforce unhelpful stereotypes.

RESEARCH BOX 9.2   Doctors' attitudes to mental illness

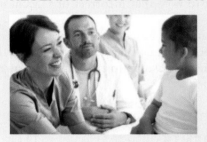

Source: Selmaemiliano, June 2007,
Public Domain

Background

Many members of the general population possess negative stereotypes and prejudices about people with mental illness. Previous research has indicated that many people with mental illnesses report unfair treatment from their doctors.

Method and findings

166 doctors working in primary care were randomly allocated to receive a letter from a 30-year-old married housewife with a 5-year-old child who wishes to be registered at the doctor's practice because since moving to the area two months previously she has been troubled by insomnia, fatigue, and nausea. The letter was altered to say that she either had (1) no previous major illnesses, or a past history of (2) schizophrenia, (3) depression, or (4) diabetes. For options 2–4 it was made clear that the illness was well controlled by the appropriate medication.

In spite of the clear statement that the mental illnesses were well controlled, doctors were significantly less happy to register a patient with schizophrenia than the three other patient types. Doctors who received the letter with a history of schizophrenia were significantly more concerned about the risk of violence and the child's welfare, and were more likely to say that they would personally contact the patient's previous doctor.

Significance

Schizophrenia arouses concerns in doctors that are not simply due to the fact that people have a mental illness. People with schizophrenia may have difficulty finding a doctor prepared to register them, and this can hamper the likelihood they will receive the integrated, community-based healthcare they need. These findings also suggest a need to educate doctors about the care of people with schizophrenia.

Lawrie, S.M. et al. (1998) General practitioners' attitudes to psychiatric and medical illness. *Psychological Medicine, 28*: 1463–1467.

Summary

- Group membership is an important part of individual identity.
- Different social roles entail different rights and obligations. In medicine, social roles influence the behaviour of doctors and patients (e.g. the sick role).
- People tend to conform to the expectations of the groups to which they belong.
- People often obey leaders without questioning – sometimes even when what they are being asked to do is harmful to others.
- Group decision making can be impaired by the tendency toward conformity and because alternative positions are not considered.
- Effective leadership involves the appropriate use of authority and the best use of the skills and capacities of group members.
- Stereotypes are cognitive short-cuts which are a core aspect of prejudices. They can exert important influences on behaviour, including health-related behaviour.

CLINICAL NOTES 9.3

Avoiding prejudice and careless assumptions in healthcare

- Be aware of your attitudes toward different groups of people – whether they are ethnic groups, particular types of patients, or particular professions in healthcare.
- Ensure that your attitudes do not affect your treatment of different patients.
- The fundamental attribution error means we are prone to assume that people's behaviour is due to them and not their circumstances.
- Remember that people's behaviour is often strongly influenced by their history or current social circumstances – do not assume people are intrinsically difficult or badly motivated.

9.4 ANTI SOCIAL AND PROSOCIAL BEHAVIOUR

9.4.1 AGGRESSION

Aggression involves behaviours that are enacted to cause physical or psychological harm or pain to another person. Aggression can be actual (e.g. physical attacks) or symbolic (e.g. burning flags). Different explanations of aggression are outlined below. Strategies for dealing with angry or aggressive people are covered in Chapter 18.

The frustration-aggression hypothesis (Berkowitz, 1989) argues that when we are prevented from achieving our goals we become frustrated and this can lead to aggression.

Although frustration may be important in the lead-up to aggression, it cannot be the sole answer. For example, if someone is frustrated because a library book they want has not been returned they do not automatically become violent, because they know that the library is not an appropriate place for aggressive behaviour. The cue-arousal theory of aggression therefore argues that frustration is more likely to lead to aggression if there are situational cues that aggression is appropriate (Geen & O'Neal, 1969). In medical contexts, such situational cues may include rude or aggressive behaviour that is exhibited by other patients or medical professionals. Other important situational factors include the effects of alcohol and other drugs, which may impair cognition or reduce inhibitions against violent behaviour.

A review of research revealed that patient aggression and violence are prominent occupational hazards for medical professionals: half of all healthcare professionals working in general hospitals have experienced verbal assaults, and one-quarter have experienced physical assaults (Hahn et al., 2008). These assaults can have a serious negative impact on staff wellbeing (Schablon et al., 2012). Aggression and violence may be more common in particular settings, such as inpatient geriatric care settings, and younger staff may be more vulnerable to assault (Schablon et al., 2012). It has been suggested that people who are anxious or in pain pay more attention to threatening stimuli and that aggression may be a response to increased feelings of threat (Winstanley, 2005).

The likelihood of aggressive behaviour appears to be influenced by organisational procedures, such as prolonged waiting times, which can increase patient frustration, and by medical procedures that induce pain or anxiety (Hahn et al., 2008). Training staff to deal better with aggressive or violent people can reduce the risk that they will experience verbal or physical assaults, and it can reduce the negative emotional impact of assaults that do occur (Schablon et al., 2012).

People with certain conditions may be more likely to become aggressive. This can be particularly likely in dementia or psychiatric conditions characterised by cognitive impairments, delusions, or disinhibition (see Chapter 16). However, situational factors are important because not all people with such conditions will become aggressive or violent. The fundamental attribution error referred to earlier is also evident in that healthcare professionals tend to attribute aggressive behaviour among people with psychiatric diagnoses to internal characteristics such as delusional thoughts or stress, whereas people tend to attribute their aggressive behaviour to external or situational factors such as being provoked, teased, or 'bugged' by staff (Nolan et al., 2009).

Summary

- Several different theories of aggression have been put forward. Although there is support for most theories, no single theory explains all acts of aggression.
- Aggressive behaviour appears to be a combination of individual tendencies toward aggression, the psychological state of the individual at a particular time, and situational cues or stressors.

9.4.2 PROSOCIAL BEHAVIOUR

Although social psychology often focuses on why people engage in undesirable behaviours like aggression and prejudice, many researchers focus on positive social behaviours such as helping and altruism. Such prosocial behaviours include the activities of medical professionals and other healthcare workers (although people might not engage in such behaviours for purely altruistic reasons).

Altruistic behaviours are prosocial behaviours that we engage in without expecting to be rewarded – although the feeling of 'doing good' that arises from altruistic behaviours may be a form of reward in itself. Some people would argue that our capacity for empathy explains why we do help others: we can imagine what it would be like to be in their position, so we try to help them (Batson et al., 1981). Others would argue that we choose to help others to relieve our own distress at seeing someone in need of help (Cialdini et al., 1987). It is also possible that people engage in seemingly altruistic behaviours because they expect a reward or recognition in the future (e.g. we may do voluntary work because we think it will look good on our CV). Consenting to donate one's organs can be seen to be purely altruistic because there is no possibility of a reward for such behaviour. However, the knowledge that we will be helping others after we die can also be construed as a reward.

In more mundane everyday circumstances, the likelihood that we will help others is influenced by our perceptions of the costs and benefits of helping. We are more likely to help others if we perceive that doing so will not be too taxing for us in terms of time, effort, and emotion (Piliavin et al., 1969). For example, we are less likely to help someone get their cat out of a tree if we are rushing to a job interview. This principle helps to explain mobile blood donation services. Such services eliminate some of the time and money costs associated with donation, thereby increasing the attractiveness of this behaviour.

In addition to being influenced by perceived personal costs and benefits, the likelihood of helping others is influenced by our perceptions of whether other people are helping. Social learning and modelling concepts (see Chapter 10) suggest that we are more likely to help if we can see others doing so, and less likely to help if we see others not getting involved. In situations where nobody helps this can be because of a diffusion of responsibility. Each individual assumes that somebody else will take responsibility for helping, with the net result that nobody does so (Latané & Darley, 1970). This can be illustrated by the fact that people are more likely to help when they are not in groups. For example, if a person has an epileptic seizure, people are more likely to help if they are the only bystander, but the likelihood of helping will decrease as the number of inactive bystanders increases. A review of published research indicated strong evidence for the bystander effect, but also found that this effect was weaker in dangerous emergency situations (Fischer et al., 2011).

Social cues to helping can be used to encourage prosocial behaviour (just as social cues may encourage aggression). Examples include the coloured badges, ribbons, and wristbands worn to demonstrate support for various charities. These are in some part symbolic of a material exchange – e.g. you donate money so you get a reward. They are also a public demonstration of commitment and a signal to others that they should also consider supporting the cause.

Summary

- Altruistic behaviours are helping or prosocial behaviours that people do for others with no expectation of a personal reward.
- The likelihood of helping appears to be influenced by the personal costs and benefits of helping.
- The behaviour of others is also a cue for helping behaviour. We are more likely to help if we can see others helping, or if there are no other people available to offer help.

FURTHER READING

Hogg, M.A. & Vaughan, G.M. (2013) *Social Psychology* (7th edition). Harlow: Pearson Prentice Hall. A good introduction to a wide range of social psychology topics. However, this book is designed for psychology students, so it lacks a specific focus on the application of key concepts to health contexts.

Stroebe, W. (2011) *Social Psychology and Health* (3rd edition). London: McGraw-Hill Education. This book discusses health and related interventions from a social psychological perspective.

REVISION QUESTIONS

1. What is meant by the term 'cognitive dissonance'? How can it be used to encourage healthy behaviour?

2. Outline the characteristics of messages and messengers that will increase the likelihood that people will respond to them in positive ways.

3. How does the clothing doctors wear affect people's perceptions of them? Why is this the case?

4. How can perceived discrepancies between people's actual and ideal selves prompt behaviour change? Give one healthy example and one unhealthy example.

5. What is meant by the 'fundamental attribution error'? Give two health-related examples of this phenomenon.

6. What is meant by the term 'sick role'? What does it mean to say that doctors are 'gatekeepers' of the sick role?

7. How well does the proverb 'Many hands make light work' apply to medical decision making? Discuss with reference to the concepts of conformity and groupthink.

8. What is a stereotype? What is the link between stereotypes and prejudice?

9. Why is the cue-arousal theory likely to be a better explanation of aggression than the frustration-aggression hypothesis?

10. Describe the characteristics of situations that make it more likely that people will help others.

10 PERCEPTION, ATTENTION, LEARNING, AND MEMORY

(Continued)

LEARNING OBJECTIVES

This chapter is designed to enable you to:

- Describe perceptual processes and give examples of how these are relevant to medical settings.
- Understand the processes of attention and how they contribute to medical errors.
- Describe classical and operant conditioning and discuss how these can be used in clinical practice.
- Understand the characteristics of short- and long-term memory.
- Use this information to help devise effective ways to revise for exams.

Learning to be a medical professional involves the accumulation of knowledge, clinical, and surgical skills – all of which are driven by cognitive processes of perception, attention, learning, and memory. Understanding how these processes work can help us in a wide variety of ways. We can find better ways to learn, be more alert to the conditions under which medical errors might occur, and help people to change behaviours, such as helping children with eczema to stop scratching. In this chapter we shall look at perception, attention, learning, and memory, with examples of how these are relevant to medicine.

10.1 PERCEPTION

Perception involves the way information from our environment is transformed via our senses (sight, hearing, smell, touch, and taste) into experience. It is helpful to clarify the difference between perception and attention, which we shall look at in the next section. **Attention** refers to those aspects of our environment we focus on and process.

Let us start with visual perception because, on the surface at least, this appears quite straightforward. Light from the environment is projected onto our retina and transformed into electrical impulses by the rods, cones, and ganglion cells of the retina. These impulses are transmitted via the optic nerve to the visual cortex where we 'see' the image. However, the mind has a strong influence on how we interpret stimuli. Activity 10.1 is an example of this.

ACTIVITY 10.1

How many F and T letters are there in this sentence?

'INFERTILITY TREATMENT IS THE RESULT OF YEARS OF SCIENTIFIC STUDY COMBINED WITH THE EXPERTISE OF CLINICIANS'

Many get the task in Activity 10.1 wrong because we tend to process small and frequently used words, such as 'the' and 'of', as single units. This makes it much harder to 'see' the individual letters in these words. Visual perception is therefore a combination of visual stimuli (bottom-up processing) and our existing knowledge (top-down processing). Other examples of top-down processing are size and shape constancy and depth perception. In size and shape constancy, an object is perceived as remaining the same despite the

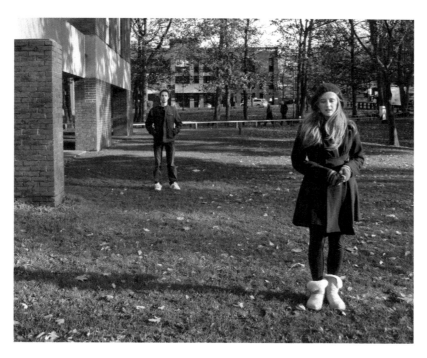

FIGURE 10.1   Size constancy and depth perception

fact that it appears larger as we move toward it and changes shape depending on the angle we see it from. Our mind knows that most objects do not change shape, so therefore concludes that we are moving and seeing it from different perspectives.

This knowledge is used in the perception of depth. For example, we know that people are approximately similar in size. In Figure 10.1 we can therefore see that the person in the background is further away from the camera. In this instance, our previous knowledge about people's size gives us clues about depth. Our interpretation of it happens very rapidly at an unconscious level. This effect is so strong it can even override our conscious perceptual processes. Compare the size of the image of the person in the background with the image of the person in the foreground. How much smaller would you say the person in the background is, compared to the person in the foreground? Now look at Figure 10.2, in which the image is actually brought forward in the picture. You probably would not have judged the image to be this small because size constancy and depth perception automatically biased your judgement.

The study of perception has established that not only are we unable to realise the extent of some true differences (such as the difference in size between the two people in Figure 10.2), but that we are also quite selective and biased in what we perceive. The underlying concept here is that of perceptual sets, where the influence of attention, previous experience, and motivation is combined so we perceive information that is relevant to us, both as humans and individuals. A perceptual set is influenced by the factors summarised in Box 10.1. Threshold for perception is where one stimulus has a lower or higher threshold for perception than others. If someone shouts 'Fire' it is more likely to get your attention than if they shout 'Air'. Similarly, in a noisy environment where lots of people are talking, you might suddenly become aware that someone across the room has said your name. This is because you will naturally have a lower threshold for 'hearing' your name.

The influence of past experience is evident through the effects of size constancy and depth perception. Past experience, expectations, and individual values will combine to influence perception in more subtle ways as well. For example, poor children and adults overestimate the size of coins compared to more affluent people (Ashley et al., 1951). In healthcare contexts, experiments of symptom perception show that just telling people a stimulus might be painful makes them more likely to report pain in response to it (Colloca et al., 2008). The placebo and nocebo effects provide classic examples of the role of expectations and learning in the perception of symptoms (see Chapter 4). Research suggests that expectancies influence pain intensity processing in the central nervous system (Atlas & Wager, 2012).

Current drive state affects what we perceive in different ways. First, our level of arousal determines how much attention we will pay to our environment. When we are sleeping we do not consciously perceive much, if anything, of our external environment unless there is a large change, such as a loud noise or a change in temperature. The processes through which people perceive stimuli when in a low level of consciousness are important in anaesthesia. Anaesthesia aims to remove conscious awareness, yet approximately 1% of people report some perception during surgery (see Research Box 10.1). Second, our motivational state will also determine what we pay attention to in our environment. For example, when we are hungry we are more likely to notice food-related stimuli (Seibt et al., 2007).

BOX 10.1   **Factors that influence perceptual sets**

- Threshold for perception
- Past experience
- Current drive state
- Emotions
- Individual values
- Environment
- Cultural background and experience

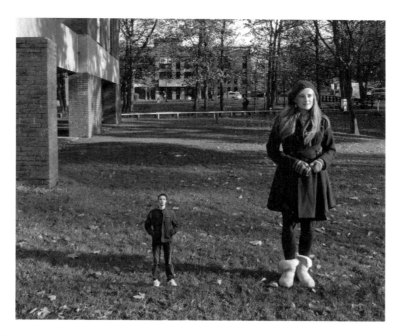

FIGURE 10.2   Size constancy and depth perception

Emotions affect what we attend to and perceive. It has been well established that anxiety results in an increased perception of threat and a narrowing of attention onto threatening stimuli (Ouimet et al., 2009). Perceptual changes can also be seen for positive emotions. Classic studies of young children's perception of Santa Claus found that before Christmas children's drawings of Santa Claus were much larger and more elaborate than after Christmas – suggesting children's emotional state influenced their perception and representation of Santa Claus (Sechrest & Wallis, 1964).

RESEARCH BOX 10.1   Awareness and memory during anaesthesia

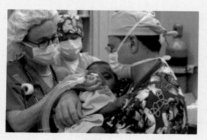

Photo courtesy of U.S. Navy photo by Mass Communication Specialist Seaman Joseph Caballero

Background

Epidemiological research has shown that awareness during anaesthesia is more likely during some types of surgery, in people who have a history of awareness, are obese, use central nervous system depressant drugs, and who are younger – particularly children. This study looked at awareness and memory in children during surgery.

Method and findings

184 children aged 5–18 were tested for awareness and memory during surgery via various means:

1. During surgery children were told to squeeze their hand if they could hear (awareness).
2. During surgery words were played 20 times then children were tested after surgery for their increased recognition of these words (implicit memory).
3. After surgery children were asked if they remembered anything from the surgery (explicit memory).

Children could not explicitly recall the events of surgery or recognise the words played during surgery. However, two children (1%) showed awareness during surgery by responding to the command to squeeze their hand. These two children were similar to the rest of the sample in terms of type of surgery, anaesthetic technique, and previous history.

Significance

This study added to existing evidence by using in-surgery techniques to measure awareness and memory in children. The 1% of children who showed awareness during surgery is similar to that reported by adults. However, it is interesting that these children had no implicit or explicit memory for surgical events.

Andrade, J., Deeprose, C. & Barker, I. (2008) Awareness and memory function during paediatric anaesthesia. *British Journal of Anaesthesia, 100*(3): 389–396.

The environment provides the external stimuli that we interpret into experience. Despite top-down influences and our perceptual set, most of us are remarkably accurate in what we see. This is partly due to our previous experiences of the environment which can help us interpret what is happening. However, sometimes our knowledge of the environment can override what we see and result in a distorted perception. A classic example of this is the Ames room – a specially constructed room where the walls, window, and floor are faked to look like a square room when the back wall is in fact on the diagonal. This means that if a person in the room walks from one corner to the other they appear to shrink or grow. In reality this is because they are walking further away. However, to a viewer, the perceptual cues that the room is square can override this so they 'see' the impossible, i.e. that the person shrinks or grows as they walk (there are many examples of the Ames illusion on www.youtube.com).

Cultural factors influence perception less than might be expected. Many aspects of visual perception are consistent across cultures. One of the strongest effects of culture on perception is that we are quicker and better at recognising people of our own ethnic group compared to people of another ethnic group (Meissner & Brigham, 2001). This can influence how healthcare professionals interact with people of different ethnicity. A review of cultural influences on doctor–patient communication found that consultations with people from ethnic minorities involve less emotional expression by the doctor and patient, and less verbal expression by patients. The authors concluded that perceptual biases contributed to culture-related communication difficulties in medical consultations (Schouten & Meeuwesen, 2006).

So far we have discussed the influence of perceptual sets on normal visual perception. However, we also need to understand abnormal perceptual processes. These are relevant to many disorders, including autism and schizophrenia. For example, people with autism and people with anti social characteristics both have poor perception of facial expressions of emotion (Marsh & Blair, 2008). Schizophrenia and other psychotic experiences are particularly interesting because they involve the perception of illusory events as real. Research suggests that psychotic-type thinking is more likely when people with schizotypal characteristics are put in situations of perceptual ambiguity and overload (Grave et al., 2017; Tsakanikos, 2006). This type of research could eventually help us to understand more about the conditions that trigger psychotic symptoms, which in turn could inform the treatment and management of schizophrenia.

Summary

- Perception is the way information from our environment is transformed and interpreted into experience.
- Perception is the combination of environmental stimuli (bottom-up processing) and existing knowledge (top-down processing).
- A perceptual set is where attention, previous experience, and motivation determine the information each person perceives.
- Perceptual sets can be influenced by thresholds for perception, past experience, individual values, current drive state, emotions, environment, and culture.

10.2 ATTENTION

Attention is the ability to select information in the environment to attend to and process. Attention is therefore an important part of perception, learning, and performance – particularly in situations where we need to multitask (i.e. divide our attention between different tasks). What we attend to and how much attention we pay to it is influenced by our physical arousal, motivation, and emotion. Attention can also be biased by these factors. Knowledge of how attention works can therefore help us understand errors in medicine, such as giving wrong drug dosages or making surgical errors.

Attention involves many different mental processes and it would be wrong to think in terms of a single attentional system. For example, studies of people with brain damage show they often have problems with some aspects of attention but not all (Posner & Petersen, 1990). Attention can be voluntary, such as when we concentrate on learning or doing a task, or involuntary, such as when a loud noise or sudden movement grabs our attention. Attention has been likened to a spotlight or filter that can have either a broad or narrow focus. When attention is focused, central information is processed in detail but peripheral information may be ignored or lost. To be able to function well in various situations, we need to be able to:

- Focus our attention on a particular stimulus.
- Remove or disengage our attention from a stimulus.
- Shift attention between different stimuli.

Attention is intertwined with cognitive processes of perception and memory (see Figure 10.3). **Sensory buffers** are short-term stores of incoming information that can be used to select which information to attend to consciously. Auditory sensory buffers register all incoming sounds for a few seconds, so this information is potentially recoverable during this time. A good example of this is when we 'tune out' of a conversation for a few seconds but can then replay what was just said in our head. This is especially useful if we are accused of not listening to what someone has just said!

Many theories of attention propose that we have a **limited capacity processor** that restricts the amount of information we can consciously attend to. Research has broadly confirmed this, although capacity is not as fixed as this implies. There is evidence that we can still unconsciously perceive information not attended to and that our capacity to

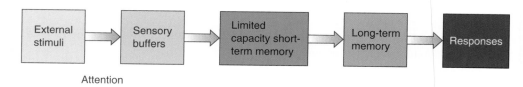

FIGURE 10.3 Cognitive processes

process information or to multitask increases as tasks become more practised or automatic and hence demand less conscious attention. For example, neuroimaging research indicates that even when we do not consciously attend to stimuli, there is similar but weaker neurological activation in the same parts of the brain that are activated during conscious attention (Talsma et al., 2010; Vuilleumier, 2005).

10.2.1 ATTENTION AND CLINICAL SKILLS

Clinical skills are essential for medical practice. During your training you will learn skills such as clinical interviewing, physical examinations, and medical procedures. Skill acquisition draws on the processes illustrated in Figure 10.3. Learning a new skill demands our concentrated attention, short-term memory, cognitive motor processes, and effortful responses. Initially, attention is needed for both perception and response stages. As we learn and practise a skill it gradually becomes easier and requires less of our attention or concentration. There are three broad stages in skill acquisition (Adams, 1971):

1. *Cognitive stage* – development of a mental representation of the skill and how to perform it. At this stage learning usually relies on explicit instruction through teaching from an expert, demonstration, and self-observation (e.g. relying on a senior colleague to tell you what to do when taking blood).
2. *Associative stage* – an effective motor programme has been developed so the person is able to carry out the broad skill but lacks the ability to perform finer subtasks with fluency. Development is guided by knowledge or feedback (e.g. able to drive but consciously aware of actions such as turning the wheel and changing gear).
3. *Autonomous stage* – the skill is largely automatic and relies on implicit knowledge and motor coordination, rather than explicit instruction (e.g. able to drive automatically without conscious effort).

Studies of skill acquisition show that practice is more important than aptitude. For example, hours of practice are the strongest predictor of musical ability – more so than musical aptitude, parents' musical ability, and social class (Sloboda et al., 1994). If learning or practice is spaced out over time it also improves learning (see the section on Memory). In the healthcare context, similar principles appear to apply – practice, with appropriate supervision and feedback, is crucial to developing expertise (Ericsson, 2004).

Multitasking is easiest when the skills are automatic and the tasks are not too similar or complex. You might write an essay while listening to music or talk to someone while driving a car. However, even under easy conditions, multitasking entails competing processes which will influence how each task is carried out. For example, using a phone while driving results in slower response times, a reduced ability to notice when the car in front slows down, and less attention to sensory inputs. This effect on driving appears to occur regardless of whether the phone is hands-free (Briggs et al., 2016). Studies of attention have shown that incorrect actions or mistakes are most likely:

- When the correct response is not the strongest or most habitual.
- When our full attention is not given to the task.
- Under conditions of stress and anxiety.

The advantage of developing a skill to the autonomous stage is that it frees up our attention for multitasking (although other tasks will still impinge on the automatic one). The disadvantage is that automatic behaviour is no longer consciously controlled so it is possible to make mistakes. This is particularly relevant to medicine: it is estimated that in the USA alone over 200,000 patients die every year from preventable mistakes (Ferner & McDowell, 2006). Studies of manslaughter cases against doctors over the last century indicate that the majority of cases arise from errors in administering or prescribing medication. Other types of error are wrong treatment or diagnosis and surgical errors (see Research Box 10.2).

RESEARCH BOX 10.2   Medical mistakes and manslaughter

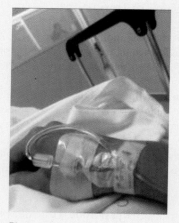

Photo courtesy of Leo Carbajal, February 2013

Background

Medical errors sometimes lead to patient death. It is therefore important to identify the causes the of medical errors and to find ways to prevent them from happening.

Method and findings

Newspapers and journal archives in the UK were searched to identify legal cases where doctors were charged with manslaughter to examine the causes of death. Between 1795 and 2005, 85 doctors were charged with manslaughter, with a large increase in prosecutions since 1990. The majority of doctors were acquitted: only 29% were convicted or pleaded guilty. The main causes of manslaughter were as follows.

Mistakes (44%): errors in planning

For example, a 20-year-old man with muscular dystrophy died after circumcision. The surgeon guessed the man's weight and inadvertently gave three times the recommended dose of lidocaine. He was charged with manslaughter but acquitted.

Slips (20%): errors due to distraction or a failure of concentration

For example, a 6-week-old boy died after cardiac arrest during surgery for pyloric stenosis. The anaesthetist injected air into the bloodstream instead of the nasogastric tube. The anaesthetist was charged with manslaughter but acquitted.

(Continued)

Violations (19%): deliberate violation of medical practice

For example, a 2-year-old boy died from hypoxia that occurred during a hernia operation. The anaesthetist had deliberately inhaled anaesthetic before and during the operation. He was charged with manslaughter and found guilty.

Technical errors (4%): failure to carry out an action successfully even though the plan of action and technique were appropriate

For example, a 16-year-old girl being treated for leukaemia died after an attempt to insert a Hickman line (central venous catheter) caused cardiac rupture. The surgeon was charged with manslaughter but acquitted.

Significance

Nearly two-thirds of patient deaths brought to prosecution are due to unconscious errors (mistakes or slips) that could be a direct consequence of automatic behaviour. The authors argue that the prosecution of individual doctors would not improve patient safety as much as changing healthcare systems to incorporate checks that reduce such errors.

Ferner, R.E. & McDowell, S.E. (2006) Doctors charged with manslaughter in the course of medical practice, 1795–2005: A literature review. *Journal of the Royal Society of Medicine*, 99: 309–314.

Skilled surgeons will carry out surgery relatively automatically at the same time as doing other things, such as listening to music (which is quite common). Although music can be quite calming emotionally and physically, research into attention suggests that if something goes wrong and quick decisions or actions are required, music will interfere with our ability to focus attention on the emergency situation and responses. Research suggests this is particularly the case for novice surgeons. Miskovic et al. (2008) examined surgical skill in junior doctors who carried out simulated (virtual reality) laparoscopies with no music, calming music, or lively music. Junior doctors who did not listen to music were almost three times better at the simulated laparoscopy than those listening to music. This difference was less obvious once junior doctors had had more practice, illustrating the effect of practice and automaticity. Other research into surgical skill showed that student and junior doctors' performance was strongly affected by the context and that adverse events were usually preceded by individual errors, often in response to contextual factors, as summarised in Figure 10.4.

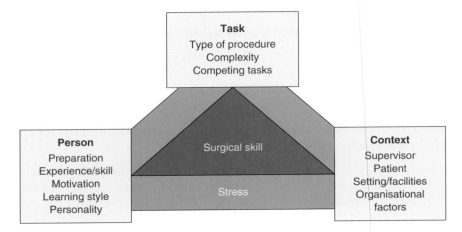

FIGURE 10.4   Influences on surgical skill (adapted from Schout et al., 2010)

10.2.2 BIASED ATTENTION

As with perception, attention is biased toward certain stimuli. Normal and abnormal biases have been found. Normal biases include being more likely to attend to faces and emotional stimuli. For example, infants will spend more time looking at faces or face-shaped stimuli than other shapes (Dannemiller & Stephens, 1988). Studies of reaction times to different objects have shown we are quicker to pay attention to emotional items and take longer to disengage from them. Neuropsychological research shows emotional stimuli will produce stronger neurological responses than neutral stimuli regardless of whether they are visual or auditory. In other words, if we see emotional expressions or hear emotional voices, we will have stronger neurological responses than we do to neutral expressions or voices (Vuilleumier & Huang, 2009).

Attention is biased in some psychological disorders. People with eating disorders are more likely to attend to stimuli that are food, body, or weight related (Aspen et al., 2013). Anxious people are more likely to attend to threat-related stimuli and may be hypervigilant for particular stimuli. This is the case in generalised anxiety disorder, obsessive-compulsive disorder, post-traumatic stress disorder (PTSD), and phobias. For example, a person with a blood phobia will continually scan the environment for signs of blood, which takes up cognitive processing and attentional resources. In other psychological disorders, normal biases may be disrupted. For example, a review of studies of pregnant women and new mothers revealed that compared to non-depressed women, mothers with depression or anxiety are more likely to identify negative emotions such as sadness in infants' faces and less accurate at identifying positive emotions such as happiness (Webb & Ayers, 2015).

Emotions are also important in how attention is directed and focused. Positive emotions are associated with a broadening of attention and negative emotions with a narrowing of attention onto particular stimuli (Vuilleumier & Huang, 2009). This can have various repercussions. On the one hand, narrowing our attention in emergency situations is useful because it helps us focus on the problem and what actions are needed to resolve it. On the other hand, this narrow focus means subsidiary or peripheral information is potentially ignored or less likely to be picked up. There are many examples of accidents that have occurred because vital information has been missed and mistakes made (Esgate & Groome, 2005). Knowledge of attention processes shows that, to a certain extent, slips and mistakes are inevitable parts of being human. It is therefore important to recognise the role of systems and organisations in such circumstances. If adequate systems of checking and monitoring are in place, then individual errors are more likely to be caught and corrected before they have severe consequences. The World Health Organisation has produced such a checklist for surgical safety (WHO, 2009c).

Summary

- Attention concerns the ability to select information in the environment to attend to and process.
- Attention influences the way in which we perceive, process, and respond to stimuli.
- Learning new skills involves concentrated attention, short-term memory, cognitive motor processes, and effortful responses.
- There are three stages involved in learning skills: cognitive, associative, and autonomous.
- At the autonomous stage, skilled behaviour can be carried out without conscious or effortful control.
- Multitasking requires divided attention and is easiest when one or both tasks are practised and automatic.
- Mistakes are most likely when the correct response is not strongest or habitual, when our full attention is not given to the task, and in conditions of stress or anxiety.
- Attentional biases include a bias toward emotional expressions and voices and the influence of emotions on the breadth of attentional focus.
- Abnormal biases are found in some psychological disorders where people show a bias toward stimuli that are relevant to that disorder.

10.3 LEARNING

Learning can be defined as the acquisition of knowledge or skills through experience, observing, studying, or being taught. **Associative learning** is how we learn the relationship between two events that occur together. For example, if one event occurs at the same time as another it indicates a temporal relationship; if one event always follows another it indicates a causal (and temporal) relationship. Different learning processes have a range of implications for healthcare, both in terms of your own learning and helping patients to recover and change their behaviour. Key learning processes include classical conditioning, operant conditioning, modelling, and imitation. Conditioning processes are particularly useful when working with young children or people with cognitive impairments who are less likely to change their behaviour in response to verbal reasoning.

10.3.1 CLASSICAL CONDITIONING

Classical conditioning is best known and illustrated by the work of Pavlov and his dogs. Dogs have a normal reflex to salivate when food is presented. Food is therefore an unconditioned stimulus and salivation is an unconditioned response because it occurs naturally without learning. Pavlov noticed that his dogs began to salivate at other times, such as when he entered the room, because they had learned that he was associated with being fed. Pavlov formally demonstrated classical conditioning by ringing a bell just before feeding the dogs. The bell was initially a neutral stimulus because it was not associated with food and did not produce salivation. However, after a short while the dogs began to salivate when they heard the bell. The bell had therefore become a conditioned stimulus and salivation to the bell a conditioned response because the dogs had learned the association between the bell and food.

Many other characteristics of classical conditioning have been identified. For example, the *nature of the stimulus* is important, as some stimuli are more easily conditioned than others. Novel food or drinks are more readily associated with physical symptoms such as nausea. This is probably due to biological mechanisms that encourage learning in situations that may be dangerous – in this case to prevent us eating poisonous foods. Therefore, if a novel food is associated with illness or vomiting most of us will develop an aversion to that food.

ACTIVITY 10.2

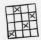

- Is there a food that you particularly dislike and will not eat? What learning processes do you think this might be due to?

The *order and timing of the stimulus* will also determine whether conditioning takes place. The neutral stimulus (e.g. a bell) must be presented very shortly (e.g. half a second) before the unconditioned stimulus (e.g. the food) for conditioning to occur. If it is presented afterwards very little or no conditioning will take place.

Finally, conditioning can be blocked or unlearned. Once classical conditioning has occurred, then attempts to condition a third stimulus can be blocked. In other words, once dogs learn that the bell predicts food they will not always respond if a third stimulus is introduced, such as a flashing light, but may continue to rely on the bell. Conditioning can be *extinguished* or undone by presenting the conditioned stimulus (e.g. bell) repeatedly without the unconditioned stimulus (e.g. food).

Classical conditioning and physical symptoms

Many physical responses can be classically conditioned, including immune and neuroendocrine responses (Figure 10.5), allergy symptoms, and nausea. Classical conditioning is therefore highly relevant to medicine and occurs in many clinical situations, especially where illness or treatment involves pain or other adverse symptoms. The sights, sounds, or smells associated with hospitals may induce physical and emotional responses such as anxiety, or nausea. A good example of classical conditioning involves chemotherapy. Cytotoxic drugs can often have strong side effects, such as nausea and vomiting, and up to 30% of people undergoing chemotherapy will experience anticipatory nausea and vomiting by the fourth session of chemotherapy (Kamen et al., 2014). This is because some aspects of the hospital environment become associated with symptoms of nausea and vomiting through classical conditioning. Thus, when people are re-exposed to the hospital stimulus associated with chemotherapy they will feel nauseous or vomit.

Our understanding of classical conditioning can be used to reduce symptoms or induce positive physical responses. For example, we know that physical symptoms are more easily conditioned in response to novel food or liquid. We also know that once conditioning has occurred it can block a third stimulus becoming conditioned. Research has confirmed that giving people a novel drink before each chemotherapy infusion prevents anticipatory nausea and even shortens the time that nausea is experienced during chemotherapy because they associate nausea with the drink and not the hospital context (Stockhorst et al., 1998). This has also been demonstrated with allergy symptoms. If people are given a novel drink just before taking antihistamine drugs for five days, the drink alone will start to trigger the same drop in basophil activity and improvement in symptoms as the antihistamine drug (Goebel et al., 2008). Classical conditioning therefore plays an important role in placebo effects (see Chapter 4) and may underpin many of the effects of complementary and alternative therapies.

Classical conditioning and psychological problems

Classical conditioning can be involved in the development of psychological problems such as phobias. A traumatic experience can lead to a particular object becoming associated with severe anxiety and fear. Subsequent exposure to this object can then trigger severe anxiety and, if the person then avoids the object, a phobia may develop. An example of this is needle phobia, which can develop following a negative experience of an injection or blood test. To treat phobias we need to extinguish the learned association by exposing the person to the

Decreasing and enhancing the immune function using classical conditioning

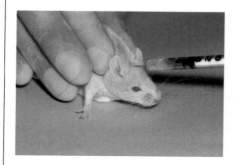

The immune system can be conditioned using classical conditioning to decrease or improve the immune function with a previously neutral stimulus. Studies typically pair a drug that suppresses or enhances the immune system with a new taste, such as saccharin, then re-administer the saccharin at a later date without the immune altering drug, to see if the immune function is affected.

The immune system can be suppressed or enhanced in this way through classical conditioning, although the effects are small (Ader, 2003). Research in humans has shown a similar conditioning of symptoms, such as anticipatory nausea before chemotherapy.

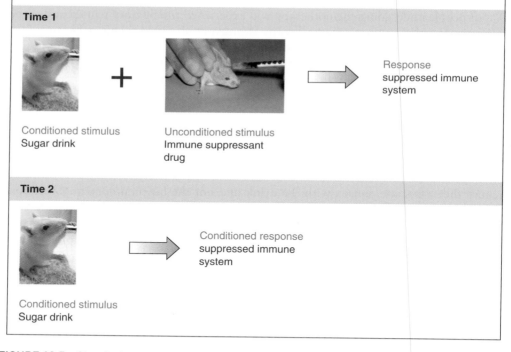

Time 1

Conditioned stimulus
Sugar drink

Unconditioned stimulus
Immune suppressant drug

Response
suppressed immune system

Time 2

Conditioned stimulus
Sugar drink

Conditioned response
suppressed immune system

FIGURE 10.5 Classical conditioning and placebo. Photograph of mouse drinking reproduced courtesy of © Edstrom. Photograph of mouse being injected reproduced courtesy of the Comparative Biology Centre, Newcastle University

object while reducing or minimising the conditioned response. This is usually done through flooding or systematic desensitisation, which are based on the fact that strong anxiety responses cannot be sustained indefinitely. Flooding therefore involves exposing a person to the feared stimulus for a long enough time so that their anxiety reduces and the association between the stimulus and anxiety is extinguished. However, this is very hard for people with phobias to accomplish because it is an extreme way to face their fear.

Systematic desensitisation is a more gradual procedure where people are taught relaxation techniques and gradually exposed to stronger versions of the feared object or situation. For example, a person with a needle phobia might be asked to imagine a needle while relaxing. Once they are relaxed in this situation they might repeat it while looking at a picture of a needle, then a real needle, then perhaps a nurse giving someone else an injection. Thus they can learn to relax when exposed to the feared stimulus and the association is gradually extinguished. Research shows that both flooding and systematic desensitisation are highly effective treatments for phobias (Wolitzky-Taylor et al., 2008). Advances in technology mean that information technology can be used to deliver systematic desensitization programmes for medically-relevant phobias (Armfield & Heaton, 2013).

10.3.2 OPERANT CONDITIONING

Operant conditioning is learning from the consequences of our behaviour and reinforcement. In operant conditioning, behaviour is shaped by whether it results in positive reinforcement (e.g. a reward) or negative reinforcement (e.g. a punishment). In particular, behaviour is very quickly learned if it is followed by positive reinforcement, such as food or praise. Primary reinforcers are those needed for survival, such as water, food, sleep, and sex. Secondary reinforcers are those that acquire value through experience, such as money, praise, and attention. People's behaviour can therefore be 'shaped' by reinforcement. Different patterns of reinforcement are given in Box 10.2 and vary in effectiveness. Variable ratio patterns of reinforcement usually lead to the strongest responses and are hardest to extinguish. This may partly explain why gamblers often find it hard to stop. It also has repercussions for drug abuse treatment. For example, methadone blocks the positive effects of heroin, but if it is used intermittently and the drug user gets occasional highs from heroin, they are on a variable ratio pattern of reinforcement and may find it even harder to stop.

BOX 10.2   Patterns of reinforcement

- Fixed ratio: behaviour is always rewarded after a fixed number of times (e.g. bonuses when you reach a target).
- Variable ratio: behaviour is usually rewarded after an average number of times but this varies (e.g. gambling).
- Fixed interval: behaviour is rewarded after a fixed time interval (e.g. once a week).
- Variable interval: behaviour is rewarded but at varying time intervals.

In contrast to positive reinforcement, negative reinforcement reduces or extinguishes behaviours. Negative reinforcement can occur in two ways. The first is if the behaviour results in the removal of an aversive stimulus. For example, taking drugs that relieve pain will reinforce the use of painkillers. This kind of reinforcement is highly relevant to avoidance or escape behaviours where people learn to avoid situations that hurt them or make them anxious. The second form of negative reinforcement is punishment where the behaviour results in aversive consequences. Research has shown that punishment is much weaker than positive reinforcers and any effect of punishment is short-lived. In fact, it has been argued that punishment only suppresses a response, rather than leading to new learning. This may explain why a hangover is not enough to stop people drinking again! Given this knowledge, it is odd that our society places so much emphasis on punishment, from disciplining children to our penal system (Eysenck, 2000).

Operant conditioning and medicine

Operant conditioning shows that to learn and improve at any task, including medicine, we need feedback on our performance – preferably immediately – and this feedback is most powerful if it is positive. Operant conditioning can be used by healthcare professionals to encourage adaptive behaviours and is particularly useful with children or people with cognitive impairments (see Case Study 10.1). Research with people with severe learning disabilities shows that behaviours such as destructive outbursts or refusing to eat can be changed very effectively by positively reinforcing an alternative behaviour (Petscher et al., 2009). Operant conditioning can also be useful for families caring for ill relatives. For example, chronic pain behaviours can be reinforced if families are overly sympathetic, or urge the person to lie down or rest and do everything for them. Although the family may believe they are doing the right thing, in the long term it will lead to more pain behaviour. Hence, families need to learn to ignore pain behaviour and respond positively to non-pain behaviour.

10.3.3 MODELLING AND IMITATION

Social learning theory has shown that we also learn by observing and imitating others. In a series of famous experiments, Bandura showed that when children observed an adult being aggressive toward a life-size doll they were more likely to do the same when playing with the doll (Bandura et al., 1961). A meta-analysis of research conducted using various experimental designs found that whereas playing violent video games increases aggression and aggression-related variables and decreases prosocial outcomes, playing prosocial video games has the opposite effects (Greitemeyer & Mügge, 2014). However, social learning cannot account for all of our behaviour, because we do not imitate the behaviour of everyone we encounter. Social learning is more likely to take place if the person is seen to be rewarded, is high status (e.g. a teacher, a medical consultant), is similar to us (e.g. colleagues, family), or friendly (e.g. friends).

Modelling and imitation is an integral part of healthcare professionals' education where students learn from observing and (selectively) imitating the behaviour of senior staff. Positive role models can be used in other settings to promote positive behaviours, such as health promotion campaigns, patient support groups, and helping people prepare for surgery. The importance in health promotion of using models that are perceived as similar or relevant is illustrated by the anti-smoking campaign in Chapter 19 (see Figure 19.3).

CASE STUDY 10.1   Conditioning and paediatric pain

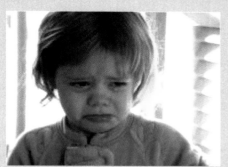

How could you use conditioning to help?

Jessica is a 3-year-old girl who has third-degree burns to her legs. She needs physiotherapy and must wear uncomfortable splints on her legs. Treatment is not progressing because Jessica gets increasingly upset until therapy is stopped. Her mother tries to comfort her but finds it very difficult and is starting to question whether therapy is really necessary.

The physiotherapist sometimes tries offering Jessica sweets to pacify her but she seems to be getting worse rather than better. When Jessica is put into bed she struggles until she has removed the splints. If she can't get them off her crying intensifies to the point of screaming and she remains sobbing well into her sleeping time until she falls asleep or staff come and distract her.

Jessica has learned that the more she cries and struggles the more likely it is that:

- Her mum will cuddle her.
- She will be offered sweets.
- The splints will be removed.
- The physiotherapy will stop.
- Staff will come and distract her.

Some of these reinforcements are occasional so these may be a variable ratio pattern of reinforcement which leads to the strongest responses and is hard to extinguish.

To help Jessica we need to stop reinforcing the negative behaviour and positively reinforce the behaviour that helps her recover. This could include:

(Continued)

- Star charts, praise, and treats to reward her when she keeps her splint on for a period of time, does physiotherapy exercises, etc.
- Preventing distress by using distraction and encouragement at critical times (e.g. the beginning of physiotherapy and bedtime) can also help.
- Teaching her ways to relax or cope during physiotherapy or when in bed that may reduce the pain felt.
- Ignoring the distress as much as possible and using a decreasing schedule of contact. For example, when she first cries in bed a staff member might check her and with minimal words or contact tell her it is OK and she must keep the splint on. Jessica could then be left for increasingly longer intervals with minimal or decreasing interaction at each point. The splints must be put back on if she removes them.
- Physiotherapy should not be ended because of Jessica's distress. However, this needs to be managed sensitively. It might help to ensure there is adequate pain relief and reduce the length of physiotherapy initially to help Jessica to cope with this.

Summary

- Associative learning occurs when we learn the relationship between two events that happen together.
- Classical conditioning occurs where a neutral stimulus (e.g. a bell) is paired with an unconditioned stimulus (e.g. food) to produce a conditioned response (e.g. salivation to the bell).
- Physical responses can be classically conditioned – including immune and neuroendocrine responses, allergy symptoms, and nausea.
- Classical conditioning can be used to create placebo effects and may underpin some of the effects of alternative therapies.
- Phobias can be a result of classical conditioning and are treated using extinguishing methods – i.e. flooding or systematic desensitisation.
- Operant conditioning occurs when we learn through the consequences of our behaviour – namely positive or negative reinforcement.
- Positive reinforcement is an effective way to encourage adaptive behaviour.
- Modelling and imitation can also influence behaviour, but people are selective in whose and what behaviour they imitate.

10.4 MEMORY

How and why we remember things affects every aspect of our lives from day-to-day functioning to exam performance. The importance of memory is most apparent in the devastating impact of disorders such as dementia and amnesia. Understanding memory processes can help us improve our own memory and also the way we give information to patients so they are more likely to remember it. Research suggests that people immediately forget around 50% of information they are told in consultations (Kessels, 2003). Furthermore, the greater the amount of information that is given, the worse recall is (Selic et al., 2011). This section addresses the basic organisation and characteristics of memory and the relevance of this to medicine – namely effective revision techniques and clinical applications.

10.4.1 ORGANISATION AND CHARACTERISTICS OF MEMORY

Learning and memory involve three stages of encoding, storage, and retrieval. Encoding takes place when the stimuli are presented and memory traces are created. Storage involves memory stores where information is organised and stored. Retrieval involves how we access and recall stored information. Memory problems can occur at any of these stages – information can be encoded wrongly (or not at all), storage may be partial, or retrieval may fail.

Memory is thought to be broadly structured, as shown in Figure 10.3. Initially, information is held in sensory buffers. Some of this information is then processed by our short-term memory and the relevant or learned information will go on to be stored in our long-term memory.

The short-term or working memory is used to manipulate and temporarily hold incoming information. Examples of using our working memory are when we first learn a patient's history, make a diagnosis, or calculate drug dosages. The working memory has visual and auditory components, both with a limited capacity. For example, the auditory loop will usually only hold as many words as we can read aloud in two seconds. This is consistent with early research that established the average short-term memory span is 7±2 pieces of information (Miller, 1956). However, if the information has meaning or is chunked together our memory span can be significantly increased. An everyday example of this is chunking telephone numbers. It is much easier to remember 0141 337 4501 than 0-1-4-1-3-3-7-4-5-0-1.

Other characteristics of working memory are primacy and recency effects. The recency effect means people are most likely to remember information that has been most recently presented, such as the last few words on a list. This is probably because this information is most accessible in our working memory. The primacy effect means people are more likely to remember items at the beginning of a list compared to the middle. This is probably because of the extra time they have had to rehearse these items. Thus, when giving information, we need to present the most important information first and last and chunk information so that more is remembered.

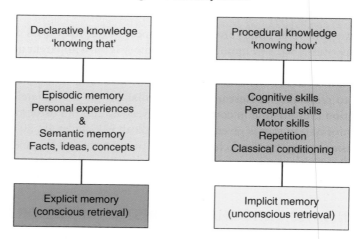

FIGURE 10.6   Long-term memory stores (adapted from Eysenck, 2000)

The long-term memory holds information for future retrieval and is dependent upon the formation of associations between nodes when information is active in our working memory. Different types of long-term memory are shown in Figure 10.6 and many theories have been put forward about how long-term memory stores work. The known characteristics of our long-term memory are shown in Box 10.3.

BOX 10.3   Characteristics of memory

- Distinctiveness: distinctive or unique information is more likely to be remembered.
- Elaboration and processing: if information is elaborated in terms of meaning it will be processed more deeply and remembered better.
- Categorisation: information is stored in semantic categories (e.g. animals, food, people), which influences how quickly new information is processed and recognised.
- Spacing and chunking: chunking information increases the amount that can be learned and spacing out learning over time improves memory and retrieval.
- Construction of memories: memories are actively constructed and can be influenced by subsequent events (e.g. eyewitnesses' memory is notoriously subject to distortion).
- Context dependent: memories are associated with the context in which they were encoded – this includes environment and mood. Retrieval is therefore better in the context in which it was first encoded.
- Power of retrieval: the more frequently information is retrieved the better it is remembered – probably because the neural trace is strengthened.

10.4.2 MEMORY AND STUDYING MEDICINE

Given what we know about memory, it is peculiar that many students do not revise effectively. With a few rare exceptions, studies of people with an outstanding memory have shown it is down to practice and using strategies, such as mnemonics, rather than being innately gifted. Memory is improved through (Chase & Ericsson, 1982):

- Meaningful encoding – e.g. relating information to knowledge you already have.
- Structured retrieval – e.g. adding as many different cues as possible to the information to help retrieval.
- Practice – to make memory processing quick and automatic.

Successful encoding of information involves understanding the meaning rather than learning things by rote. Elaborating and organising information means it is processed more deeply and integrated into existing knowledge. Effective revision strategies include summarising your notes and reorganising the information into different categories, thinking about connections between new information and the things you already know, finding personal relevance or a connection, adding visual images or drawing diagrams or mind maps. Encoding is better if it is spaced out rather than crammed into one long session. Research clearly shows that spacing learning over time results in better memory and retrieval (Esgate & Groome, 2005; Groome & Eysenck, 2016). The most effective strategy is to gradually increase the time between each session.

Using visual imagery can increase our learning because it means both the auditory and visual aspects of our working memory are being used; and it adds further associations in the long-term memory. Visual imagery has been shown to increase memory performance, particularly if objects are pictured together (Esgate & Groome, 2005; Groome & Eysenck, 2016). For example, if you have to remember to get a suture kit, a sandwich, and patient records for Ms Alade, you might visualise Ms Alade with a sandwich that has been sutured up balancing on her head. This is a visual mnemonic. Mnemonics are strategies that can help you remember lists of information that have little connection or meaning. Mnemonics are effective at increasing memory and are widely used in medical education for things like the cranial nerves or how to perform examinations for pain (see Clinical notes 10.1).

CLINICAL NOTES 10.1

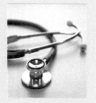

SOCRATES examination for pain

- Site – where is the pain?
- Onset – when did the pain start? Was the onset sudden or gradual?
- Character – what is the pain like?
- Radiation – does the pain radiate anywhere else?
- Associations – any other signs or symptoms associated with the pain?
- Time course – does the pain have a pattern over time?
- Exacerbating/relieving factors – does anything help the pain? Make it worse?
- Severity – how bad is the pain?

RESEARCH BOX 10.3   Using smartphone apps to boost memory

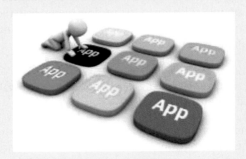

Background

The term 'formative testing' refers to using tests to increase retention of information and enhance understanding. This approach results in better knowledge retention than simply studying the material for an equal amount of time. Furthermore, testing can be used to structure revision and to focus on areas of weakness. This study examined whether formative testing using smart-phone apps would (i) be attractive to students, (ii) improve study behaviour, and (iii) improve study performance.

Method and findings

336 medical students and 125 biomedical sciences students who registered for the course 'Circulation and Respiration' at a university in the Netherlands were invited to participate in this study. The app (available here: www.physiomics.eu/app) invited students to complete seven formative tests throughout the four-week course. Each of the seven tests was available for 3–4 days to encourage students to distribute their study activities throughout the four-week course. Wrong answers were met with feedback to direct students to material that could correct their misunderstanding.

72% of the students used the app and rated it favourably. These students obtained significantly higher grades during the final exam for the course and were less likely to fail the exam. More intensive users of the app also reported significantly longer study time. The students who benefitted most from using the app were those who had performed less well in previous courses.

Significance

This study shows that a smartphone application to facilitate and encourage formative testing is an attractive and effective intervention among (bio) medical students.

Lameris, A.I. et al. (2015) The impact of formative testing on study behaviour and study performance of (bio)medical students: A smartphone application intervention study. *BMC Medical Education*, *15*: 72.

Research has shown that students who use strategies like these to improve their revision and memory do better in exams (Lahtinen et al., 1997). In particular, summarising notes and drawing mind maps are very effective. If you want to find out more about how to improve your revision technique see the Further Reading at the end of this chapter.

Retrieval in exams can be improved using the characteristics of memory previously outlined (see Box 10.3). First, the more times you retrieve a piece of information the more you will remember it. Therefore, doing practice exams, testing yourself and others, or talking about topics are all good strategies to help remember information better. Smartphone applications for testing knowledge are an attractive, accessible, and effective way to improve knowledge among students (see Research Box 10.3) (Lameris et al., 2015). Second, memory is context-dependent. In other words, you are more likely to remember information if the context in which you learned it and then recall it remains the same. Therefore, try to revise under exam conditions. If you get writers' block in an exam, try imagining yourself in the lecture theatre or the place where you revised. Focus on cues such as what was around you, the PowerPoint slides, the paper you wrote on, books, etc. This can help retrieve the information you need.

CLINICAL NOTES 10.2

How to revise effectively for exams

- Summarise lecture notes and draw diagrams or mind maps.
- Concentrate on the meaning of the information rather than rote learning.
- Elaborate information as much as possible – how does it fit with what you already know? How does it relate to your personal experience? How can you use it clinically?
- Chunk information into meaningful groups or categories.
- Use mnemonics to remember lists – distinctive mnemonics are more easily remembered.
- Space out your learning – do not cram revision into one long session.
- Recall the information regularly through testing yourself and doing mock exam papers.
- Work with other people in revision groups where you can explain or discuss different topics.
- If you are stuck in exams, think back to the context in which you learned the information.
- Use websites and smartphone apps to help you organise your revision (e.g. www.reviseaid.com; www.brainscape.com; www.oxfordmedicaleducation.com).

Clinical applications

There are many clinical applications of understanding memory, not least in trying to treat memory disorders such as Alzheimer's disease, or understanding why most of us don't remember anything from the first two or three years of our life. Particularly vivid memories are commonly reported by people after shocking or extreme events, such as traumatic events, car accidents, and a myocardial infarction (Catarino, 2015; Tedstone & Tarrier, 2003). These 'flashbulb' memories usually occur in response to events that involve strong emotion. Re-experiencing these memories through flashbacks can be a symptom of PTSD. Research has shown that in situations of strong emotion people tend to remember emotions at the expense of facts. For example, if a doctor appears worried, then patients may well think the situation is more severe, become more anxious themselves, and remember fewer facts from the consultation (Shapiro et al., 1992). However, doctors' use of affective communication – by being empathic, reassuring, and supportive – can reduce people's physiological arousal and result in better recall of information (Sep, 2014).

The most common clinical situation where memory is important is giving information to patients. From our understanding of memory and other cognitive processes in this chapter, there are a number of things we can do to improve the likelihood a patient will remember what we tell them (see Clinical notes 10.3). It also helps to avoid distractions, use written and visual information aids, ask people to say in their own words what they have been told, correct any inaccuracies, and to be aware of the impact of emotions on the consultation (Watson & McKinstry, 2009).

CLINICAL NOTES 10.3

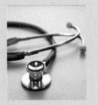

Giving information in consultations

- Put important information first and last.
- Emphasise the information that is important.
- Chunk information into meaningful groups or categories.
- Make the categorisation explicit – e.g. 'now I am going to tell you: what is wrong with you, what tests are needed, and what you must do'.
- Use repetition.
- Make the information salient to the person.
- Use simple words and short sentences.
- Be specific.
- Avoid overloading people by giving them too much information (Ley, 1997).

Summary

- Learning and memory involve three stages of encoding, storage, and retrieval.
- Memory involves sensory buffers, the short-term or working memory, and long-term memory stores.
- Short-term or working memory manipulates and temporarily holds incoming information.
- Long-term memory stores hold information for future retrieval.
- Memory is improved through meaningful encoding, structured retrieval, and practice.
- Characteristics of memory can be used to improve revision techniques and memory performance.
- Memory is context dependent – this includes the physical and emotional context.
- We can use our understanding of memory to give information to people in ways that make it more likely they will remember it.

FURTHER READING

Llewellyn, C.D. et al. (eds) (2018) *The Cambridge Handbook of Psychology, Health and Medicine* (3rd edition). Cambridge: Cambridge University Press. Includes short chapters on cognitive dysfunction in intellectual and developmental disability, dementias, amnesia, aphasia, head injury, and stroke.

Groome, D. & Eysenck, M. (2016) *An Introduction to Applied Cognitive Psychology* (2nd edition). Hove: Psychology Press. An introduction to how cognitive theory and evidence relate to things like everyday memory, biological cycles, performance, and decision making.

Cottrell, S. (2013) *The Study Skills Handbook* (4th edition). Basingstoke, UK: Palgrave Macmillan. This is a useful guide to study skills that is very action-oriented, with plenty of activities based on the principles discussed above. It has a useful companion website.

REVISION QUESTIONS

1. What is a perceptual set? Discuss the evidence for three factors that influence our perceptual set.

2. How do we learn skills? Outline the three stages involved in learning skills.

3. Discuss the conditions under which people can multitask. What are the implications of these for clinical practice?

4. Discuss two biases of attention and their implications for clinical practice.

5. What is classical conditioning? How can it be used to create a placebo effect?

6. Describe operant conditioning. What are the most effective forms of reinforcement?

7. Describe modelling and imitation and the three characteristics that make it more likely children will imitate someone's behaviour.

8. What are (a) short-term and (b) long-term memory? What characteristics do they possess?

9. From your understanding of memory, discuss five techniques that can be used when giving information in consultations.

10. How can our understanding of memory help improve revision techniques and memory performance?

SECTION III

BODY SYSTEMS

11 IMMUNITY AND PROTECTION

LEARNING OBJECTIVES

This chapter is designed to enable you to:

- Understand the effect of stress and emotion on the immune system.
- Describe the role of psychological factors in immune disorders.
- Describe aspects of psycho-dermatology.
- Outline the psychosocial risk factors for cancer.
- Explain how psychological factors might affect the progression of cancer.

Do you get sick around exam time? Your greater susceptibility to infections at such times may be related to inadequate sleep, a lack of exercise, a poor diet, and may also be affected by stress. Links between emotions and health have long formed a part of medical thinking. Pre-modern medical thought was based on the beliefs that optimal health depended on a balance of the four humours (blood, yellow bile, black bile, phlegm) and that imbalances influenced disease and behaviour. For example, the depressive melancholic personality is named after the Latin words for black bile.

Our understanding of disease is now very different, but modern medicine continues to find evidence of intricate links between psychological and physical wellbeing. In a classic early study, Ishigami (1919) found decreased phagocyte function among people with tuberculosis when they were emotionally agitated. Since then, our understanding of the links between psychological states and immune function has increased. Over the same period, there has been increasing evidence of pathogenic involvement in diseases previously not thought to involve the immune system (e.g. *Helicobacter pylori* infection is often implicated in peptic ulcers and myocardial infarctions) (see Chapters 12 and 13).

Psychoneuroimmunology (PNI) examines how psychological states affect our immune function. Although most PNI research has focused on negative psychological states such as stress and depression, recent research has examined the beneficial

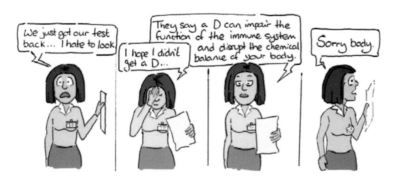

effects of positive moods. In this chapter we shall first look at the effect of psychological factors on the immune system and immune disorders. The next section looks at our main protective organ – the skin. Finally, the large body of knowledge on psychosocial factors and cancer is examined as an illustration of how immune impairment can ultimately lead to disease.

11.1 INFECTION, INFLAMMATION, AND IMMUNITY

The presence of protein molecules called antigens on the surface of each cell allows the immune system to distinguish body cells from potentially harmful foreign cells.

There are two broad types of barriers to infection – non-specific and specific. The non-specific barriers include mucous membranes, which destroy many foreign micro-organisms, and phagocytes, which consume and destroy foreign micro-organisms and debris.

The specific immune barriers involve the action of specialised white blood cells called lymphocytes. There are two components to this type of immune response. The **cell-mediated immune response** involves T lymphocytes. The **antibody-mediated immune response** (also called the humoural response) involves B lymphocytes. In each case, a response to an immune challenge is usually reflected in an increase in proliferation of T lymphocytes and B lymphocytes.

11.1.1 STRESS AND IMMUNE FUNCTION

Stress has measurable effects on our immune function, susceptibility to infections, severity of infections, response to vaccinations, and wound healing (Glaser & Kiecolt-Glaser, 2005; Segerstom & Miller, 2004; Zorrilla et al., 2001). Whether these effects are beneficial or detrimental is determined by the duration of stress.

Acute stress produces improvements in the immune function – particularly non-specific barriers – with this reverting to normal levels fairly quickly after the stressor ends (Dhabhar, 2013). Thus, stressful events such as public speaking or an athletic competition may temporarily enhance our immune function. If threats are brief stressors that invoke the fight-or-flight response, there is evidence of the body preparing adaptively to deal with potential infection and/or injury arising from that threat. The immune response to stress is affected by activation of the sympathetic nervous system and hypothalamic-pituitary-adrenal axis (HPA axis) (see Chapter 3). There is a complex interplay between the nervous, endocrine, and immune systems so it is difficult to determine which factors are more or less important. The sympathetic nervous system increases immune system activity, particularly large granular lymphocyte activity such as natural killer cells. However, the HPA axis suppresses some immune activity through the production of cortisol, which has an anti-inflammatory effect and reduces both the number of white blood cells and the release of cytokines.

Chronic stress tends to impair our immune function. Chronic stress can arise from various causes: work, unemployment, difficult relationships, caring for sick relatives. More severe and longer lasting stressors are associated with more global immunosuppression – initially in our cell-mediated immunity and then across the spectrum of immune functions. Immune down-regulation associated with chronic stress can lead to impaired wound healing, poorer responses to infectious diseases, autoimmune diseases, and the progression of cancer (Dhabhar, 2013).

A different pattern can be seen in people who have been exposed to traumatic events, such as natural disasters, war or terrorism, particularly those who also develop symptoms of post-traumatic stress disorder (PTSD). In these instances, exposure to a severely traumatic event is associated with increased immune measures such as antibodies, lymphocytes, interleukins, and natural killer cell activity which may persist many years after the traumatic event. Thus it appears that trauma and PTSD are associated with a long-term enhanced immunity. This is an intriguing contrast to the effect of chronic stress and other negative effects (e.g. depression): it may be explained by the observation that PTSD leads to a dysregulation of the HPA axis and reduced cortisol responses (Bachen et al., 2007). Paradoxically, despite an enhanced immune function, people with PTSD report increased symptoms of illness and greater use of medical services (Ramchand et al., 2008).

Substantial evidence of the effect of stress on the immune system has led to interest in whether interventions that alleviate stress can counter the stress-related suppression of immune function. There is some evidence that emotional disclosure (e.g. writing about negative emotions and experiences), hypnosis, and conditioning can produce positive changes in our immune function (Miller & Cohen, 2000; Morgan et al., 2014; Tekampe et al., 2017). The evidence for the efficacy of stress-management or relaxation programmes, however, is less convincing. It should be noted that many studies involve small samples from specific groups of people. Therefore, in addition to developing more effective approaches to stress management, there is a need to conduct research which allows more valid statistical conclusions and generalisations to be made.

11.1.2 EMOTIONS AND IMMUNE FUNCTION

Negative emotions

Negative emotions like depression are associated with impaired immune function (Herbert & Cohen, 1993; Kiecolt-Glaser & Glaser, 2002). The effect of negative emotions on the immune system may be the common pathway between negative emotions and illnesses such as cardiovascular disease, rheumatoid arthritis, Type 1 diabetes, and some cancers. There is substantial evidence that negative emotions are associated with a dysregulation of the immune system, an increased susceptibility to infections, and slower wound healing.

Depression is associated with several changes in the immune function (see Box 11.1) as well as changes in clinical outcomes. For example, depressive symptoms have been linked with the more rapid progression of disease among people with HIV/AIDS (Leserman, 2008) and heart disease (Chapter 12). However, not all studies find the same results. It must also be acknowledged that the links between depression and impaired immune function may be influenced by less healthy behaviours among depressed people, including poorer adherence to treatment (Gonzalez et al., 2011).

ACTIVITY 11.1

- The last time you were ill, what was the relationship between your physical symptoms and emotions?
- Do you think one caused the other, that they influenced each other, or that they were separate?

BOX 11.1   Changes in immune function associated with depression

- Lower total numbers of lymphocytes.
- Reduced proliferation of lymphocytes in response to mitogens that usually promote lymphocyte production.
- Reductions in the numbers and functioning of natural killer cells.
- Increased CD4/CD8 ratios.
- Changes in pro-inflammatory cytokines.
- Increases in interleukin-6 (an important mediator of fever and inflammation).

Given the association between depression and immune function, it is not surprising that psychotherapy for depression can also affect the course of immune disorders. Moreover, interventions that improve psychological wellbeing can lead to improvements in immune disorders (Antoni, 2013; Nanni et al., 2015).

Positive emotions

There is some evidence that positive moods and personalities are associated with enhanced immune function (Brod et al., 2014; Pressman & Black, 2012). For example, optimism, emotional expressiveness, and extraversion are associated with greater numbers of helper T lymphocytes and greater natural killer cell cytotoxicity (Segerstrom et al., 1998). Such results suggest that our mood may be an important moderator of the links between stress and immune function. Whereas some studies have examined optimism as a dispositional characteristic of individuals, other studies have examined the effect of positive psychological experiences. For example, watching humorous films can produce significant improvements in several parameters of immune function (Berk et al., 2001). Some of these effects may last for several hours.

Whereas hundreds of studies have examined the effects on our immune function of negative psychological states (allowing for the publication of meta-analyses), fewer studies have examined the links between positive emotions and immune function. It is therefore more difficult to be sure about the immune benefits of positive moods and positive experiences. More research is required to determine the causal mechanisms through which positive moods might affect immunity. However, some studies have made interesting comparisons of the effects of positive and negative moods on immune function (see Research Box 11.1).

RESEARCH BOX 11.1   Positive and negative emotions and immune function

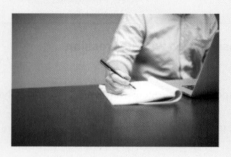

Background

The aim of this study was to examine how day-to-day changes in psychological states could affect our immune function.

Method and findings

Ninety-six healthy married men completed a diary of events and emotions every day for three months. On each day, participants indicated their experience of various emotions provided on a checklist (e.g. determined, distressed, inspired, irritable, nervous, and upset). They also indicated their daily experience of a range of positive and negative events in various domains (e.g. work, friends, household, activities, finances). The men's reports were corroborated with those of their wives.

The men were then given an orally ingested pathogen and their immune responses to this pathogen were recorded via an analysis of daily-collected saliva samples. Production of antibodies to the orally ingested antigen was higher on days when men reported more positive moods and lower on days when they reported more negative moods. The strongest positive immune effects were found for experiences of desirable leisure and household events. The strongest negative effects were found for undesirable work events. There was some evidence that positive experiences and moods had longer-lasting effects than negative experiences.

Significance

This study demonstrates that positive and negative experiences and emotions have opposite effects on immune function. The study shows that daily variations in affect have observable effects on the single immune parameter that was assessed. In the years since this study, more evidence has accrued to support these findings, although more research is required to provide a fuller understanding of the mechanisms involved.

Stone, A.A., Neale, J.M., Cox, D.S., Napoli, A., Valdimarsdottir, H. & Kennedy-Moore, E. (1994) Daily events are associated with a secretory immune response to an oral antigen in men. *Health Psychology*, 13: 440–446.

11.1.3 IMMUNISATIONS

Immunisations are an important part of tackling disease and promoting health in our society. Immunisations prime the immune system to respond to a disease by giving a small, usually disabled, form of the virus or bacteria. The ability of vaccines to protect against the disease depends on the strength of the immune response to the vaccine. Given the relationship between stress and immune functioning, it is perhaps not surprising that people who are stressed, upset, or anxious have weaker, delayed, or less lasting responses to vaccines (Glaser & Kiecolt-Glaser, 2005).

In recent years there has been some controversy over vaccines for young children, and this has led to reduced uptake: for example, the uptake of measles/mumps/rubella (MMR) immunisation has fallen to below 70% in some areas. Whether parents decide to immunise their child is determined by beliefs about the perceived risks associated with the disease and with vaccination – and such beliefs can be shaped by misinformation (Flaherty, 2011). Parents are less likely to immunise children if they think there are dangers associated with the vaccine, have doubts the vaccine will be effective, believe they can protect their children from exposure, or think their children are unlikely to catch the disease (de Visser & McDonnell, 2008; Sturm et al., 2005).

Vaccinations and other medical procedures involving needles can cause substantial anxiety and distress in children, adolescents, and some adults. Many children and parents consider needle-procedures to be one of the most traumatic experiences of hospitalisation (Taddio et al., 2009). Needle-related distress and anxiety has adverse short- and long-term psychological effects, including anticipatory nausea, insomnia, eating problems, PTSD, and avoidance behaviour (Kennedy et al., 2008; Young, 2005). Furthermore, needle-related distress can escalate with successive procedures. Effective management of needle distress in children is therefore critical. Pharmacological management involves analgesics during or after the injection, which can be topical (applied to the skin) or oral. However, parents and healthcare professionals can have a strong influence on children's distress during needle procedures (Kajikawa et al., 2014). Perhaps counter-intuitively, being empathic, reassuring, or critical is associated with increased distress in children. Conversely, using humour, talking about other things, and instructing the child to cope by using distraction or other adaptive means are associated with decreased distress (Mahoney et al., 2010). Learning (and unlearning) fear of needles is covered in Chapter 10.

11.2 PSYCHOLOGICAL ASPECTS OF IMMUNE DISORDERS

So far we have focused on how psychological states can affect immune function. Of course, the reverse is also true: changes in immune function can lead to changes in psychological wellbeing. Many of us find that when we have a cold or other illness our mood can also be affected. In the case of more serious and/or chronic infections, the psychological consequences can be more severe. Research indicates that depression tends to be more common among people with chronic illnesses than in the broader population (Clarke & Currie, 2009; Ryu et al., 2016). In general, self-reported quality of life also tends to be lower among people with chronic autoimmune diseases (e.g. Cohen, 2002). Such experiences of depression, stress, and anxiety resulting from disease may in turn impair the immune function.

Autoimmune diseases occur when the body's immune system mistakenly identifies self-cells as foreign cells and mounts an immune response against initially healthy tissues. Some examples of autoimmune diseases are given below. Others include coeliac disease and lupus erythematosus. The mechanisms involved in many immune diseases are not fully understood. Thus, people may have no hope of a cure, and must adjust physically and psychologically to the long-term management of symptoms (see Chapter 6).

Rheumatoid arthritis is a chronic systemic inflammatory autoimmune disorder which can affect many tissues and organs, but principally attacks the synovial lining of joints. There is no known cure for rheumatoid arthritis, but different treatments may be used to alleviate symptoms, including pain, and/or to try to prevent future joint destruction. People with rheumatoid arthritis are more likely than healthy controls to report anxiety and depression (Barton et al., 2010; Margaretten et al., 2011). Longitudinal research indicates that greater anxiety and depression are associated with increased perceptions of pain, and higher levels of pain and/or disability in turn predict higher levels of distress. These findings suggest a reciprocal relationship between psychological wellbeing and experiences of pain or disability (Odegård et al., 2007).

There is a paradox in the role of stress in inflammatory diseases like rheumatoid arthritis. Physical responses to stress involving the HPA axis and autonomic nervous system can play a vital role in inflammation. As we have seen, the release of cortisol via the HPA axis should reduce inflammation. Thus, in theory, stress should improve the symptoms of rheumatoid arthritis. However, stress actually results in worse immunological markers, physical symptoms, and disability (de Brouwer, 2010; Geenen et al., 2006). This seems to be due to a physical hypo-responsiveness to stress: people with rheumatoid arthritis have consistently reduced autonomic nervous system responses to stressful events. HPA responses to stress also appear blunted and out of proportion to corresponding immune activity. There is a need for further longitudinal prospective research (i.e. research that follows people over time) with larger samples to determine the effects of different kinds of stressors on the autonomic nervous system, HPA axis, and immune function (de Brouwer, 2010).

Type 1 diabetes mellitus (also called insulin-dependent diabetes mellitus) is an autoimmune disease in which the insulin-producing cells of the pancreas are destroyed by an inappropriate immune response. As a result, the body is unable to regulate blood sugar levels. There is no known cure for Type 1 diabetes, and people must use insulin replacement therapy to avoid potentially fatal diabetic ketoacidosis. The prevalence rate of depression is more than three times higher in people with Type 1 diabetes than in the general population (Roy & Lloyd, 2012). Among people with diabetes, hyperglycaemia resulting from poor glycaemic control is linked to depression (Lustman et al., 2000), but the mechanisms and casual links are not fully understood (Moulton et al., 2015).

A synthesis of published research has revealed that experience of diabetes-related complications, including retinopathy, neuropathy, renal disease, coronary artery disease, and sexual dysfunction, is associated with depressive symptoms (de Groot et al., 2001). Depressive symptoms are also associated with lower levels of treatment adherence so it is important to address the psychological wellbeing of people with diabetes (Gonzalez, 2008).

CASE STUDY 11.1   Living with HIV

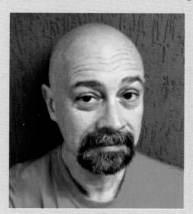

The following comes from an interview with Jose, a 42-year-old bisexual man who was diagnosed with HIV seven years before the interview. HIV had had a marked influence on Jose's plans for the future. He had initially worried about an early death, but he is now more concerned about the prospect of living with a chronic condition and managing antiretroviral therapy.

> Before I found out I was HIV positive, I was determined to live forever – and live life accordingly. I had great expectations of making a bloody fortune with the company I was running.

At first, I thought that the diagnosis meant I was dying. I hadn't really thought about it before, and I didn't know much about what treatment was available. But then I learnt about the treatments that are available now.

Now I do feel that I have a future, but I also just live day to day because these drugs I'm on are not the answer. Resistance could develop, and if resistance develops, then I'm not sure what my treatment options might be. I do also worry about what taking these drugs might be doing to my body in the long term.

I'm a person obviously living with a disease that our medical science can't deal with. And there's no prospect of them curing it in the near future – or even in my lifetime. However, long or short that may be.

(Adapted from Ezzy, 2000)

Unlike the autoimmune diseases discussed above, **HIV/AIDS** is an acquired immune deficiency. There is clear evidence that the course and development of HIV/AIDS is affected by psychosocial factors such as stress, depression, and social support

(Schuster et al., 2012). Longitudinal studies show that a faster progression to AIDS occurs among men with higher stress levels and less support (Leserman et al., 1999). Depression is more common among people with HIV/AIDS than among the general population, probably because of the impacts of the virus on people's health and social lives (Ciesla & Roberts, 2001). HIV can have profound and long-lasting impacts on health, work, finances, and sexual relationships (e.g. Ezzy et al., 1999; Groß et al., 2016). This affects how people experience their current health and wellbeing, and how they plan for the future (see Case Study 11.1). The net effect is that people with HIV/AIDS tend to have a lower quality of life. However, it is important to note that interventions designed to treat depression or to help people manage stress result in better outcomes for people with HIV/AIDS (Arseniou et al., 2014; Brown & Vanable, 2008).

Summary

- Acute stress leads to enhanced immune responses, but chronic stress impairs immune functioning.
- Negative emotions, such as depression, are associated with reduced immune functioning.
- Conversely, positive emotions appear to have a positive effect on immune function.
- Immune disorders are associated with a reduced quality of life, increased anxiety, and increased depression.
- There is a reciprocal relationship between negative mood, pain, and disability.
- Some psychological interventions, such as disclosure and conditioning interventions, may result in improved immune function in disorders such as HIV/AIDS.

11.3 SKIN

The skin is a key protective organ that is made up of many layers of epithelial tissues. It protects the body against pathogens, insulates the body, prevents dehydration, and protects the internal organs, muscles, etc. against damage from external sources. The impact of psychological factors on skin has mainly been examined in relation to wound healing and skin disorders.

11.3.1 WOUND HEALING

Wound healing research typically carries out punch biopsies or suction blisters on volunteers and monitors immune activity and healing over time. It has consistently shown that stressed people heal 20–40% slower than people who are not stressed, apparently because of an interaction between glucocorticoids (e.g. cortisol) and proinflammatory cytokines (Walburn et al., 2009). For example, Marucha, Kiecolt-Glaser and Favagehi (1998) made small punch biopsy wounds in students' oral hard palates: once during the summer vacation and once just before exams. In the exam period, students took 40% longer for their wounds to heal and had 68% less interleukin 1ß messenger RNA than during the vacation, because they were more stressed at exam time.

Wound healing is slower when we experience difficult circumstances, such as caring for chronically ill people or having relationship difficulties. However, wound healing is not only affected by stress. Wounds also heal more slowly in people who are depressed, anxious, or have poor anger control (Gouin et al., 2008). Positive factors that speed up wound healing include emotional disclosure, close personal relationships, and exercise (Emery et al., 2005).

The prospective experimental design of wound healing studies makes it possible to establish a causal link between stress and healing. This is relevant to many areas of medicine, but particularly surgery. There is substantial evidence that negative emotions such as fear and anxiety are associated with worse outcomes after surgery, including more post-operative distress, pain, use of analgesia, a longer hospital stay, and a slower return to normal functioning. Similarly, research shows that preparing people for surgery by providing more information, coping skills, or relaxation techniques can result in lower post-operative pain, shorter hospital stays, and better psychological outcomes (Powell et al., 2016). This is an area of medicine where psychological preparation has the potential to make a real difference to clinical outcomes, but there is a need for more robust evidence about what works, and how.

CLINICAL NOTES 11.1

Immunity, vaccinations, and surgery

- Negative emotions are associated with poorer immune function. This is especially important for people who have serious health conditions.
- It is therefore important to address negative emotions via appropriate psychosocial interventions.
- You can have a strong influence on people's distress during invasive procedures – use distraction, humour, and give them strategies to help them cope.
- Empathy, reassurance, and criticism are more likely to increase children's distress during invasive procedures.
- Wound healing is slower when people are stressed.
- Surgical outcomes are better if people feel prepared for surgery and are relaxed. Anxiety and distress lead to worse outcomes.
- Give people undergoing surgery as much information as they want, help them develop coping skills, and encourage them to use relaxation techniques.

11.3.2 SKIN DISORDERS

The field of psychodermatology acknowledges that many dermatological disorders have a psychosomatic or behavioural aspect, and that the skin and the mind are linked through psychoneuroimmunoendocrine mechanisms and behaviours that can strongly affect the onset or progression of skin disorders (Shenefelt, 2011). Psychological factors can affect the course of dermatological disorders in several ways. First, stress is associated with increased symptoms in disorders such as psoriasis, atopic dermatitis, alopecia areata, and urticaria (Picardi & Abeni, 2001). This is likely to be due to physiological mechanisms such as those detailed above and changes in behaviour that are also associated with stress, such as scratching and increased tobacco or alcohol use. Scratching can exacerbate symptoms and cause further skin damage and is usually a conditioned response (see Chapter 10). Early research showed that people with skin conditions such as eczema develop conditioned scratching responses more quickly, and are slower to unlearn them than people without skin disorders (Robertson et al., 1975).

Second, people with various skin disorders have higher than average levels of anxiety, depression, and dysfunctional coping strategies, such as avoidance. A pan-European study of people undergoing outpatient treatment for various dermatological conditions revealed that they were more likely than a control group to have clinical depression (10% of patients), clinical anxiety (17% of patients), and suicidal ideation (13% of patients) (Dalgard et al., 2015). The likelihood of depression or anxiety was especially high for people with psoriasis, atopic dermatitis, hand eczema, and leg ulcers. However, there is little prospective research into the causal relationship between negative emotions and symptoms of skin disorders. It is therefore difficult to know whether negative emotions make physical symptoms worse or whether worse physical symptoms cause people to become more anxious or depressed. The severity of skin disorders is not associated with the level of distress a person feels. Instead, distress and quality of life are more closely related to physical appearance, disfigurement, fear of negative evaluation, and social stigma (Harcourt, 2017).

ACTIVITY 11.2

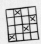

- If scratching is partly a conditioned response, how might you go about reducing scratching behaviour in someone with eczema?

Psychological interventions can be very effective in the clinical management of skin disorders (Shenefelt, 2010). Interventions draw on a variety of techniques, such as education, relaxation training, biofeedback, cognitive restructuring, and social skills training to manage stigma (see Chapters 6 and 19). The most important part of these interventions appears to be improving self-control of scratching through habit-reversal training. This involves helping people to:

- Recognise scratching cues or triggers.
- Interrupt and prevent the automatic scratching response.
- Use a competing response, such as relaxation, to reduce the itching sensation.

Providing relaxation techniques helps reduce stress and is a good substitute for scratching. Relaxation techniques include progressive muscle relaxation and using calming or healing imagery. Research shows that improving the self-control of scratching and using relaxation techniques are both effective for reducing the symptoms of skin disorders (Stangier, 2007).

Summary

- Stress and negative emotions are associated with slower wound healing.
- Distress and anxiety are associated with poorer psychological and physical recovery from surgery.
- Stress is also associated with increased symptoms of skin disorders.
- A substantial minority of dermatological outpatients report psychiatric symptoms, which are less influenced by the severity of the skin disorder than physical appearance, disfigurement, the fear of a negative evaluation, and social stigma.
- Psychological interventions add significantly to the effectiveness of the clinical management of skin disorders, resulting in less psychiatric and physical symptoms.

11.4 CANCER

There are over 100 different types of cancer and it has been estimated that up to half of all people born after 1960 will develop cancer at some point in their life (Ahmad et al., 2015). The development of cancerous tumours is a complex process that involves a cascade of events that is a bit like cellular anarchy. At least three different types of gene damage or mutation are necessary for cancer to develop. Cancer cells have to avoid the normal process of programmed cell death (apoptosis) that usually protects against the proliferation of abnormal cells. Normal cells have a fixed capacity of division and growth, but cancer cells manage to divide indefinitely. As the tumour grows, it requires nourishment and the removal of waste products, so it has to encourage blood vessel growth around it. The tumour also has to be able to invade other areas of the body. This requires the inactivation of a whole series of factors that will usually restrict cells to a specific site. In the later stages of the disease, cancer cells may break off (metastasise) and migrate to other areas of the body.

Psycho-oncology examines (i) psychosocial risk factors that influence the development of cancer, (ii) responses to cancer, and (iii) interventions for people with cancer. These are looked at in turn.

11.4.1 PSYCHOSOCIAL RISK FACTORS FOR CANCER

Cancers are often caused by the interplay between environmental factors such as toxins, viruses, and lifestyle, and internal factors, such as genetic vulnerability and hormones. Psychosocial factors that influence cancer onset include:

- Demographic factors.
- Lifestyle and health behaviour.
- Social support.
- Coping and adjustment (see section 11.2).

Demographic factors that influence cancer include ethnicity, country of residence, and socio-economic status. For example, malignant melanoma (skin cancer) is more common in white people; breast cancer is more common in Northern European and white American women but relatively rare in Asians; Japanese people are up to ten times more likely to get stomach cancer than white Americans or Europeans. Figure 11.1 shows the most common cancers for men and women living in different countries. For many cancers, people who have poor socioeconomic status are more at risk, although this is not true for all cancers. For example, studies in France and England have revealed that although various cancers in men and women are more likely to occur among people of lower socioeconomic status, melanoma is more likely to occur among people of higher socioeconomic status (Bryere, 2014).

The observed differences in cancer rates for people from different ethnicity, socioeconomic status, and country of residence are often due to differences in lifestyle. For example, higher rates of stomach cancer in Japan are associated with the high salt content of the Japanese diet: if Japanese people move to the USA, their risk of stomach cancer decreases compared to people who remain in Japan, but their risk of breast cancer increases (Keegan et al., 2007; Tsugane, 2005). This suggests that behavioural patterns in the country of residence affect a person's health risks. Similarly, higher rates of melanoma in people from higher socioeconomic groups may reflect the fact that they can afford vacations in sunny locations, but do not properly protect their skin.

Lifestyle factors include *health behaviours* such as smoking, diet, exercise, and alcohol use. They also include *exposure to toxins or infections* such as asbestos (lung cancer), *H. Pylori* (stomach cancer) and human papilloma virus (cervical cancer). As shown in Figure 11.1, tobacco, diet, and infections alone are thought to be responsible for 54% of cancers in developed countries. Changing people's behaviour so that they live healthier lifestyles could prevent up to 60% of cancer deaths, particularly smoking-related and gastro-intestinal cancers (Institute of Medicine, 2005). Risk factors vary for different cancers and many cancers have multiple risk factors. For example, risk factors for breast cancer include genetic vulnerability, greater age, the early onset of periods, being childless or not having children until over 30, using hormone replacement therapy, and greater alcohol consumption.

It has been proposed that stress contributes to the progression of some cancers through its effect on the immune system (Lutgendorf & Sood, 2011). This suggestion is mainly supported by animal research where increased tumour growth and metastases are observed in non-human animals that have been implanted with tumour cells and then put in

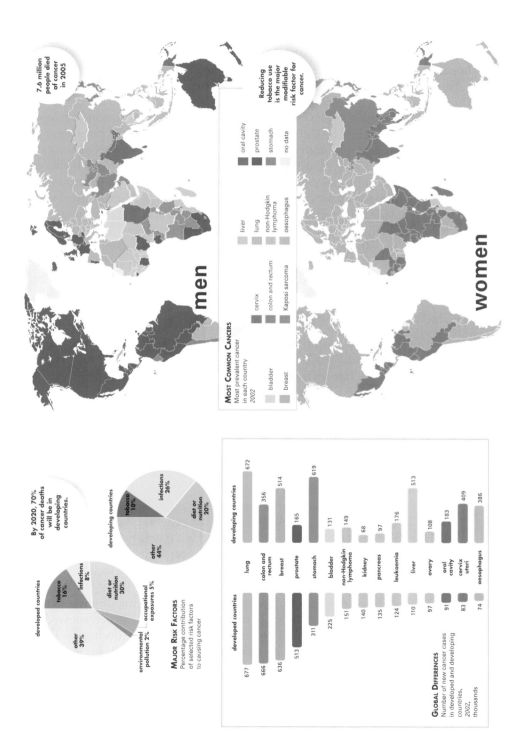

FIGURE 11.1 Most common cancers across the world

Reproduced from *The Atlas of Health*, by Diarmuid O'Donovan, 'Most common cancers', pp. 44–45, Earthscan 2008. Copyright © 2008 Myriad Editions Ltd/ www.MyriadEditions.com

stressful situations. Research in humans is less consistent: the evidence suggests that stress has more of an effect on cancer progression than cancer onset (Chida et al., 2008).

Social support is important for psychological health and adapting to chronic illness (see Chapter 6). Thus, it is not surprising that support can influence the onset and progression of cancer. One meta-analysis revealed that the risk of premature cancer mortality was 25% lower in people with high levels of perceived social support and 20% lower in people with larger social networks (Pinquart & Duberstein, 2010). Cancer mortality rates were also 12% lower among married people, with never married people at greater risk of premature death than those who were widowed, divorced, or separated. Stronger beneficial effects of social support were found in people with leukaemia and lymphomas, and stronger effects of network size were found for breast cancer. Another meta-analysis of longitudinal studies revealed strong evidence for a link between better social support and slower progression of breast cancer, but less convincing evidence of the benefits of social support for other types of cancer (Nausheen et al., 2009). Further research is required to fully determine the causal links between social support and cancer mortality for different cancers at different stages.

11.4.2 PSYCHOLOGICAL RESPONSES TO CANCER

Cancer poses a severe threat to health that requires extensive adjustment on the part of individuals and their loved ones (see Chapter 6). A diagnosis of cancer therefore has to be given carefully and sensitively (see section 18.4). Many people with cancer report significant levels of anxiety, depression, or PTSD (Abbey et al., 2015; Watts et al., 2014). The likelihood of developing psychological disorders is related to medical factors such as cancer type, severity, and prognosis, and partly due to individual factors, such as a younger age, history of psychological problems, life stress, and poor support (Abbey et al., 2015; Arden-Close et al., 2008; Kangas et al., 2002). The vulnerability-stress model is a useful framework for thinking about how individual vulnerability interacts with medical factors to determine a person's distress (see Figure 3.4).

Although anxiety is more common than depression in response to cancer diagnosis (Arden-Close et al., 2008; Watts et al., 2014), the relationship between cancer and depression has been more widely studied. Depression is associated with cancer onset and mortality, but it is difficult to tease out whether depression causes cancer or is a response to cancer. Prospective studies suggest that people with a history of depression have a slightly increased risk of getting some cancers, but not others (Chang et al., 2015; Gross et al., 2010; Oerlemans et al., 2007). However, depression probably plays a more important role in the *progression* of cancer. A prospective study of over 15,000 men and women showed that people with a history of cancer were almost two times more likely to die during the 10-year observation period if they had high levels of psychological distress at baseline (Hamer et al., 2009). The study did not control for the severity of cancer at baseline, but the effect of psychological distress remained when people who died in the first year of the study were excluded (as a proxy for cancer severity).

CASE STUDY 11.2 Managing the stress of cancer

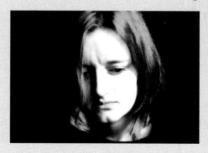 Hannah is a 32-year-old woman who was diagnosed with breast cancer six months ago. She had a double mastectomy two months ago, but there were indications the cancer might have spread, so Hannah has started chemotherapy. She is frightened of cancer, tearful, and does not feel she is coping. She thinks she is going to die, has stopped going out, and does not want to talk about it. Hannah is convinced that no man will want to be in a relationship with her now because she's had a mastectomy. Chemotherapy makes her feel worse and she can't bear the thought of losing her hair. She has missed her two most recent chemotherapy appointments.

Stress management

Stress management involves education about stress and coping, exploring the person's ways of coping, and facilitating more adaptive coping. Stress management has many forms. In this example we use the transactional model (see Chapter 3) to examine the role of perceived demands, resources, appraisal, and coping:

Demands: explore the demands of cancer on Hannah so they are explicit

- What are the triggers to this situation (e.g. breast cancer, chemotherapy)?
- What demands does it place on her (e.g. cancer threatens her life, identity, attractiveness)
- How real are these demands? Are they based on fact or fears?

Appraisal: examine her appraisals and how they affect her feelings and coping

- When she is feeling overwhelmed and unable to cope, what is she thinking?
- How can she think differently to help her feel and cope better?

    o For example, 'Many women go through breast cancer and chemotherapy and are fine.'
    o For example, 'Breasts are not the only quality that make women attractive.'

Resources to cope: explore the resources she has to cope

- What support does she have available to her?
- How has she coped with previous stressful situations?
- How can she use these strategies to cope now?
- What new ways of coping might help her now?

(Continued)

Drawing on the previous stages, you can explore practical steps and strategies that would help Hannah manage her cancer and chemotherapy both now and in the future. This is very individual. For example, if talking to people in the same situation helped her in the past, she might join a support group. Or she might realise that in the past she was able to think differently and talk herself out of her fears.

The relationship between depression and cancer is bidirectional and involves physiological and behavioural mechanisms. First, neuroendocrine and immune changes that accompany depression may contribute to the progression of cancer. Second, depression may interact with lifestyle to contribute to the onset and progression of cancer. For example, one 12-year study of over 2,000 people found that smokers were 1.6 times more likely than non-smokers to develop any cancer. However, smokers who were depressed were 2.5 times more likely to develop cancer and 18.5 times more likely to develop smoking-related cancers (Linkins & Comstock, 1990). Third, having cancer may contribute to or exacerbate a depressed mood.

The coping strategies people use are influenced by their appraisal of cancer. As noted in Chapter 3, our appraisal of events determines the extent to which we find them stressful and how we attempt to cope with them. This is also the case in response to cancer (see Case Study 11.2 and Chapter 6). People who appraise the cancer as a threat or challenge are more likely to use problem-focused coping strategies, such as information gathering, problem solving, accepting responsibility, and seeking support. People who appraise the cancer as involving harm or loss are more likely to use avoidant strategies, such as denial, distancing, wishful-thinking, and substance use (Franks & Roesch, 2006).

Coping strategies can be either adaptive or maladaptive, depending on the individual and the context. For example, a review of the use of denial by people with cancer found that it was more likely to be used by elderly people or those in the terminal phase of cancer. The effect of denial on physical and psychological function was inconsistent, although passive-escape strategies were associated with increased distress (Vos & de Haes, 2007). However, as with depression, it is difficult to determine the direction of causality of this relationship. Furthermore, there may be reciprocal relationships between quality of life and coping strategies among people with cancer (Danhauer et al., 2009).

Although the way people cope influences their emotional response to cancer, the role of coping in cancer progression is less obvious. Meta-analyses have shown there is little consistent evidence that coping styles play an important part in cancer survival or cancer recurrence (Petticrew et al., 2002).

This does not mean we should dismiss coping as completely unimportant. Coping is important in promoting psychological wellbeing and self-help behaviour. For example, one qualitative study of people with incurable cancer who had outlived their diagnosis by 2–12 years found they had common coping styles of:

- Authenticity – a clear understanding of what was important in their lives.
- Autonomy – a perceived freedom to shape their lives around what they valued.
- Acceptance – more peaceful, joyful experiences and greater emotional closeness to others.

These people were also more involved in their own self-help soon after diagnosis than those who did not survive (Cunningham & Watson, 2004).

Responses to cancer are not always negative. There is increasing evidence that many people experience positive personal changes in response to cancer (Koutrouli, 2012). One review found six important components of psycho-spiritual wellbeing (Lin & Bauer-Wu, 2003):

- Self-awareness.
- Coping and adjusting effectively with stress.
- Connectedness with others.
- A sense of faith.
- A sense of empowerment and confidence.
- Living with meaning and hope.

A meta-analysis of research with people with cancer and HIV showed that personal growth is associated with lower levels of distress, better mental health, and better self-ratings of physical health (Sawyer et al., 2010). Furthermore, the positive aspects of personal growth increased over time: people who believed their cancer had led to positive changes in their life continued to do well in terms of their mental health and perceived physical health.

11.4.3 INTERVENTIONS FOR CANCER

Research generally confirms that psychological interventions can increase psychological and physiological adaptation in people with cancer, but less is known about the extent to which these positive effects influence tumour growth, cancer recurrence, or survival (Antoni, 2013; McGregor & Antoni, 2009). Various psychosocial interventions for cancer can be used, including counselling, cognitive behaviour therapy, mindfulness interventions, and support groups (see Chapter 19).

Cognitive behavioural therapy (CBT) for cancer usually focuses on reducing stress and negative emotions, helping people manage pain, fatigue, appetite control, and the side effects of treatment. This can be done through individual or group programmes and usually involves education, an examination of stress and coping styles, and the use of cognitive and behavioural techniques to improve coping with the difficult and stressful aspects of cancer and its treatment. Research shows that CBT interventions can lead to improved quality of life, reduced distress, and reduced fatigue (Gielissen et al., 2007). In recent years, research has begun to examine the long-term effects of online CBT programmes for people with cancer (Abrahams et al., 2015).

There has been increasing interest in the use of **mindfulness** interventions (see Chapter 19), which encourage people to experience life fully by paying attention to moment-to-moment experiences. People are encouraged to be aware of the world, other people, their own thoughts and emotions, and to accept these emotions and thoughts without judgement. Because mindfulness focuses on the present, it is a good way to prevent people ruminating about the past or future. Mindfulness-based interventions (MBIs) include education and training about mindfulness and meditation. Evaluations of MBIs in people with cancer have shown promising results, suggesting that it may contribute to reductions in psychological distress, sleep disturbance, and fatigue, and may help to promote personal growth. MBIs can also have positive effects on activity in the immune system, HPA axis, and ANS, but it is not yet clear whether these always translate into clinically relevant health benefits (Rouleau et al., 2015).

Support interventions include individual support, telephone support, support groups, and internet support. The support is often provided by a peer, but may instead be a healthcare professional. Early research into support interventions suggested they could prolong survival (Spiegel et al., 1989). However, later research has been mixed. Reviews of research indicate that although support interventions are positively evaluated and lead to high levels of satisfaction, the evidence for significant psychological and physical benefits is mixed (Hong et al., 2012). Mixed findings are probably due to a wide variation in support interventions and individuals. Support groups do not appeal to everyone: 20–40% of people with cancer will refuse to attend or drop out. People with less severe cancer may be more distressed by attending support groups with people who are at the end-stages of the disease. Support interventions are therefore only likely to be beneficial for a subgroup of people, such as those with high levels of distress, poor personal resources, and not much support. People who *do* choose to attend support groups usually report improved psychological wellbeing and quality of life (Hong et al., 2012).

Other interventions have been used with positive results. These include physical exercise programmes, which help to improve quality of life, physical functioning, and emotional wellbeing, and reduce fatigue (May et al., 2009; Mustian et al., 2017). Massage therapy has been found to reduce pain, nausea, distress, and fatigue (Ernst, 2009).

CLINICAL NOTES 11.2

Coping with cancer

- Psychosocial factors influence the onset and progression of many cancers.
- Encourage people to change risk factors, such as lifestyle, stress, emotions, and psychological problems.
- It is important to treat psychological disorders in people with cancer.
- Encourage the partners and relatives of people with cancer to engage actively in discussions about cancer to find constructive ways of coping with it.
- Generally it is not helpful if the partners of people with cancer hide their concerns.
- Support groups are helpful for some people with cancer, but be aware that many people do not find them to be beneficial.

Summary

- Psychosocial risk factors for cancer include demographic factors, lifestyle, stress, and support.
- Tobacco use, diet, and infections are responsible for up to half of all cancers.
- Poor social support and depression are associated with the onset and progression of some cancers, but it is unclear whether depression causes cancer or is a response to cancer.
- Many people with cancer report clinically significant levels of anxiety, depression, or PTSD.
- Psychosocial interventions for cancer include cognitive behavioural therapy, mindfulness-based interventions, and support groups.
- These interventions usually improve quality of life and psychological wellbeing but there is little consistent evidence that they affect physical outcomes.

FURTHER READING

Llewellyn, C.D. et al. (eds) (2018) *Cambridge Handbook of Psychology, Health and Medicine* (3rd edition). Cambridge: Cambridge University Press. Includes short chapters on psychoneuroimmunology, immunisation, and many specific skin disorders and cancers.

Glaser, R. & Kiecolt-Glaser, J.K. (2005) Stress-induced immune dysfunction: Implications for health. *Nature Reviews: Immunology*, 5: 243–251. An excellent, authoritative overview of research into the impact of stress on the immune system.

Breitbart, W.S., Jacobsen, P.B., Loscalzo, M.J., McCorkle, R. & Butow, P.N. (eds) (2015) *Psycho-Oncology* (3rd edition). New York and Oxford: Oxford University Press. A comprehensive book covering all aspects of psycho-oncology, including lifestyle factors and risk, screening, responses to treatment, psychiatric comorbidity, psychosocial intervention, cancer in special groups such as children, and those with other special needs.

Bewley, A., Taylor, R.E., Reichenberg, J.S. & Magid, M. (eds) (2014) *Practical Psychodermatology*. Chichester, UK: Wiley. This book provides a practical guide to the management of people with psychocutaneous conditions. It considers issues from the perspectives of dermatologists and psychiatrists.

REVISION QUESTIONS

1. How do the immune effects of acute stress differ from those of chronic stress?

2. Describe the links between negative emotions and immune function.

3. Describe the links between positive emotions and experiences on immune function.

4. How does stress affect responsiveness to vaccinations?

5. Compare the prevalence of depression in people with immune disorders to the prevalence in the general population. How can we explain the observed differences?

6. What do the results of wound healing studies tell us about the impact of negative psychological states on immune function?

7. Why are psychological interventions useful for treating skin disorders?

8. Outline the important psychosocial risk factors for cancer onset.

9. How do psychosocial factors like coping and social support affect cancer progression?

10. 'Every person with cancer should join a support group'. Give arguments for and against this statement.

12 CARDIOVASCULAR AND RESPIRATORY HEALTH

(Continued)

> **Research boxes**
>
> 12.1   Stress-induced ischaemia in people with coronary artery disease
> 12.2   The psychological impact of CHD
> 12.3   A mobile phone intervention to increase asthma medication adherence

LEARNING OBJECTIVES

This chapter is designed to enable you to:

- Understand the role of psychosocial factors in the development of cardiovascular disease.
- Outline the various pathways through which psychosocial factors impact on cardiovascular disease.
- Describe the role of psychosocial factors in respiratory infections and asthma.
- Discuss the efficacy of psychological interventions for cardiovascular and respiratory disorders.

The first part of this chapter examines how psychosocial factors can affect the development and progression of heart disease. Cardiovascular health is affected by a range of psychosocial risk factors, including lifestyle, stress, emotions, and social circumstances. These factors can affect the development of heart disease, as well as the prognosis in people who already have heart disease. Coronary heart disease (CHD) is life-threatening and so requires extensive adjustment and changes in lifestyle. Unsurprisingly, CHD may result in high levels of fear, distress, anxiety, and depression, which in turn may affect both health and prognosis. Cardiac rehabilitation supports people after the onset of heart disease and may help them to reduce their risk of future illness.

The second part of this chapter examines psychological factors and respiratory health. Breathing and emotions are strongly interlinked. Furthermore, psychosocial factors can influence the onset and progression of respiratory disorders. Given the range and variety of respiratory disorders, it is not possible to cover them all. Here we focus on common examples of respiratory infections and asthma to illustrate the role of psychological factors in acute and chronic respiratory disorders.

12.1 CARDIOVASCULAR HEALTH

Psychosocial factors affect heart disease through four pathways:

- Lifestyle factors such as smoking, diet, and exercise affect the risk of atherosclerosis and CHD.
- Psychosocial factors can trigger acute cardiac events in people with existing coronary pathology.

- Sociodemographic factors are associated with risk and the accessibility of services.
- Beliefs influence the use of healthcare services by people with cardiovascular disease.

This section examines the key psychosocial risk factors that influence CHD: lifestyle, stress, depression, hostility or anger, and social isolation.

12.1.1 PSYCHOSOCIAL RISK FACTORS FOR HEART DISEASE

Numerous research studies have identified chronic and acute risk factors for CHD. Chronic risk factors exert their influence over longer periods and include things like smoking, hypertension, and high cholesterol. Acute risk factors are transient physical changes that occur following exposure to physical or psychological triggers, such as exercise or stress, which cause clinical events such as ischaemia, infarction, or sudden death. Chronic and acute risk factors combine to increase the overall risk of a cardiac event. In other words, people with high chronic risk (e.g. a smoker with a family history of CHD) have the greatest risk of a problem occurring when acute risk factors arise (e.g. intense exercise or stress). Table 12.1 shows the main chronic and acute risk factors for CHD.

Many physical and psychosocial risk factors overlap, so separating out the impact of physical, lifestyle, and psychological risk factors can be a challenge. For example, a study

TABLE 12.1   Chronic and acute risk factors for coronary heart disease (Barth et al., 2010; Benjamin et al., 2017; Edmin et al., 2016; Peters et al., 2014; Steptoe & Kivimäki, 2013)

	Chronic risk	**Acute risk**
Physical	Family history	Cardiovascular reactivity
	Cholesterol	
	Hypertension	
	Diabetes	
Demographic	Age (older)	
	Sex (male)	
	Socioeconomic status	
Lifestyle	Smoking	Intense exercise
	Obesity	
	Sedentary lifestyle	
Psychosocial	Stress	Intense stress
	Hostility/anger	Intense anger
	Depression	
	Anxiety	Anxiety
	Social isolation	

that followed 2,272 men over 10 years found that those with the lowest incomes were three times more likely to die of any cause and more than twice as likely to die of CHD (Lynch et al., 1996). However, the effect of socioeconomic status on CHD was due to 23 different risk factors. These included:

- Physical factors (e.g. fibrinogen, cholesterol, triglycerides, blood pressure, and body mass index).
- Lifestyle factors (e.g. smoking, alcohol use, and physical activity).
- Psychosocial factors (e.g. depression, hopelessness, and social support).

It is therefore important to consider all areas of risk in the prevention and treatment of CHD.

Lifestyle and health behaviours

Lifestyle has a powerful impact on cardiovascular health. A study of more than 20,000 men and women over 10 years identified four behaviours that made a dramatic difference to mortality, particularly deaths from cardiovascular causes. People who did not smoke, were physically active, had moderate alcohol intake, and ate five or more servings of fruit or vegetables a day were four times less likely to die prematurely than people who did none of these behaviours (Khaw et al., 2008). This difference remained even after taking into account age, sex, body mass index, and socioeconomic status. In fact, the impact of doing these four health behaviours was equivalent to being 14 years younger.

Changes in lifestyle factors can therefore account for a large proportion of the reduction in CHD over recent decades (Ezzati et al., 2015). Figure 12.1 shows the contribution of medical treatments and lifestyle to CHD mortality in the UK at the end of the last century: decreases in smoking, hypertension, and high cholesterol made a large contribution to reducing CHD. Reductions in smoking alone had a greater impact than all the advances in medical treatments during this time (Ünal et al., 2005). Smoking is therefore the single most important lifestyle risk factor to address. Smokers are twice as likely to die from CHD and 2–4 times more likely to have a sudden cardiac arrest or myocardial infarction (MI). If people with CHD stop smoking their risk of death drops by 36% and risk of another MI drops by 32% compared to those who continue to smoke (Critchley & Capewell, 2004).

Diet and exercise are important – especially so given the trend for increasing obesity and physical inactivity, which is adversely affecting rates of CHD, as shown in Figure 12.1. Governmental agencies and non-governmental organisations recommend that people's diets should be characterised by:

- A variety of fruit and vegetables every day
- Two portions of fish per week – particularly salmon, mackerel, or other fish rich in omega-3 fatty acids
- Whole grains such as brown rice, and wholemeal bread or tortillas
- Low fat intake – with as little saturated fat as possible
- Low salt intake

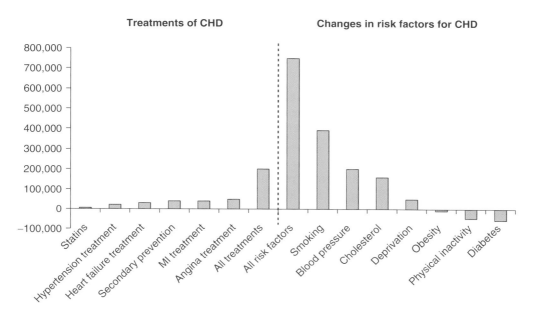

Number of life years gained through treatment of CHD and reducing risk factors

FIGURE 12.1 Effect of treatment and risk factors in the decline in CHD (England and Wales, 1981–2000) (adapted from Ünal et al., 2005)

It is commonly thought that moderate alcohol consumption reduces the risk of cardiovascular disease, but more recent analyses do not provide clear evidence of the protective effects of moderate alcohol consumption (Roerecke & Rehm, 2014a, 2014b). Regular moderate exercise reduces the risk of CHD, and is effective as part of efforts to reduce weight, body fat, blood pressure, and cholesterol, and to improve psychological wellbeing (Reiner et al., 2013).

Being aware of a person's risk factors and helping them to stop smoking, exercise more, and eat healthily are important parts of cardiac disease prevention and rehabilitation. However, one study found that fewer than 20% of cardiology notes covered all the major risk factors (Gravely-Witte et al., 2008). Critical risk factors of smoking and cholesterol were reported in 80% of the notes, but other risks, such as obesity and family history, were reported in less than 50% of notes. Careful screening of risk behaviour is an important first step toward reducing CHD and improving the prognosis in people with CHD. Various evidence-based techniques for health behaviour change can contribute to effective intervention and rehabilitation (see Chapter 5).

Stress

The physical and lifestyle risk factors referred to above account for about half the variance in new cases of heart disease, but they leave much of the risk unaccounted for.

Researchers have therefore focused on other potential risk factors, such as stress and differences in cardiovascular responses to stress, emotions, and social isolation.

ACTIVITY 12.1

- When you are stressed, how does this affect your lifestyle (e.g. health behaviours like smoking, drinking, diet, sleep, and exercise)?
- How do you think we can separate the effect of stress from the effects of lifestyle?

There is substantial evidence from epidemiological, experimental, and animal studies that stress affects CHD onset and cardiac events (Steptoe & Kivimäki, 2013). Epidemiological studies show that stressors such as natural disasters, war, terrorism, and even sporting events can be associated with increased cardiac morbidity and mortality. For example, a national survey in the USA showed that diagnosed CHD increased by 53% after the 9/11 terrorist attacks, even after taking into account existing risk factors (Holman et al., 2008). Football matches can have similar effects. Hospital admissions for cardiac emergencies are more common on World Cup match days, especially in the hours during and after matches (Wilbert-Lampen et al., 2008).

Experimental studies have shown that stressful tasks like giving a public speech increase both heart rate and blood pressure and can trigger ischaemia (restricted blood flow to the heart) in people with CHD (Steptoe & Kivimäki, 2013). Ischaemia is easily provoked, reversible, and clinically important, so it is a good way to study the effects of stress on the heart. Studies of naturally occurring ischaemia show that it is more likely to occur during intense physical activity, stressful mental activity, or when people feel angry. Research Box 12.1 describes one such study.

RESEARCH BOX 12.1 Stress-induced ischaemia in people with coronary artery disease

Background

The association between stress and cardiovascular disease is well established. This study was designed to examine the links between myocardial ischaemia induced by mental stress and exercise-induced ischaemia.

Method and findings

The study involved 79 people with coronary artery disease whose earlier completion of a treadmill test indicated that they experienced exercise-induced ischaemia. All patients

(Continued)

completed a stressful mental arithmetic task and a task in which they recalled an annoying and/or frustrating event from their lives. After a rest period, they then completed an exercise stress task on a treadmill. Performance on this exercise stress test was compared to the earlier exercise stress test.

Of the patients, 61% showed ischaemia during the mental stress test. The results of the exercise stress tests revealed two important and statistically significant findings: (i) participants who developed ischaemia in the mental stress tests had shorter average times to onset of ischaemia in the treadmill test; (ii) all participants had shorter average times to onset of ischaemia in the treadmill test after they had completed the mental stress tests (regardless of whether they developed ischaemia in the mental stress test).

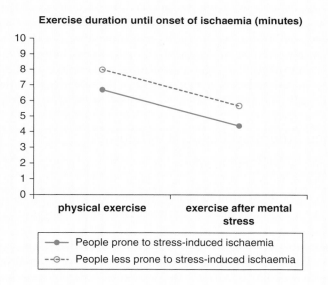

Exercise duration until onset of ischaemia (minutes)

Significance

This study confirms that mental stress can induce myocardial ischaemia in people with coronary artery disease. This study also demonstrates that mental stress can make myocardial ischaemia during physical activity more likely.

Stepanovic, J., Ostojic, M., Beleslin, B., Vukovic, O., Djordjevic-Dikic, A., Giga, V., Nedeljkovic, I., Nedeljkovic, M., Stojkovic, S., Vukcevic, V., Dobric, M., Petrasinovic, Z., Marinkovic, J. & Lecic-Tosevski, D. (2012) Mental stress-induced ischemia in patients with coronary artery disease: Echocardiographic characteristics and relation to exercise-induced ischemia. *Psychosomatic Medicine, 74*: 766–772.

Hostility and anger

The study of hostility and anger originated from research into the association between CHD and Type A behaviour pattern. Type A personalities are characterised by excessive competitiveness, impatience, time-consciousness, and hostility or aggression. Early research in the 1950s found that Type A men were more at risk of CHD. However, later research revealed that hostility and anger were the most important components of Type A in the development and prognosis of CHD. Meta-analyses show that anger and hostility are associated with an increased risk of CHD in healthy people, particularly men, and with a poor prognosis in people with CHD, even after taking into account the severity of the disease (Chida & Steptoe, 2009).

Anger and hostility are therefore chronic risk factors for CHD. Anger is also a potent trigger of acute cardiac events. In two large studies of MI in the USA and Sweden, anger was found to be a particularly strong trigger. People were between two and four times more likely to have an MI after an angry episode compared to when they were not angry (Steptoe & Brydon, 2009). Interview studies of people after MI show that between 2% and 17% of them reported being angry in the two hours before their MI symptoms. Newton (2009) places the role of anger and hostility in a social context – namely, through social dominance and submissiveness. Dominant people have been shown to react more strongly to stress and recover more slowly, particularly if the stressor is a social challenge.

Depression and other psychosocial difficulties

As with stress, there is substantial evidence that depression is associated with CHD onset and prognosis, and that CHD is in turn associated with depression. It has been argued that we should consider depression to be a major modifiable risk factor for cardiovascular disease in the same way that smoking, hypertension, and hyperlipidaemia are (Dhar & Barton, 2016).

Up to 40% of people who have experienced a major cardiac event meet the diagnostic criteria for major depressive disorder, and rates may be higher among those who undergo cardiac surgery (Dhar & Barton, 2016). Depression seems to be more common in people with CHD who are younger, female, socially isolated, experience greater pain or disability, or have a history of psychological problems (Bennett, 2007a).

People with depression after CHD have a worse prognosis (Gathright et al., 2017). Many studies show a clear dose–response relationship between the severity of depression and cardiac morbidity. This relationship is evident even after physical risk factors are taken into account. Depression after an acute cardiac event lowers quality of life and increases the risk of premature morbidity or mortality (Dhar & Barton, 2016).

The link between depression and CHD may be due to both physical and behavioural pathways (see Table 12.2). People with depression after CHD show physiological changes that increase their vulnerability to future cardiac problems. For example, studies have shown depression can be associated with HPA axis dysfunction, increased platelet activation and inflammatory responses, and impaired vascular function (Lichtman et al., 2008). An interesting review of twin studies found that nearly 20% of the variability in symptoms of depression and CHD was due to common genetic factors (McCaffery et al., 2006).

Thus there may be common genetic determinants of CHD and depression, possibly via inflammatory pathways and serotonin responses.

Given the links described above, it is important to identify and treat depression in people with CHD. The American Heart Association recommends that all people with CHD are screened for depression. Those with mild symptoms should be followed up during subsequent routine visits. Those with moderate or severe symptoms should be referred for comprehensive evaluation and treatment by a mental health professional (Lichtman et al., 2008). However, many cardiologists do not routinely ask people about depression, and even when depression is identified, it is not always treated (Feinstein et al., 2006). Although there is currently no consensus on the optimal screening tool for depression in people with CHD, there is a clear need to increase the use of any of the existing screening tools (Ren et al., 2015). Table 12.3 shows a brief screening questionnaire that can be used with people with CHD to identify depression and other forms of psychological distress.

TABLE 12.2 Mechanisms through which depression affects the prognosis of CHD

	Chronic risk
Biological	Hypothalamic-pituitary-adrenal (HPA) axis dysfunction
	Reduced heart rate variability
	Increased inflammatory response
	Impaired vascular function
	Increased platelet activation
Behavioural	Poor adherence to medication and treatment regimes
	Lack of participation in cardiac rehabilitation
Lifestyle	Smoking
	Diet
	Sedentary lifestyle
Psychosocial	Social isolation
	Chronic stress
	Comorbid anxiety disorders

RESEARCH BOX 12.2   The psychological impact of CHD

Background

The importance of lifestyle modification among people with CHD is well known, but only 50% of people adhere to recommended lifestyle changes. There is a clear need to understand why people do or do not engage with secondary prevention activities.

(Continued)

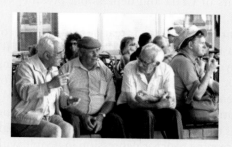

Photo courtesy Pedro Ribeiro Simões, July 2009, CC BY 2.0

Method and findings

Qualitative methods can provide useful insights into people's experiences and understanding of health and illness, but individual studies often have small samples. Meta-synthesis of the findings of multiple qualitative studies can highlight important similarities and differences across samples. In this study, the authors analysed the accounts of over 500 people with CHD from 27 studies in eight countries.

Results revealed that all participants experienced a change from their 'familiar' identity to an 'unfamiliar' identity. The change required them to 'find new limits' and find 'a new normal' in a lifestyle that was also considered to be 'a life worth living'. These major changes to identity often led to people having to 'reassess past, present, and future lives'. In the context of major changes to identity, patients saw behaviour modification as one extra change that they were being asked to make.

Significance

This meta-synthesis highlights people's desire for normality in the context of a major change to their health and identity. People's ability to adhere to recommended lifestyle changes is likely to be affected by how large and manageable these changes are in the context of other major life changes.

Astin, F., Horrocks, J. & Closs, S.J. (2014) Managing lifestyle change to reduce coronary risk: A synthesis of qualitative research on people's experiences. *BMC Cardiovascular Disorders*, 14: 96.

Over the last two weeks, how much have you been bothered by:

TABLE 12.3 Screening tool for psychosocial distress (STOP-D)

Feeling sad, down, or uninterested in life?	Not at all	0	1	2	3	4*	5	6	7	8	Extremely
Feeling anxious or nervous?	Not at all	0	1	2	3	4*	5	6	7	8	Extremely
Feeling stressed?	Not at all	0	1	2	3	4	5*	6	7	8	Extremely

(Continued)

| Feeling angry? | Not at all | 0 | 1 | 2 | 3 | 4 | 5* | 6 | 7 | 8 | Extremely |
| Not having the social support you feel you need? | Not at all | 0 | 1 | 2 | 3 | 4 | 5* | 6 | 7 | 8 | Extremely |

* Recommended cut-off indicating those people who need referral to psychological services for further assessment and treatment for psychological distress.

Reproduced courtesy of Quincy Young from Young et al. (2007)

Social isolation and support

The effect of social support, negative interpersonal relationships, and isolation on cardio-vascular disease has been well established (Barth et al., 2010). For example, physiological studies indicate that cardiac reactivity to acute stress is greater when people are prompted to think about negative or ambivalent relationships (Carlisle et al., 2012).

Research conducted over the last 40 years has revealed better cardiovascular outcomes for married people, with single men tending to have worse patterns of cardiovascular risk factors and cardiovascular disease (Manfredini et al., 2017). Although attention has often been given to the benefits of relationships for men, a study of over 700,000 British women found that those who were married or living with a partner had a significantly lower risk of ischaemic heart disease mortality (Floud et al., 2014). However, it is not just being in a relationship that is important: relationship quality matters. For example, meta-analysis of 126 studies involving over 72,000 people showed that greater marital quality is related to lower cardiovascular reactivity during marital conflict (see section 12.1.2) (Robles et al., 2014). This influence of marriage and social support on CHD is partly due to single people being more likely to have unhealthy lifestyles and increased distress. For example, a study of over 13,000 Scottish adults showed that 59% of the risk of dying of cardiovascular causes was explained by health behaviours, metabolic dysregulation, and distress (Molloy et al., 2009).

Social isolation is highly pathogenic: it is associated with morbidity and mortality in healthy people and people with CHD. For example, a study of 430 people with CHD found that people who had fewer than four close friends or family were more than twice as likely to die from CHD or other causes – even after controlling for disease severity, age, hostility, smoking, and psychological distress (Brummett et al., 2001). The increased risk associated with extreme social isolation is at least as great as the risk of other major factors, such as smoking (but there are no differences in risk between people with medium or large support networks).

In sum, psychosocial factors such as stress, depression, anger, and social isolation are influential risk factors for cardiac morbidity and mortality. Depression and social isolation in particular are equivalent to other major risk factors, such as smoking. The physical processes through which stress, emotions, and social isolation can affect CHD are believed to include stress-induced autonomic nervous system dysfunction, haemodynamic responses, neuroendocrine activation, inflammatory responses, and prothrombotic responses (notably platelet activation). These factors contribute to coronary plaque disruption, ischaemia, cardiac dysrhythmias, and thrombus formation (Steptoe & Brydon, 2009). The role of cardiovascular reactivity and other haemodynamic responses is therefore examined in the next section.

12.1.2 CARDIOVASCULAR REACTIVITY

Efforts to understand the links between psychosocial factors and CHD focus increasingly on cardiovascular responses to stress and how these are moderated by other risk factors. There is now a wealth of evidence that people vary in the magnitude of their cardiovascular responses to stress. Such research typically involves monitoring changes in blood pressure, heart rate, ischaemia, or endothelial function while people complete stressful tasks like those described in Research Box 12.1. Cardiovascular reactivity appears to be an enduring individual trait: people's responses are fairly consistent over time and with different stressors. The key question is whether hyper-reactivity causes future heart disease or whether it serves as a marker of future risk (without necessarily being causal). A review of prospective studies found that people with hyper-reactive responses to stress were more likely to develop hypertension in subsequent years (Treiber et al., 2003). Hyper-reactivity may also be associated with atherosclerosis and left ventricular mass, which may be precursors to CHD (Treiber et al., 2003). However, hyper-reactivity was not associated with the development of CHD in healthy populations. This was different in people with CHD, where hyper-reactivity was associated with subsequent cardiac morbidity.

Cardiovascular reactivity therefore differs between people and is associated with long-term risk factors for CHD and a higher clinical risk in people with CHD. However, reactivity is influenced by a number of other factors, including physical fitness, family history, and support. A review of research evidence indicated that aerobic and resistance training to enhance fitness can attenuate cardiovascular reactivity to stress, and may reduce the incidence of stroke and myocardial infarction (Huang et al., 2013). Research also shows that having a friend or ally present when performing stressful tasks can reduce cardiovascular reactivity, particularly if the friend is female (Christenfeld & Gerin, 2000).

Another area of interest is vascular endothelial reactivity. Endothelial function contributes to vessel tone, dilation, platelet aggregation, and inflammation. Stressful situations typically result in a reduction in endothelial-dependent vasodilation, whereas positive emotions, such as laughing, result in increases. In one study, people who watched a comedy film had a 22% increase in vasodilation whereas those who watched a harrowing war film had a 35% decrease (Miller et al., 2006). Thus, it has been proposed that vascular reactivity may be the critical link that explains the impact of positive and negative emotions on cardiovascular health.

12.1.3 IMPACT OF HEART DISEASE

MI is a sudden, unexpected, and potentially life-threatening event that can have a severe impact on a person's wellbeing and lifestyle. As noted earlier, up to 30% of people report depression in the first year after an MI. In addition, 12% develop clinically relevant symptoms of post-traumatic stress disorder (PTSD). PTSD is bad enough in itself, but it also doubles the risk of subsequent acute cardiac events (Edmondson et al., 2012). As with most illnesses, there is little association between the severity of CHD and psychological distress, with the exception of end-stage heart failure when people are likely to be highly distressed. For example, one study found that the following factors were strong predictors of the development of PTSD:

- History of psychological problems.
- Belief that the MI had negative consequences (e.g. problems in relationships or dealing with medication and self-care).
- Dysfunctional coping techniques (e.g. trying to numb emotions, distract themselves from upsetting thoughts).

These factors were more strongly associated with PTSD than the perceived severity of the MI (Ayers et al., 2009).

The effect of psychological problems is compounded by the fact that they often occur together. For example, people with PTSD after MI are also more likely to have symptoms of anxiety, depression, and social dysfunction (Ayers et al., 2009). A review of studies of people with CHD revealed that hospital readmission rates were increased in those who had depression, anxiety, or PTSD. The results indicated that comorbid psychological conditions in people with CHD result in greater healthcare use and higher overall and outpatient health care costs (Baumeister et al., 2015). Symptoms of anxiety, such as a racing heart or palpitations, may be a particular issue because they mimic the symptoms of cardiac problems. Much of this is due to worry and health concerns rather than cardiac problems.

Psychological problems therefore affect people's wellbeing, quality of life, and use of health services. They may also affect whether people change unhealthy behaviours. Some studies have shown that people with CHD who are depressed are less likely to stop smoking or exercise, and that depression and PTSD are associated with medication non-adherence. For example, a recent study of people with CHD revealed that those with more severe symptoms of depression were less likely to adhere to complex medication regimens (Goldstein et al., 2017).

However, the effect of heart disease on psychological wellbeing is not always negative. Positive changes can also occur after illnesses such as MI. Studies have revealed that in the months after MI some people report a greater appreciation of life, improved close relationships, and healthy lifestyle changes (Petrie et al., 1999).

12.1.4 TREATMENT AND REHABILITATION

The prognosis following MI is much better if treatment is obtained quickly. However, many people take several hours to go to hospital for treatment. It is interesting to note that the amount of pain a person feels does not affect how quickly they obtain treatment (Walsh et al., 2004). Women and single people are slower to attend hospital, whereas people who believe a heart attack has serious consequences and those who have active or problem-focused coping styles are quicker to attend hospital (Perkins-Porras et al., 2009; Walsh et al., 2004).

CLINICAL NOTES 12.1

Treating cardiovascular disease

- Careful screening of risk behaviour is an important step toward reducing CHD and improving the prognosis in people with CHD.
- When taking a cardiovascular history it is important to ask about:
  - Lifestyle factors of smoking, physical activity, alcohol intake, and diet.
  - Current stress, depression, anxiety, anger, relationship quality, and social isolation.
- These factors can be as important as physical risk factors in the progression of illness.
- Depression occurs in 30% of people with CHD and increases the risk of death. Anxiety and PTSD are also prevalent.
- Depression is more likely in younger, female, socially isolated people or those with a history of psychological problems.
- Guidelines recommend screening for depression and referring moderately or severely depressed people for appropriate treatment.
- Cardiac rehabilitation reduces mortality but attendance is poor. Make sure you refer all patients and strongly encourage them to attend.
- You may want to consider using a home-based psychological rehabilitation programme that can be facilitated by a specialist nurse, such as the Heart Manual.

Cardiac rehabilitation

Rehabilitation programmes vary widely between countries and regions. Programmes may give different attention to diet, exercise, or other factors. They may also vary in the extent to which they focus on psychological variables known to improve adherence to therapeutic advice. It is therefore important to identify which programmes and their component parts are more effective. A meta-analysis of 23 trials involving over 11,000 people with CHD revealed that lifestyle modification programmes can lead to significant improvements in diet and exercise – particularly when programmes incorporate self-regulation techniques such as goal setting, self-monitoring, planning, and feedback techniques. Such changes in lifestyle are associated with reductions in all-cause mortality, cardiac mortality, cardiac readmissions, and non-fatal reinfarctions (Janssen et al., 2013).

A key issue is that attendance at rehabilitation programmes and adherence to recommended lifestyle changes are poor. Lower attendance is seen in people with ischaemic heart disease, older people, women, and people from ethnic minority groups. Beliefs about the illness can also influence attendance and other measures of recovery. A systematic literature review that examined the relationship between illness perceptions and attendance at cardiac rehabilitation in over 900 people found that people are more likely to attend rehabilitation if they view their condition as more controllable, as more symptomatic, as having more severe consequences, and if they feel that they understand their condition more (see section 4.4) (French et al., 2006). How severe a person believes the consequences of CHD are also influences how quickly they return to work, levels of disability, and social impairment – although it is difficult to determine how much of this is due to the actual severity of CHD (Petrie et al., 1996).

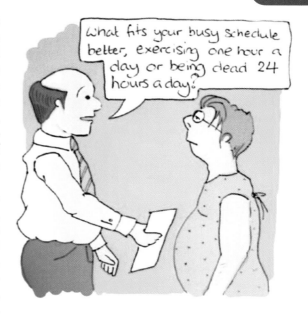

Despite the importance of beliefs and emotions in whether people attend rehabilitation, adhere to treatment, and recover, there is mixed evidence about the use of psychological intervention in rehabilitation programmes. Various rehabilitation programmes with psychological components have been proposed, such as the MULTIFIT programme in the USA (Taylor et al., 1997) and the Heart Manual in the UK (Lewin et al., 1992). These are home-based programmes administered by a trained facilitator. They use CBT or self-efficacy approaches for positive coping, changing maladaptive beliefs, stress management (see Chapter 3), self-management (see Chapter 4), and relaxation training (see Chapter 19). An example of this kind of programme is given in Case Study 12.1. Evaluations of these interventions are broadly positive: people prefer them to hospital-based programmes and are less likely to drop out (Lewin, 2007), and such programmes are as effective as hospital-based rehabilitation on numerous psychological, behavioural, biological, service, and cost outcomes (Clark et al., 2011). A systematic review concluded that psychological interventions provide a moderate protective effect against cardiac mortality, but found no convincing evidence that psychological intervention reduces the risk of premature death from any cause, revascularisation, or non-fatal infarction (Whalley et al., 2011). However, psychological interventions do result in significant improvements in depression and anxiety.

CASE STUDY 12.1   Cardiac rehabilitation

Omar was 42 when he had an MI and surgery to insert a stent into the blocked artery. Since then he has been on aspirin, an ACE inhibitor, and statins to reduce the likelihood it will occur again. He is married with a daughter and manages a regional finance office.

(Continued)

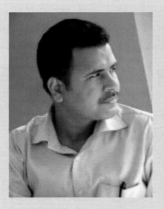

After Omar was discharged from hospital, he participated in a home-based rehabilitation programme using the Heart Manual, with regular check-ups with a nurse to facilitate his progress. The programme was a six-week course based on CBT principles that involve working through manuals and audio recordings to increase understanding and promote lifestyle changes.

First, Omar was assessed by a nurse to find out what his needs were with regard to medication adherence and lifestyle changes. Unhealthy behaviours and maladaptive beliefs were explored and Omar was encouraged to challenge these throughout his rehabilitation.

- Part 1 of the Heart Manual provides information and education about heart attacks and heart health. Omar listened to a CD of interviews about heart attacks with doctors, patients, and carers. Part 1 also includes information on common psychological reactions to heart attacks and how to manage distress or seek help if necessary.
- Part 2 of the Heart Manual is a six-week rehabilitation programme, which includes an exercise programme, health education, risk factor reduction, stress management, and sections on low moods, sleep problems, anxiety, and depression. During these six weeks, Omar used a diary to monitor his lifestyle and set his own weekly goals. He was also encouraged to recognise and write down any barriers and benefits to attaining these goals. He also used a CD of relaxation exercises.
- Part 3 of the Heart Manual gives facts and advice to help recovery. Topics include medicines, tests, revascularisation procedures, chest pains, anxiety, stress, and depression.

Omar's wife was involved throughout the rehabilitation programme and encouraged to help Omar achieve his goals and change. She was given a carer's booklet about the impact of a heart attack on relationships, how best to support Omar, and common effects on intimacy and sex. This was particularly useful because Omar admitted taking some of his anger and frustration out on his wife. Being able to recognise this and change it helped their relationship.

Omar met the nurse every week for the first few weeks and then continued to complete the Heart Manual programme on his own. He was followed-up two months later so that any depression or unhealthy behaviour could be picked up on.

Summary

- Psychosocial factors affect heart disease through three pathways: (i) the impact of health-related behaviours, (ii) direct or chronic physiological changes that contribute to heart disease, and (iii) accessing medical care and treatment.
- The main psychosocial risk factors for heart disease are lifestyle (smoking, exercise, diet), stress, depression, hostility/anger, and social isolation.
- People differ in their cardiovascular reactivity to stress. Reactivity may be a critical link between stress/emotion and cardiovascular health.
- Heart disease is associated with psychological disorders: many people develop depression or anxiety, or experience PTSD.
- Psychological problems are associated with a reduced quality of life, a reduced uptake of rehabilitation programmes, poor adherence to treatment, and the increased use of health services.
- Cardiac rehabilitation programmes significantly reduce cardiac mortality, but are not attended by the majority of people who are referred to them.
- Psychological interventions for heart disease can reduce non-fatal reinfarctions, depression, and anxiety, but does not influence mortality.

12.2 RESPIRATORY HEALTH

In the rest of this chapter we shall consider how psychological factors can contribute to different respiratory disorders and intervention. It is not possible to cover *all* respiratory disorders. Here we will focus on two common examples – acute respiratory infections and chronic asthma – which differ widely in terms of their management and prognosis. These disorders illustrate the different applications of psychological knowledge to respiratory disorders.

12.2.1 BREATHING AND EMOTIONS

Breathing is closely linked to our psychological state: it is the only vital bodily function that can be controlled voluntarily or by reflexes. Controlled slow breathing is the basis for many relaxation exercises and meditation techniques and can reduce physiological arousal, tension, and distress. Fast breathing and hyperventilation are common when we are stressed, anxious, or panicked. Our emotions, thoughts, and behaviour therefore both influence breathing and are influenced *by* breathing. For example, if people are asked to breathe quickly – to hyperventilate voluntarily – they will report a significant increase in anxiety, showing that how we breathe affects our emotions and vice versa.

ACTIVITY 12.2

- Take short, shallow breaths – at least 30 per minute – for five minutes.
- What symptoms did you notice? How did you feel physically and emotionally?

Hyperventilation may play a role in panic disorder. Symptoms of hyperventilation (e.g. shortness of breath) are common during panic. Exaggerated respiratory responses are associated with spontaneous panic attacks and people with panic disorder will often have low arterial carbon dioxide (CO_2) caused by chronic hyperventilation. Experimental studies in which people are given CO_2 show that people with panic disorder or a family history of panic disorder respond with greater anxiety (Zvolensky & Eifert, 2001). This effect remains even when they are compared with people with a generalised anxiety disorder or other mood disorders. Thus it may be that people with panic disorder are more sensitive to CO_2. Physical vulnerability to panic is compounded by psychological factors, particularly thoughts and the interpretation of physical symptoms. Panic disorder is strongly associated with anxiety sensitivity – a relatively stable characteristic where people are frightened, worried, or embarrassed by physical symptoms of anxiety.

The reciprocal relationship between breathing and emotion means that controlled breathing can be useful when treating stress-related disorders and panic. It can also be useful in promoting emotional wellbeing in chronic lung diseases such as asthma and emphysema (Timmons & Ley, 1994).

12.2.2 UPPER RESPIRATORY TRACT INFECTIONS

Upper respiratory tract infections (URI) such as colds and influenza account for 50% of all acute illnesses and are a major cause of morbidity and mortality worldwide. Colds are the most common URI and are caused by over 200 viruses (Marsland et al., 2007). The economic impact of the common cold is enormous – this includes not just the direct costs of treatment, but indirect costs associated with people taking time off work.

Exposure to a virus does not necessarily mean people will develop the clinical symptoms and illness that go with it. In fact, only one in three people exposed to a cold virus will develop a cold (Cohen, 2005). The most obvious variables to consider are the degree of exposure to a virus and the strength of someone's immune system and overall health. For example, the fact that colds are most prevalent in children may be due to their increased exposure to viruses through contact with other children at school or nursery and a relative lack of resistance. Contrary to folklore, catching a cold is not affected by cold weather. Evidence shows that putting people in cold conditions has little or no effect on the development or severity of a cold, unless these are extreme conditions.

Nor is susceptibility related to factors such as exercise, diet, or enlarged tonsils or adenoids. The use of mega doses of vitamin C does not prevent people catching colds, but can have a small effect on speeding up recovery (Hemilä et al., 2013).

Psychosocial factors associated with susceptibility to URIs include stress, social relationships, sleep, emotions, and socioeconomic status. The evidence is most convincing for stress. The impact of stress on immune function is well established (see Chapter 3), but it seems to be particularly related to a susceptibility to upper respiratory tract infections. For example, one study assessed medical students at several points over a year and found that during stressful exam periods students had worse immune function and more health problems, most of which were URIs (Glaser et al., 1987). In another series of well-controlled studies, volunteers were given a cold virus by a nasal spray and then quarantined for a number of days. Measures were taken of subjective ratings of illness (e.g. self-reported symptoms) as well as the objective indicators of illness (e.g. immune function and mucus production). Stress was consistently associated with an increased risk of developing a cold: the longer the duration of stressful events, the greater the risk of becoming infected. This effect remained even when controlling for factors such as age, weight, time of year, allergic status, pre-existing immune function or resistance, smoking, diet, and exercise (Cohen, 2005; Marsland et al., 2007).

Social relationships affect our susceptibility to URIs. Interpersonal stress such as conflict with family, friends, or colleagues increases the susceptibility to colds. Furthermore, people with good social networks (both in terms of size of network, integration, and sociability) seem to be protected from the development of colds. It is notable that more sociable people appear to be less at risk of developing colds. Although the contact hypothesis suggests that increased exposure to other people increases the risk of contracting a virus, sociability appears to be more important than this.

12.2.3 ASTHMA

Asthma is one of the most common chronic diseases in the world and is the most common chronic disease among children in developed countries. The World Health Organisation estimates that 300 million people worldwide have asthma (WHO, 2007). The highest prevalence can be found in the UK, Ireland, New Zealand, and Australia – and these rates are increasing. Asthma attacks incur large economic costs in terms of lost productivity, medical treatment, and social security costs. In the past, asthma was thought of as a psychosomatic disease – i.e. due to, or influenced by, psychological factors. We now know that several factors can contribute to the condition, including a genetic predisposition, diet, and lifestyle factors, as summarised in Table 12.4. It can be seen that, in comparison to the CHD risk factors in Table 12.1, there are fewer lifestyle and psychosocial causes of asthma. In fact, the role of psychosocial factors is largely limited to triggering asthma attacks in people who already have the disease.

Genetic vulnerability and parental smoking are strong risk factors for the initial onset of asthma. Although there is no specific gene that causes asthma, a combination of genes

TABLE 12.4 Risk factors for developing asthma or triggering asthma episodes

	Development of asthma	Factors that trigger asthma attacks or exacerbate symptoms
Physical	Genetic vulnerability (family history)	Allergens, e.g. pollen, dust mites
		Food allergies, e.g. nuts, shellfish
		Chest infections
		Chemical fumes
		Cold weather
Demographic	Age (younger)	
	Sex (male)	
	Socioeconomic status	
	Ethnic minority	
	Maternal age (younger)	
Lifestyle	Maternal smoking in pregnancy	Smoke
	Maternal anxiety	Pollution or vehicle exhaust fumes
	Smoking in the home	Intense exercise
	Violence in the home	
Psychosocial		Stress
		Anxiety

passed from parents to children approximately doubles the likelihood of children having asthma. Lifestyle factors are also important, primarily smoking and exposure to other pollutants. For example, if a woman smokes during pregnancy her child has a 35% increased risk of being wheezy or having breathing difficulties. Children whose parents smoke are 1.5 times more likely to develop asthma. Reducing parental smoking is therefore one of the most important, modifiable, risk factors for the development of asthma. Psychological knowledge can be useful in targeting health promotion to encourage parents to give up smoking (see Chapter 5).

Stressful life events may be involved in triggering asthma symptoms (Lietzén et al., 2011). There is substantial evidence that symptoms in people who already have asthma are exacerbated by stress (e.g. Liu et al., 2013; Sandberg et al., 2000). Research has also shown that children who are exposed to conflict report more symptoms and have an increased risk of complications (Tobin et al., 2015). The core pathological process of inflammation of the airways has led to the proposal that stress-induced changes in immune responses may contribute to this exacerbation and triggering of asthma (see Chapter 3). For example, in one study children with and without asthma were asked to make a speech and do mental arithmetic in front of an audience (Buske-Kirschbaum et al., 2003). The children did not differ in their heart rate responses to this stress, but those with asthma showed a significantly reduced cortisol response. Cortisol is anti-inflammatory so dysregulation of the cortisol response may be important in chronic asthma. There are similar findings for other chronic inflammatory diseases, such as rheumatoid arthritis (see Chapter 11).

In the previous section (12.2.2), we saw that chronic stress makes people much more vulnerable to respiratory infections. The role of respiratory tract infections in triggering asthma is well established: this is another important pathway between stress and asthma attacks (Cohen & Rodriguez, 2001). Section 12.2.1 highlighted the links between breathing and emotions, particularly anxiety. However, there is a lack of clear evidence that breathing training for asthma leads to improved outcomes – partly because breathing training is often presented as part of a broader intervention programme (Freitas et al., 2013; Macêdo et al., 2016).

There is evidence that anxiety disorders can exacerbate asthma symptoms. For example, a study of self-reported asthma attacks after the 9/11 terrorist attacks showed that among people with asthma, those who also had PTSD were three times more likely to have symptoms and visit their doctor and six times more likely to visit Accident and Emergency departments. This increased risk was irrespective of pre-9/11 asthma symptoms, demographic characteristics, or the amount of physical exposure to the attacks (Fagan et al., 2003). It therefore appears that anxiety disorders are important in the triggering and perception of asthma symptoms. A meta-analysis found that people with asthma were more likely than the rest of the population to have anxiety disorders (Weiser, 2007).

CLINICAL NOTES 12.2

Treating respiratory disorders

- Smoking and passive smoking are among the most important, modifiable risk factors.
- Most people cannot reliably detect changes in their lung function. It is important to confirm people's self-reports with physical measures such as a spirometer.
- Anxiety is strongly implicated in respiratory symptoms. Symptoms can be triggered or exacerbated by stress and anxiety.
- Symptoms are strongly affected by anxiety and beliefs about illness – these factors are more predictive of health outcomes than objective physical health.
- Self-management programmes are very effective at helping people manage their illness better.
- Self-management programmes involve education, the self-monitoring of lung function and triggers, using action plans to cope during episodes, and exploring and changing people's beliefs about illness.
- Guidelines state that self-management programmes should be incorporated into regular medical care.

Although psychological factors are not strongly implicated in the onset of asthma, they are very important when it comes to managing it. People with asthma are expected to monitor their symptoms and use inhaler medication when they need it. However, many people with asthma are unable to reliably detect changes in their lung function (Kendrick et al., 1993). The perception of symptoms and medical outcomes is associated with various psychological factors, including anxiety, pessimism, and perceived stigma. Compared to objective measures of asthma symptoms, these factors are better predictors of outcomes, such as the number of times a person is hospitalised for asthma, how long they stay, and their medication prescription. Thus there is a strong role for psychological factors in the management of asthma symptoms and their consequences. This is illustrated in Case Study 12.2, which shows how people's illness representations affect how they manage their symptoms (see section 4.4).

CASE STUDY 12.2   Illness representations and asthma symptoms

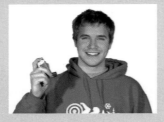 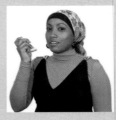

Illness Identity cause	Asthma is a mild condition. Caused by infections and a pet allergy.	Asthma is a severe condition. I inherited it from my dad.
Timeline	It's a remitting condition that some people grow out of.	It'll never go away.
Control	I can control the symptoms and exposure to triggers.	I can't control it.
Consequences	It is unlikely to kill me.	If it gets bad it could kill me.
Management	Relaxed attitude but avoids triggers where possible; will increase medication when he has an infection. Low anxiety, so will only visit the doctor when his own attempts to manage his symptoms do not work.	Tense and anxious about asthma symptoms. Has not thought about what might trigger her asthma, so is constantly worried and hypervigilant. Takes regular preventive medication and visits her doctor at the first sign of breathlessness.

RESEARCH BOX 12.3   A mobile phone intervention to increase asthma medication adherence

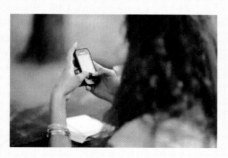

Background

To best manage asthma, people must take at least 80% of their preventive doses of inhaled corticosteroid medication. People with asthma often fail to meet this requirement. Lower levels of adherence are related to beliefs about key aspects of their illness (e.g. symptoms, cause), long-term implications, duration, and the extent to which it can be controlled by medication and lifestyle changes. It is therefore important to identify ways to promote healthier beliefs among people with asthma.

Method and findings

An 18-week SMS text message intervention was developed to modify illness beliefs. In New Zealand, 216 people with asthma completed a baseline questionnaire. Their responses enabled researchers to develop individually-tailored programmes of messages that were most likely to increase their medication adherence. Messages were sent at a frequency of two per day for the first six weeks, one per day for the next six weeks, and once every three days for the final three weeks. At the end of the intervention, when compared to people in a control group, those randomly allocated to the intervention realised the greater necessity of preventer medication, had greater belief in the long-term nature of their asthma, had greater perceptions of control over their asthma, and significantly improved adherence.

Significance

Text messaging is a cheap and effective way of changing illness and treatment perceptions to promote greater adherence to asthma medication. Text messaging may be an efficient way to deliver interventions to people who find it difficult to engage with face-to-face interventions.

Petrie, K.J. et al. (2012) A text message programme designed to modify patients' illness and treatment beliefs improves self-reported adherence to asthma preventer medication. *British Journal of Health Psychology, 17*: 74–84.

Psychological interventions to help people manage asthma include: education, self-monitoring of lung function and triggers, developing an action plan to help the patient know what to do during an asthma episode, and exploring and modifying illness beliefs. There is evidence that patient-centred self-management interventions are highly effective and result in reduced hospitalisation, fewer visits to health professionals, and fewer days off school or work (Qamar et al., 2011). Other positive outcomes include increased self-efficacy in children and reduced nocturnal asthma episodes in adults. Guidelines for asthma therefore explicitly state that self-management should be incorporated into regular medical management and that health professionals should encourage people to use self-management techniques (Global Initiative for Asthma, 2017).

Summary

- The reciprocal relationship between breathing and emotion means that controlled breathing can be useful when treating stress-related disorders and panic.
- Susceptibility to URIs is affected by stress, social relationships, sleep, emotions, and socioeconomic status. The effect of stress and social relationships on susceptibility to URIs is probably mediated by changes in immune function.
- Traditionally, asthma has been viewed as a psychosomatic illness but the evidence shows the initial onset is mainly determined by biological factors (genetic vulnerability, age, sex) and parental factors (e.g. being exposed to smoking or violence in the home).
- Anxiety is strongly implicated in respiratory symptoms. In those who have asthma, symptoms can be triggered or exacerbated by stress and anxiety.
- Although psychological factors are not hugely implicated in the onset of asthma, they are very important when it comes to managing it. Self-management interventions are highly effective and can result in less hospitalisation and fewer visits to the doctor or days off.

CONCLUSION

This chapter has examined the role of psychosocial risk factors in cardiovascular and respiratory disease. There are similarities and differences in the role of psychosocial factors in disorders of these two body systems. Psychosocial factors are extensively associated with heart disease: lifestyle, stress, and negative emotions are critical in the development of disease and the subsequent prognosis. Emotions of depression and anger/hostility are particularly implicated in heart disease. Respiratory disorders are also affected by lifestyle, stress, and emotions, but research shows that anxiety is especially important. In the respiratory disorders addressed here, psychosocial factors are less implicated in the development of pathology but are implicated in triggering or exacerbating symptoms. Of course, we have only looked at URIs and asthma and it is true to say that lifestyle factors – particularly smoking – are critical in the development of other respiratory diseases such as Chronic Obsructive Pulmonary Disease (COPD) and lung cancer.

Psychological intervention in cardiac or pulmonary rehabilitation has various effects. In cardiac rehabilitation, psychological intervention improves psychological wellbeing, and can reduce overall mortality, but it does not affect specific cardiac outcomes. In chronic respiratory disorders there is strong evidence that interventions that include psychological components can improve symptom management and healthcare use in disorders that involve significant self-management.

FURTHER READING

Llewellyn, C.D. et al. (eds) (2018) *Cambridge Handbook of Psychology, Health and Medicine* (3rd edition). Cambridge: Cambridge University Press. Includes short chapters on cardiovascular disease, coronary heart disease, and hypertension, as well as specific respiratory disorders (asthma, lung cancer, COPD, colds).

Levenson, J.L. (ed.) (2011) *The American Psychiatric Publishing Textbook of Psychosomatic Medicine: Psychiatric Care of the Medically Ill* (2nd edition). Arlington, VA: American Psychiatric Association Publishing. A 1,200-page book with very broad coverage of the topics covered in this and other chapters, including chapters on heart disease, lung disease, and oncology.

REVISION QUESTIONS

1. Describe three pathways by which psychosocial factors will influence the onset and progression of heart disease.

2. Outline the major psychosocial risk factors for cardiovascular disease and the magnitude of their effect on CHD risk.

3. How do individual differences in a cardiac reactivity to stress affect the risk of cardiovascular disease?

4. Describe the common psychological responses to cardiovascular disease. Outline the impact of psychological interventions on physical and psychological wellbeing.

5. Outline the factors associated with delays to seeking treatment for CHD and non-adherence to treatment regimens.

6. How is the relationship between breathing and emotions reciprocal? What is the clinical relevance of this observation?

7. Describe how psychosocial factors influence the susceptibility to upper respiratory tract infections.

8. Compare the relative importance of psychological and biological factors for asthma onset and episodes.

9. Outline why self-management interventions are effective in treating asthma.

10. Compare and contrast the role of psychosocial factors in cardiovascular and respiratory disease.

13 GASTROINTESTINAL HEALTH

(Continued)

LEARNING OBJECTIVES

This chapter is designed to enable you to:

- Outline the physiological basis for the relationship between psychological factors and GI health.
- Describe the role of stress in GI function and illness.
- Consider the impact of diet and alcohol use on GI health and illness.
- Outline the role of psychosocial factors in specific GI disorders.

There are clear links between psychology and the gastrointestinal (GI) system. This close relationship is illustrated in common language. Common expressions of psychological states include (to follow the sequence of the GI tract) *choking* on information, not *digesting* difficult news, having butterflies in the *stomach*, someone making us *sick*, having a *gut* feeling, or being scared *shitless*. Direct bi-directional physiological links exist between the brain, autonomic nervous system, and enteric nervous system. This is called the brain–gut axis. The four main links between psychological states and the GI system are:

1.   Brain–gut axis.
2.   Effect of stress on GI function.
3.   Effect of lifestyle – e.g. diet, alcohol use, smoking.
4.   Psychological impact of GI disorders.

The relative importance of these links varies. Functional GI disorders, such as Irritable Bowel Syndrome and dyspepsia, are more likely to be affected by factors such as stress and symptom perception. Organic disorders, such as cirrhosis or cancer, have stronger associations with lifestyle factors such as diet, drug, and alcohol use. GI medicine is therefore an area that certainly requires a biopsychosocial approach to prevention and treatment.

We start this chapter by examining how psychological factors interact with GI functioning through the brain–gut axis and the role of stress. We shall then examine the role of lifestyle factors on GI health, concentrating on diet and alcohol use. Finally, disorders of the GI system are examined to illustrate the complex interplay between psychology and the gut, and the profound impact of GI disorders.

13.1 PSYCHOLOGICAL FACTORS AND THE GI SYSTEM

Physiological responses to stress involve the central nervous system (CNS), autonomic nervous systems (ANS), and immune and neuroendocrine responses (see Chapter 3). All of these are implicated to varying degrees in GI function or disorders (van Oudenhove & Aziz, 2009; Muscatello et al., 2014).

13.1.1 THE BRAIN–GUT AXIS

The **brain–gut axis** comprises the CNS, ANS, and enteric nervous system (see Figure 13.1). The sympathetic and parasympathetic branches of the ANS innervate GI organs such as the stomach, liver, spleen, pancreas, and bowel. Under stress, the sympathetic nervous system and subsequent release of adrenaline (epinephrine) will reduce blood flow and peristalsis and inhibit the contraction of the rectum. Sympathetic activation is also associated with reduced food intake and weight loss. Under normal conditions, the parasympathetic nervous system restores blood flow and peristalsis to the usual functioning when the stressor is removed.

The **enteric nervous system** is embedded in the lining of the GI system and has been referred to as the '*brain of the gut*' or '*second brain*' because it is large and complex (approximately 100 million neurons) and uses the same neurotransmitters as the CNS. Although it is connected with the CNS, it is able to operate independently. It controls all the functions of the GI tract. Sensory information is sent from the enteric system to the CNS via the vagal nerve, which is thought to comprise 80% afferent fibres (Goyal & Hirano, 1996).

The existence and influence of the brain–gut axis means that psychological and gastric phenomena influence each other (Keightley, 2015; Muscatello et al., 2014; Van Oudenhove & Aziz, 2013). For example, placebo pills and suggestion may increase or decrease GI activity (Meissner, 2009), and the symptoms of nausea and vomiting can be classically conditioned, such as when people having chemotherapy develop anticipatory nausea (see Chapter 10). People with functional GI disorders are more likely to have psychological disorders or to have had past traumatic experiences. Furthermore, a high

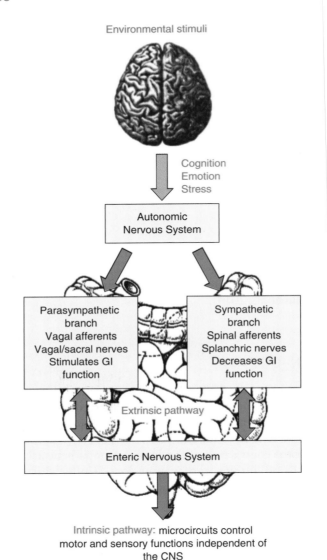

Environmental stimuli

Cognition
Emotion
Stress

Autonomic
Nervous System

Parasympathetic
branch
Vagal afferents
Vagal/sacral nerves
Stimulates GI
function

Sympathetic
branch
Spinal afferents
Splanchric nerves
Decreases GI
function

Extrinsic pathway

Enteric Nervous System

Intrinsic pathway: microcircuits control
motor and sensory functions independent of
the CNS

FIGURE 13.1 The brain–gut axis

prevalence of functional GI disorders is found in people with mental health problems, especially depression and anxiety disorders.

This reciprocal relationship between emotions and GI function is found not only in people with GI disorders. For all of us, emotions such as anxiety and disgust are linked with GI symptoms. Disgust tends to be accompanied by physiological movements that mimic retching or vomiting. Products of the GI system (e.g. vomit, faeces) are universal triggers of disgust across cultures (Rozin et al., 2000). Anxiety is associated with changes in GI function. In one study, healthy volunteers were asked to recall experiences that had made them feel neutral or anxious. These were recorded and then played back to them while they underwent various tests of gastric function. When listening to the recording of their anxious experience, volunteers had reduced gastric function and more reports of bloating and fullness (Geeraerts et al., 2005).

In functional GI disorders the brain–gut axis may become dysregulated. This is analogous to ANS and HPA-axis dysregulation in stress disorders (see Chapter 3), or dysregulation of immune responses in autoimmune disorders (see Chapter 11). Dysregulation of the brain–gut axis leads to altered sensation, symptoms, motility, and other aspects of GI function. Other alterations include an increased sensitivity to GI symptoms and altered pain pathways. Permanent changes may occur to the distribution of neurons in the enteric nervous system in chronic disease such as Crohn's disease or ulcerative colitis (Villanacci et al., 2008).

13.1.2 STRESS AND THE GI SYSTEM

As the brain–gut axis is intricately connected with stress responses it is not surprising that stress affects GI function in healthy people and exacerbates existing GI disorders, particularly functional disorders such as Irritable Bowel Syndrome (IBS) or ulcers (Fink, 2011; Leza & Menchen, 2008). Around 70% of the general population report changes in bowel function in response to stress (Drossman et al., 2002), and experimental studies indicate that stress can produce changes in bowel function (see Research Box 12.1) (Pritchard et al., 2015). Stress leads to a number of changes in the gut, including increased motility, altered ion secretion, increased intestinal permeability, low-grade inflammation, epithelial abnormalities, and enteric neuron dysfunction. In people with GI disorders, stress can contribute to gastric erosions and ulcers and increase the severity of colitis (Fink, 2011). Stress may interact with pathogens such as *Helicobacter pylori* or non-steroidal anti-inflammatory drugs (NSAIDs) to increase the likelihood of GI disorders (Caso et al., 2008; Fink, 2011).

The relationship between stress and GI function is complex because stress is also associated with psychological factors, such as an increased sensitivity to GI sensations and symptoms, decreased pain tolerance, and changes in behaviour that can affect GI function (Jennings et al., 2014). For example, one study found that people with functional GI disorders reported more stress and were more likely to perceive major life events as negative or stressful (Hui et al., 1999). Emotional distress, increased sensitivity, and an increased perception of symptoms may play a role in this. For example, in addition to reporting more anxiety, depression, and reduced quality of life, people with constipation are also more likely to monitor symptoms, are more sensitive to rectal distension and urge sensations, and are less tolerant of bowel volume (Chan et al., 2005).

Although the relationship between stress and GI symptoms is well established, the exact causal mechanisms through which this occurs are complex and likely to involve many factors, including physiological changes, emotional wellbeing, sensitivity, and symptom perception (see Figure 13.2 and Research Box 13.2 below). Stress may interact with

RESEARCH BOX 13.1　Stress and bowel function

Background

Stress is known to affect GI function and can lead to exacerbation of GI disorders such as Irritable Bowel Syndrome (IBS). This study used an experimental approach to determine the effect of two different forms of stress on bowel function in healthy people.

Method and findings

Thirty-six healthy adults were allocated to one of two groups. One group was exposed to stress in the form of a cold water hand immersion challenge or a non-stress control condition in the form of a warm water hand immersion. The second group was

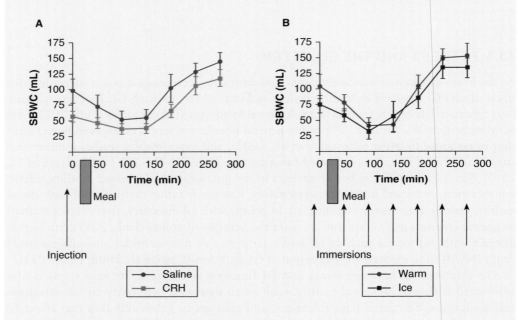

exposed to stress hormones via the intravenous administration of corticotrophin releasing hormone (CRH) or non-stress in the form of intravenous saline. Participants were monitored following consumption of a standard test meal of rice pudding.

Exposure to both stressors was followed by significant reductions in small intestine water content. The cortisol injection was followed by significant increases in ascending colon volume, but the cold water stress exposure did not produce a significant change.

(Continued)

Significance

This study provides evidence that stress – in response to cold immersion or CRH – accelerates the transfer of water from the small intestine to the large intestine. The results reflect the common experience that stress makes one's guts churn.

Pritchard, S.E. et al. (2015) Effect of experimental stress on the small bowel and colon in healthy humans. *Neurogastroenterology & Motility*, *27*: 542–549.

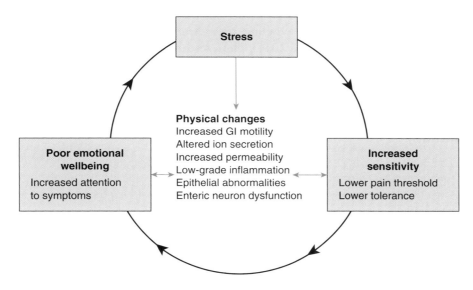

FIGURE 13.2 Stress and GI function

other factors such as an exposure to pathogens, lifestyle, and individual differences in coping style. This means that treating GI disorders can be particularly challenging: healthcare professionals must assess which physical and psychosocial factors are contributing to the disorder and then treat these appropriately.

13.1.3 A BIOPSYCHOSOCIAL APPROACH TO GI DISORDERS: THE CASE OF PEPTIC ULCERS

One clear example of the need to take a biopsychosocial approach is the history of our understanding of peptic ulcers. In the early 1980s Robin Warren and Barry Marshall conducted Nobel Prize-winning research which identified the role of the bacterium **Helicobacter Pylori** in stomach ulcers. Marshall used himself as a guinea-pig and infected himself with *H. pylori*, after which he developed gastritis. This discovery changed our understanding of what causes peptic ulcers. Since then, research has shown that *H. pylori* can be associated with a range of GI problems, including dyspepsia (heartburn, bloating, and nausea), gastritis, ulcers, and stomach cancer. Treatment of *H. pylori* with antibiotics has resulted in a steady decline in the incidence of peptic ulcers.

However, not all people with *H. pylori* develop disease, and up to 20% of people with ulcers do not have *H. pylori*. It is now thought, therefore, that *H. pylori* alone does not cause ulcers, but interacts with other factors, including dietary intake, to create the conditions in which disease may develop (Amieva & Peek, 2016). Other contributing factors include a genetic vulnerability, excess stomach acid, and the use of NSAIDs. Moreover, it has been estimated that psychosocial factors such as stress and lifestyle contribute to 30–65% of ulcers, regardless of whether these are caused by *H. pylori* or NSAIDs (Levenstein, 2000; Levenstein et al., 2015). Thus, research into *H. pylori* and peptic ulcers illustrates how we have moved from a purely biological explanation to a biopsychosocial explanation of peptic ulcer disease.

Summary

- The brain–gut axis comprises the CNS, ANS, and enteric nervous system, which means psychological and GI states influence each other quickly and easily.
- The enteric nervous system is connected with the CNS but is able to operate independently.
- In functional GI disorders the brain–gut axis may become dysregulated.
- The relationship between stress and GI function and symptoms is well established, but the relationship is complex and likely to involve many physiological and psychological factors.
- Stress leads to changes in GI motility and physiology. Stress is also associated with decreased pain tolerance, an increased sensitivity to GI sensations, a greater perception of symptoms, and changes in lifestyle that may further impact on GI function.
- A biopsychosocial approach is vital in GI medicine, as illustrated by the interaction between *H. pylori* and psychosocial factors in peptic ulcers.

13.2 LIFESTYLE AND GI HEALTH

Lifestyle factors such as diet, smoking, alcohol use, and exercise affect GI health. Smoking is associated with an increased risk of Crohn's disease, peptic ulcers, and cancers of the upper GI tract, but a reduced risk of ulcerative colitis. What we eat influences our risk of developing many disorders, including cancer, diabetes, and the intermediate outcomes of obesity: it is estimated that approximately 30% of cancers in developed countries are caused by unhealthy diets (see Figure 11.1). Alcohol use is a risk factor for liver disorders and six cancers of the GI tract (cancer of the oropharynx, larynx, oesophagus, liver, colon, and rectum) as well as breast cancer (Connor, 2017). In this section we shall therefore examine diet and alcohol use in more detail.

13.2.1 HEALTHY AND DISORDERED EATING

Diet and GI health

Diet is important to GI health. However, the links are complex because our diet consists of different nutrients that can affect our health directly or in combination with each other. Various aspects of diet are important to health (see Box 13.1). Although there are some areas where evidence is incomplete or inconsistent, the following aspects of diet are known to be important for GI health:

- **High fibre** reduces bowel cancer risk by up to 40%. This may be due to the effect of fibre on bowel function (i.e. stools spend less time in the bowel), so there is less time for food-related chemicals and antigens to damage the bowel lining. Alternatively, it may be due to the creation of short-chain fatty acids when fibre is broken down, which may make it harder for tumours to develop.
- **Fruit and vegetables** reduce the risk of cancers, particularly of the upper GI tract. This may be because they are a good source of fibre (as above) or because they provide vitamins A, B, and C, which may protect against cancer.
- **Oily fish** such as salmon and mackerel decrease the risk of cancer and heart disease.
- **Salt** is associated with an increased risk of stomach cancer, which is more prevalent in countries that have a very salty diet, such as Japan (see Figure 11.1).
- **Red meat** increases the risk of stomach and bowel cancer, particularly if the meat is processed (e.g. bacon, salami). This increased risk is thought to be due to chemicals contained in red meat, such as haem, that will damage the bowel when broken down. Carcinogens are also created when meat is cooked at high temperatures.

BOX 13.1   Guidelines for a healthy diet

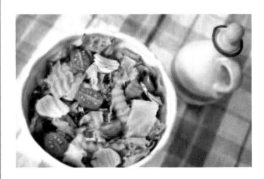

- Diet should be high in fibre: it should include foods such as fruit, vegetables, pulses, rice, and wholegrain foods.
- Eat 5+ portions of fruit and vegetables per day.
- Eat 2+ portions of oily fish a week.
- Decrease the intake of red or processed meat.
- If you drink alcohol, do so in moderation.
- Decrease salt intake.
- Avoid refined sugar.
- Avoid saturated fats.

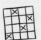

ACTIVITY 13.1

- How does your diet compare to the recommendations given in Box 13.1?
- What kind of factors influence the type of food you eat and when?

Why do we eat what we eat?

Given the evidence outlined above, it is a public health concern that many people do not have a healthy diet. For example, along various dimensions, the diets of people across Europe generally do not conform to guidelines for healthy eating (White et al., 2011). It is important to note, however, that although there is some variation in diets across Europe, globalisation has also resulted in an increasing homogenisation of diets. Whatever the norm for a particular country, women usually eat more fruit, vegetables, fibre, and less saturated fat than men. This appears to be because women have more concerns about weight and more healthy attitudes and beliefs about food.

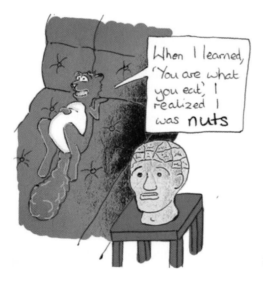

With obesity increasing, it is important to understand how poor dietary habits can develop. Research suggests that we are not born with a tendency to overeat or have a poor diet. Studies of infants and young children suggest that if they are offered a variety of healthy food and allowed to eat what they want, they will naturally choose a balanced diet (Tanofsky-Kraff et al., 2007). Poor dietary habits therefore appear to be learnt. This occurs through processes of exposure, reinforcement, modelling, and imitation during childhood (see Chapter 10). Dietary habits are also influenced by attitudes, beliefs, and weight concerns in adolescence and adulthood. Children will eat the food they are exposed to and will prefer those foods they are exposed to regularly. Therefore the more that unhealthy food is available and accessible in the environment (e.g. fast food), the more likely it is that children will eat and prefer this. Eating habits are also shaped through imitating friends and family. Modelling good eating behaviour can be used to promote healthy eating. Studies in several countries have assessed the impact of 'food dudes' – older children who were filmed enthusiastically eating healthy food – and found that exposure to such modelling can successfully change children's preferences for foods and increase their fruit and vegetable intake (Laureati et al., 2014; Wengreen et al., 2013).

The meaning of food in interactions between children and parents can shape children's eating behaviour. Food used as a reward or treat will be liked more and preferred over food that is seen as a non-reward. This means that strategies such as telling children they can only have pudding if they eat their vegetables may result in children learning to prefer pudding and dislike vegetables even more! Parental control over what children eat may have different effects depending on how the control is exercised. Hidden or covert control, such as making sure unhealthy food is not available in the child's environment, is associated with less snacking on sweets or energy-dense foods, and can lead to lower BMI (Ogden et al., 2006; Rodenburg et al., 2014). Overt control, such as telling the child what they can and cannot eat, is associated with an increased intake of healthy foods like fruit (Ogden et al., 2006). However, parental restrictions may lead to a child eating more 'bad' foods when not in the home environment or under parental control.

In adolescence and adulthood, diet is increasingly affected by body dissatisfaction and weight concerns. One longitudinal study of adolescents and young adults in the USA revealed that at least 20% of men and 50% of women had been on a diet in the last year – with dieting defined as 'changing the way you eat so you can lose weight' (Neumark-Sztainer et al., 2011). In one study of almost 16,000 university students in 22 low, middle, and emerging economy countries, 27% of those whose BMI indicated that they were not overweight were, nevertheless, trying to lose weight (Peltzer & Pengpid, 2015).

Dietary restraint or restrained eating does not always lead to weight loss or reduced weight gain in people who are overweight or of healthy weight (Clark, 2015; Lowe et al., 2013; Tucker & Bates, 2009). It is therefore important to note that restrained eating outside validated weight-loss programmes is often associated with a range of negative psychological states, including body dissatisfaction, food cravings, preoccupations with food, guilt about food/eating, over-estimating body size, low self-esteem, anxiety, and depression (Hawks et al., 2008; Schaumberg et al., 2016). Dietary restraint may also contribute to eating disorders such as anorexia and bulimia. Conversely, disinhibited or uncontrolled eating – where people find it hard to control their eating in response to environmental cues – may play a role in overeating and obesity. Some research has examined whether restrained eaters are more or less likely to become disinhibited eaters after they eat a high calorie snack. The results are inconsistent, but for some individuals the combination of restrained eating with difficulty in controlling their eating behaviour may lead to overeating and fluctuations in weight.

The following sections take a biopsychosocial approach to different eating disorders, but it is important to note the effect that emotions can have on the eating behaviour of people of normal weight who do not have eating disorders. For example, a meta-analysis revealed that stress, depression, and sadness tend to elicit eating behaviours that are unhealthy because of the foods that are chosen and/or the amount of food that is consumed (Devonport et al., 2017).

Disordered eating: anorexia, bulimia, and binge eating

Paradoxically, as food has become more widely available, there has been an increase in disordered eating: anorexia nervosa, bulimia nervosa, and binge eating disorder. Estimates of lifetime prevalence are less than 1%, but many more people may have symptoms of eating disorders without meeting the full criteria for diagnosis. Eating disorders are associated with an increased risk of other psychiatric problems, such as phobias, anxiety disorders, and substance misuse (Levinson et al., 2017). For example, in the USA comorbid anxiety disorders occur in 48% of people with anorexia, 81% of people with bulimia, and 65% of people with binge eating disorder (Hudson et al., 2007). Eating disorders can lead to a variety of physical problems, especially GI tract disorders such as gastric reflux, peptic ulcers, and constipation. Severe cases can lead to other problems, such as cardiac arrhythmias or cardiac arrest.

Anorexia nervosa is a refusal to maintain a healthy body weight. Anorexia has a lifetime prevalence of approximately 1–2% of women and 0.3% of men and cases are increasing (Smink et al., 2012). It is most likely to occur in women during their teenage years or early adulthood, and it is rare for new cases to occur after age 25 (see Case Study 13.1). White women from wealthy families are most at risk. Anorexia is also more prevalent in certain occupational groups, such as models and dancers, where there is pressure to be thin. Anorexia has the highest mortality rate of any psychiatric disorder, with suicide a common cause of death (Smink et al., 2012).

Many theories have been developed to explain why anorexia occurs, including a genetic vulnerability, biological abnormalities in noradrenaline or serotonin systems, mood disturbances, a need for control, low self-esteem, perfectionism, the internalisation of thin body ideals, dysfunctional family dynamics, and childhood sexual abuse. Although these factors have been found to be *associated* with anorexia, there is little prospective research that allows us to determine whether such factors are the causes or consequences of anorexia (Stice & Shaw, 2007). Twin studies indicate that genetic and environmental factors are both important (Bulik et al., 2016; Mazzeo et al., 2009).

Bulimia nervosa is characterised by binge eating followed by compensatory behaviours. These usually take the form of purging (e.g. self-induced vomiting or the use of laxatives) or non-purging (e.g. excessive exercising or fasting). Bulimia nervosa affects around 1–2% of women and 0.5% of men (Smink et al., 2012). Most people with bulimia are of average weight so this can often go undetected. Most evidence supports a social-cognitive explanation of bulimia where the promotion of thin body-ideals in the media leads to increased body dissatisfaction, negative feelings, and low self-esteem. These negative feelings can trigger dieting and bulimic behaviours. Bingeing and purging are thought to be used by bulimics to deal with or distract from their negative feelings and thoughts. This then becomes self-reinforcing because it temporarily removes negative feelings. Evidence supports this explanation. Research also confirms that binge eating is usually preceded by negative emotions, such as anxiety, depression, or loneliness (see Research Box 13.2).

Binge eating disorder (BED) (see Research Box 13.2) or **uncontrolled eating** is increasing. The prevalence of BED is around 2–4% of women and 1–2% of men (Smink et al., 2012). People with BED report poor social adjustment, impaired functioning, worse physical health, and more psychological disorders than people without BED (Palmeira et al., 2016; Wilfley et al., 2003). BED differs from other eating disorders in a number of ways. In contrast to anorexia, new cases of BED occur throughout adulthood – even up to age 60 (Hudson et al., 2007). However, it also tends to last longer than anorexia and bulimia

(Pope et al., 2006). Furthermore, sex differences are less marked than for other eating disorders. People with BED are not necessarily obese, although BED is slightly more common in obese people than in the general population. Its aetiology is unclear, but it is thought to be due to factors similar to those associated with bulimia. Prospective studies suggest that initial increases in weight can lead to body dissatisfaction, dietary restraint, negative emotions, and emotional eating, which will increase risk of BED (Stice & Shaw, 2007). Experimental studies indicate that the eating behaviour of people with BED is more likely than that of other people to vary in response to stress, suggesting that food intake may be varied as part of efforts to regulate negative emotions (Laessle & Schulz, 2009; Russell et al., 2017).

CASE STUDY 13.1   Anorexia nervosa

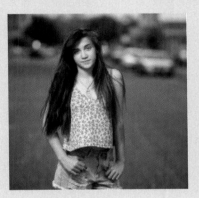

Andrea developed anorexia nervosa at the age of 15 and suffered from it for four years before finally returning to a healthy weight. Although she was always slim, Andrea said she felt 'deeply uncomfortable about my body and under-confident about who I was'. Comparing herself to girls at school and models in magazines, she felt overweight and became determined to get thin. She started to restrict her food intake and exercise excessively. Eventually her weight fell to less than 4.5 stone (29 kilos). Her BMI was 10.8.

The anorexia led to heart palpitations. Tests showed extreme malnutrition, so Andrea was admitted to hospital. After inpatient treatment Andrea's weight increased to six stone and she was allowed home. She said being ill and in hospital 'was a turning point as it made me realise the damage I was doing to myself. I had to help myself'. Andrea had several months of psychotherapy to help her develop a better relationship with food, a healthier and more realistic view of her body, and a more critical view of media representations of women.

RESEARCH BOX 13.2   Regulating distress by eating

Background

Theories of bingeing and purging argue that it is used by people with eating disorders to deal with and regulate negative emotions.

(Continued)

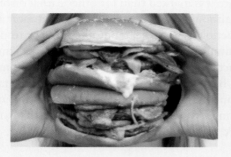

Photo courtesy of Paul Townsend, July 2013, CC BY-ND 2.0

Method and findings

This study examined factors that may be used to predict bingeing behaviour in 130 people with bulimia nervosa. The study used interviews and questionnaires to measure a wide range of factors, including impulsivity and people's tendency to act quickly and rashly to avoid negative emotions without thought of the consequences (negative urgency).

Negative urgency was the only variable that predicted binge eating when other factors were controlled for, including anxiety, depression, mood, age, sex, ethnicity, education, premeditation, and functioning.

Significance

This study demonstrated a strong association between the need to act rashly to regulate negative emotions and binge eating in people with bulimia, even after taking into account negative moods such as anxiety and depression.

Anestis, M.D., Smith A.R., Fink, L.E. & Joiner, T.E. (2009) Dysregulated eating and distress: Examining the specific role of negative urgency in a clinical sample. *Cognitive Therapy Research, 33*: 390–397.

ACTIVITY 13.2

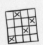

- When are you most likely to overeat and consume a large number of highly calorific foods?
- What factors do you think are important in triggering overeating?

Preventing and treating eating disorders

To be effective, the prevention of eating disorders should be based on our understanding of what causes these disorders. Simple educational approaches are not effective; it is also important to encourage attitude change and to develop skills. Prevention programmes are most likely to be effective if they are interactive, involve more than one session, promote body acceptance, address personal, familial, and social factors, and are facilitated by a healthcare professional (Ciao et al., 2014).

Treatment of eating disorders varies according to the disorder. It may involve psychotherapy, medication, exercise, physical activity, relaxation, or yoga. The ability to draw strong conclusions about intervention efficacy is hampered by a lack of good-quality studies (Vancampfort et al., 2014). Of course, programmes are most likely to have a beneficial effect if people complete them. However, a systematic review of treatment of outpatients with anorexia nervosa revealed that dropout was mostly in the range of 20–40% (Dejong et al., 2012). This is an important statistic in itself, but it also hampers the ability to draw strong conclusions about the efficacy of interventions for eating disorders. Physical therapy in the form of aerobic and resistance training may increase weight in people with anorexia nervosa (Vancampfort et al., 2014). Aerobic exercise, massage, basic body awareness therapy, and yoga may also improve psychological and physical quality of life in people with anorexia. There is some evidence that family therapy may be effective when measured in terms of anorexia remission (Fisher et al., 2010). There is no conclusive evidence that antipsychotic medication is an effective treatment for anorexia (Kishi et al., 2012).

Reviews of the research evidence indicate that cognitive behavioural therapy (CBT) and self-help strongly based on CBT can be effective for bulimia and BED (Hay et al., 2009). Such programmes counter dysfunctional thoughts about weight and body shape to reduce binge–purge cycles and enhance self-esteem. Antidepressants can also reduce the symptoms of binge eating and purging in the short term, although this may be a placebo effect. CBT for bulimia and BED results in reduced bingeing, dietary restraint, and depression, but not weight loss (Striegle-Moore & Franko, 2008). A review of research indicates that aerobic exercise, massage, basic body awareness therapy, and yoga may improve psychological and physical quality of life in people with bulimia (Vancampfort et al., 2014).

Summary

- What we eat affects our risk of many disorders, including cancer, diabetes, and the intermediate outcomes of obesity.
- A healthy diet includes high fibre, fruit, vegetables, and oily fish, and reduced salt, red meat, sugars, and saturated fat.
- Poor dietary habits are learned during childhood though modelling, exposure, reinforcement, and family interactions.
- In adolescence and adulthood, dieting and body dissatisfaction is common, even in those who are not overweight.
- Restrained eating is associated with body dissatisfaction, food cravings, preoccupations with food, guilt, overestimating body size, low self-esteem, anxiety, and depression.
- Eating disorders occur in approximately 3% of the population and include anorexia nervosa, bulimia nervosa, and binge eating disorder.
- Bulimia and binge eating disorder are influenced by a social pressure to attain the thin-ideal, increased body dissatisfaction, negative emotions, and low self-esteem. Less is known about the causes of anorexia.
- CBT is currently the most effective treatment for bulimia and binge eating disorder.

13.2.2 OBESITY

Obesity has been labelled an epidemic by health organisations. It is defined using the body mass index (BMI) (see Table 13.1) and is associated with an increased risk of chronic diseases, including Type 2 diabetes, cardiovascular disease, and cancer. The prevalence of being overweight or obese has increased in recent decades (World Health Organisation, 2014c). Globally, the prevalence of obesity nearly doubled between 1980 and 2014. In 2014, 38% of adult men and 40% of adult women were overweight and 11% of men and 15% of women were obese. This amounts to more than half a billion adults worldwide. Figure 13.3 shows that being overweight or obese are most common in the Americas, Europe, and the Eastern Mediterranean region, but they are also increasing in Africa and Asia.

TABLE 13.1   Levels of obesity

Classification	BMI (kg/m²)	Treatment
Overweight	BMI 25 – 29.9	Self-directed diet and exercise; behavioural weight-loss programmes
Obese (I)	BMI 30 – 34.9	Behavioural weight-loss programmes
Obese (II)	BMI 35 – 39.9	Pharmacotherapy; very low calorie diet
Obese (III)	BMI ≥ 40	Bariatric surgery

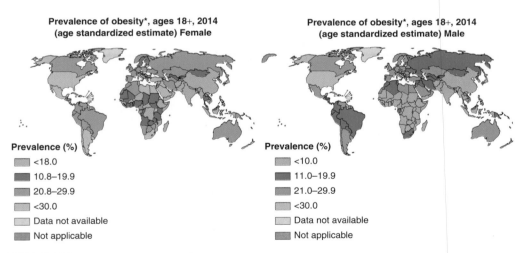

Prevalence of obesity*, ages 18+, 2014 (age standardized estimate) Female

Prevalence of obesity*, ages 18+, 2014 (age standardized estimate) Male

Prevalence (%)
- <18.0
- 10.8–19.9
- 20.8–29.9
- <30.0
- Data not available
- Not applicable

Prevalence (%)
- <10.0
- 11.0–19.9
- 21.0–29.9
- <30.0
- Data not available
- Not applicable

FIGURE 13.3   Global rates of obesity

Reprinted from Prevalence of obesity ages 18+, 2014 (age standardized estimate) Female, World Health Organisation, WHO © 2016

A basic explanation of weight gain is that it occurs because the intake of energy is greater than the energy expended. This balance is influenced by a complex system of physiological, psychological, and social factors. Such factors include:

- **Genetic vulnerability:** a number of genes have been identified that are associated with obesity. It is thought these genes predispose people to weight gain and interact with other physiological feedback systems, such as the hormone leptin, which is released by adipose tissue and has a role in appetite regulation. Genes are important, but they are not the most important influence on obesity, and gene–environment interactions must also be considered (Huang & Hu, 2015).
- **Physiological appetite control:** processes of homeostasis should regulate food intake according to need – as seen in the eating behaviour of infants and young children. However, it is clear that many people eat more than they need. This is probably due to food cues in the environment overriding physiological cues.
- **Early development and parental obesity:** parental obesity is strongly associated with children's obesity. This is likely to be due to a combination of genetic and environmental factors. Birth weight and development in early infancy are important in later chronic diseases such as diabetes and heart disease. Rapid weight gain in early childhood is associated with adult obesity.
- **Eating behaviour:** eating behaviour is determined by motivation (see Chapter 2) and the availability of food. Animal research shows that internal drives (i.e. satiety) are overridden when a variety of palatable food is available. In our society, the wide availability of various palatable foods (in large portions) creates an environment where people are more likely to overeat.
- **Diet:** the risk of obesity increases if a person's diet includes foods with high energy density, high fat, sugary drinks, or low fibre. Alcoholic drinks are often high in calories.
- **Lack of physical activity:** changes in transport, technology, and work patterns mean there has been a steady reduction in the energy we expend in our daily lives. Global data indicate that 27% of women and 20% of men do not achieve the recommended level of physical activity: 150 minutes per week of moderate intensity physical activity (WHO, 2014c). The proportion of people who are insufficiently physically active is highest in the Americas and the Eastern Mediterranean region, and in areas that are better off in economic terms.
- **Work patterns:** increased working hours are associated with obesity; and increased income is associated with spending more on take-away food or dining out.
- **Attitudes and beliefs:** patterns of eating and exercising are influenced by attitudes and beliefs (see Chapter 5). Therefore models of health behaviour can be used to promote more healthy attitudes, beliefs, and eating behaviour (Akbar et al., 2015; Riebl et al., 2015).
- **Economic factors:** the cost of food as a proportion of our total expenditure has steadily decreased over the last 50 years. In addition, unhealthy foods that are high in sugar or fat tend to be cheaper than healthy foods such as fruit or vegetables.
- **Obesogenic environment:** a range of social, cultural, and infrastructural factors create an environment where obesity is more likely. These include the availability of high energy foods, the design of buildings and workspaces to minimise physical exertion, effort-saving devices, and increases in sedentary entertainment.

Case Study 13.2 illustrates how some of these different individual, social, and environmental factors might interact to promote obesity. The relative contribution of different causes of obesity may differ between individuals so any treatment should be tailored appropriately. A stepped-care approach should be taken to obesity.

Lifestyle modification, consisting of improving diet and facilitating physical activity as part of broader behavioural therapy can be effective for reducing weight, with pharmacotherapy a possible supplement if necessary (Carvajal et al., 2013; Vetter et al., 2010). A course of 20 weekly group sessions based on CBT principles results in around a 9% reduction in body weight; pharmacotherapy results in a 7–10% reduction in body weight, which is superior to placebos. Continued physical activity is one of the best predictors of maintaining weight loss (Thomas & Brownell, 2007). Surgery is only used in severe cases and leads to dramatic and sustained weight loss. However, treating obesity by focusing on individuals ignores the wide range of environmental and social factors that contribute to the epidemic. Prevention is a priority and must tackle social influences, food production and consumption, psychological factors, individual activity, and environmental barriers to activity.

CASE STUDY 13.2   Psychosocial factors and obesity

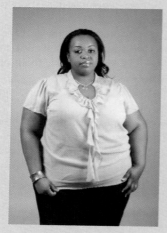

Photograph © Monteleone/ Fotolia

Kayla knows that she needs to lose weight, but she finds it difficult to do so. She is 32 years old and is morbidly obese at 118kg (24 stone, BMI = 40.8). Kayla is unable to work and is largely confined to the home. She finds it hard to be physically active. She has chronic pelvic pain, Type 2 diabetes, and hypertension. She is also being seen by psychiatric services for recurrent depression.

Kayla does not seem highly motivated to lose weight. The doctor suspects that there are complex reasons why Kayla and her husband find it hard to engage in weight reduction programmes. Kayla was sexually abused as a child and started putting on weight during this time. She has not had many relationships but recently got married to a man she met through her church.

Kayla receives government disability benefits and her husband Carlos is her full-time carer. Carlos is also overweight. Their diet is very poor – with lots of high fat and sugar-rich foods. They enjoy take-away food and do this at least three times a week. Carlos says he is supportive of Kayla's desire to lose weight, but he seems to undermine any attempts at weight loss or changing their diet.

CLINICAL NOTES 13.1

Overweight and obesity

- Treating overweight and obese people is challenging because weight regain is common.
- Pharmacological treatment results in weight loss but this is often regained when drugs are stopped.

(Continued)

- Lifestyle changes of diet and exercise are more likely to lead to a sustained weight loss.
- Combined lifestyle and pharmacological approaches may be more effective.
- People should be encouraged to build physical activity into their daily lives – e.g. walking instead of driving, taking the stairs instead of the escalator.
- Programmes for obese and overweight children can be effective and are increasingly available (e.g. www.mendprogramme.org; www.cdc.gov/bam)
- Where possible, families should be involved in weight reduction programmes to address familial influences on eating behaviour.

Summary

- Obesity is defined as a BMI ≥ 30 and is associated with an increased risk of chronic diseases. Its prevalence has increased in recent decades.
- Obesity is caused by a combination of factors, including a genetic vulnerability, physiological appetite control, early development, family context, eating behaviour, attitudes and beliefs, a lack of physical activity, and environmental factors.
- Current interventions include behavioural weight loss programmes, pharmacotherapy, and surgery – all of which vary in effectiveness and cost.

13.2.3 ALCOHOL USE

Excessive alcohol use is widespread, and it has an enormous health impact. Globally, 6% of all deaths and 5% of the burden of disease is attributable to alcohol consumption (World Health Organisation, 2014b). Alcohol misuse is associated with a wide range of health problems and pathologies, including liver damage, hypertension, stroke, seven types of cancer, accidents, sexually transmitted infections, memory loss, anxiety disorders, personality disorders, depression, and drug use. Alcohol-related problems are on the increase: between 1990 and 2010, alcohol changed from being the eighth to the fifth most important causes of death and disability worldwide (WHO, 2014b). Whereas a common belief is that moderate alcohol use can have some health benefits, recent analysis shows that any benefits occur only for very low-level drinking, and for most adverse health outcomes any increase in alcohol intake puts people at more risk of harm (Rehm et al., 2017). Many people lack the knowledge, motivation, or skills required to adhere to government alcohol intake guidelines, but some interventions that help people to monitor their alcohol intake have been shown to have benefits (de Visser, 2015; de Visser et al., 2017a).

Alcohol affects the liver in a number of ways. Alcohol is a toxin so even small amounts put a strain on the liver. Acute alcohol poisoning is caused by heavy episodic drinking ('binge drinking') and can be fatal. Chronic alcoholic liver disease starts with inflammation (hepatitis), then a fatty liver, both of which are potentially reversible if alcohol use is stopped. The final stage of alcoholic liver disease is cirrhosis, where the scarring of the liver is largely permanent. Symptoms will often only arise when liver disease is advanced. They include abdominal pain, tenderness, thirst, fatigue, jaundice, a loss of appetite, fever, mental confusion, weight gain, and nausea. Alcoholic liver disease is the main reason for liver transplants in many developed countries.

Screening for alcohol use in primary care is important, and simple screening tools such as the AUDIT (see Box 13.4) are available for this. Alcohol *dependence* has physical, psychological, and social components. It usually involves an increased physical tolerance, withdrawal symptoms when intake is stopped, the increasingly dominant role of alcohol in a person's life, difficulty in controlling alcohol intake (e.g. consuming more than intended, unsuccessful attempts to reduce intake), and continued drinking despite the knowledge that this is a problem (Sayette, 2007). Alcohol *abuse* is present when a person has at least one of the following behaviours:

- Continued drinking that interferes with a major role or obligation, such as work.
- Continued drinking despite legal, social, or interpersonal problems related to alcohol use.
- Recurrent drinking in situations where intoxication is dangerous.

ACTIVITY 13.3

- How much do you think someone has to drink to become dependent on alcohol?
- Do you think this varies between individuals?

Alcoholism is determined by an interaction of genetic, psychological, and cultural factors. Twin and family studies confirm that the children of alcoholics are at greater risk of developing alcohol problems. This may be partly due to a greater sensitivity to the positive effects of alcohol or a decreased sensitivity to its negative effects (Hägele et al., 2014; Sayette, 2007). Explanations of alcoholism also draw on learning theory (see Chapter 10): alcohol use is reinforced by increasing positive emotions (positive reinforcement) or decreasing negative emotions (negative reinforcement). Alcohol use may become associated with a particular social context or cues, which can make it hard for individuals to abstain when exposed to these cues.

Treatments for alcohol disorders should therefore address the physical, psychological, and social aspects of the disorder. Pharmacotherapy can be used to reduce the positive effects of alcohol, increase negative effects, or reduce craving. Effective psychological interventions include motivational interviewing (see Case Study 2.2), skills training, CBT, self-help groups, and couples therapy. The importance of addressing social factors is illustrated by the finding that, for married or cohabiting people, couples therapy is more

BOX 13.2   Screening for alcohol problems (AUDIT)

Read questions as written. Record answers carefully. Begin AUDIT by saying 'Now I am going to ask you some questions about your use of alcoholic beverages during this past year'. Explain what is meant by 'alcoholic beverages' by using local examples of beer, wine, vodka, etc. Code answers in terms of standard drinks. Place the correct number in the box at the right.

TABLE 13.2   Screening for alcohol problems (AUDIT)

1. How often do you have a drink containing alcohol? (0) Never [Skip to Qs 9–10] (1) Monthly or less (2) 2 to 4 times a month (3) 2 to 3 times a week (4) 4 or more times a week	4. How often during the last year have you found that you were not able to stop drinking once you had started? (0) Never (1) Less than monthly (2) Monthly (3) Weekly (4) Daily or almost daily
2. How many drinks containing alcohol do you have on a typical day when you are drinking? (0) 1 or 2 (1) 3 or 4 (2) 5 or 6 (3) 7, 8, or 9 (4) 10 or more	5. How often during the last year have you failed to do what was normally expected from you because of drinking? (0) Never (1) Less than monthly (2) Monthly (3) Weekly (4) Daily or almost daily
3. How often do you have six or more drinks on one occasion? (0) Never (1) Less than monthly (2) Monthly (3) Weekly (4) Daily or almost daily *Skip to Questions 9 and 10 if Total score for Questions 2 and 3 = 0*	6. How often during the last year have you needed a first drink in the morning to get yourself going after a heavy drinking session? (0) Never (1) Less than monthly (2) Monthly (3) Weekly (4) Daily or almost daily

(Continued)

7. How often during the last year have you had a feeling of guilt or remorse after drinking?

(0) Never

(1) Less than monthly

(2) Monthly

(3) Weekly

(4) Daily or almost daily

9. Have you or someone else been injured as a result of your drinking?

(0) No

(2) Yes, but not in the last year

(4) Yes, during the last year

8. How often during the last year have you been unable to remember what happened the night before because you had been drinking?

(0) Never

(1) Less than monthly

(2) Monthly

(3) Weekly

(4) Daily or almost daily

10. Has a relative or friend or a doctor or another health worker been concerned about your drinking or suggested you cut down?

(0) No

(2) Yes, but not in the last year

(4) Yes, during the last year

Total scores >8 indicate harmful or hazardous drinking (a cut-off score of 10 provides greater specificity but at the expense of sensitivity).

Total scores between 8 and 15 suggest a need for simple advice focused on the reduction of hazardous drinking.

Total cores between 16 and 19 suggest a need for brief counselling and continued monitoring.

Totals scores >20 indicate possible alcohol dependence and suggest a need for further diagnostic evaluation.

Babor, T.F., Higgins-Biddle, J.C., Saunders, J.B. & Monteiro, M.G. (2007) *AUDIT: The Alcohol Use Disorders Identification Test: Guidelines for Use in Primary Care* (2nd edition). Geneva: World Health Organisation (available at: http://whqlibdoc.who.int/hq/2001/WHO_MSD_MSB_01.6a.pdf)

effective than individual therapy in reducing short- and long-term alcohol intake and increasing relationship functioning (O'Farrell & Clements, 2012). Reviews show that the outcome of treatment is also better if the initial alcohol dependence is less severe and if the individual has no comorbid psychopathology, greater self-efficacy, a greater motivation to quit, and a treatment goal (Adamson et al., 2009; Kadden & Litt, 2011).

CLINICAL NOTES 13.2

Helping people with alcohol problems

- The AUDIT can be used to screen people for alcohol problems (Box 13.2):

   - (i) AUDIT scores of 8–15: give advice on alcohol use, the health risks, and importance of staying within recommended limits.
   - (ii) AUDIT scores of 16–19: refer for counselling and monitoring of alcohol use.
   - (iii) AUDIT scores of 20+: refer to specialist alcohol services for evaluation and treatment.

- Remember that people will often under-report their alcohol use.
- People with a history of alcohol dependence should be treated at lower levels of use.
- Use your clinical judgement if what the patient reports is not consistent with other evidence.

Summary

- Alcohol misuse is associated with a wide range of health problems, including liver damage, hypertension, strokes, cancer, accidents, sexually transmitted infections, and psychological disorders.
- Acute alcoholic hepatitis is caused by heavy episodic drinking, and can be fatal. Chronic alcoholic liver disease includes inflammation (hepatitis), a fatty liver, and cirrhosis.
- Alcohol dependence involves an increased physical tolerance, withdrawal symptoms, a dominant role for alcohol in a person's life, difficulty in controlling alcohol intake, and continued drinking despite the knowledge that it is a problem.
- Alcohol abuse occurs when drinking interferes with a person's major roles or obligations; causes legal, social or interpersonal problems; or continues in situations where intoxication is dangerous.
- Alcoholism is caused by the interaction between genetic, psychological, and cultural factors.
- Couples therapy is an effective treatment for alcoholism but the outcome of treatment is partly determined by the severity of alcohol dependence, comorbid psychopathology, alcohol-related self-efficacy, and a motivation to quit.

13.3 GI DISORDERS

13.3.1 IRRITABLE BOWEL SYNDROME

Irritable Bowel Syndrome (IBS) is a functional bowel disorder that is diagnosed when no organic disorder is identified. It is one of the most common GI disorders – prevalence estimates in most countries range from 10–20%, but this variation may reflect differences in definitions of the condition (Sperber et al., 2016). Physiological risk factors include genetic vulnerability, being female, and dietary/intestinal microbiota, low-grade inflammation of the bowel, and disturbances in the bowel's neuroendocrine system, but do not include food allergies or intolerances (El-Sally, 2012, 2015). Symptoms are shown in Box 13.3.

BOX 13.3   Rome-IV criteria for Irritable Bowel Syndrome (Lacy et al., 2016)

The following elements must have been present for the last three months, with symptom onset at least six months before diagnosis:

- Recurrent abdominal pain, on average, at least one day/week in the last three months, associated with two or more of the following criteria:

  o   Related to defecation
  o   Associated with a change in frequency of stool
  o   Associated with a change in form (appearance) of stool.

IBS is associated with increased stress, psychological disorders, and experiences of physical or sexual abuse in childhood or adulthood (van Oudenhove & Aziz, 2009). People with IBS have an increased prevalence of depression, generalised anxiety disorder, panic, phobias, and somatisation disorders. They are also hypersensitive to GI symptoms such as rectal distension. This appears to be due to a greater vigilance for these symptoms and a greater likelihood of labelling such symptoms as negative or painful (Hauser et al., 2014). Functional MRI studies show that people with IBS do not have the same pattern of cortical response to painful stimuli. Most notably, they have increased activation in areas of the brain associated with emotional processes such as anxiety and hypervigilance (Johns & Tracey, 2009). Such findings have led some to conclude that IBS is best conceptualised as a hyper-reactivity of the brain–gut axis that can be triggered by psychological or biological factors (Hauser et al., 2014).

The role of psychological factors in IBS is illustrated by the fact that it is responsive to placebo and suggestion. One study used a placebo 'analgesia' gel during rectal distention and found it led to less pain and less cortical activity in the neural pain matrix. This reduced activity was the same as if the rectal distention was smaller (Price et al., 2007).

Reviews of the research evidence indicate that effective treatment of the physical symptoms of IBS is provided by antidepressant medication, CBT, hypnotherapy, multicomponent psychological therapy, and dynamic psychotherapy (Ford et al., 2014). For example, one study of individuals who did not respond to initial medication found that the addition of six sessions of CBT to their medication regimen led to a greater improvement in IBS symptoms up to six months later (Kennedy et al., 2006). Treatment of physical symptoms is clearly important, but so too is the treatment of psychological distress: people with IBS are more likely than people with inflammatory bowel disease or healthy people to consider or attempt suicide: the risk of suicide is positively correlated with more severe or chronic IBS (Spiegel et al., 2007).

13.3.2 INFLAMMATORY BOWEL DISORDERS

Inflammatory Bowel Disorders (IBD) include Crohn's disease and ulcerative colitis, which are chronic diseases characterised by periods of remission and relapse. Main symptoms include abdominal pain, vomiting, blood in stools, weight loss, and diarrhoea. IBD is thought to be caused by an interaction between the environment and a genetic susceptibility that leads to immune dysfunction in the GI tract.

The majority of people with IBD think lifestyle and psychological factors such as diet and stress are important for the course of their IBD (Sajadinejad et al., 2012). Although the role of stress in the onset of IBD is yet to be established definitively, there is clear evidence that stress can trigger and exacerbate symptoms of IBD (Sajadinejad et al., 2012). The influence of stress on IBD may be due to any of the physical effects of stress on the GI system (see Figure 13.2), but a key pathway appears to be through triggering increased mucosal inflammation in people with IBD.

Lifestyle factors are important, but the role they play is unclear. Smoking is associated with an increased risk of Crohn's disease but with a decreased risk of ulcerative colitis. Use of oral contraceptives increases the risk of IBD. Diet is generally thought to be important because food-related antigens in the gut may trigger inflammatory responses: high dietary intake of fats, polyunsaturated fatty acids, omega-6 fatty acids, and meat increase the risk of Crohn's disease and ulcerative colitis. However, dietary interventions have not been found to have large effects on disease progression (Yamamoto, 2013).

IBD can have a profound impact on self-esteem and quality of life (Grodzinksy et al., 2015). In one Europe-wide study of people with IBD, most respondents reported that symptoms affect their work (66%) and leisure activities (75%) (Ghosh & Mitchell, 2007). In a prospective pan-European study, quality of life was found to be most impaired in people reporting IBD symptoms at the 10-year follow-up, people receiving a disability pension due to IBD, and people on sick leave (Huppertz-Hauss et al., 2015). The relationship between IBD and psychological distress is not as strong as in functional disorders, such as Irritable Bowel Syndrome. However, anxiety increases as IBD gets worse (Nahon et al., 2012). The progressive nature of IBD means many people require surgery – around one-third of people with ulcerative colitis will have a colectomy (Hanauer, 2008). Although surgery reduces the severity of symptoms, it can lead to other difficulties, such as faecal incontinence, pouch failure, and female infertility.

Adjusting to IBD is a significant challenge. However, comparatively little attention has been paid to this in the psychological literature. One study found that if people blamed themselves for IBD they were more likely to use avoidant coping (i.e. to avoid thinking or talking about it), which in turn was related to poor adjustment (Voth & Sirois, 2009). In contrast, taking responsibility for IBD resulted in less avoidance and better adjustment. People with most severe IBD were more likely to use avoidance and have poor adjustment. It is difficult to know whether the disease severity leads to avoidance or vice versa. However, this study suggests that encouraging people to take responsibility and not blame themselves or use avoidant coping might be helpful.

Psychological interventions for IBD include CBT, stress management, and support groups. There is inconsistent evidence that these interventions affect the physical symptoms of IBD. However, they do help people manage their symptoms better. Psychological interventions based on CBT, psychodynamic approaches, and hypnosis may lead to reductions in symptom-related stress, disease-related worries, depression, anxiety, and pain (Knowles et al., 2013). Interventions that combine psychological and physical care may be even more effective but there is insufficient evidence at present. As for other conditions, there is interest in whether the psychological impact of IBD may be treated using online interventions (Stiles-Shield & Keefer, 2015). It is important to determine the efficacy of such interventions, because some studies suggest that people with IBD may be more willing to participate in computerised psychological interventions than face-to-face interventions (McCombie et al., 2014). There is some evidence that antidepressant medication may have a beneficial impact on the course of IBD (Macer & Prady, 2017).

13.3.3 CANCER OF THE GI TRACT

Gastro-intestinal cancers are common and deadly. Globally, cancer of the lower GI tract (colon and rectum) is the second most common cancer among women and the third most common cancer overall (Stewart & Wild, 2014). Cancer of the upper GI tract (oesophagus, stomach, pancreas) is less common but has high mortality rates because it tends to be asymptomatic in the early stages. Survival rates therefore tend to be low. Symptoms and challenges of cancer in the upper and lower GI tract differ. Cancer of the upper GI tract may lead to problems eating, swallowing, dysphagia, nausea, and vomiting, whereas cancer of the lower GI tract leads to symptoms associated with bowel function and treatment may involve an ostomy (a surgically-created opening between the intestines and the abdominal wall).

Cancer of the upper GI tract

Cancer of the upper GI tract is associated with being male, being older, *H. pylori* infection, dietary factors, and smoking. In addition, genetic vulnerability may play a role in some stomach and pancreatic cancers. Cancer of the upper GI tract is more common in older adults and men. Epidemiological research shows that diets high in salt and processed meat increase the risk of stomach cancer, whereas a high fruit intake can reduce the risk (Jeongseon et al., 2014; Vingeliene et al., 2016). As noted earlier in section 13.2, alcohol consumption increases the risk of oesophageal cancer. There may be important gene–diet interactions that greatly increase some people's risk of cancer of the upper GI tract.

The prognosis is poor because there are very few symptoms in the early stages of upper GI tract cancer. It is common for the cancer to have metastasised before diagnosis. Six-month survival rates for stomach and oesophageal cancer therefore range from 15% to 65% depending on the stage of the cancer. Treatment nearly always involves surgery, such as a partial or total removal of the oesophagus or stomach. These surgical procedures are difficult and can have a range of side effects. Symptoms and side effects include pain, difficulty in swallowing, weight loss, malnourishment, acid reflux, and abdominal discomfort. Unfortunately, curative surgery is often not an option for people with gastric cancer. These people are offered palliative care to manage the pain and surgical intervention to manage perforation or obstruction.

Given the poor prognosis, it is understandable that many people experience anxiety and depression. The relationship between depression and cancer is particularly strong in pancreatic cancer, where survival rates are approximately 5% over five years. Many people with pancreatic cancer have severe depression (Mayr & Schmid, 2010). This fact, and the fact that the cancer often progresses without symptoms, means that depression may be listed as a presenting symptom of pancreatic cancer.

Studies of quality of life show that physical functioning, work, and home life are strongly affected by upper GI tract cancers. Quality of life generally decreases immediately after surgery, but may improve in the long term, especially if treatment is curative. Quality of life is better in people who have less invasive or toxic treatments and who feel involved in decision making about their treatment (Kim et al., 2008). However, one aspect of quality of life that is not consistently affected is emotional functioning (Conroy et al., 2006). This may reflect individual differences in emotional responses to stress (see Chapter 3). Psychological wellbeing and coping are important in adjusting to disease and can affect disease outcomes (e.g. Tian et al., 2009; see also Chapter 6). Quality of life is commonly considered an outcome of diagnosis or treatment, but it is notable that in one study, better quality of life predicted survival after chemotherapy among people with advanced gastric cancer (Park et al., 2008). There is a need for better conceptualisation, assessment, and treatment of these dimensions of patient experience (Tzelepis et al., 2014).

Cancer of the lower GI tract

Cancer of the lower GI tract is associated with genetic vulnerability, older age, diet, smoking, being sedentary and overweight. It is estimated that lifestyle changes such as being physically active, eating healthily, and maintaining a healthy body weight could at least halve the risk of GI cancers (Cummings & Bingham, 1998; Khan et al., 2010).

Exercise and body weight have a dose–response effect on bowel cancer. For example, compared to people with a healthy BMI, obese people are 33% more likely to develop colon cancer (Ma et al., 2013). Many studies have shown that physical activity decreases the risk of developing bowel cancer and improves the prognosis in people who have bowel cancer. The underlying mechanisms are unclear, but may involve increased insulin-like growth factor-binding protein and reduced prostaglandins. Exercise in people with bowel cancer is associated with better quality of life and reduced mortality from cancer and other causes (Trojian et al., 2007).

Much of the literature on quality of life in colorectal cancer focuses on the impact of ostomy surgery. This shows that ostomies can have a significant impact on emotional wellbeing, quality of life, sexuality, and body image (Brown & Randle, 2005). Most people will experience a sharp decline in their body image after surgery, but this then gradually improves over time. People with ostomies are more likely to be depressed than people with the same illness but without ostomies, particularly if they are younger, female, less educated, or have poor support. For many aspects of quality of life, the effect of ostomies is bimodal: people are either not very affected or severely affected (Brown & Randle, 2005). This highlights the importance of individual differences in coping and levels of support in helping people adapt to ostomies and accept changes in their body image (Torquato & Decesaro, 2014).

CLINICAL NOTES 13.3

Working with GI disorders

- People with GI disorders such as IBS or GI cancers, are at a high risk of psychological problems.
- Be alert for people who have psychological and/or social problems because these are associated with poor quality of life and may influence the course of the disease.
- Although IBS is strongly associated with psychological factors, it is not helpful to portray it as 'all in the mind'.
- Explaining the brain–gut axis can help people understand the impact of psychological, lifestyle, and physical factors.
- It may be helpful to encourage people not to blame themselves or to use avoidant coping, but instead to take responsibility for the course of their illness.
- Encouraging lifestyle changes such as increased exercise, healthy diet, and reduced alcohol use can improve people's emotional wellbeing and in some cases improve the prognosis.
- Screen for psychological disorders and offer support or psychological intervention where appropriate.

Summary

- Irritable Bowel Syndrome (IBS) is one of the most common GI disorders, affecting 3–18% of the population. It is associated with stress, psychological disorders, and past psychological trauma.
- Psychological intervention and antidepressants can result in some improvement in IBS symptoms.
- Inflammatory Bowel Disorders (IBD), including Crohn's disease and ulcerative colitis, are caused by an interaction between the environment and a genetic susceptibility that result in immune dysfunction in the GI tract.
- Stress is associated with relapse in IBD. Psychological and social problems predict quality of life and whether symptoms will worsen over time.
- Psychological interventions for IBD reduce symptom-related stress, disease-related worries, depression, anxiety, pain, and the use of anti-inflammatory drugs.
- GI cancers are strongly associated with lifestyle factors, including diet, smoking, physical activity, and weight.
- Anxiety and depression are common in people with GI cancer. This is particularly the case for pancreatic cancer, where depression is a possible presenting symptom.
- Ostomies can have a significant impact on emotional wellbeing, quality of life, sexuality, and body image, but there are large individual differences in how people cope and adjust.

FURTHER READING

Llewellyn, C.D. et al. (eds) (2018) *Cambridge Handbook of Psychology, Health and Medicine* (3rd edition). Cambridge: Cambridge University Press. Includes short chapters on many relevant topics, including cancers of the digestive tract, obesity, eating disorders, Irritable Bowel Syndrome, Inflammatory Bowel Disorders, gastric and duodenal ulcers, etc.

Levenson, J.L. (ed.) (2011) *The American Psychiatric Publishing Textbook of Psychosomatic Medicine: Psychiatric Care of the Medically Ill* (2nd edition). Arlington, VA: American Psychiatric Association Publishing. A 1,200-page book with very broad coverage of the topics covered in this and other chapters, including chapters on gastrointestinal disorders and oncology.

Toner, B.B. et al. (2000) *Cognitive-Behavioral Treatment of Irritable Bowel Syndrome: The Brain–Gut Connection*. New York: Guilford Press. A guide to individual and group CBT for IBS.

REVISION QUESTIONS

1. Describe the brain–gut axis.

2. What is the relationship between stress and GI function?

3. Why is a biopsychosocial approach important in GI illness? Illustrate your answer with reference to one specific GI illness.

4. How does diet affect health?

5. What constitutes a healthy diet?

6. Outline three eating disorders and discuss what causes them.

7. How do we define obesity? Outline five different types of causes of obesity.

8. How does alcohol use and misuse affect health?

9. What is the difference between alcohol dependence and alcohol abuse?

10. Discuss the role of psychosocial factors in one GI disorder.

14 REPRODUCTION AND ENDOCRINOLOGY

LEARNING OBJECTIVES

This chapter is designed to enable you to:

- Outline the psychological and mood changes associated with the menstrual cycle and menopause.
- Discuss the role of psychosocial factors during pregnancy and birth.
- Describe the main psychological problems that can occur during pregnancy and after birth.
- Outline the major links between endocrine disorders and psychosocial wellbeing.
- Consider the ethical issues associated with the use of hormonal treatment.

In this chapter we shall consider reproduction and endocrinology together, primarily through focusing on reproductive events and disorders. We shall also consider (in section 14.2) non-reproductive endocrine disorders. The emphasis of the chapter is on the psychological, behavioural, and social factors that can influence, and are influenced by, the reproductive and endocrine systems.

14.1 REPRODUCTION

Reproductive events include the onset of menstruation (menarche), conception, pregnancy, miscarriage, childbirth, and menopause. Although these events mostly focus on physical changes in women, they also involve issues that affect both men and women, such as sexual dysfunction and infertility. Procedures and treatments associated with reproduction that are particularly common include contraception, cervical smear tests, hysterectomy, and hormone replacement therapy (HRT). Reproductive issues raise unique ethical dilemmas such as: when terminating a pregnancy is morally defensible; the rights of donor parents and the children of donors; the use of assisted reproductive techniques for pregnancy in older women; and whether a subsequent pregnancy should be used by parents to provide a child with the right genetic make-up to be an organ or tissue donor for a sick older sibling.

These events can be viewed from a biomedical, psychological, social, and cultural perspective. Which perspective we take affects both our understanding and treatment of disorders (see Chapter 1). For example, a biomedical perspective would see premenstrual syndrome as caused by fluctuations and imbalances in hormones associated with the menstrual cycle. Treatment would therefore involve pharmacological methods to counteract hormonal imbalances or influence mood. A psychological perspective of premenstrual syndrome (PMS) might examine how women's patterns of stress and behaviour contribute to worsening mood around menstruation, such as noticing particular triggers and maladaptive responses. Treatment might involve identifying and changing maladaptive thinking or behaviour, and finding coping strategies to help women respond in a more adaptive way. A social perspective of premenstrual syndrome might examine women's sociodemographic circumstances and levels of support, or cultural beliefs and narratives about premenstrual syndrome. This might lead to treatment providing practical or emotional support to women during critical times, or public health campaigns to change cultural beliefs and narratives.

It is clear that none of these perspectives on their own provides an adequate explanation for, or treatment of, PMS. Therefore it is important to take a **biopsychosocial approach** where we consider all the different perspectives outlined above. This in turn will lead to a more informed and holistic approach to consultation and treatment.

In this chapter it is not possible to examine the wide range of reproductive and endocrine events and disorders. We shall therefore concentrate on menstruation, menopause, pregnancy, and childbirth. We then look at a selection of endocrine disorders. You will also find relevant information in other chapters covering such subjects as puberty (Chapter 8), Cushing's syndrome (Chapter 3), and diabetes (Chapter 11).

14.1.1 MENSTRUATION AND MENOPAUSE

The age at which girls start menstruating – **menarche** – has fallen markedly throughout the twentieth century. This change is thought to be due to better health and basic nutrition, but also to increased weight and obesity in young girls (see Chapters 8 and 13). Figure 14.1 shows biological events and changes during the menstrual cycle.

The effect of the **menstrual cycle** has been examined in relation to a range of behaviours such as sexual behaviour, sleep, and diet. The follicular phase prior to and during ovulation has been associated with an increased libido (DeBruine et al., 2010; Gangstead & Thornhill, 2008). From an evolutionary perspective, increased sexual behaviour at this time increases a woman's chances of conception. The menstrual cycle may also influence our choices of mate: women in the fertile phase of the menstrual cycle have a greater preference for men with more typically masculine characteristics (e.g. taller, with more masculine faces and bodies) (DeBruine et al., 2010; Gangstead & Thornhill, 2008). However, this is only the case when women are asked to rate or choose men for short-term relationships, and not when they are instructed to choose men for long-term relationships (Little et al., 2007).

The menstrual cycle may affect sleep. There is evidence that the proportion of time spent in different stages of sleep (e.g. REM, slow-wave sleep) varies across the menstrual cycle but mostly after ovulation (the luteal phase) (Driver et al., 2008). Women report poorer sleep quality just before and during menstruation, although the proportion and timing of sleep is relatively stable around menstruation. However, a study in which women kept detailed daily sleep records found that women rated their quality of sleep as worse in

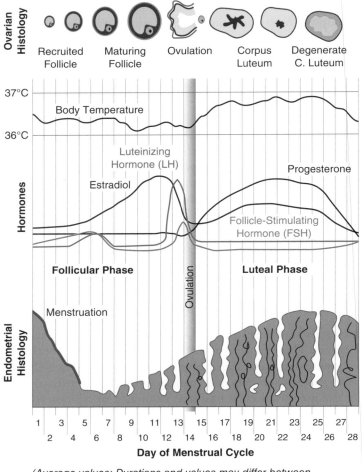

FIGURE 14.1 Physiological events of the menstrual cycle

the days before and during menstruation, despite there being no actual difference in the amount of sleep or waking time recorded during the night (Baker & Driver, 2004). The menstrual cycle may also interact with sleep and circadian rhythms. A review of research found that after ovulation (luteal phase) markers of circadian rhythms (cortisol and melatonin) are not as large in amplitude. When circadian rhythms are disrupted, such as when women do shift work, women are also more likely to have irregular or longer menstrual cycles (Baker & Driver, 2007).

The menstrual cycle does not affect diet as much as is commonly believed. Research suggests that changes in food preferences are more strongly influenced by cultural norms than biological changes. For example, chocolate cravings during the menstrual cycle differ strongly between cultures and do not decrease substantially after menopause when the menstrual cycle has stopped (Hormes & Rozin, 2009; Zellner et al., 2004). This suggests that any effect of the menstrual cycle on food preferences is more likely to be due to psychosocial factors rather than hormonal ones.

Premenstrual Syndrome (PMS)

Psychological symptoms often occur just before menstruation in the late luteal stage. These symptoms are commonly referred to as **premenstrual tension** (**PMT**) or **premenstrual syndrome** (**PMS**). PMS includes a range of emotional and behavioural symptoms that occur just before menstruation and have a significant impact on a woman's quality of life. Common symptoms are irritability, depression, anxiety, mood swings, feelings of loss of control, and tiredness. Physical symptoms of abdominal bloating, tender breasts, headaches, and muscle aches are also reported (Rapkin & Lewis, 2013). PMS is reported by up to 30% of women and is most common among those aged 25–35.

Around 1–2% of women experience a severe form of PMS, referred to as premenstrual dysphoric disorder (PMDD). A study of 1,246 women in the USA found that 1.3% met diagnostic criteria for PMDD, which include disturbances in home life, social life, and work due to significant changes in sleep, appetite, energy, concentration, mood, and anxiety, which appear during most of the week prior to menstruation and disappear the week after menstruation (American Psychiatric Association, 2004). PMDD is not simply the exacerbation of an existing mood disorder during the premenstrual period; it is supposed to be 'switched on' during certain days within the menstrual cycle and 'switched off' for the remainder of the cycle. However, women with a past history of depression are more likely to suffer from PMDD, and PMDD is also associated with poor overall health.

PMS and PMDD have a considerable impact on women's quality of life and functioning. A review of 44 studies of the menstrual cycle and suicidal behaviour found evidence of higher rates of suicide attempts in the late luteal phase, particularly in women with PMS (Saunders & Hawton, 2006).

The relative contribution of physical, psychological, and cultural factors to PMS and PMDD is unclear and the diagnosis remains controversial. The timing of symptoms suggests fluctuations in hormone levels play some causal role in the psychological symptoms (Rapkin, 2003). The increased vulnerability of women with a history of depression suggests that predisposing psychological vulnerability can be exacerbated by the menstrual cycle. In addition, cultural differences in PMS show that the interpretation of symptoms is influenced by cultural norms. For example, a study of 3,856 women from ethnic minority groups in the USA found that women who were born abroad or moved to the USA after the age of 6 were less likely to have PMDD. The longer a woman had lived in the USA the more likely she was to suffer from PMDD (Pilver et al., 2011).

Thus, in order to understand PMDD we therefore need to incorporate physiological, psychological, and cultural factors. One explanation that does this is the Material-Discursive-Intrapsychic model (Ussher, 2010), which suggests that PMS and PMDD are due to the interaction between three factors:

- Material factors – e.g. hormones, physiological arousal, life stresses, relationship or marital context.
- Intra-psychic factors – e.g. the mode of evaluating and coping with changes, expectations of self, and defence mechanisms.
- Discursive factors – e.g. cultural constructions and the discourse of PMS, reproduction, and gender.

This approach suggests that all these factors combine to produce emotions, bodily sensations, and behaviours which are labelled as PMS by the woman, and diagnosed as PMS or PMDD by a clinician (Ussher, 2018).

A range of treatments for PMS and PMDD have been developed. Biomedical interventions, such as antidepressants or hormone treatments, can be effective in reducing symptoms but do not address the other factors involved in PMS and PMDD. Reviews and meta-analyses show there is good evidence to support the use of antidepressants but that progesterone or progestogen treatment is not clinically effective (Ford et al., 2006; Wyatt et al., 2001; Wyatt et al., 2002). Despite this, practices still vary between countries. The recommended treatment of PMS in the UK and USA is antidepressants. A study of patterns of PMS and PMDD in different countries found that very few practitioners actually diagnosed these syndromes (Weisz & Knaapen, 2009). When women were diagnosed, they were most commonly treated with medication. Practitioners in the USA, the UK, and Canada favoured antidepressants, French practitioners favoured hormone and analgesic treatment, and German doctors favoured complementary medicine.

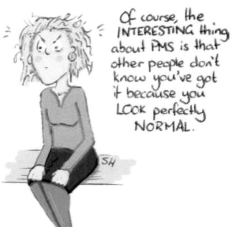

Of course, the INTERESTING thing about PMS is that other people don't know you've got it because you LOOK perfectly NORMAL.

Psychological interventions for PMS are effective. Meta-analyses of intervention trials show that education and monitoring are of limited use, but cognitive behaviour therapy (CBT) and CBT-based interventions can result in reduced depression and anxiety, less interference of symptoms on daily functioning, and more positive behaviour changes (Busse et al., 2009). There is some evidence that CBT is as effective as antidepressants in reducing distress in the short term and more effective in reducing long-term distress (Hunter et al., 2002a, 2002b). Standard intervention packages are now available. Case Study 14.1 gives an example of an eight-session intervention. One trial found this intervention to be as effective as antidepressants over six months and more effective over the first year (Hunter et al., 2002a).

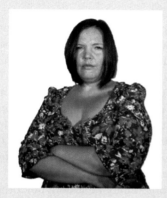

CASE STUDY 14.1   Narrative therapy for premenstrual syndrome

Margo's PMS symptoms are intolerance, impatience, and angry outbursts. Everything annoys her when she has PMS. Anger alternates with feelings of vulnerability, insecurity, depression, and the guilt of knowing she has hurt others. She does not 'own' her PMS self, whom she strongly dislikes. It makes her feel like a Jekyll and Hyde character: she is normally gentle and loving, but PMS makes her angry and aggressive. She is very open about having PMS and uses it to explain her aggressive behaviour. She thinks PMS is due to hormones and diet, but she recognises that the symptoms can be worse if she is stressed or feeling down.

Margo had eight sessions of psychotherapy as follows:

Session 1: Margo's history of PMS and the effect it has on her life. Develop a working model of her PMS that includes physical factors (hormones, diet), psychological factors (mood, stress, relationship issues), and narrative factors (blaming PMS, seeing her PMS-self as someone else).

Session 2: The influence of stress as a trigger for angry outbursts. Relaxation exercises to help cope with stress.

Session 3: Relationships and PMS: how relationships are affected by, or contribute to, maladaptive patterns of behaviour. How to respond assertively instead of aggressively.

Session 4: Self-care: the importance of expressing needs and doing things she enjoys. Develop an activity schedule and discuss the importance of diet and exercise.

Session 5: Thinking positively and 're-writing' her PMS experience so she feels more in control.

Sessions 6 & 7: Consolidation: continuing to redefine her PMS, use positive thinking, and more adaptive coping.

Session 8: Review of therapy: how Margo has changed and what she learned that will help in the future.

After therapy Margo felt more in control, her relationships and self-esteem had improved, and she was more aware of how her behaviour was affecting other people. She also felt more ownership of her PMS: *'I have a lot of relief knowing that it's all under my control really; that it isn't something apart from me'*. Her symptoms were also not as intense.

(Adapted from Ussher et al., 2002)

Menopause

Menopause is defined as the last menstrual period. There is variation in when this occurs but it is usually between 45 and 55 years of age. The physical changes of menopause result in an increased risk of diseases like osteoporosis. Menopause has been associated with a variety of symptoms that vary between cultures. Between 50% and 70% of women in western cultures experience symptoms such as hot flashes (also known as hot flushes) and night sweats. Other symptoms include poor memory, a loss of libido, irritability, problems with skin or hair, vaginal dryness, anxiety, and headaches. Reporting of menopausal symptoms in cultures such as Japan has increased as cultural awareness of the menopause, or *kônenki*, has also increased (Melby et al., 2005). Thus, as noted for PMS, cultural discourses influence the interpretation of menopause symptoms.

In terms of mental health, there is some evidence that women may be more vulnerable to depression during this time. Epidemiological studies suggest women have an increased risk of depression during menopause, compared to before or after menopause. A review concluded that fluctuations and declines in ovarian hormones are associated with this increased risk, particularly for women with a previous history of depression (Deecher et al., 2008). Ovarian hormones are known to have specific modulatory effects on the serotonergic and noradrenergic systems, both of which are involved in depression. Reviews and meta-analyses suggest that **hormone replacement therapy (HRT)** with women who are severely depressed may improve mood and facilitate the efficacy of antidepressants (Miller, 2003; Zweifel & O'Brien, 1997).

However, there are likely to be multiple physical, psychological, and cultural causes of depression during menopause. For example, an Australian study found that depressed mood in menopausal women was strongly influenced by a history of depression, a history of premenstrual complaints, negative attitudes toward ageing or menopause, poor health, more frequent symptoms, and daily hassles (Dennerstein et al., 2004). In cultures where menopause is viewed positively and increases the prestige of the women concerned, much lower levels of symptoms are reported (Freeman & Sherif, 2007). In western cultures, however, it has been found that concurrent stressful events are important predictors of women's wellbeing during menopause. Menopause often coincides with significant role changes, such as children leaving home. A multidimensional approach, such as the biopsychosocial or Material-Discursive-Intrapsychic approach, is necessary to provide a better understanding of wellbeing during menopause.

The use of HRT to treat the symptoms of menopause has been controversial and is a good illustration of the importance of research methods when examining treatment effects. Early studies of HRT were methodologically weak (e.g. they did not control for the baseline health status or have a placebo group as a comparison). However, in recent large-scale placebo-controlled clinical trials, use of HRT was stopped early when it became apparent that it was associated with an increased risk of breast cancer and thromboembolism and did not protect against heart disease as originally thought (Women's Health Initiative, 2009).

Summary

- The menstrual cycle is associated with changes in behaviours and mood, but these vary between cultures.
- PMS and PMDD are psychological symptoms associated with the luteal phase of the menstrual cycle. PMS affects up to 30% of women and PMDD up to 2%.
- Physical, psychological, and cultural factors affect PMS/PMDD, but the specific influence of each is unclear.
- Psychological intervention for PMS/PMDD can be as effective as antidepressants.
- Menopause is often associated with hot flashes and a range of other physical and psychological symptoms.
- There is some evidence that menopause can be associated with depressed mood, which is probably due to physical, psychological, and cultural factors.

14.1.2 PREGNANCY AND BIRTH

Pregnancy, birth, and becoming a parent are a time of great physical and psychosocial change for women and their partners. Childbirth is a pivotal life event that can be challenging, may involve pain, and evokes positive and negative emotions. Physiologically, childbirth involves systems and hormones that are affected by psychological factors, such as the HPA axis, cortisol, endogenous opioids, and oxytocin. Unpleasant psychosocial factors such as stress and anxiety in pregnancy are associated with poor outcomes, such as preterm birth and low birth weight. Healthy behaviours during pregnancy are important contributors to the health of women and the developing foetus. Poor health behaviours, such as poor diet and use of substances, are associated with a range of adverse outcomes for the child.

Psychological theories and evidence are therefore highly relevant to understanding the experience, behaviour, and outcomes of pregnancy and birth for women and their families. These include theories of health beliefs, health behaviour, measurement, interventions, and implementation. Health-related theories range from broad frameworks for understanding health, such as the biopsychosocial or diathesis-stress models, to specific theories of behavioural and psychological phenomena. Despite this, a lot of perinatal research has been atheoretical. A search of research on postpartum depression found that only 16% of research papers included the word 'theory' and only 3% of papers mentioned 'theory' in the title, abstract, or keywords (Ayers & Olander, 2013). This suggests that very little perinatal research explicitly draws on psychological theory, despite its relevance (Ayers & Olander, 2013; Saxby, 2017).

The biopsychosocial approach shows that pregnancy outcomes are influenced by biological, psychological, social, and macrocultural factors (Suls & Rothman, 2004). At the macrocultural level, pregnancy and birth are influenced by cultural norms and rituals that affect women's expectations and experiences (Iravani et al., 2015; Jordan, 1993). For example, maternal mortality and morbidity is much less likely in high-income countries compared to low-income countries. Surgical intervention in the form of caesarean sections has increased the safety of birth and the World Health Organisation estimates that caesarean sections are necessary in 10–15% of births to reduce mortality and morbidity for women and/or their babies (World Health Organisation, 2015). However, there are large cultural differences in the rates of caesarean section (Betrán et al., 2016), with the USA and the UK increasing from 4% to over 25% over the last 60 years. Rapidly developing countries, such as Brazil and China, have seen even greater increases with no significant improvement in perinatal outcomes (McCourt et al., 2007).

There are many possible reasons for the increase in caesarean sections: changing cultural beliefs and norms; an increase in biological risk factors such as increasing maternal age or obesity; convenience for medical staff or women of scheduled births (Palmer et al., 2015); institutional, legal and economic factors; and an increase in maternal requests for caesarean sections. This illustrates how the likelihood of a woman having a caesarean birth may be influenced by macrocultural, psychological, and social factors, as well as by biological complications and risk.

Pregnancy

Women's physical and psychological health in pregnancy is important for them and for the developing foetus. Research on the developmental origins of health and disease finds associations between pregnancy/birth outcomes and adult disease in offspring. This is most established in terms of physical health, such as poor nutrition during pregnancy and low birth weight being associated with a greater risk of developing cardiovascular disease as an adult (Wadhwa et al., 2009). However, evidence indicates that psychological factors during pregnancy can also affect the developing foetus. The strongest evidence is for the links between stress and anxiety in pregnancy and a greater risk of a range of adverse outcomes for the child (Glover, 2016).

The effect of stress in pregnancy on the infant is due to a combination of epigenetic and environmental factors. As noted in Chapter 16, the likelihood of a child developing psychological disorders such as schizophrenia may be influenced by a genetic predisposition *and* experiences during pregnancy/birth, early childhood, or later life. Similarly, material presented in Chapter 8 shows how the cognitive potential children inherit in their genes can be optimised or impaired by psychosocial experiences in childhood. The field of **epigenetics** has provided increased understanding of how environmental factors, such as stress in pregnancy, may regulate the activity and expression of genes in the foetus and child (Wadwa et al., 2009).

The effect of stress in pregnancy on the infant is thought to occur through epigenetic neurobiological **foetal programming**. The evidence for foetal programming mostly comes from animal and epidemiological research. For example, studies of women who were pregnant during the Quebec ice storm in 1998 found that exposure to stress during pregnancy was associated with a range of adverse outcomes for the child, including the baby being more likely to be fussy/difficult, dull, and needing attention (Laplante et al., 2016); poorer child development (Laplante et al., 2008); and greater metabolic changes such as central adiposity and obesity (Cao-Lei et al., 2015). The study in Research Box 14.1 shows that both women's exposure to the ice storm (i.e. objective stress) and their appraisal of the ice storm as positive or negative (i.e. subjective stress) were associated with altered patterns of DNA methylation in their children 13 years later (Cao-Lei et al., 2015). This is consistent with theories of stress which emphasise the importance of appraisal (see Chapter 3), and illustrates how appraisal of stress in pregnancy possibly influences the genome of the unborn child.

RESEARCH BOX 14.1   Stress in pregnancy and DNA changes in offspring

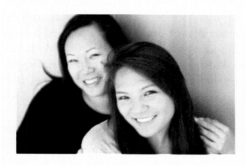

Background

Studies of humans and animals have shown that stress in pregnancy can impact on a range of child outcomes that may persist into adulthood. These effects occur through epigenetic changes, such as DNA methylation, in the foetal genome. However, it is not clear whether this is due to objective stress (i.e. severity of the stressor) or subjective stress (i.e. a woman's appraisal).

Method and findings

Project Ice Storm is a long-term follow-up of 218 women who were pregnant during the 1998 Quebec ice storm and their children. When the children were age 13 this study looked at their DNA methylation and compared those whose mothers had rated the storm as negative (n = 12) in 1998 with those whose mothers rated the storm as neutral or positive (n = 22).

Results revealed significant differences in DNA methylation between adolescents whose mothers appraised the storm as positive or negative. Differences were found in the methylation levels of 2,872 child genome sites. These sites are affiliated with 1,564 different genes and 408 different biological pathways that are prominently featured in immune function.

Significance

This study suggests that pregnant women's cognitive appraisals of a stressor may have widespread effects on DNA methylation across the entire genome of their unborn children that are detectable during adolescence.

Photograph © J.K. Califf, www.flickr.com

Cao-Lei, L., Elgbeili, G., Massart, R., Laplante, D.P., Szyf, M. & King, S. (2015) Pregnant women's cognitive appraisal of a natural disaster affects DNA methylation in their children 13 years later: Project Ice Storm. *Translational Psychiatry, 24*(5): e515.

There is also evidence from epidemiology and animal research that environmental influences such as greater adversity or a lack of nurturing can lead to physiological changes that are then passed from parents to children and grandchildren. This is often referred to as the **intergenerational transmission of vulnerability**. This is attributable to both epigenetic transmission (see Chapter 8) and shared aspects of the environment that increase the likelihood of poor child outcomes, such as exposure to intimate partner violence. However, it is worth highlighting that although stress in pregnancy and the early years is associated with a greater risk of adverse outcomes, most children are not affected. The mechanisms that determine which children are affected, and in which ways, are not yet well understood (Glover, 2016).

Another way in which psychological factors are important in pregnancy is through beliefs and health behaviour. A study of beliefs in late pregnancy, based on the self-regulatory model (see Chapter 4), found that women's beliefs about personal control, consequences, coherence, and emotional representations of pregnancy explained a large proportion of the variance in women's physical and psychological health in pregnancy (Jessop et al., 2014). Health behaviours like smoking, alcohol and substance use, exposure to toxins, diet, and exercise also affect the woman and developing foetus in a number of ways. For example, the overuse of alcohol during pregnancy is associated with miscarriage, stillbirth, and foetal alcohol syndrome.

Theories of health behaviour change can therefore be used to guide health promotion and intervention during pregnancy. The COM-B framework may be particularly useful for perinatal interventions (Olander et al., 2016). This framework was developed from a synthesis of 19 theories of health behaviour change and suggests change is a function of Capability, Opportunity, and Motivation (Michie et al., 2011). These are likely to fluctuate during pregnancy and after birth because of changes in physical, psychological, and social factors. Therefore, although women may be more motivated to change during pregnancy, they also need the capability and opportunity to change, which can vary across the perinatal period.

Birth

Birth is a significant life event for women and their partners, and women often have detailed expectations of labour and birth. Social norms and women's expectations influence women's choices about where to give birth, how they give birth, and the use of pain relief. The widespread provision of antenatal classes in developed countries is partly based on an assumption that there is a causal relationship between a woman's expectations and her experience of birth. Proponents of natural childbirth, such as Dick-Read (Dick-Read, 1993, 2004), believed that expectations of pain cause fear, and that fear consequently results in increased tension and pain during labour. Dick-Read argued that if women are educated so that they change their expectations and learn relaxation techniques to combat tension, then pain will be reduced. Although research does not provide unequivocal evidence that attendance at antenatal classes leads to a reduction of pain in labour (Gagnon & Sandall, 2007), the incorporation of antenatal classes is now an accepted part of antenatal care.

The greatest social change in experiences of childbirth has been the context and type of birth. Births have moved from home to hospital and, as outlined earlier, caesarean births are increasing. For example, in the UK, caesarean rates have risen from under 5% in the 1950s to almost 30% today. The suggestion that this increase is partly due to more women wanting caesareans is not supported by research evidence. An Australian study found that only 6% of pregnant women wanted a caesarean delivery – and most of these women had obstetric complications or a previous complicated delivery (Gamble & Creedy, 2001). Most caesareans are performed as emergency deliveries after labour has started, suggesting that the rise in caesarean sections is due to increased complications during labour and/ or an increased tendency for clinicians to carry out caesareans rather than continue with non-operative births. There is some evidence to support this. A UK study of 64,538 healthy women with low-risk pregnancies showed that only 58% of women who gave birth in hospitals had a 'normal birth', compared to 76% of women who gave birth in midwifery units, and 88% of those who planned to give birth at home (Birthplace in England Collaborative Group et al., 2011). 'Normal birth' was defined as a birth without induction of labour, epidural or spinal analgesia, general anaesthesia, forceps or ventouse delivery, caesarean section, or episiotomy.

Discourses and ideologies around birth and maternity care are culturally determined, but also vary within cultures. For example, within a society, individuals may have contrasting views that birth is risky and care should be highly medicalised, or that birth is a natural process where interference is harmful (Malacrida & Boulton, 2012). Maternity services and practitioners usually have internalised or embraced a set of ideologies around birth and, for hospital birth, this is likely to be driven by a biomedical approach. Differences in beliefs and notions of risk between healthcare professionals and pregnant women may result in conflict and misunderstandings. Giving birth in a hospital may be reassuring, informed, technologically advanced, and 'safe' to women with a biomedical view of birth, but may feel cold, stressful, and perilous to women with different assumptions (Miller & Shriver, 2012). For example, a study from Australia, where hospital birth is highly medicalised, found that women who chose a home birth against medical advice or without trained health professionals were well educated about the risks of birth. However, they perceived hospital care to be more risky than staying at home, with 17 out of 20 having had a previous birth experience and four women being midwives themselves (Jackson et al., 2012). Women in this study had therefore intensely scrutinised, or personally experienced, the risks inherent in giving birth in a hospital, and decided that the harmful activities of healthcare providers and organisations were more risky than the birth process itself. Other studies show that around 10% of women would prefer a home birth – most of them because they think they will have more control (Davies et al., 1996). However, research in the Netherlands, where approximately 30% of women give birth at home, suggests that the place of birth makes no difference to the proportion of women who find birth traumatic (Stramrood et al., 2011).

Women's expectations of birth are complex and dynamic. Research shows that most women have well-formed expectations of many aspects of childbirth, the baby, being a mother, and their partner's role. Women have positive and negative expectations of different aspects of birth, such as emotions, control, pain, and obstetric events. These expectations can be refined with new information and experiences (Gupton et al., 1991). Women's expectations are broadly associated with birth experiences. Positive expectations of birth are associated with experiencing greater control in birth, greater satisfaction, and emotional wellbeing. Conversely, negative expectations are associated with finding birth less fulfilling, being less satisfied with birth, and reporting less emotional wellbeing after birth (Ayers & Pickering, 2005; Green et al., 1998). These associations may partly be due to other factors, such as anxiety or self-efficacy.

Fear can have a strong effect on women's expectations and experiences. Fear of childbirth occurs in 7–26% of pregnant women (Laursen et al., 2009), with a small proportion developing severe fear of birth (tokophobia) (Nieminen et al., 2009). Symptoms include high levels of anxiety about pregnancy and birth, fear of harm or death during birth, and poor sleep and somatic complaints. A study of 7,200 women in six European countries found that there are significant differences between countries, with the prevalence of severe fear of childbirth ranging from 2% to 14% (Ryding et al., 2015; van Parys et al., 2012). Fear of childbirth is multifactorial and associated with having a first baby (nulliparous), poor mental health, younger age, lower education, and low self-efficacy (Laursen et al., 2009; Rouhe et al., 2009; Salomonsson et al., 2013). Although fear of childbirth is more common in nulliparous women, women who have a negative or traumatic experience of birth are five times more likely to report fear of childbirth in a subsequent pregnancy (Størksen et al., 2013). The importance of traumatic birth experiences and fear of childbirth is apparent from large epidemiological studies that find that women who fear childbirth are more likely to want interventions such as epidural analgesia and caesarean sections (Nieminen et al., 2009; Rouhe et al., 2009).

The birth of a baby is usually thought of as a positive event. However, evidence shows 20–30% of women in western countries find giving birth traumatic, and 4% develop post-traumatic stress disorder (PTSD). Women who have assisted deliveries or caesarean sections are more likely to develop PTSD, but it is not a straightforward relationship: individual risk factors interact with what happens during birth to determine whether women find it traumatic. A meta-analysis of 55 studies showed the strongest risk factors for PTSD are fear of birth, depression, previous trauma, poor health or complications in pregnancy, negative birth experiences, lack of support during birth, and dissociation (where people feel detached from reality) (Ayers et al., 2016). The symptoms of PTSD following birth include flashbacks to the birth, intrusive thoughts about what happened, avoidance of reminders of the birth, hyperarousal (e.g. hypervigilance, anger, irritability), and negative cognitions and mood (American Pyschiatric Association, 2013). Women who have severe complications during pregnancy or birth, such as pre-eclampsia or preterm babies, are particularly at risk, with 19% reporting PTSD (Dikmen-Yildesz et al., 2017). An example of CBT treatment for a woman with PTSD and depression after birth is given in Case Study 19.1.

Support from others during labour has a critical influence on birth outcomes and psychological wellbeing. Women are more likely to have PTSD if they feel poorly informed, not listened to, inadequately cared for, and have little support from staff or their partner (Ayers & Ford, 2015). The provision of support for women during labour is not standard in many poorly resourced countries. This means that experimental studies have been possible where women are randomly allocated a person to support them or not. An example of one of these studies is given in Research Box 14.2. A meta-analysis of these studies shows that simply providing a lay person (a 'Doula') to support a woman during labour results in better physical outcomes for both mother and baby, including shorter labours, less analgesia, fewer assisted or operative deliveries, and higher maternal satisfaction with the birth experience (Hodnett et al., 2013).

In terms of medical care, the factors outlined above have a number of implications. One is that providing good support during labour may prevent a number of women being traumatised. Another is that reducing fear, stress, and anxiety in pregnancy may improve maternal and infant outcomes. For example, providing antenatal counselling to women with a severe fear of childbirth can reduce requests for elective caesarean deliveries (Halvorsen et al., 2008).

Another implication is the impact of stress on female healthcare professionals who are pregnant. As we have seen, stressful and physically demanding jobs are related to adverse outcomes. Research shows female healthcare professionals are at increased risk of pregnancy complications, especially in late pregnancy. During pregnancy, female doctors working in hospitals report that the physical demands of the job (e.g. night shifts, standing for long periods) are stressful and there is poor support from colleagues. Institutional support for female healthcare workers during pregnancy is lacking and needs to be properly examined (Finch, 2003).

In summary, pregnancy and birth are a time of great change and transition when biological, psychological, social, and macrocultural factors all influence pregnancy outcomes for the woman and her child. Psychological theories and evidence are highly relevant. We illustrated this by examining how stress and anxiety in pregnancy affect the developing foetus, and how expectations and fear of childbirth influence birth.

CLINICAL NOTES 14.1

Antenatal care

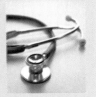

- It is important to identify pregnant women with high levels of distress or anxiety and offer appropriate intervention.
- Reducing stress and anxiety in pregnant women benefits the wellbeing of women and their unborn babies.
- Reducing stress and anxiety in pregnancy may also lead to fewer requests for elective caesarean sections.
- Referral to perinatal psychology services may be appropriate. They can provide psychological support for women and their families in pregnancy and after birth.
- Such services are increasing as health services realise the long-term impact maternal health in pregnancy and after birth has on both the mother, and the health and development of children.

RESEARCH BOX 14.2   Support in labour

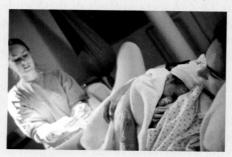

Background

Experimental studies in countries where women do not usually have a companion with them during labour clearly show that providing a lay person to support women results in better outcomes for both mother and baby. However, it is not ethically possible to replicate these kinds of studies in countries where women usually have a partner or other supportive person with them during labour.

Method and findings

This study included 16,610 women giving birth in the same year, excluding women who had planned caesarean sections. A range of health and psychosocial variables were measured during pregnancy, birth, and the postnatal period.

Women who did not have anyone accompanying them during labour were more likely to have a preterm birth, an emergency caesarean section, pain relief, a short labour, and low satisfaction with life nine months after the birth. Their babies had a lower birth weight, were more likely to be in intensive care, and had delayed motor development.

Women were less likely to have a supportive companion during labour if they were single, from ethnic minority groups, from poor households, and with low levels of education.

Significance

Support during labour is as critical for women in western countries as in non-western countries where experimental research has been done. This study identified groups of women who are at a greater risk of being alone and unsupported while giving birth. Such women may benefit from more support from healthcare professionals during labour and after birth.

Photograph © Raphaël Goetter, www.flickr.com

Essex, H. & Pickett, K. (2008) Mothers without companionship during childbirth: Analysis within Millennium cohort study. *Birth*, 35: 266–276.

14.1.3 HIGH RISK PREGNANCIES AND BIRTH

Pregnancy and birth can be high risk for a number of reasons. Pregnancy loss can be particularly difficult and includes miscarriage, termination of pregnancy, and stillbirth.

Approximately one in five pregnancies end in miscarriage. Although often thought of as a lesser event than stillbirth, miscarriage can be distressing for women and result in depression or PTSD, with between 10% and 50% of women reporting symptoms of depression (Lok & Neugebauer, 2007) and around 11% reporting symptoms of PTSD (Daugirdaitė et al., 2015).

Worldwide, every year 2.6 million babies are stillborn after 24 weeks of pregnancy. In the majority of cases the reason for death is unexplained. Studies unanimously find this is an intensely painful loss for parents, with reports of intense grief, marital difficulties, feelings of worthlessness, isolation, shame, and guilt. Around a third of women report high levels of anxiety, depression, and/or PTSD (Campbell-Jackson & Horsch, 2014). Current medical practice offers parents a chance to see and hold their dead infants on the assumption that it will help the grieving process. However, the evidence for this is inconsistent and some research suggests that, although parents appreciate the opportunity to do this, they may have poorer mental health in the long term. Stigma and reduced chances to talk about the stillbirth and baby appear to contribute to poor mental health in the long term (Crawley et al., 2013).

14.1.4 MENTAL HEALTH IN PREGNANCY AND AFTER BIRTH

The transition to parenthood is a time of great change and adjustment, which for some new parents can exacerbate existing mental health problems or lead to the development of new mental health problems. It has been estimated that up to 20% of women develop some form of mental health problem in pregnancy or after birth. In addition to affecting women's wellbeing, this has a substantial cost to society. For example, it is estimated that perinatal mental health problems cost the UK £8.1 billion for every annual cohort of women giving birth. A substantial proportion of this cost (72%) is due to the long-term impact on the child (Bauer et al., 2014). There is also evidence that men can be affected, with up to 10% of fathers having depression in the perinatal period and up to 18% having anxiety disorders (Cameron et al., 2016; Leach et al., 2016; Paulson & Bazemore, 2010).

A range of mental health problems can occur during pregnancy and after birth, such as anxiety, depression, PTSD, puerperal psychosis, and bonding disorders. The most common psychological problems are anxiety and depression, which occur in pregnancy or after birth in approximately 10–20% of women. Other possible problems include PTSD, obsessive compulsive disorder (OCD), and stress-related conditions such as adjustment disorder. Puerperal psychosis is a rare but very severe disorder which is one of the leading indirect causes of maternal death (Knight et al., 2014). Puerperal psychosis occurs in one in every 1,000 women and puts the woman and her baby at high risk of harm, including infanticide and suicide, so it requires immediate hospitalisation. Puerperal psychosis typically has a rapid onset, within hours or days of birth, and is more likely to occur in women with a personal or family history of bipolar or psychotic disorders. A high degree of comorbidity is often found among perinatal affective disorders. For example, between 25% and 50% of women with OCD also have depression (Fairbrother & Abramowitz, 2016).

How mental health or illness is conceptualised is important in perinatal mental health (see Chapter 16). It is possible that diagnosis and estimates of prevalence are affected by normal perinatal factors such as fatigue and anxiety about the baby's wellbeing. It has been argued that some anxiety is normal during pregnancy and after birth (Matthey, 2016). A focus on diagnostic criteria also means that many women who have symptoms that do not fit diagnostic criteria or meet thresholds for treatment will be missed. These symptoms might still be distressing for women and potentially have long-term consequences for them and their child. For example, in one survey of 1,500 women in the UK with self-identified perinatal mental health problems, a range of symptoms were reported (see Figure 14.2). These included less commonly recognised symptoms such as anger and changes in appetite. It also showed that 22% of women in this survey had thought about suicide (Boots Family Trust Alliance, 2013).

One important issue with postnatal mental health problems is determining whether these are present before the birth. For example, women with anxiety or depression in pregnancy are more likely to have postnatal depression. In addition, research suggests that the prevalence of depression during pregnancy is not significantly different from depression after birth. Thus, some people would question whether the notion of 'postnatal' mental health problems is appropriate. It may be that pregnancy, birth, and adjusting to parenthood can exacerbate or initiate a wide range of different mental health problems, similar to those observed after other stressful events, such as bereavement or divorce.

Risk and resilience

A number of risk factors make it more likely that women will develop perinatal mental health problems. Some of these risk factors are remarkably consistent across different disorders and cultures. For example, mental health problems are more likely to occur if women live in circumstances of social adversity (e.g. deprivation, low socioeconomic status, domestic violence), have a history of psychological problems or childhood adversity, and have poor support available to them. In addition, if women are anxious or depressed during pregnancy this is likely to continue or worsen postpartum.

Nonetheless, the majority of women are psychologically healthy during pregnancy and after birth, so we need to look at what characterises health during pregnancy and the factors associated with resilience. A study of over 1,300 women in the USA found that women who were resilient were characterised by low depression and stress and high support and self-efficacy. These women were also less likely to have risky health behaviours in pregnancy and were more likely to have better birth outcomes. In contrast, vulnerable women were characterised by high depression and stress and poor support and self-efficacy. Vulnerable women were more likely to have an unintended pregnancy, risky health behaviours, and have their baby preterm (Maxson et al., 2016).

The impact of perinatal mental health problems

Perinatal mental health problems are important because of the potential for them to negatively affect women, children, and families. The impact on women and children varies according to the type of mental illness and timing: whether it occurs in the pre- and/or

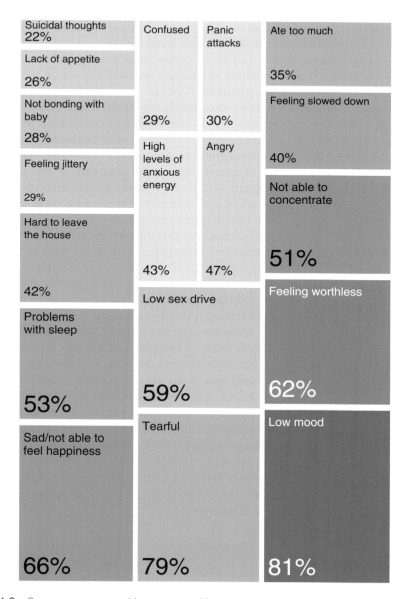

FIGURE 14.2 Symptoms reported by women with postnatal mental health problems (Boots Family Trust Alliance, 2013)

Reproduced with permission by the Boots Family Trust Alliance, Perinatal mental health: Experiences of women and health professionals (2013)

postnatal period, and whether it is acute (short-lived) or chronic (enduring). Overall, the evidence shows that perinatal mental health problems can have a severe impact on women and their families, particularly for depression.

As we have seen, stress and anxiety during pregnancy are associated with increased risk of a range of adverse outcomes for women and their children, including preterm birth (Ding et al., 2014), which is one of the major causes of morbidity and mortality in children. After birth, mental health problems can have a negative impact on the relationship between the mother and baby, and her partner (Delicate et al., 2018). Women with mental health problems may be less sensitive to their baby's emotional state and display less optimal parenting, such as being withdrawn and unavailable to the baby or over-intrusive (Murray et al., 2010). The impact of postpartum mental health problems on the child has been mostly researched in relation to postpartum depression. This shows that depression is associated with poor development and mental health problems in children (Murray et al., 2010). Poor parental mental health is also one of many factors associated with child maltreatment. However, it must be noted that maltreatment is a rare occurrence, and the majority of parents with mental health problems do *not* maltreat their children. Nonetheless, these are some of the mechanisms through which mental health problems and social adversity can be transmitted from one generation to the next in the intergenerational transmission of vulnerability.

Treatment and interventions at this time are important to prevent the transmission of social adversity and mental health problems between generations. Progress in this regard is patchy for a number of reasons. First, only a small proportion of women with perinatal mental health problems come to the attention of health services, and fewer of these women receive treatment (Khan, 2015). This is due to a range of factors, which include a lack of screening (or ineffective screening), barriers to women seeking help during this time, clinician barriers to diagnosis and treatment, lack of perinatal psychology services, and limited evidence on effective treatments. In the UK, a survey showed that very few cities or regions have adequate perinatal psychology services (www.everyonesbusiness.co.uk). In terms of effective treatments, there is most evidence for the treatment of postnatal depression with CBT or interpersonal therapy. Clinical guidelines are available that recommend effective psychotherapies on the basis of current evidence (National Institute for Clinical Excellence, 2014; Scottish Intercollegiate Guidelines Network, 2012). Despite this, recent reviews of diagnosis and treatment of perinatal depression by primary care physicians suggest antidepressants are often the first line of treatment.

CLINICAL NOTES 14.2

Postnatal care

- Birth can be experienced as traumatic and some women develop PTSD following difficult births.
- Watch out for high levels of anxiety and the re-experiencing of symptoms such as nightmares, intrusive thoughts, and flashbacks.

(Continued)

- Postnatal PTSD is usually successfully treated if women are referred to psycho-therapy in the first few months after birth.
- Be vigilant for signs of postnatal depression, but be aware that many women have depressive symptoms prior to, or during, pregnancy.
- Women may develop a range of other anxiety disorders, such as OCD, panic, or social phobia.
- Puerperal psychosis is very severe and women should be given *immediate* inpatient treatment – preferably in a mother–baby unit so the infant can go as well.
- Make sure you are aware of the availability of psychological interventions for women with postnatal mental health problems, particularly puerperal psychosis which requires fast action and referral.

Summary

- Antenatal stress and mental health problems are associated with a range of adverse outcomes for women and their babies.
- The context and type of birth has changed historically with more women given birth in hospitals and an increasing number of caesarean section deliveries.
- Supporting women during labour results in better physical outcomes and maternal psychological wellbeing.
- The transition to parenthood is associated with increases in depression, anxiety, and psychotic disorders. Anxiety disorders may be more prevalent than depression but are remarkably under-recognised.
- Psychological problems following a birth can have an adverse impact on the woman, their relationships, and the infant.
- High-risk pregnancies, miscarriage, and stillbirth are associated with high levels of distress, such as depression and PTSD.

14.2 ENDOCRINE DISORDERS AND PSYCHOSOCIAL WELLBEING

Psychoneuroendocrinology is the study of how psychological states are influenced by changes in hormone secretion. It is playing an increasing role in the diagnosis and treatment of affective disorders and anxiety disorders. One of the most obvious reasons for this change is the observation that people with primary endocrine disorders are more likely than the general population to experience psychiatric morbidity. Alongside this observation, there is increasing understanding of the synergies between the neural and endocrine systems and the differing roles of hormonal and neuronal control of the function of the pituitary (which is often referred to as the 'master gland') by the hypothalamus. Dysfunction in brain regions such as the hypothalamus can affect the functioning of the endocrine system, which is in turn associated with psychiatric symptoms.

The notion of the 'psychopharmacological bridge' has also guided work in this area. If a drug produces a therapeutic effect (e.g. relieving symptoms) and has specific biochemical actions (e.g. modifying hormone secretion), then this suggests a causal link between the therapeutic effects, the biochemical changes, and the cause of the syndrome. For example, if a drug known to treat cortisol hypersecretion also reduces the psychiatric symptoms of depression, this suggests that cortisol hypersecretion is a casual factor in the onset and progression of the depression.

Hypothalamic-Pituitary-Adrenal axis (HPA)

There is a wealth of research evidence documenting HPA axis hyperactivity in people with depression who are not taking medication. Changes in HPA axis in depressed people include elevated corticotrophin releasing hormone (CRH) in cerebrospinal fluid, enlarged pituitary and/or adrenal glands, and increased production of adrenocorticotropic hormone (ACTH) and/or cortisol during periods of depression. It is not completely clear whether these HPA changes are a cause or symptom of depression. For example, dysregulation of the HPA axis can occur after periods of chronic or severe stress. This is also observed in other stress-related illnesses, such as PTSD, where conversely there is a reduced cortisol response (see Chapter 3).

Cortisol hypersecretion (Cushing's syndrome)

Common psychiatric aspects of cortisol hypersecretion include depression and irritability. In the initial description of his eponymous syndrome, Cushing (1932) described a relationship between cortisol hypersecretion and psychological symptoms. People with Cushing's syndrome often have a consistent constellation of psychological symptoms, predominantly impaired affect. Around three-quarters are depressed and 90% are irritable. Fatigue is universal and may be explained by common insomnia. Many people also report decreased libido. Cognitive symptoms include decreased concentration and poor problem solving and memory. These factors combine to influence social withdrawal, which may also be affected by changes in physical appearance, such as truncal obesity, a round face, and a 'buffalo hump'.

In people with cortisol hypersecretion there may be problems of **differential diagnosis**: without thorough investigation, it may be difficult to determine whether a patient with hypercortisolemia has primary depression or early Cushing's syndrome.

Cortisol hyposecretion (Addison's disease)

The major behavioural manifestations of cortisol hyposecretion are lethargy and apathy. Other behavioural manifestations include irritability, crying, and impaired sleep. People may also have problems with memory and concentration, and report tachycardia.

In people with cortisol hyposecretion there may be problems of differential diagnosis because the patient may show non-specific symptoms that wax and wane. In addition, periods of stress exacerbate symptoms – because the adrenal glands are called on to increase secretion (see Chapter 3) – and these symptoms decrease when the stress abates. These presenting symptoms mean hypocortisolism can be misdiagnosed as a primary psychiatric condition. For example, tachycardia, dizziness, and complaints of lethargy may be seen as signs of anxiety disorders or may be misdiagnosed as chronic fatigue syndrome.

For both of the cortisol-related syndromes just described, there is evidence that changes in cortisol levels produce the original psychiatric symptoms (Hunt et al., 2000; Sonino & Fava, 2001). Effective treatment of cortisol hypersecretion is associated with improvements in mood and cognitive function. Effective treatment of cortisol hyposecretion leads to an alleviation of psychological and behavioural symptoms.

ACTIVITY 14.1   DIFFERENTIAL DIAGNOSIS

- What is meant by differential diagnosis?
- Why may differential diagnosis be difficult in people with cortisol hyposecretion or hypersecretion?

Hypothalamic-Pituitary-Thyroid axis (HPT)

The link between thyroid function and behaviour was first documented nearly 200 years ago. Parry (1825) noted that hyperfunction of the thyroid was associated with 'various nervous affectations' and symptoms such as restlessness, hyperactivity, and impaired concentration. A causative role of hypothyroidism in psychopathology was demonstrated by Asher (1949): a case series indicated that administration of desiccated thyroid alleviated psychological symptoms of depression and psychotic symptoms. Abnormal thyroid function is more common among people with psychiatric illnesses than in the general population. However, part of this difference is iatrogenic: various psychotropic medications (e.g., lithium, neuroleptics, and antidepressants) will disturb the HPT axis function to varying degrees.

In recent decades, there has been an increase in understanding of links between thyroid function and psychological wellbeing. Most people with thyroid disorders complain of a psychological disturbance that is alleviated on correction of the thyroid illness. This indicates the involvement of the HPT system in psychological states.

Hyperthyroidism

The behavioural states observed in hyperthyroidism include intense dysphoria, usually with pronounced anxiety. Other common complaints include nervousness, emotional lability, restlessness, and impaired concentration. Insomnia and fatigue are common and people may feel too weak and tired to carry out planned activities. Decreased concentration and impaired memory are correlated with thyrotoxicosis.

Hypothyroidism

Hypothyroidism is the most common clinical disorder of thyroid function. The most common psychiatric symptoms can be grouped into cognitive dysfunction (impaired memory, inattentiveness, slower and poorer problem solving) and mood changes (predominantly depressed mood, but also anxiety, insomnia, irritability, and confusion). Psychosis may be present in severe hypothyroidism.

For both the thyroid-related syndromes just described, there is evidence that psychological symptoms abate following effective treatments of the hormonal abnormality (Sonino et al., 2007). This indicates that the hormonal imbalance causes the psychological symptoms. In hyperthyroidism, scores on measures of mood, anxiety, and cognitive function often return to normal after a return to euthyroid status. Similarly, in hypothyroidism, psychiatric symptoms are alleviated following effective treatment of the thyroid disorder. However, it is important to note that many people have impaired quality of life even after thyroid hormone levels have returned to within the normal range, often because of an altered relationship to their body (Nexø et al., 2015).

Growth hormone

Excess secretion of growth hormone (GH) results in gigantism in children and acromegaly in adults. The most common cause of GH hypersecretion is pituitary adenoma. Physical symptoms are usually obvious – e.g. abnormal growth of the hands and feet, changes in bony and soft tissue, including an altered facial appearance. Psychiatric symptoms are rare, although depression may occasionally occur. Although clinical psychiatric symptoms are rare, people with acromegaly have lower scores on measures of quality of life and self-esteem, which appear to be related to changes in body image (Webb & Badia, 2016). These changes can lead to social withdrawal, disruption in interpersonal relations, mood swings, and a loss of initiative and spontaneity. In addition to medical or surgical treatment to address the cause of GH hypersecretion, there may be benefits from exercise therapy to improve quality of life and self-esteem (Hatipoglu et al., 2014). It is interesting to note that treatment of excessive secretion of GH to cure acromegaly can lead to improvements to quality of life (Wexler et al., 2009). The remainder of this section examines the psychosocial impact of GH deficiency.

GH deficiency causes an absence or delay in the lengthening and widening of the skeletal bones. In some cases, the onset of the disorder occurs antenatally and in others the condition occurs months or years later. Clinical psychiatric symptoms of growth hormone deficiency are rare. However, it has clear impacts on self-esteem and a distorted body image. Children with GH deficiency have higher rates of anxiety, depression, social phobia, and attentional dysfunction than their peers. In adults, quality of life is lower in

RESEARCH BOX 14.3   Psychological aspects of treated endocrine disorders

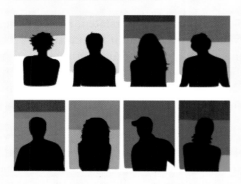

Background

Many people with endocrine disorders complain of disturbances to psychological wellbeing and quality of life. The close links between psychological wellbeing and endocrine function mean that there may be value in expanding the concept of recovery in endocrine disorders to give greater consideration to psychosocial issues.

Method and findings

The sample consisted of 146 consecutive outpatients aged 18–65 who had primary endocrine disorders, but who were cured or had been in remission for at least six months following successful surgical and/or pharmacological treatment. They were assessed for psychiatric disorders according to DSM-IV criteria. Psychosomatic conditions were assessed using Diagnostic Criteria for Psychosomatic Research (DCPR).

The results data revealed that 62% of patients had at least one psychiatric diagnosis. When assessed in relation to DSM-IV diagnostic criteria, 29% of patients had generalised anxiety disorder, 26% had major depressive disorder, and 8% had agoraphobia. When assessed in relation to DCPR diagnostic criteria, 46% of patients had irritable mood, 34% experienced demoralisation, and 21% had persistent somatisation (a tendency to experience psychological distress as bodily physical symptoms). The vast majority of patients (81%) had at least one psychiatric or psychosocial disorder. The patterns of diagnoses and symptoms matched those that would be expected within each (untreated) patient group (e.g. depression in patients with cured/treated Cushing's syndrome).

Significance

This study shows that a purely biomedical approach to treating endocrine disorders is not sufficient. It highlights the need for ongoing attention to the psychological wellbeing of people who have been cured of, or successfully treated for, the physiological aspects of endocrine disorders.

Sonino, N. et al. (2004) Persistent psychological distress in patients treated for endocrine disease. *Psychotherapy and Psychosomatics*, *73*: 78–83.

those with growth hormone deficiencies (Hull & Harvey, 2003). This may be displayed as social phobia, fear of negative evaluation, decreased interest or pleasure in activities, depression, fatigue, and irritability. In addition, there are lower marriage rates and higher rates of unemployment.

Some of the psychological impacts of GH deficiency are height-related, especially for men (Swamia et al., 2008). However, the observed differences cannot be explained solely on the basis of short stature. Comparisons among adults of a very short stature show that people who are short but do not have a GH deficiency have fewer psychosocial problems than people who have GH deficiencies (Hull & Harvey, 2003). Furthermore, effective treatment of a GH deficiency in adults does not increase height, but can improve quality of life (Ahmid et al., 2016; Mo et al., 2014).

The close links between psychological wellbeing and endocrine function have prompted some to suggest that the concept of recovery in endocrine disorders should be expanded to give greater consideration to psychosocial issues (Sonino & Fava, 2012). The need for this attention to psychological impacts is illustrated in Research Box 14.3.

CLINICAL NOTES 14.3

Endocrine disorders

- Given the common occurrence of psychological symptoms in endocrine disorders, it is important to make an accurate diagnosis.
- Don't assume that psychological symptoms are 'just psychological' – they may be the result of endocrine disorders.
- A differential diagnosis is important for ensuring that appropriate treatment is administered.
- Even when physiological aspects of endocrine disorders are successfully treated, there may be a need for ongoing psychosocial support.

Sex hormones and psychosocial wellbeing

Testosterone has two effects on the body: androgen effects (the development and maintenance of secondary male sexual characteristics) and anabolic effects (the promotion of muscle growth). **Anabolic androgenic steroids** (AAS) are synthetic compounds structurally related to testosterone. Bodybuilders and many athletes use AAS to develop a more muscular physique. This practice is generally banned in competitive sports because of concerns that competition should be fair and based on natural ability.

Long-term AAS use can have serious consequences for physical and psychological wellbeing. It can lead to irreversible toxicity in the cardiovascular system and organ systems including the liver (van Amsterdam et al., 2010). AAS misuse also appears to be associated with psychosocial problems such as dependence syndromes, mood disorders, psychotic syndromes, and progression to other forms of substance abuse (Kanayama et al., 2008; van Amsterdam et al., 2010). Although psychological problems may be a contributor to AAS misuse, it should be noted that people who have low self-esteem or mood disturbances, or those who have experienced negative or adverse events during childhood, may be more likely to misuse AAS. Most research has focused on young men, but attention is also being given to AAS use among women (Onakomaiya & Henderson, 2016).

In men, use of AAS has unwanted physical side effects, such as testicular atrophy, reduced sperm production, acne, and the development of abnormally large mammary glands (Thiblin & Petersson, 2004; van Amsterdam et al., 2010). There is also concern about the psychological side effects of using androgenic anabolic steroids, particularly the phenomenon colloquially known as 'roid rage', as illustrated in Case Study 14.2. Reviews of research provide some evidence of increased rates of hypomania and increased aggressiveness and violence among steroid users, but it is important to note that the underlying personality traits of aggression and hostility among a specific

CASE STUDY 14.2 'Roid rage': the impact of steroids on behaviour

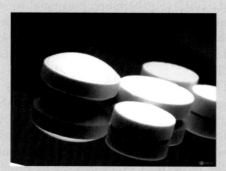

The story of DB is cited as an example of 'roid rage' – aggression and violence linked to the use of anabolic steroids. In 2004 *The Times* newspaper carried a report on how DB's misuse of steroids resulted in 'a trail of lives shattered by an American dream turned sour'.

DB came from a comfortable middle-class background and was remembered by his school friends as happy and even-tempered. In his late teens, DB began using steroids, ostensibly to make him a stronger footballer. The drugs changed DB's physique, but also altered his temper. A little over 10 years after he began using steroids, DB was responsible for the contract killing of a business rival, the attempted murder of a former lover, and violent assaults against a string of girlfriends. Some people – including DB's father – blamed steroid misuse for his violent behaviour.

subgroup of AAS misusers may be relevant (Lundholm et al., 2015; van Amsterdam et al., 2010). Furthermore, as noted in the section on aggression, there is no simple explanation for all aggressive or violent behaviour (see Chapter 9). Research in this area is hampered by the fact that because non-prescribed steroid use is illegal it is difficult to estimate the size of the population at risk, or to recruit large numbers of steroid users into controlled trials.

14.2.1 ETHICAL ISSUES IN HORMONE THERAPY

The sections above highlight how the treatment of hormonal abnormalities can improve psychological wellbeing. However, it is also true that hormonal treatment can be used to treat problems that do not have a hormonal cause. Such use of hormones is often accompanied by ethical and moral concerns. One example of this is illustrated by an Australian study of girls who had been treated with oestrogen in order to reduce their adult height. The treatment was found to reduce adult height, and it was administered to reduce the supposed negative psychosocial impacts of being 'too tall'. The study revealed that the assessment and treatment procedures carried out during the sensitive period of adolescence were a negative experience for many of the girls involved (Pyett et al., 2005). Furthermore, hormonal treatment increased the likelihood of fertility problems in adulthood (Venn et al., 2004), and it did not lead to better psychosocial wellbeing (Bruinsma et al., 2006).

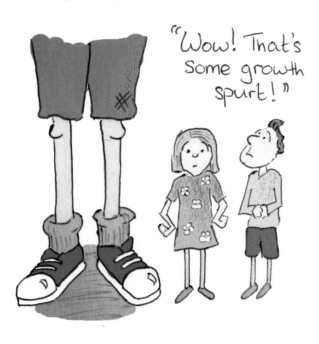

The use of hormonal treatment raises a range of other ethical issues. For example, in our society, tallness is usually desirable and the treatment of growth hormone deficiencies can be used to increase final adult height. However, its potential use by people without growth hormone deficiencies raises important questions about where we draw the line between medical therapy and psychosocial enhancement.

Another domain in which endocrinology and hormonal treatment raises ethical issues is fertility control. Many people have concerns about the use (or the timing of use) of hormonal contraception, emergency post-coital contraception (often called the 'morning-after pill'), and hormonal methods to terminate unwanted pregnancy.

14.2.2 STRESS AND ENDOCRINE FUNCTIONING

As well as considering how changes in endocrine function can affect psychological wellbeing, it is important to note that psychological states can affect endocrine function. A key focus of research in this domain is the study of responses to stress. All stressors – be they physical threats or psychological stress – produce a two-phase pattern of endocrine response (Pinel, 2014). In the first phase, stress prompts adaptive changes in the endocrine system to help the person (or other animal) to deal with physical threats – e.g. the mobilisation of energy resources, the inhibition of inflammatory responses, and increased resistance to infections. However, where stress is prolonged or repeated, it can produce maladaptive changes in the endocrine system, such as enlarged adrenal glands.

Prolonged stress can lead to the dysregulation of endocrine function and increased strain on systems regulated by the endocrine system, labelled allostatic load (see Chapter 3). Prolonged stress can also lead to impaired immune function because of interactions between the endocrine and immune systems: cortisol inhibits the production of pro-inflammatory molecules by macrophages and other immune cells, and adrenalin and noradrenalin can modulate the production of cytokines by immune cells (Griffin & Ojeda, 2011). The influence of stress on immunity is covered in detail in Chapter 3.

Summary

- Psychoneuroendocrinology is the study of how psychological states are influenced by changes in hormone secretion.
- Disorders of the HPA axis, thyroid function, and sex hormones all have associated psychological symptoms, suggesting some biological basis for these symptoms.
- Growth hormone disorders are less associated with psychological symptoms.
- Use of hormonal treatment reduces psychological symptoms, suggesting a biological basis.
- Use of hormonal treatment for social problems, such as height, raises a range of ethical issues, especially if it does not improve psychological wellbeing.
- Endocrine function is strongly affected by stress, which can result in dysregulated responses such as those observed in depression and PTSD.

FURTHER READING

Llewellyn, C.D. et al. (eds) (2018) *Cambridge Handbook of Psychology, Health and Medicine* (3rd edition). Cambridge: Cambridge University Press. Includes short chapters on many topics, including HRT, antenatal screening, pregnancy and birth, birth complications, perinatal mental health, endocrine disorders, growth retardation, hyperthyroidism, etc.

Martin, C. (ed.) (2010) *Perinatal Mental Health*. Keswick, Cumbria: M&K. A comprehensive, up-to-date book that covers a wide range of psychological disorders in pregnancy and after birth.

Schatzberg, A.F. & Nemeroff, C.B. (eds) (2017) *American Psychiatric Association Publishing Textbook of Psychopharmacology* (5th edition). Arlington, VA: American Psychiatric Association Publishing. At over 1,400 pages, this textbook has broad coverage of many topics and includes a chapter on psychoneuroendocrinology.

REVISION QUESTIONS

1. Describe the psychological and cultural factors that affect symptoms of menstruation, premenstrual syndrome (PMS) and premenstrual dysphoric disorder (PMDD).

2. What strategies can be used to help women manage PMS or PMDD?

3. Describe the psychosocial impact of menopause.

4. Discuss psychosocial factors important in pregnancy outcomes.

5. Discuss which factors are important in women's experiences of birth.

6. Outline women's psychological responses to miscarriage and stillbirth. Why do these responses occur?

7. Describe the main psychological problems that can arise during pregnancy and after birth.

8. Choose one endocrine disorder. Outline its common psychosocial symptoms.

9. Consider the evidence that 'Anabolic steroid use makes men more violent'.

10. How might prolonged stress lead to endocrine disorders?

15 GENITOURINARY MEDICINE

(Continued)

Case studies

15.1   A sexually transmitted infection
15.2   Prostate cancer diagnosis and treatment

Figure

15.1   The ABC of safe sex: a billboard in South Sudan

Research boxes

15.1   Does promoting sexual abstinence work?
15.2   Improving adherence among people undergoing dialysis

LEARNING OBJECTIVES

This chapter is designed to enable you to:

- Understand sexual health from a biopsychosocial perspective.
- Outline psychological approaches to limiting the spread of sexually transmitted infections.
- Appreciate how concerns about personal reputation, embarrassment, and gender identity can affect the experience of illness and help-seeking behaviour in genitourinary medicine.
- Outline patient experiences and concerns in kidney disease.

Genitourinary medicine is an umbrella term that covers aspects of andrology (men's reproductive health), gynaecology (women's reproductive health), and urology. Genitourinary medicine is primarily related to diagnosing and treating **sexually transmitted infections** (STIs). Thus, much of this chapter will focus on STIs. First, however, we shall consider broader issues related to sexual health. The closing sections of this chapter will look at problems in the urinary and renal systems.

15.1 SEXUAL HEALTH

People commonly equate **sexual health** with **reproductive health** (see Chapter 14). However, sexual health is much broader. If we were to equate 'sexual health' with 'reproductive health', we would exclude a consideration of the sexual health needs of people who (a) are infertile, (b) choose not to reproduce, (c) are post-reproductive, or (d) are not heterosexual. The WHO definition of health (see Chapter 1) has therefore been adapted to define sexual health as:

> A state of physical, emotional, mental and social well-being in relation to sexuality; it is not merely the absence of disease, dysfunction or infirmity. Sexual health requires a positive and respectful approach to sexuality and sexual relationships, as well as the possibility of having pleasurable and safe sexual experiences, free of coercion, discrimination and violence. (World Health Organisation, 2006)

This is a broad, biopsychosocial conceptualisation of sexual health which includes a consideration of three domains of sexual freedom, sexual pleasure, and sexual safety. These three domains are outlined below.

15.1.1 SEXUAL FREEDOM

Following on from the definition of sexual health given above, sexual freedom can be considered to be characterised by having pleasurable and safe sexual experiences that are free of coercion, discrimination, or violence Unfortunately, **sexual coercion** and abuse are widespread: 20% of women and 5% of men report that they have had unwanted sexual activity because of actual or threatened force (de Hans et al., 2012; de Visser et al., 2014b). Experience of sexual coercion is related to a range of subsequent difficulties. People who have been coerced have poorer psychological wellbeing, poorer physical health, greater health anxiety, and use health services more. They are more likely to engage in health-compromising behaviours, such as smoking, heavy drinking, and illicit drug use, and are more likely to have been diagnosed with an STI. They are also more likely to experience sexual problems, such as a fear of intimacy, a lack of sexual pleasure, and anxiety about sexual performance. Research reveals that any sexual coercion – not just early, repeated, or more severe coercion – leads to poorer health and less healthy patterns of behaviour (de Visser et al., 2007). It is clear there is a need for support services for people who experience sexual coercion in order to minimise its impact.

Treating the aftermath of sexual coercion or abuse requires sensitivity and excellent communication skills (see Chapter 18). More broadly, healthcare professionals need to be aware that people's understandings of sex and related issues may differ (see Box 15.1). People may report a diverse array of sexual orientations and sexual behaviours. As long as these behaviours are consensual and legal, any judgemental attitudes or discrimination from healthcare professionals are inappropriate and may be a barrier to promoting sexual health.

BOX 15.1   What is sex?

Although people will usually assume that 'sex' means 'vaginal intercourse', it is important when taking a medical history to be very clear about what people mean when they talk about sex.

During his presidency, Bill Clinton was questioned several times about whether he had had a sexual relationship with White House intern Monica Lewinsky. Clinton publicly stated 'I did not have sexual relations with that woman', but later revealed that his use of the term 'sexual relations' excluded his receiving oral sex. It is interesting to note that many people agree with Bill Clinton that oral sex does not count as sex (Rissel et al., 2003; Sanders & Reinisch, 1999).

ACTIVITY 15.1   HOW DO WE TALK ABOUT SEX?

- Take a few minutes to write different colloquial or 'slang' terms for different sexual behaviours.
- Now write down the terms that you would use if you were talking to a medical professional about your own sexual behaviour.
- It is important to be aware of the terms that people may use to refer to sexual behaviour. Some may prefer slang terms. Others may prefer euphemisms or will refer indirectly to their sexual behaviour.

15.1.2 SEXUAL PLEASURE AND SEXUAL PROBLEMS

The vast majority of adults believe that an active sex life is important for their overall wellbeing and relationships (de Visser et al., 2014a). Unfortunately, **sexual problems** or **sexual dysfunctions** are remarkably common and many become more common with age. A large population-based study in Australia found that over 70% of women and nearly 50% of men reported at least one sexual problem in the previous year (de Visser et al., 2017a; Mitchell et al., 2016). Some sexual problems have an organic cause, while others are primarily psychological in nature. Whatever their causes, sexual problems can impair quality of life. For example, many people report that they feel anxious about their sexual performance or do not find sex pleasurable.

Many men report that they achieve orgasm too quickly and many experience problems in achieving or maintaining an erection. Rapid ejaculation has a strong psychological component and psychological interventions can therefore be effective treatments. Erectile dysfunction may be caused by psychological factors, but commonly has an organic cause. The likelihood of erectile dysfunction is significantly greater in older men, particularly if they have cardiovascular disease, diabetes, or undiagnosed hyperglycaemia

(Binmoammar et al., 2016; Gandaglia et al., 2014). It is notable that after treatments for erectile problems became available in the late 1990s, the number of men reporting erectile dysfunction appeared to increase (Kaye & Jick, 2003). It was suggested that this was due to pharmaceutical companies marketing drugs designed to treat erectile problems as 'lifestyle' drugs that may be desirable to all men (Lexchin, 2006). Such findings indicate that a biopsychosocial approach (see Chapter 1) is just as important in genitourinary medicine as in other medical domains.

ACTIVITY 15.2   HOW YOUNG IS TOO YOUNG? HOW OLD IS TOO OLD?

- What would you think – and what would you say – if a 15-year-old patient asked you for a prescription for oral contraception?
- What would you think – and what would you say – if an 80-year-old patient asked you for a prescription for medication to treat erectile dysfunction?

Common sexual problems among women include vaginal dryness and pain during intercourse or an inability to orgasm (de Visser et al., 2017b; Moureau et al., 2016). Some of these problems are more common among older women, particularly vaginal dryness, which is influenced by hormonal changes associated with menopause (see Chapter 14). However, others, such as painful intercourse are more common in younger women.

When treating sexual problems it is often useful to distinguish between Desire for sex, Arousal once sex is initiated, and obtaining Orgasm (DAO). Dysfunction is often limited to one of these stages and an accurate diagnosis can aid the appropriate targeting of treatment. Sexual difficulties are an important focus of treatment because they are related to less satisfaction with physical and emotional aspects of relationships and a lower level of general happiness (Richters et al., 2003b). However, it is important to note that many people do not seek treatment, even for long-lasting problems that they report have a major impact on their lives – often because patients and healthcare professionals find it difficult to discuss sexual wellbeing (de Visser et al., 2017b; Gott et al., 2004).

Chronic Pelvic Pain

Chronic Pelvic Pain (CPP) is not a diagnosis of a single disease; rather, it is a symptom which may be the result of underlying processes in one or more different organ systems. CPP is defined as constant or intermittent pain in the pelvis or lower abdomen not associated with menstruation, pregnancy, or sexual intercourse. It is believed to affect around 15–20% of women (Ayorinde et al., 2017). However, the actual prevalence may be higher because many women accept the symptoms as part of being female and when they do seek medical help the lack of a clear cause of CPP means that it may be diagnosed in different ways. Numerous potential causes of CPP in different organ systems have been proposed (Howard, 2003; Vercellini et al., 2009):

- Gynaecological (e.g. endometriosis, chronic pelvic inflammatory disease).
- Gastrointestinal (e.g. Irritable Bowel Syndrome, Inflammatory Bowel Disorder).
- Urological (e.g. interstitial cystitis).
- Musculoskeletal (e.g. fibromyalgia, pelvic floor abnormalities).
- Psychoneurological (e.g. nerve entrapment).

Women with CPP are more likely than other women to have a history of sexual abuse. They are also more likely to experience depression, anxiety, and catastrophic thinking. These psychological phenomena could be implicated in CPP as either causes or consequences. Whatever their role is in CPP, it should be noted that such negative states influence the perception of pain (see Chapter 4), and that they should be addressed by suitably qualified professionals.

It has been argued that CPP is a symptom rather than a disease, and that it rarely reflects a single pathologic process (Vercellini et al., 2009). However, women who experience CPP will usually want a diagnosis or explanation of their symptoms. This may not always be easy if it is possible. Because of the complex nature of CPP and the large number of different causes with similar or overlapping symptoms, it is important to conduct a thorough patient history which will allow a differential diagnosis and the selection of the appropriate treatment. This can be time-consuming and demanding, particularly given the need to focus on experiences of sexual abuse as potential aetiological factors. However, gaining women's trust and developing a strong patient–practitioner relationship is of utmost importance for the long-term outcome of care.

Treatment for CPP is directed more toward managing symptoms than curing the disease. There is a lack of solid evidence about the efficacy of different treatments for CPP. A systematic review revealed support for the efficacy of progestogen (Cheong et al., 2014). Pain has been shown to be alleviated among women who undergo reassurance ultrasound scans accompanied by counselling (compared to women treated with a standard 'wait and see' approach), and among women who undertake disclosure writing therapy (compared to a non-disclosure group).

Although much of the research into CPP has focused on women, men may also experience chronic pelvic pain and this is often a symptom of prostate cancer (see section 15.3.1) (Suskin et al., 2013).

15.1.3 SEXUAL SAFETY

Sexual safety is important: it protects against unwanted pregnancy and STIs. Teenage birth rates in many developed countries are high: they are higher in the USA, the UK, and other English-speaking countries than elsewhere in European nations (World Health

Organisation, 2016b). Teenage birth rates are markedly higher in most developing countries. Although some teenagers are happy to become parents, most teenage pregnancies are unplanned. Teenage motherhood is associated with fewer educational qualifications and poor employment prospects (UNICEF, 2001). When teenage birth rates are combined with the high rates of termination of pregnancy in teenagers, it is clear that many young people do not take adequate precautions to avoid an unintended pregnancy. A failure to practise **safer sex** consistently also explains why STIs are widespread. We shall examine this in the following section.

Summary

- Sexual health is broader than reproductive health and includes sexual freedom, sexual pleasure, and sexual safety.
- A substantial minority of women and men have experienced sexual coercion or abuse. This is associated with poor psychological and physical wellbeing, increased health anxiety, increased health service use, and more health-compromising behaviours.
- Sexual problems are remarkably common, with the majority of adult women and men reporting at least one sexual problem in the previous year.
- Chronic Pelvic Pain may arise from dysfunction in several different organ systems. Because its underlying causes may be difficult to determine, it may not be possible to give people the accurate diagnosis or effective treatment they are seeking.
- Sexual risks include unwanted pregnancies and contracting STIs, both of which can be avoided by practising safer sex.

15.2 SEXUALLY TRANSMITTED INFECTIONS

15.2.1 HIV/AIDS

Human Immunodeficiency Virus (HIV) is a retrovirus which causes **Acquired Immune Deficiency Syndrome (AIDS)**. The predominant mode of transmission is unprotected sexual activity. It is estimated that approximately 37 million people worldwide are infected with HIV, with over 2 million new infections per year: the vast majority of these are in sub-Saharan Africa (World Health Organisation, 2017c). The prevalence of HIV infection varies widely between regions, and is markedly higher in sub-Saharan Africa than elsewhere.

In many regions, sex between men and women is the primary route of transmission. Heterosexual transmission is an important contributor to the spread of HIV, even in areas where sex between men and injection drug use have been, or continue to be, the major transmission routes. For example, in Europe in 2008 approximately 32% of new infections with a known cause were attributed to heterosexual activity (WHO, 2017c).

Although the virus was identified in the early 1980s, no vaccine or cure has been developed. Since the mid-1990s highly-active antiretroviral therapies (HAART) that suppress viral replication have been available. For many people, HIV/AIDS is now a chronic illness rather than a terminal illness. However, these medications are expensive and so are often unavailable in the poorer countries which have been hardest hit by the global AIDS epidemic. Although antiretroviral medications are effective at prolonging life, the treatment regimens can be quite complicated and burdensome in terms of the timing of doses and changes to food and fluid intake. This means that adherence is often a problem. Meta-analysis has revealed that interventions can improve adherence and produce lower viral loads (Mbugabaw et al., 2015; Simoni et al., 2006). The data suggest that effective programme components include: adherence counselling; web-based or face-to-face cognitive behavioural intervention; home visits by nurses; text-message reminders; contingency management; modified directly observed therapy; and a once-daily (rather than twice-daily) drug regimen. It is also important to provide information about the importance of adherence and to discuss people's beliefs, motivations, and expectations about treatment (see Chapter 19).

The complexity of antiretroviral medication regimens together with impaired health and uncertainty about the future often combine in ways that worsen the quality of life in people living with HIV (e.g. Brandt et al., 2017; Ezzy, 2000; Langius-Eklöf et al., 2009). The psychological impacts of HIV infection are addressed in Chapter 11 on immunology and include higher rates of depression than in the general population (Ciesla & Roberts, 2001). Interventions designed to treat psychological distress among people with HIV/ AIDS are effective at both reducing depression and improving immune function (Antoni et al., 2006; Brown & Vanable, 2008).

Until recently, safer sexual behaviour was the only way to contain the further spread of the epidemic because there is no vaccine or cure for HIV infection. However, the development of HAART and its application mean that viral load can be reduced to such an extent that the risk of transmission is virtually eliminated. As a result, rates of mother-to-child transmission have been reduced (Siegfried et al., 2011). HAART can also be used to prevent sexual transmission of HIV either through post-exposure prophylaxis (PEP) immediately after high-risk events or pre-exposure prophylaxis (PrEP) for people who engage in recurrent high-risk behaviours (Krakower et al., 2015). Although such medical interventions are effective at preventing HIV, it is important to note that they do not protect against other sexually transmissible infections.

Behavioural means for preventing the sexual transmission of HIV are the same as those for other STIs. The epidemiology, psychosocial impacts, and prevention of STIs are addressed in the following section.

15.2.2 SEXUALLY TRANSMITTED INFECTIONS

The terms sexually transmitted infections (STI) and **sexually transmitted diseases (STD)** are used interchangeably, but it is important to note that these two acronyms can refer to quite different things. The term STD refers to disease, and physical manifestations of infection. An STD-focused sexual health programme would only target those people who had physical manifestations of disease. In contrast, all people infected or at risk of infection would be the targets of an STI-focused programme. This distinction is important because asymptomatic STIs may still damage the reproductive organs.

After notable declines during the late 1980s and early 1990s, in many countries the prevalence and incidence of numerous sexually transmitted infections (STIs) have risen and continue to rise or show no signs of marked decline in many developed countries (European Centre for Disease Prevention and Control, 2015). However, these increases have not been observed in all countries. The large cross-national differences cannot be explained by differences in rates of sexual behaviour *per se*, but reflect instead differences in patterns of preventive behaviours, cultural attitudes toward sex, and provision of sexual health services.

In population-representative samples, around 15% of adults report ever having been diagnosed with an STI, and 2–3% test positive for STIs or were diagnosed with an STI in the previous year (Grulich et al., 2014; Sonnenberg et al., 2013). However, many more people have STIs that are undiagnosed because of a lack of knowledge or consultation. Young people are particularly likely to have undiagnosed STIs. For example, the UK National Chlamydia Screening Programme, which consists of the opportunistic screening of under-25s, found that 13% of men and 10% of women tested positive for chlamydia. Many STIs can be prevented by the consistent and correct use of condoms. However, as we shall see in the next section, rates of condom use are not as high as is desired by health professionals.

Although young people are a key focus of STI prevention activities, the sexual health of older people should not be overlooked. Older people are now more likely than in past generations to be single or undergoing relationship change, and changes to dating and relationships facilitated by technology mean that their sexual network may be broader than those of previous generations. The availability of drugs to treat erectile dysfunction may also contribute to greater levels of sexual activity and a corresponding increase in the likelihood of STI transmission. An important influence on the quality of sexual health care for older people is that healthcare professionals and older people often find it embarrassing to talk about sexual issues (Hinchliff et al., 2011).

Treatment with antibiotics is available for many bacterial STIs (e.g. Chlamydia, gonorrhoea). However, cures for viral STIs are not available, although symptomatic treatment is available (e.g. sores due to genital herpes). Untreated STIs can lead to serious complications, including infertility in women. Many STIs can be asymptomatic for some time. This explains why the proportion of people treated for STIs is often lower than the prevalence rates found in population-based screening. Furthermore, people may delay seeking treatment because of embarrassment about talking to others about their sexual behaviour (de Visser & O'Neill, 2013).

15.2.3 PROMOTING CONDOM USE

In the absence of vaccines or curative treatments for HIV and many other STIs, it is vital to encourage those behaviours that will limit the spread of STIs between people. These are sometimes split into the **'ABC' of STI prevention**: Abstaining, Being faithful and using Condoms (see Table 15.1).

Most attention within public health and health promotion has been given to Part C (using condoms), because A and B require more fundamental changes in sexual behaviour. Indeed, research into abstinence-based sexual health programmes indicates that they have no overall impact on the delay of initiating sex, limiting sexual partners, or the increasing use of condoms or other contraception. Indeed, there is concern that abstinence-only programmes may be counterproductive in the long run, because such programmes do not teach people how to have safer sex if they cease to abstain from sex (see Research Box 15.1).

Although the vast majority of people do use condoms sometimes, rates of consistent condom use are low. For example, when people are asked about their most recent sexual experiences, fewer than 25% report that they used a condom (de Visser et al., 2014c). Furthermore, among people who do use condoms, around one in seven do not put the condom on before genital contact, thereby exposing themselves to infection with a range of STIs. It is therefore necessary to promote correct and consistent condom use.

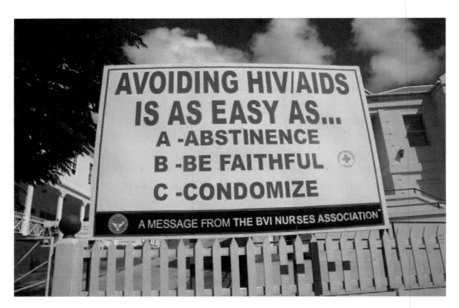

FIGURE 15.1   The ABC of safe sex: a billboard in South Sudan

Photo courtesy of Allan Rae, accessed: https://crossingenres.com/dispatches-from-south-sudan-195d70d38919

TABLE 15.1   The ABC of safe sex

A	Abstain from sex	If you don't have sex, then you cannot get an STI
B	Be faithful	If you are in a monogamous relationship with a partner who has no STIs, you cannot get an STI
C	Use condoms	If you use condoms, the risk of acquiring an STI is reduced

RESEARCH BOX 15.1   Does promoting sexual abstinence work?

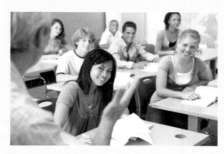

Background

During the Bush administration in the United States, sexuality education programmes were eligible for special funding if they agreed to promote the message that abstinence was the only certain way to avoid pregnancy and STIs, and agreed not to promote the use of contraception or provide instructions in using contraception.

Method and findings

This study aimed to determine whether abstinence-only programmes run using the special funding had the intended positive effects on young people's sexual health. Four different abstinence-only programmes run in four States were evaluated: 1,209 adolescents were randomly allocated to abstinence-only programmes and 848 were assigned to control-group programmes. Follow-up data were gathered 4–6 years after the programmes began.

The results revealed that abstinence-only programmes did not reduce sexual activity among adolescents. Indeed, the average age at first sexual intercourse and the average number of sexual partners were the same regardless of which education programme the teenagers received. There was no evidence that the abstinence-only programmes had better outcomes related to the risks of teenage pregnancy or STIs. Adolescents in all programmes (abstinence-only or control) had poor knowledge about healthy sexual behaviours.

Significance

Abstinence-only programmes provide outcomes that are no better or worse than conventional sexuality education. However, given the high levels of STIs and unplanned pregnancies among teenagers and young adults, comprehensive sexuality education programmes aimed at improving knowledge and skills are likely to provide the best long-term outcomes.

Photo © Monkey Business/Fotolia

Trenholm, C. et al. (2008) Impacts of abstinence education on teen sexual activity, risk of pregnancy, and risk of sexually transmitted diseases. *Journal of Policy Analysis and Management*, 27: 255–276.

Impact of behavioural interventions

Research based on social cognitive models of behaviour (see Chapter 5) shows that people's condom use may be predicted from their attitudes, subjective norms, self-efficacy, and intentions to use condoms (Albarracín et al., 2001; Sheeran et al., 1999). Condom use tends not to be influenced by knowledge about HIV/STIs, perceived susceptibility to infection, or the perceived severity of infection. Thus, scare campaigns are likely to be ineffective in promoting condom use (Kirby, 2006; Ruiter et al., 2014; Witte & Allen, 2000). It is better to focus on attitudes, beliefs, skills, and confidence. Indeed, because condom use involves more than one person, it is important that people develop the skills to communicate about condom use with their sexual partners. Interventions to promote condom use are more effective when they include a skills component rather than only focusing on changing individuals' knowledge and attitudes (Albarracín et al., 2003). A Cochrane review found that significant reductions in HIV risk behaviours among homosexually active men can be achieved via behavioural interventions, be they individual interventions (e.g. promoting personal skills), small group interventions (e.g. group counselling), or community-level interventions (e.g. community-building empowerment activities) (Johnson et al., 2008).

The observed low rates of condom use among heterosexual people are influenced by the availability of hormonal contraception. People tend to be more concerned about unplanned pregnancy than STIs and will often make a trade-off between condoms and other contraception (Morroni et al., 2014). This means that if people are using the contraceptive pill to prevent pregnancy, then they tend not to use condoms. Among young couples, the shift from condoms to the pill is often a marker of the seriousness of the relationship and mutual trust. Condom use is much less common between regular partners than between new partners or in 'one night stands'. Reasons for condom use differ in these different contexts – people tend to be less worried about STIs with regular partners (de Visser & Smith, 2001). However, the decision not to use condoms in regular relationships is not always based on accurate knowledge of partners' STI status.

CLINICAL NOTES 15.1

Sexual behaviour and contraception

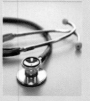

- Many people feel embarrassed talking about sexual behaviour and sexual problems. Let people know that you are comfortable talking about these issues in a non-judgemental way.
- When prescribing oral contraception, ensure that people are aware that non-barrier methods do not offer protection against STIs. Encourage individuals and their sexual partners to be tested (and treated) for STIs.
- People are more likely to use condoms if you address their attitudes and beliefs. However, it is also important to help people develop the skills needed to negotiate condom use with sexual partners.

Rates of condom use may continue to decline in response to the increasing availability and use of the oral contraceptive pill, long-lasting hormonal contraception implants, and post-coital contraception (the 'morning-after pill'). Because hormonal contraception offers no barrier to STI transmission, it can be argued that it is irresponsible to

CASE STUDY 15.1   A sexually transmitted infection

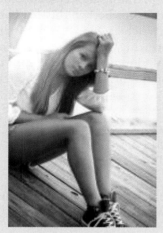

Lucy is a 19-year-old student who recently approached a specialist sexual health service for the first time. Several months ago she met Tom through a dating app, and they ended up going back to his house and having intercourse. They did not use a condom. Lucy was using oral contraception, and she didn't want to spoil the moment by asking Tom to use a condom. She was worried he would think she was suggesting he might have an STI.

A few weeks later, Lucy noticed discharge from her vagina and a soreness/itchiness when urinating. She was embarrassed about this and even more embarrassed about seeing her usual doctor, so she waited for a few days hoping that the symptoms would clear up. When they didn't, she decided to visit a specialist STI clinic.

> I was a bit embarrassed going in to get tested... I was worried that there would be real matron-type nurses telling me off for being stupid... or dirty old men in the waiting room. I didn't want to see anyone I knew, because it wouldn't be good for my reputation. So I didn't make eye contact with anyone in the waiting room. I think most other people there felt the same way.

She said that it was very reassuring to be treated by staff who did not judge her but simply addressed the facts and offered reassurance. Lucy was diagnosed with gonorrhoea and treated with a single dose of antibiotics.

Lucy was relieved that treatment was so quick and effective, but the information she was given by the clinic staff made her more concerned about other STIs and the impact they could have on her reproductive capacity:

> It did get me thinking about condoms, but it's hard when you're getting carried away. I know that I need to get better at asking guys to use condoms. One tip a friend gave me was to say that you aren't on the pill even if you are. That way you can get a guy to use a condom without saying anything about diseases.

prescribe the pill without also giving condoms to protect against STI transmission. However, it has also been found that few people using the pill also use condoms, so there is a need to find out how to encourage condom use among people who use hormonal contraception.

Given that unplanned pregnancy and STIs are both attributable to sexual activity without adequate precautions, it makes sense to address both outcomes in settings which traditionally addressed only one of these outcomes, for example family planning services or STI clinics. However, reviews of research revealed that there is a need for better integration of STI and HIV within family planning services, and conclude that there is too little research available to determine whether this leads to better outcomes for people (Church & Mayhew, 2009; Wilcher, 2013). One potential pathway for integrated care is adding HIV/STI testing to family planning services; another is to add contraceptive services to HIV clinics. Whether either or both of these approaches is taken, different domains for the integration of services have been identified:

- Provider level – healthcare professionals offering both family planning and STI services.
- Facility level – internal referral between family planning specialists and STI specialists.
- Referral services – external referrals from family planning to STI services and vice versa.

Within primary care, brief interventions can be an efficient way of addressing sexual health issues in people who may not otherwise attend specialist sexual health services.

Summary

- In addition to its physical effects, HIV has detrimental effects on psychological well-being and quality of life. Quality of life can also be affected by complex treatment regimens which can suppress viral replication, but do not offer a cure.
- Rates of STIs have increased in recent years in many countries. This increase has not been limited to young people, but has also occurred among older adults.
- Although condoms offer effective protection against HIV, other STIs, and unwanted pregnancy, only a quarter of people regularly use condoms.
- Among heterosexual people there is often a trade-off between condom use and oral contraceptives.
- Condom use can be increased by targeting people's knowledge and attitudes. However, it is also important to equip people with the necessary skills to negotiate and use condoms.

15.3 PROSTATE AND TESTICULAR CANCER

Cancers of the prostate and testicles are common and may affect, and be affected by, men's views of masculinity or sexuality. Many men endorse and embody traditional definitions of masculinity, according to which men are supposed to be 'strong silent types'. Such beliefs help to explain why men are less likely to use healthcare services (de Visser & McDonnell, 2013). Men's reluctance to seek screening and treatment may be particularly marked for health conditions which affect sexual potency, because sexual potency is a central aspect of many people's definitions of strong masculinity.

15.3.1 PROSTATE CANCER

Epidemiology and screening

The prostate gland surrounds part of the urethra of men and produces a fluid component of semen. **Prostate cancer** is one of the most common cancers in men, accounting for about a quarter of all diagnosed cancers among men in developed countries (see Figure 11.1). It is becoming more common. Although the causal mechanisms involved in prostate cancer are not precisely known, risk factors include greater age, African heritage, and a family history of prostate cancer or breast cancer. Specific concerns related to prostate cancer include its potential impact on masculinity and sexuality (de Sousa et al., 2012; Kunkel et al., 2000).

At the time of diagnosis with prostate cancer, many men are asymptomatic. Symptoms become more prominent when the cancer is advanced. A common symptom is urinary incontinence. Pain in the lower back, hips, or thighs may be experienced if the cancer has metastasised. Diagnosis of prostate cancer may lead to anxiety or depression that may arise from an unmet desire for information about the prognosis, and uncertainty about treatment options and their potential side effects. However, anxiety and depression often go unnoticed and many men feel that their psychological needs are not met by the services available to them.

Healthcare professionals must be aware of the psychological aspects of screening, diagnosis, and treatment for prostate cancer. **Prostate Specific Antigen** (**PSA**) levels are a widely used marker for prostate cancer. However, PSA screening is somewhat controversial because it may not always detect cancer or reduce mortality, but may increase anxiety and lead to over-treatment (Ilic et al., 2013). Digital rectal examination is another form of screening where a physician feels for abnormalities that may indicate prostate cancer. However, many men find rectal examinations difficult because of perceived links between anal penetration and homosexuality: indeed, rectal examinations are perceived more negatively than colonoscopies, and many men find the insertion of a finger more difficult than the insertion of a piece of equipment (Christy et al., 2014).

Treatment

Treatment options vary depending on whether the cancer is restricted to the prostate or has metastasised. Men with low-risk localised tumours may be offered active monitoring or 'watchful waiting' rather than treatment. Higher risk localised cancers may be treated by a radical prostatectomy – surgery to remove the prostate gland, external radiotherapy, or internal radiotherapy.

Surgery, radiation, and hormone treatment commonly have side effects which reduce quality of life. Radical prostatectomy and radiotherapy often lead to transient or permanent urinary incontinence and impotence. Urinary incontinence is experienced by the majority of men post-surgery and can lead to embarrassment, a loss of a sense of control, depression, and reduced social interactions (Ko & Sawatzky, 2008; see also section 15.4.1). The impact of impotence is influenced by men's pre-surgery levels of sexual activity and their partners' levels of concern about impotence (Kirschner-Hermanns & Jakse, 2002). Nerve-sparing surgery can reduce the likelihood and severity of urinary incontinence and impotence. Furthermore, research suggests that after prostatectomy psychoeducational interventions can improve urinary incontinence and sexual difficulties (Lassen et al., 2013).

It is important to discuss concerns about urinary incontinence and sexual function when decisions are made about surgery, radiation therapy, or watchful waiting. The choice of therapy is not simple, because there is a lack of conclusive evidence that any single approach consistently offers better long-term prospects. This means that it may be particularly important to consider the impact of different treatments on quality of life. For example, men's willingness to undergo a radical prostatectomy may be influenced by the extent to which they are concerned about potential impairments to sexual function due to nerve damage. The adverse psychosocial impacts of diagnosis and treatment for prostate cancer can be reduced via effective psychological intervention (see Case Study 15.2). Counselling and providing erectile aids or medication may be beneficial.

If a tumour has spread beyond the capsule surrounding the prostate, then surgery or radiotherapy may be combined with a course of hormone treatment – the growth and function of the prostate is affected by testosterone, so some treatments work by reducing the testosterone levels. A systematic review of research revealed that androgen-ablation therapy is associated with significant (but subtle) declines in cognitive capacity (McGinty et al., 2014; Nelson et al., 2008). Research with animals and studies of older men also indicate that lower levels of testosterone are related to cognitive impairments.

CASE STUDY 15.2   Prostate cancer diagnosis and treatment

Vishal is a 69-year-old retired teacher who was diagnosed with prostate cancer two years ago. His experiences highlight a number of important psychosocial issues related to the care and treatment of men with prostate cancer.

(Continued)

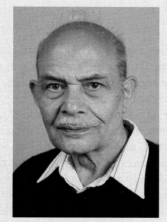

Vishal found some of the screening processes and tests difficult. This was partly due to the uncertainty of some of the test results. It was also because some of the tests were challenging, particularly when the doctor inserted a gloved finger into Vishal's rectum to feel for lumps, hardness, or other abnormalities in the prostate gland:

> Some parts of the whole diagnosis process were pretty strange. I mean, having another man put his finger up your back passage is not something that had happened to me before... and I won't be rushing back to do it again!

The experience of diagnosis was made worse by the insensitivity of some staff. There were times when unknown staff walked in and out of the room without introducing themselves or having any apparent reason to come in when he was (and felt) so exposed.

Once the diagnosis had been made, Vishal found it hard to make a decision about treatment – surgery, radiotherapy, or 'watchful waiting'. The outcomes and side effects associated with each option were quite varied. Furthermore, he felt he was having to deal with probabilities rather than certainties:

> A friend of mine is hyper-logical and he suggested I draw up a table of different pros and cons and give each treatment option a score and decide that way... but I mean, how can you really weigh up the different options? What's more important – living, having sex, or not wetting myself? I was tempted to take the 'wait and see' approach just to avoid having to decide.

Vishal found it useful to attend a group support network. Although he was apprehensive about talking to other men about his concerns, he appreciated the benefits after attending a few sessions:

> It was great because all the people there had prostate cancer, and some were worse off than me, but they were all very genuine. They weren't so concerned any more about how much money they earned, or what car they drove, or those kinds of things. Everyone was on a very genuine level. This made it easier to join the group. It gave me a lot of support and helped me decide on which treatment to undertake.

Photo © YellowCrest/Fotolia

15.3.2 TESTICULAR CANCER

Epidemiology and screening

The testicles produce sperm so are vital for men's reproductive capacity. They also produce testosterone, which is the principal male sex hormone. **Testicular cancer** is relatively rare, accounting for around 1% of cancers in men. However, it is most common among men in their twenties and thirties, and it is one of the most common cancers among young men. It is more common in Caucasian men than men with Asian or African ethnic backgrounds.

Testicular self-examination (TSE) is an important element of diagnosing and treating testicular cancer because (as for other cancers) early detection and treatment are associated with better outcomes. Because it is unusual to develop cancer in both testicles at the same time, men can compare one testicle to the other to identify any lumps or swellings which should be checked by a medical professional. Although TSE may be an important part of monitoring, very few men practise this behaviour and many are unaware of the importance of TSE (Rovito et al., 2015; Saab et al., 2016).

There is a clear need to increase awareness of the importance of TSE, and to identify effective strategies to increase rates of TSE. A review of the research in this area indicated that the Health Belief Model and Theory of Planned Behaviour (see Chapter 5) are effective frameworks for TSE-promotion interventions, but that not all interventions have a strong theoretical foundation (Rovito et al., 2015). One study of young men revealed that rates of TSE could be improved significantly by a brief intervention which encouraged men to develop **implementation intentions** specifying 'when', 'where', and 'how' they would perform TSE (Steadman & Quine, 2004).

Treatment

It is sometimes possible surgically to remove small tumours from a testicle. However, the most common surgical response is removal of the affected testicle (an orchidectomy or orchiectomy). This procedure reduces the risk that pre-cancerous cells may remain in the testis and is possible because men with only one testicle can maintain their fertility and hormone production. Modern treatments can cure most people with testicular cancer, and may involve an orchidectomy with or without radiotherapy or chemotherapy (Huddart et al., 2005).

Although most people treated for testicular cancer are cured, treatment side effects include impairments to sexual function and fertility. These issues are important to consider given the epidemiology of testicular cancer – diagnosis and treatment often occur before men have become fathers and at an age when sexual activity is important to them. Men may be concerned that the removal of a testicle will make them impotent (i.e. unable to get or maintain an erection) and infertile (i.e. unable to produce children). However, a man with one healthy testicle can still have normal erections and produce healthy sperm. Nevertheless, problems with impotence and fertility do often occur in men post-orchidectomy.

A meta-analysis of outcomes of testicular cancer treatment found that the prevalence of sexual problems varied widely (Jonker-Pool et al., 2001). The most common problem was ejaculatory dysfunction (45% of men), and this was clearly related to surgery in the retro perineal region. At least 10% of men reported erectile problems or decreases in sexual desire, sexual activity, orgasm intensity, or sexual satisfaction. Although erectile disorders were the least common of these problems (12% of men), they were significantly related to reductions in satisfaction, sexual activity, desire, and orgasmic intensity. The authors of this meta-analysis concluded that physiological outcomes (impaired ejaculation and erection) were clearly related to treatments that affect the neurological systems involved. In contrast, psychological outcomes (desire, activity, orgasm, and satisfaction) did not vary according to treatment modality. Thus, although sexual problems appear to be more common among men treated for testicular cancer, not all of the observed impairments can be attributed to disease or treatment factors. Instead, psychosocial factors are important. The symbolic importance men and society in general give to men's genitals mean that removal of a testicle can be a challenge to their perceived masculinity (Carpentier et al., 2011; Gurevich et al., 2004).

In addition to the impact of testicular cancer on men, it is important to consider its impact on relationships, and to consider how supportive relationships may affect men's adjustment to testicular cancer. Being in a stable relationship appears to reduce the likelihood that men will experience sexual problems, and sexual and marital satisfaction among men and their partners are mutually correlated (Jankowska, 2011).

CLINICAL NOTES 15.2

Prostate and testicular health

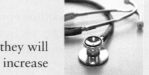

- Encouraging men to say exactly how, when, and where they will perform testicular self-examination is a simple way to increase self-screening behaviour for testicular cancer.
- When diagnosing and treating cancers of the prostate and testicles, be aware of how men's beliefs about their masculinity may be affected by the cancer itself and symptoms and side effects such as urinary incontinence and impaired sexual functioning.

Summary

- Prostate cancer is one of the most common cancers in men.
- Treatment options for prostate cancer depend on how advanced the cancer is and men's evaluations of the side effects of treatment.
- Many men experience transient or permanent urinary incontinence and erectile problems following surgery or radiotherapy. The importance of maintaining normal functioning in these domains may influence men's decision to be treated or to undertake 'watchful waiting'.

(Continued)

- Testicular cancer is not as common as prostate cancer. However, it is more common among younger men than older men.
- Treatment of testicular cancer often involves removal of the affected testicle. Although this need not affect men's sexual or reproductive capacity, men often experience impairments in these domains after treatment. Psychological factors are important because of beliefs about intact genitalia, sexual potency, and masculinity.
- Psychological interventions can be effective in treating the psychological distress arising from the diagnosis and treatment for cancers of the prostate and testicles. This includes psychological treatment for the common impairments to sexual wellbeing.

15.4 URINARY INCONTINENCE AND RENAL FAILURE

This section will outline two common disorders of the renal and urinary systems. The first (urinary incontinence) is not life-threatening, whereas the second (renal failure) often is. In both cases, psychosocial factors must be considered in treatment and management plans.

15.4.1 URINARY INCONTINENCE

Urinary incontinence (UI) is the involuntary leakage of urine, which can have different causes. The population prevalence of any form of UI is 20–30% among young adults, 30–40% among middle-aged people, and 30–50% among elderly people (Buckley et al., 2010; Nitti, 2001). It is more common among women than men. The severity of urinary incontinence tends to increase with age. UI is the result of bladder dysfunction (urge incontinence) or sphincter dysfunction (stress incontinence). It is not possible to determine accurately whether people have urge-, stress-, or mixed-incontinence simply by studying the symptoms.

Urge incontinence is the involuntary loss of urine occurring for no apparent reason while suddenly feeling the need or urge to urinate. It occurs when bladder muscles inappropriately contract to expel urine, often regardless of the amount of urine that is in the bladder. It may be called 'reflex incontinence' if it results from overactive nerves controlling the bladder. People with urge incontinence may be described as having an 'unstable' or 'overactive' bladder. In addition to surgical and medical treatments, there is a role for psychological and behavioural therapies. These include exercises to strengthen the pelvic floor muscles and 'bladder training', whereby people are taught to 'hold on' to their urine for increasingly longer times and to empty their bladders at regular, scheduled intervals so that they can increase their capacity to resist the urge to void their bladders (Dumoulin et al., 2014).

Stress incontinence arises when the pelvic floor muscles have insufficient strength. It involves the loss of small amounts of urine when people cough, laugh, sneeze, exercise, or perform other movements that increase pressure on the bladder. Among women, stress incontinence is more common during pregnancy (because of greater pressure on the bladder), as well as during the premenstrual period and during menopause (because lowered oestrogen levels can lead to lower muscular pressure around the urethra). Among men, stress incontinence is a common side effect of prostatectomy. Because stress incontinence arises from muscle weakness, it can be treated via psychological and behavioural means such as pelvic floor muscle training and bladder training (Dumoulin et al., 2014).

UI may cause embarrassment, distress, and discomfort. It has measurable detrimental effects on quality of life (Coyne et al., 2012). Many people with UI report that it limits their ability to engage in activities which either increase the strain on the bladder (e.g. physical exercise) or those where the availability of toilets may be uncertain, intermittent, or restricted (e.g. long-distance travel, vacations, theatre/cinema, etc.). One interesting aid for people in this situation is the Australian Continence Management Strategy's National Toilet Map (www.toiletmap.gov.au), which aims to help people with urinary incontinence engage in social activities with less concern about being 'caught short' and unable to find a toilet. Similar maps are available in other countries (e.g. https://greatbritishpublictoiletmap.rca.ac.uk).

Discussions of problems related to urinary function and sexuality can be difficult and embarrassing for many people. Many healthcare professionals also find these issues difficult (see section 15.1). Clinical notes 15.3 outlines some important points to bear in mind when carrying out intimate examinations. Legal, cultural, and religious factors may influence what people believe to be appropriate behaviour from healthcare professionals.

CLINICAL NOTES 15.3

Carrying out intimate examinations

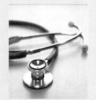

- Embarrassment and anxiety tend to be 'contagious'. The more calm and professional you are, the easier the examination will be for you and the patient.
- Guidelines for intimate examinations include:

  o Explain why the examination is necessary.
  o Explain exactly what it involves and what you will be doing.
  o Get the person's consent.
  o Offer a chaperone if appropriate.
  o Make sure the room is private and that people will not walk in during the examination.
  o Treat the person with respect and dignity (e.g. cover exposed parts of the body when you have finished).
  o Keep all discussion *relevant*. Avoid unnecessary personal comments.
  o Be prepared to stop the examination at any time if the patient asks you to.

15.4.2 RENAL FAILURE AND DIALYSIS

Chronic kidney disease (CKD) is the gradual loss of kidney function over time. The early stages of CKD may be asymptomatic, but symptoms do appear as the capacity of the kidneys to remove toxins, wastes, and excess water from the body becomes more impaired. CKD often develops into **end-stage renal disease (ESRD)**, which is when the kidneys no longer function. People with ESRD require a kidney transplant or must undergo **dialysis** to remove wastes and excess water from the body.

Kidney disease is becoming more common and is a major public health problem worldwide. A recent review of 26 population-based studies found that the median prevalence of CKD in adults is around 10% in men and women worldwide, and increases with age (Jha et al., 2013). This increase can be explained in large part by the increasing prevalence of diabetes and hypertension, which are major risk factors for CKD (Jha et al., 2013). Obesity is also associated with an increased risk of advanced CKD – in part because of its links to Type 2 diabetes and hypertension.

Psychosocial aspects of kidney disease and treatment

People with CKD and ESRD often have impaired quality of life, especially emotional well-being, but some have argued that too little attention is given to this important issue (Chong & Unruh, 2017). Particular challenges for people with kidney disease are depression arising from their current poor health and the prospect of further declines in health (Palmer et al., 2013). Depression is more common among people with CKD and ESRD than the general population. It appears to be more common or severe when illness interferes with important aspects of people's lives, such as work or family life. Poorer quality of life is important because it is an independent predictor of adverse outcomes and mortality among people with CKD and ESRD (Porter et al., 2016).

People with ESRD who experience depression may benefit from antidepressant medication, but the side effects of such medication are often difficult to tolerate. In this context, psychological interventions appear to be effective for reducing the symptoms of depression in people undergoing dialysis. A review of published research indicated evidence of the beneficial effects of regular exercise for a range of physical and psychological outcomes, including quality of life (Heiwe & Jacobson, 2011; Kaptein et al., 2010).

Treatment of kidney disease also entails restrictions to the diet and fluid intake. People with ESRD undergoing dialysis must regulate their fluid intake in order to avoid fluid overload, which can lead to congestive heart failure, hypertension, pulmonary oedema, and a shortened life span. The demands of intensive treatment regimens can impair quality of life. Time demands are particularly marked for people undergoing clinic-based dialysis, which entails 3–4 hour sessions three times per week. For these reasons, home dialysis or peritoneal dialysis (involving the use of a catheter and portable bags of dialysis fluids) may be more appealing. All people undergoing dialysis must also adjust to their dependence on artificial means for survival and a lack of control over their health (Christensen & Ehlers, 2002). For these reasons, kidney transplantation may appear more appealing than ongoing dialysis. **Kidney transplantation** should not be thought of as a cure for ESRD, but a new phase of treatment, because although transplant recipients are free from the dietary restrictions of dialysis, they must adhere to strict regimens of immunosuppressant drugs and be alert to any physical changes that may indicate infection or the rejection of the organ (Christensen & Ehlers, 2002).

A review of the evidence for ESRD treatment indicated that quality of life tends to be better among transplant recipients than among people undergoing dialysis (Purnell et al., 2013). However, when looking at different aspects of quality of life, it has been found that transplant recipients have more pain and discomfort and a poorer body image. Other studies have failed to find differences in quality of life according to treatment modality, but have highlighted the importance of psychological wellbeing and better treatment/illness knowledge for better overall quality of life (Sayin et al., 2007).

In addition to being of concern in their own right, impaired affect and quality of life are important because they may affect adherence to treatment requirements for dialysis or organ transplantation. Lower adherence may also be affected by having low self-efficacy, an external locus of control, or less social support (Christensen & Ehlers, 2002). Intervention research indicates that adherence can be improved by cognitive-behavioural strategies such as self-monitoring, forming behavioural contracts, and positive reinforcement reward systems (Christensen & Ehlers, 2002) (see Research Box 15.2) (Matteson & Russell, 2010). As for other conditions, increasing use is being made of mobile technology to improve adherence (see Chapter 17) (Welch et al., 2013).

RESEARCH BOX 15.2   Improving adherence among people undergoing dialysis

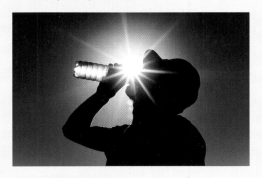

Source: Gornostay's portfolio, obtained via Shutterstock

Background

People underdoing dialysis must regulate their diets and fluid intake to avoid problems arising from electrolyte imbalances and fluid accumulation. This study was designed to address a lack of experimental evidence about effective interventions to improve adherence to fluid restrictions.

Method and findings

Twenty people undergoing dialysis took part in a behavioural intervention based on the self-regulation model (see Chapter 4). They were compared to 20 control group participants, who were matched in terms of age, sex, diabetic status, and average

(Continued)

interdialysis weight gain (a marker of adherence to fluid intake guidelines). The intervention was delivered to groups of 4–6 participants. It consisted of seven weekly hour-long sessions with homework between sessions. The contents of the intervention session were:

- Review of the importance of adherence to fluid-intake guidelines (Session 1).
- Description of the self-regulation approach and its application to dialysis (Session 1).
- Overview of behaviour of self-regulatory processes such as self-monitoring, self-evaluation, and self-reinforcement (Session 2).
- Instruction in self-monitoring skills. Initiation of homework using a diary to monitor fluid intake, mood, and behaviour (Session 3).
- Personalised goal-setting for fluid intake and weight gain between treatments (Session 4).
- Establishment of self-reinforcement strategies, including rewards (Session 5).
- Teaching stimulus control, self-instruction, and related behavioural coping skills to promote regulation of fluid intake (Session 6).
- Daily monitoring of fluid intake, which was discussed during weekly group meetings (Sessions 3–7).
- Weekly self-evaluation of fluid intake and weight gain relative to goals. Weekly review of self-regulatory coping skills and difficulties in meeting goals (Sessions 3–7).

Immediately following the intervention, there were no differences in adherence between the control and intervention groups. However, whereas adherence in the control group declined over the 8-week follow-up period, adherence improved in the group that was taught behavioural monitoring skills.

Significance

This study shows that behavioural self-regulation interventions can reverse natural patterns of worsening adherence to fluid intake restrictions over time. This study contributes to a growing body of evidence that multifaceted theory-based, group-administered behavioural interventions can improve adherence in people undergoing haemodialysis.

Photo © Picsfive/Fotolia

Christensen, A.J. et al. (2002) Effect of a behavioral self-regulation intervention on patient adherence in hemodialysis. *Health Psychology*, *21*: 393–397.

Summary

- Urinary incontinence (UI) may be caused by muscle weakness or a lack of control over an inappropriate urge to urinate.
- The prevalence and severity of UI increase with age. UI is often a cause of embarrassment and can lead people to restrict their social activities.
- Psychological and behavioural factors are important in treating UI. Treatment may involve muscle-strengthening exercises and bladder training designed to improve people's control over their urge to urinate.
- Chronic kidney disease (CKD) and end-stage renal disease (ESRD) are becoming increasingly common. Part of this increase can be explained by increases in diseases that are risk factors for CKD, such as diabetes and hypertension.
- People with ESRD rely on kidney transplants or dialysis. Transplantation is associated with a better quality of life.
- Dialysis places large demands on people's lifestyles and is associated with depression and impaired quality of life.
- Psychological interventions are effective for alleviating impairments to psychological wellbeing among people with ESRD. Psychological interventions are also effective for improving people's adherence to the dietary requirements of their treatment.

FURTHER READING

Llewellyn, C.D. et al. (eds) (2018) *Cambridge Handbook of Psychology, Health and Medicine* (3rd edition). Cambridge: Cambridge University Press. Includes short chapters on prostate cancer, contraception, HIV/AIDS, pelvic pain, sexual assault, sexual dysfunction, sexually transmitted infections, and urinary tract symptoms.

Wylie, K. (ed.) (2015) *ABC of Sexual Health* (3rd edition). London: Wiley. Developed specifically for doctors, this book covers a wide range of topics. It addresses a range of physical and psychological aspects of sexual health and sexual relationships and includes a useful chapter on taking a sexual history.

REVISION QUESTIONS

1. What is sexual health? Describe three components of sexual health.

2. What impact – according to the evidence – does sexual coercion or abuse have on people?

3. How might the increasing use of pre- and post-exposure prophylaxis for HIV affect rates of other STIs?

4. What are the possible causes of chronic pelvic pain? What impact does chronic pelvic pain have on women?

5. What psychological interventions are effective at promoting safer sex?

6. How has the prevalence of STIs changed over time? What factors may contribute to this?

7. Discuss the specific psychological challenges that may occur in men with prostate or testicular cancer.

8. Outline the psychological interventions that might be effective in the treatment of urinary incontinence.

9. What is the psychological impact of chronic kidney disease and end-stage renal disease?

10. Which psychological interventions are effective adjunctive treatments for chronic kidney disease and end-stage renal disease? What aspects of patient wellbeing and behaviour do they affect?

16 PSYCHIATRY AND NEUROLOGY

(Continued)

> **Figure**
>
> 16.1   Predisposing, precipitating, and perpetuating factors in psychiatric disorders
>
> **Research boxes**
>
> 16.1   What does consent mean in practice?
> 16.2   The influence of social support on quality of life after stroke

LEARNING OBJECTIVES

This chapter is designed to enable you to:

- Appreciate how predisposing, precipitating, and perpetuating factors influence the development of psychiatric disorders.
- Outline the major features, causes of, and treatment options for, common psychiatric and neurological disorders.
- Identify the methods for assessing psychiatric wellbeing and cognitive function.
- Describe various treatment options for psychiatric illnesses and neurological disorders.

16.1 PSYCHIATRY

Many people attend primary care with complaints that are primarily psychological rather than physical. Furthermore, as noted in previous chapters, many physical illnesses are accompanied by psychological symptoms. One large research study across 14 countries and cultures found a strong association between higher rates of psychiatric morbidity and higher numbers of physical symptoms, especially for physical symptoms that did not have a medical explanation (Kisely et al., 1997). More recent research has shown that regardless of the presence or absence of medical explanations, physical symptoms are an important component of common psychological disorders, such as depression and anxiety, and predict healthcare service use in community populations (Escobar et al., 2010). Such findings have prompted calls for us to think of somatic symptoms as being both medically explained and medically unexplained to some degree, and to recognise that somatic symptoms are multiply determined by the brain's integration of biological, psychological, and social inputs (Sharpe, 2013).

Official disease classification systems, such as the DSM-5 (American Psychiatric Assoication, 2013) and ICD-10 (World Health Organisation, 2004), define psychiatric disorders as categorical (one does or does not have the condition), distinct (the condition does not overlap with another condition), and independent (the presence of one condition should not be associated with a greater likelihood of having another specific condition). However, clinical experience and empirical research indicate that these assumptions are not justified (Krueger & Eaton, 2015). Many psychiatric disorders present combinations of similar symptoms. For example, anxiety may appear in and of itself, but is also a component of some forms of depression, schizophrenia, dementia, and personality disorders. For this reason it may be helpful to think of psychiatric disorders as syndromes rather than clear diagnostic entities, and to take a transdiagnostic approach to conceptualisation and treatment of psychological illness that is focused less on diagnosis and more on effective treatment of distressing symptoms (Harvey et al., 2004; Linton, 2013; Pearl & Norton, 2017).

ACTIVITY 16.1   WHAT IS A MENTAL ILLNESS?

- Take a few minutes to write your own definition of what a mental illness is.
- At what point does abnormal behaviour constitute illness?
- Do psychiatric disorders always have an underlying physiological cause?

16.1.1 MODELS OF PSYCHIATRIC DISORDERS

Until the 1800s in Europe and North America, witchcraft and demonic possession were common explanations for psychopathology. Such beliefs still persist in many traditional cultures. Modern medicine has a more sophisticated understanding of psychiatric disorders based on research findings. However, different explanations assign varying importance to biomedical and psychosocial factors.

Biomedical explanations

According to the biomedical model, psychiatric disorders result from dysfunctions in the biochemistry and physiology of the brain and body or damage to the brain. The implication of biomedical models is that if we identify the biological causes of psychiatric disorders, we should be able to develop effective treatments. Although this model is clearly useful for some disorders, it cannot explain all disorders. A major limitation of this model is its assumption that physical or physiological abnormalities underlie all psychiatric disorders. Some disorders (e.g. phobias) may simply be extreme forms of normal behaviour.

Psychological explanations

In contrast to biomedical models, psychological models argue that people's experiences – and responses to these experiences – may cause psychiatric disorders without there being any physiological abnormality. Three such models are (i) psychoanalysis, (ii) learning theory, and (iii) cognitive behaviour theory.

Psychoanalytic approaches explain psychiatric disorders as the result of conscious and unconscious responses to experiences rather than abnormalities in brain functioning. Therapy based on this approach would seek to identify the unconscious processes producing the symptoms and try to help the patient to manage these (see Chapter 19).

Learning theory approaches argue that many psychiatric disorders result from maladaptive learning. Treatment based on this approach would use a technique informed by operant and classical conditioning (see Chapter 10) to 'unlearn' maladaptive responses, such as phobias.

Cognitive behavioural approaches are the most commonly used psychological approaches. They are based on the idea that psychopathology arises when people acquire irrational beliefs or dysfunctional ways of thinking about themselves, their behaviour, or other people's responses to them. Cognitive behavioural therapy (CBT) is aimed at challenging and changing maladaptive patterns of thinking (see Chapter 19).

Psychosocial models

Psychiatric disorders often involve biomedical, psychological, and social factors. As a result, the biopsychosocial model (see Chapter 1) is critical in psychiatry. This approach recognises that physiological and psychosocial factors are involved in the onset and progression of psychiatric disorders (Yovell et al., 2015). For example, fMRI has been used to study psychoanalytic concepts and phenomena like repression, thereby linking medical and psychological models of normal and abnormal mental processes (Mancia, 2006). The biopsychosocial model also emphasises the importance of social responses to psychiatric disorders: do we lock 'mad' people in asylums or provide care for 'ill' people in the community?

The causes of psychiatric disorders vary between conditions, and the causes of a particular mental illness vary from person to person. Rather than assuming that all cases of particular psychiatric disorders can be explained by a single cause, it is important to think of how a range of factors can combine over time to affect the onset and course of an illness. We can think of these in terms of three Ps: Predisposing factors, Precipitating factors, and Perpetuating factors (see Figure 16.1).

Predisposing factors are things which make people more susceptible to mental illness. Genetic factors, experiences *in utero*, a difficult birth, and adverse childhood experiences such as neglect and abuse can increase the risk of some mental disorders.

Precipitating factors are events or experiences which influence whether a predisposition to a mental illness is 'activated'. Not every person with the same predisposing factors will develop a psychiatric disorder – precipitating factors may interact with predisposing factors to bring about psychopathology. A useful analogy is the interaction of genes and behaviour in lung cancer: whether a person smokes cigarettes influences whether a genetic predisposition results in the development of lung cancer. Precipitating factors known to influence the onset of psychiatric disorders include diseases such as brain tumours (Mainio et al., 2005; Starkweather et al., 2011), illicit drug use, and psychosocial factors such as traumatic events, bereavement, and social isolation or difficult relationships (Arseneault et al., 2004; Brewin et al., 2000; Espejo et al., 2012; Ksir & Hart, 2016). The interaction between predisposing factors and precipitating factors is often referred to as a **diathesis-stress model,** in which diathesis refers to predisposing factors (see Chapter 3).

Perpetuating factors act after the onset of mental illness to prolong its duration. Sometimes diseases are self-perpetuating. For example, maladaptive coping behaviours in people with anxiety disorders or depression may perpetuate the illness (McManus et al., 2008; Thompson et al., 2010). As noted elsewhere (see Chapter 17), non-compliance with treatment regimens can prolong illness, particularly if people do not understand or believe that they are unwell (Osterberg & Blaschke, 2005). Social factors may also prolong illness. For example, family members or friends may not facilitate someone's recovery. In addition, individuals may derive secondary gains, such as attention, care, and time off work, from inhabiting the sick role (see Chapter 9): a reluctance to give up these gains may prolong an illness.

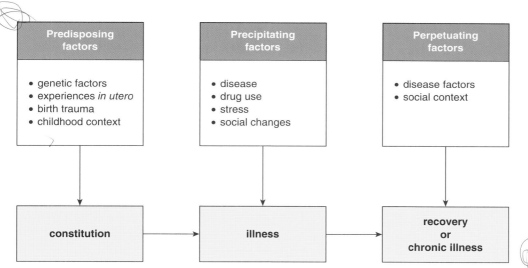

FIGURE 16.1   Predisposing, precipitating, and perpetuating factors in psychiatric disorders (adapted from Gelder et al., 2012)

16.1.2 CLASSIFICATIONS OF PSYCHIATRIC DISORDERS

Definitions of mental illness have changed over time to reflect changes in our understanding of different psychiatric disorders and their causes. Changes in social attitudes can also lead to changes in what is considered to be a mental illness (see Box 16.1).

There are two major systems for classifying mental disorders. Each is periodically updated. The *Diagnostic and Statistical Manual of Mental Disorders* (DSM) of the American Psychiatric Association is the standard classification of mental disorders used by clinicians in the United States. It is widely used in clinical practice in many other countries, and in academic research. The current version is the *DSM-5* (American Psychiatric Association, 2013).

The *International Statistical Classification of Diseases* (ICD) was developed by the World Health Organisation. It classifies all diseases, including psychological illnesses. The most recent version of this scheme is the ICD-10 (WHO, 2004), with the ICD-11 due for publication in 2018. For ease of use, the World Health Organisation has in addition produced a simplified classification of the mental disorders most commonly seen in primary care (ICD-10-PHC). The WHO primary care guidelines include checklists and brief assessment activities for identifying symptoms and developing a management plan.

BOX 16.1   What is a mental illness?

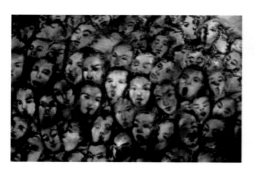

Definitions of mental illnesses are not fixed. This is reflected in the need for regular revisions to diagnostic classification systems such as the ICD and DSM. Definitions of mental illnesses often reflect contemporary social issues. For example, until 1973, homosexuality was included as a mental disorder in the American Psychological Association's classification of mental disorders. This was controversial because defining homosexuality as a disorder implied that it was something that should be cured, rather than a normal form of sexuality. Debate about pathologising homosexuality continued after 1973 because of the inclusion of a new disorder called 'Sexual Orientation Disturbance'. Part of this debate focused on whether the psychological 'disturbance' observed in some homosexual people was a consequence of the sexual orientation itself, or a reflection of the discrimination and prejudice toward homosexual and bisexual people.

16.1.3 PSYCHIATRIC DISORDERS

Here we shall introduce four common psychiatric conditions that are likely to be seen in primary care because of their prevalence or their chronicity. These are mood disorders, anxiety disorders, schizophrenia, and personality disorders. We shall outline the key features, prevalence, treatment, and prognosis. They are presented here as distinct disorders because this is how they are officially recognised in the DSM-5 and ICD-10, and how they are conceptualised for purposes such as epidemiology and insurance coverage for treatment. However, as noted earlier, the assumption that these conditions are categorical, distinct, and independent may not justified, and people's experiences may be better reflected by transdiagnostic approaches (Harvey et al., 2004; Krueger & Eaton, 2015).

Mood disorders

We all have periods of feeling down or depressed in response to losses or failures. We may also experience occasional brief periods of feeling very 'up' or 'manic'. When such changes in mood are long enough and intense enough to interfere with normal activities and relationships, they can be considered as mood disorders. The DSM-5 and ICD-10 distinguish between different manifestations of depression, mania, and combinations of **mania** and **depression** such as **bipolar disorder** (sometimes called manic depression). Depression not related to or associated with other conditions is sometimes called unipolar depression.

The key features of depressive disorders are a low mood and a loss of interest in pleasurable activities (anhedonia). Other symptoms are pessimism, a lack of energy, poor concentration, low self-esteem, and changes in sleep, appetite, and activity. The key features of mania are an elevated mood, hyperactivity, impulsive behaviour, a lack of concentration, an increased appetite, and an increased libido. Bipolar disorder consists of alternating periods of mania and depression. The changes between mania and depression can be relatively rapid (within a few hours) but usually occur over a longer period.

The global prevalence of major depression is 3.6% for men and 5.1% for women, but approximately 10% of men and 25% of women will have a major depressive episode at some point in their lives (WHO, 2017a). The population prevalence of bipolar disorder is around 1% (Merikangas et al., 2011). It has been estimated that doctors working in primary care with a registered list of 2,000 patients may see 20–30 people per year with major depression, and one or two people with an episode of mania (Gelder et al., 2012).

Mood disorders appear to result from a combination of – and interaction between – genetic, physiological, and experiential factors. Twin studies suggest a genetic predisposition to depression and bipolar disorder (Dunn et al., 2015). Studies of bipolar disorder have shown that changes in neurotransmitter levels correspond to changes from manic to depressive phases. Studies of major depression indicate the effect of reduced activity of the neurotransmitters dopamine, serotonin, and norepinephrine (Stahl, 2000). Endocrine disorders may be causally involved in some cases of depression (see Chapter 14).

Psychological factors are also important. Stressful experiences – particularly during key stages of neurobiological development – may help to explain how psychological responses to the environment affect the development of depression and bipolar disorder (Heim & Binder, 2012; Schiavone et al., 2015). There are many theories of the aetiology of depression. These include Beck's (1967) cognitive theory of depression and Seligman's (1975) theory of learned helplessness, which highlight the importance of negative thinking in the onset and progression of depression (see Chapter 19). Psychoanalytic explanations of depression view it as a response to a real or symbolic loss of a loved person or object: the individual feels worthless and hopeless and responsible for the loss.

Around half of all people who have one bout of depression will have a further depressive episode. Suicide attempts and completed suicide are considerably more common among depressed people. Various treatments for depression are available. Antidepressant

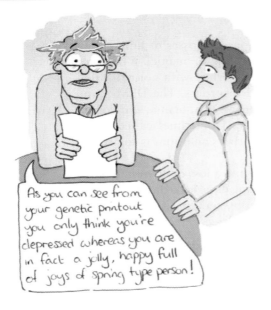

As you can see from your genetic printout you only think you're depressed whereas you are in fact a jolly, happy full of joys of spring type person!

drugs are the most widely available treatments. It is recommended that they be used only for moderate and major depression. For acute severe depression that has not responded to antidepressants, electroconvulsive therapy (ECT) may be used.

Depression responds well to psychotherapy of various forms, particularly CBT and interventions designed to enhance problem solving and social support. One approach to the treatment of moderate and severe depression may be to begin with antidepressants to alleviate immediate symptoms and then introduce psychological therapies.

People with bipolar disorder may have periods of illness separated by periods of several months of feeling well. Treatment may involve the use of an antidepressant, an anti-psychotic, or a mood stabilising drug. Psychotherapies do not appear to be as successful in bipolar disorder as they are in unipolar depression.

Anxiety disorders

The term 'anxiety disorder' is an umbrella term which incorporates various forms of abnormal and pathological fear and anxiety. An anxiety disorder may have a specific limited focus or it may be more diffuse.

Generalised Anxiety Disorder (GAD) is characterised by excessive fearful anticipation and worrying thoughts. People with GAD may have interrupted sleep and difficulty in concentrating and may also feel depressed. Physical symptoms include agitation or excitation in the gastrointestinal, respiratory, cardiovascular, urinary, and muscular systems. Because GAD is continuous and not related to individual events or circumstances, it is separate from episodic anxiety such as phobia or panic disorder.

Phobias are anxious reactions to particular situations or objects. The unpleasant physical and psychological experiences of severe anxiety accompany phobias, thus people may try to avoid the situations or objects which they fear. This may be possible for 'simple' phobias (e.g. a fear of blood or spiders), but avoidant responses can be quite debilitating when people have social phobias. **Panic disorder** is diagnosed when panic attacks occur unexpectedly and in the absence of a single identifiable trigger for an anxious response. In panic attacks the symptoms of anxiety rapidly escalate. Catastrophic thoughts (catastrophising) are common – people may think 'I'm going mad' or 'I'm going to die'.

At any point, around 3% of the general population has GAD, with a higher prevalence in women. Many people have phobias for which they do not seek treatment, but the prevalence of clinically significant simple phobias is around 5%. Social phobia and panic disorders are present in around 3% of people, and they are also more common among women (Bandelow & Michaelis, 2015; Shimada-Sugimoto et al., 2015).

Twin studies suggest that anxiety disorders have a genetic component (Shimada-Sugimoto et al., 2015). Neurochemical and brain imaging studies have provided evidence of abnormal activity in the amygdala, hippocampus, and prefrontal cortex in anxiety and panic disorders (Dresler et al., 2013). Experiences are also important. Simple phobias often develop in childhood. Social phobia often arises from a discrete experience of anxiety in a public place. The aetiology of panic disorder is less clear, but it may result from a combination of abnormal neural activity, excessive autonomic

CASE STUDY 16.1   Depression

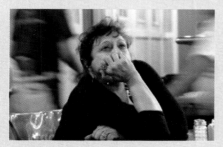

Ella is a 48-year-old woman who was diagnosed with depression at age 16. Her account reflects a biopsychosocial model of mental illness: she believes that her depression was caused by a combination of a chemical imbalance and learned behaviours. Various childhood events may have resulted in her depression: she became very introverted after her parents separated and her best friend moved schools. During adolescence, Ella also began to have trouble sleeping, and lacked energy. She feels unlucky that the doctors she saw were not attentive to her psychological symptoms.

When Ella was diagnosed at age 16, she began taking antidepressant medication. The initial side effects were unpleasant and included disrupted sleep and weight gain. However, these side effects reduced over time and she felt like she was *given my life back*. Ella feels that she can *now be a normal person*. Diagnosis and treatment had other psychological benefits for Ella: the acknowledgement that her depression was a result of serotonergic activity in her brain was a counter to people simply saying *Cheer up! Why are you so miserable?* and implying that depression was somehow her fault.

However, Ella realised that although antidepressant medication had *sorted out my brain chemistry* she was also aware that her depression was influenced by psychological factors: *you have learnt all these negative ways of looking at things, and doing things... from your parents at times.* This realisation meant that Ella saw a need for long-term therapy to help her to learn better ways of dealing with events in her life and trying to change her *total inferiority complex*. Her experiences of therapy helped her to develop a more positive approach to herself and her social interactions.

Adapted from www.healthtalkonline.org.uk © DIPEx.

nervous system responses to stress, and excessive fearful responses to the resulting autonomic arousal (Dresler et al., 2013).

Without treatment, GAD will persist for several years in over 75% of people. Phobias and panic disorders may continue for several years: phobias with a childhood onset may be particularly persistent. Medical treatments for anxiety disorders include anxiolytics (for short-term use) and antidepressants for people with GAD or phobias involving depression. Psychological therapies include relaxation training, self-help methods, and CBT designed to change maladaptive thoughts about feared situations. Combinations of psychotherapy and pharmacotherapy are often more effective than either single treatment.

CASE STUDY 16.2   Generalised anxiety disorder

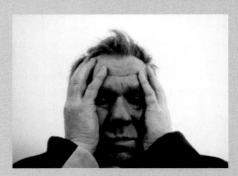

Simon is a 50-year-old freelance writer. He first developed the symptoms of a generalised anxiety disorder in his 20s. There were no specific problems related to his work, personal life, or finances. He says:

> I was just worried all the time about everything... or anything. It didn't matter that there weren't any problems, I just got worried.

The constant sense of worry began to make it hard for him to fall asleep at night. A lack of sleep led to fatigue, which combined with feelings of distraction at work, and resulted in him making 'silly little mistakes' and he lost work as a result.

Fatigue and poor performance at work made Simon irritable and angry with his friends and family. He first sought help for his anxiety from his doctor. To begin with, he was given a benzodiazepine to reduce his physical symptoms and help him to sleep. However, his doctor also referred him to a psychotherapist.

Through weekly hour-long sessions of CBT, Simon learnt more about his physiological responses to anxiety. He also learnt about how his emotional and behavioural responses to these physiological symptoms were detrimental. He developed plans for how better to deal with his anxiety when he felt it rising. He also kept a 'diary' of the thoughts and emotions that accompany his physical symptoms of anxiety to help him challenge maladaptive thoughts.

Schizophrenia

Schizophrenia is characterised by disorders of thought, mood, and anxiety. The key features of **schizophrenia** are psychotic symptoms such as delusions and hallucinations. Different subtypes of schizophrenia can be identified according to different combinations of 'positive' and 'negative' symptoms. The **positive symptoms** are additions to usual pre-existing functioning. They include thought disorders, hallucinations, and delusions. *Thought disorders* may take different forms, but all represent a variation from normal streams of thought. For example, there may be a lack of logical connections between different ideas. The most common *hallucinations* are auditory, for example, a person may imagine that they can hear the voice of another person commenting on their behaviour, or may experience a 'thought echo' in which they hear their thoughts spoken out loud. *Delusions* are false (often bizarre) beliefs which may be persecutory in nature. For example, a person may believe that the television is stealing their thoughts, or that their neighbours are spying on them for the government. The presence of such delusions without other symptoms of schizophrenia represents a delusional disorder.

The **negative symptoms** of schizophrenia are those which involve a loss of normal function. They are varied but tend to reflect impaired interpersonal and social functioning. Changes in mood may include a blunting of feeling, a reduced capacity to express emotions, and incongruous emotions (e.g. laughing in response to sad news). Reductions in attention and memory may accompany the thought disorders referred to above. Poverty of speech, depressed mood, and low motivation may combine with these emotional changes and lead to a withdrawal from normal social interactions.

The population prevalence of schizophrenia is around 0.5% and the lifetime risk is around 1% (McGrath et al., 2008). It is twice as common among men as women. It has been estimated that a doctor working in primary care with a registered list of 2,000 patients may have eight patients with schizophrenia, but that this number will be substantially higher for doctors working in urban areas with large homeless populations (Gelder et al., 2012).

Schizophrenia results from a combination of – and interaction between – genetic, physiological, and experiential factors. Twin studies indicate that some people have a genetic predisposition to this disorder (Sullivan et al., 2003). There is evidence that the lateral ventricles of the brain are enlarged in people with schizophrenia, that hippocampal volume is reduced, and that dopamine and serotonin levels may be abnormal (Picchioni et al., 2017; Shin et al., 2011). Complications during pregnancy and birth increase the likelihood of schizophrenia (Cannon et al., 2002), as do adverse childhood experiences such as neglect and abuse (Carr et al., 2013). The onset of schizophrenia often follows distressing events or periods. Early or prolonged cannabis use also increases the risk of schizophrenia (Gage et al., 2016).

The prognosis for people with schizophrenia tends to be better if positive symptoms are intermittent rather than continuous and if negative symptoms are absent or do not worsen.

Up to 10% of people with schizophrenia take their own lives. Antipsychotic medications can be effective for treating positive symptoms but do not affect the negative symptoms. Lack of adherence to medication is often a problem in schizophrenia and may be influenced by medication side effects. Psychotherapy can be a useful adjunct to medication.

Personality disorders

Personality can be defined as the enduring characteristics of an individual expressed via behaviour in different settings. **Personality disorders** are difficult to define because personality itself is an elusive concept. Unlike other psychiatric disorders, personality disorders have no clear time of onset. They consist of inflexible patterns of behaviour which deviate from social expectations and which causes distress, suffering, or harm to the individual or other people. The DSM-5 divides personality disorders into three clusters:

- Odd/Eccentric – including paranoid and schizoid personality disorders.
- Dramatic/Emotional/Erratic – including anti social and borderline personality disorders.
- Anxious/Fearful – including obsessive-compulsive disorder.

Around 5–15% of the population has a personality disorder (Quirk et al., 2016). Personality disorders are more common among younger people and among men. They may result from a complex combination of a genetic predisposition and experiential factors such as brain injury during a complicated birth, difficult parent–child interactions, or traumatic experiences.

Because personality is relatively stable, personality disorders tend not to be very responsive to treatment. Treatment often involves identifying ways to manage the person's behaviour in different social contexts, such as avoiding situations where the problem behaviour occurs and providing support to the immediate family. Comorbid psychological conditions or unhealthy patterns of alcohol and drug use should also be treated.

Summary

- Psychiatric disorders are the result of the interaction and combination of three Ps: predisposing, precipitating, and perpetuating factors.
- Biomedical and psychosocial factors can constitute predisposing, precipitating, and perpetuating factors.
- The two major systems for classifying psychiatric disorders are the *Diagnostic and Statistical Manual of Mental Disorders* (DSM), and the *International Statistical Classification of Diseases and Related Health Problems* (ICD).
- The World Health Organisation has developed a simplified classification of the mental disorders most commonly seen in primary care.
- Psychiatric disorders differ from each other in terms of the presence, nature, and intensity of disorders of thought, mood, and anxiety.

16.2 DIAGNOSIS AND TREATMENT OF PSYCHIATRIC DISORDERS

16.2.1 PSYCHIATRIC ASSESSMENT

Diagnosing a psychiatric disorder may be straightforward in some cases. However, as noted earlier, most psychiatric disorders are syndromes of symptoms that may be aspects of different disorders (Krueger & Eaton, 2015). It is therefore important to conduct a thorough examination and assessment in order to evaluate differential diagnoses. A psychiatric interview involves taking a psychiatric history and conducting a mental state examination (Gelder et al., 2012; Stevens & Rodin, 2010). It is important to note that the nature of many psychiatric disorders may make the psychiatric interview more difficult than a standard clinical interview: people may be apathetic, anxious, angry, deluded, or aggressive (see Chapter 18).

The psychiatric history should first attend to the presenting complaint and its history, including the patient's reports of the believed causes of the problem and their subjective experiences. It is also important to gain information about the patient's pre-morbid history. There may be a need to corroborate reports provided by a patient experiencing delusions or psychosis. The history should also gather information about the patient's psychiatric and medical history, including details of any medications and other treatments. Information relating to the patient's family history should identify the presence of any psychiatric disorders, drug/alcohol disorders, and causes of death.

An assessment of a patient's personal history should focus on (i) their early developmental experiences (including pregnancy and birth), (ii) their educational and occupational history, (iii) their current work and financial circumstances, and (iv) their relationship history. It is also important to collect information about their use of alcohol, tobacco, other recreational drugs, and their forensic history. Risks to consider include: (i) deliberate self-harm and suicide, (ii) aggressive behaviour directed toward others, (iii) self-neglect (i.e. a lack of self-care), and (iv) neglect or exploitation by other people.

The **Mental State Examination** (Trzepacz & Baker, 1993) can aid psychiatric diagnoses. It provides a structured way of both observing and describing several aspects of psychological functioning. It addresses the following factors:

- *Behaviour and appearance* – The focus here includes the visible signs of physical health or injury and psychological wellbeing. It also includes the style and condition of clothing and self-presentation. Behaviours to look out for include excessive or reduced physical activity, including posture, speed of movement, restlessness, gait, etc.
- *Mood* (subjective and objective) – The patient's mood is their current emotional state. As well as seeking the patient's self-assessment of their mood, medical professionals should give their own assessment of this – euthymic ('normal'), dysthymic ('down'), or hyperthymic ('up').
- *Affect* – Affect is related to mood and consists of external manifestations of emotion. If there is no apparent abnormality, affect is described as reactive (appropriate to emotional cues). In psychiatric disorders, the affect may be blunted, irritable, changeable, suspicious, perplexed, or incongruous (i.e. not appropriate for the context).

- *Speech and thought form* – The tone, speed, and volume of speech may vary in different disorders (e.g. lower, slower, and quieter speech in depression). Attend to whether the flow of ideas in speech is normal, or if it is disjointed, illogical, or repetitive.
- *Thought content* – The content of thoughts expressed in speech is also important, because someone can present in a 'normal' voice a well-connected, flowing stream of bizarre ideas. Attention should also be given to whether the patient describes feelings of guilt, depression, anxiety, hopelessness, etc. The patient may also express feelings of depersonalisation (e.g. feeling unreal, detached, or empty), or derealisation (e.g. feeling like all the world is paper), and may give evidence of delusions (beliefs which are clearly unfounded but resistant to contrary evidence).
- *Perception* – Note any illusions such as mistaking one real object for another (e.g. a bush is mistaken for a person), as well as hallucinations such as perceiving something that is not present (e.g. hearing a non-existent voice or seeing a non-existent object).
- *Insight* – The focus here is on whether or not the patient thinks that they have a psychiatric disorder or any other impairment and whether they think they need treatment.
- *Cognition* – Note whether or not there are any variations from normal memory processes (short- or long-term) and capacities for problem solving and reasoning. The 'Mini-Mental State Examination' may be helpful here (Folstein et al., 1975).

CLINICAL NOTES 16.1

Psychiatric assessments

- It is helpful to think of psychiatric disorders as syndromes rather than simple discrete illnesses. This is because many psychiatric disorders present combinations of similar symptoms.
- Make sure you understand the various components of the Mental State Examination. This may help you detect a possible psychiatric morbidity in people not presenting with psychiatric complaints.
- Brief assessments such as the Mini-Mental State Examination and Test Your Memory (TYM) can be useful for identifying cognitive impairment. Make sure you are familiar with these assessments.
- When diagnosing and treating psychiatric disorders it is important to be aware of how predisposing, precipitating, and perpetuating factors can explain the onset and maintenance of people's current symptoms.
- Be aware of how psychiatric illnesses may affect people's capacities to be involved in making decisions about their treatment.

16.2.2 MANAGEMENT AND TREATMENT OF PSYCHIATRIC DISORDERS

When treating any illness it is important to agree on a clear treatment plan with the patient and monitor their adherence and progress. Medical, psychological, and social interventions should be considered in every case. The different types of treatment are outlined below. Treatment should be planned in relation to immediate needs, short-term goals, and long-term goals.

Drug therapy

The drugs used in psychiatry can be divided into different categories (see Table 16.1). Some drugs can have more than one application (e.g. benzodiazepines have anxiolytic and hypnotic effects). Many have marked side effects. This, along with people's attitudes and beliefs about medication, may help to explain the low adherence rates among people with psychiatric disorders. Great care must be taken when considering prescribing psychotropic drugs to certain patient groups, including pregnant women (particularly during the first trimester), breastfeeding women, children, elderly people, and people with liver,

TABLE 16.1 Major categories of psychotropic drugs (adapted from Gelder et al., 2012)

Type	Indication	Drug / Class of drug
Antidepressant	depression	tricyclics
		SSRI – Specific Serotonin Reuptake Inhibitor
		MAOI – Monoamine Oxidase Inhibitor
Antipsychotic (major tranquiliser, neuroleptic)	delusions / hallucinations	phenothiazine
	mania	butyrophenone
	prevent relapse to schizophrenia	substituted benzamide
Anxiolytic (minor tranquiliser)	acute severe anxiety	benzodiazepines
		azapirone
		zopiclone
	generalised anxiety disorder	busiprone
Cognitive enhancer	dementia	anticholinesterase inhibitors
Hypnotic	insomnia	benzodiazepines
		cyclopyrrolones
		zopiclone
Mood stabiliser	bipolar disorder	lithium
	acute mood episodes	carbamazepine
		valproate
		lamotrigine
Psychostimulant	narcolepsy	amphetamine
	hyperkinetic disorder in children / ADHD	Methylphenidate

kidney, or heart disorders (National Institute for Health and Care Excellence, 2014). Care must also be taken when withdrawing or changing medication. More information about drug side effects and contra-indications is available elsewhere (Gelder et al., 2012).

In addition to addressing the presenting psychiatric disorder, it is important to address problematic drug use. Use of tobacco, alcohol, and other recreational drugs is more common among people with psychiatric disorders than among the general population (Jané-Llopis & Matytsina, 2006). There is evidence of reciprocal causal associations between these behaviours. As noted in earlier sections, some studies find that higher rates of smoking, drinking, and drug use can lead to increased risks of mental illness. Others find that increased use of cigarettes, alcohol, and other drugs are a consequence of psychiatric ill-health. Proponents of the self-medication hypothesis argue that such behaviour is used in an effort to manage psychiatric symptoms (Robinson et al., 2009).

Psychotherapy

Psychotherapy is an effective component of treatment for a variety of psychiatric disorders (Jung & Newton, 2009). As noted in Chapter 19, there are various types of 'talking cures'. Different therapies have different explanations for the causes of psychiatric disorders. However, all share the belief that there is therapeutic value in helping people to understand their past and present situation, manage their psychiatric symptoms, and develop more productive ways of thinking about themselves, their illness, and social interactions. There is substantial evidence of the efficacy of CBT for depression, anxiety disorders, phobias, and obsessive-compulsive disorders. Indeed, in some cases of depression CBT may be more effective than antidepressant drugs (Butler et al., 2006). There is also emerging evidence that self-guided online CBT is effective for various psychological conditions (Karyotaki et al., 2017).

Psychodynamic and psychoanalytic therapies are effective for some psychiatric disorders (Leichsenring & Rabung, 2011; Olthius et al., 2016). In many cases, better outcomes result from a combination of medication and counselling. For example, in anxiety disorders, anxiolytics may alleviate the immediate physical symptoms and thereby facilitate psychotherapy/counselling.

Electroconvulsive therapy

Severe depression may be treated safely and effectively using electroconvulsive therapy (ECT) (UK ECT Review Group, 2003). This procedure involves passing an electric current across a person's brain to alter its activity (e.g. to enhance monoamine function). In bilateral applications, electrodes are held on either temporal lobe to pass a current across the brain. In unilateral applications, the electrodes are placed over the non-dominant hemisphere. Although the bilateral process is more effective, it has more side effects, particularly memory loss for events just before and just after treatment. ECT tends to be used for severe depression that has not responded to medication or which threatens the wellbeing of the patient or other people (e.g. mothers with puerperal psychosis, people with a high suicide risk).

Medical decision making in mental illness

Impaired cognitive functioning associated with some psychiatric disorders may hinder people's capacities to be involved in decision making or to give informed consent to treatment. Those with thought disorders or impairments to memory and problem-solving capacities may find it hard to take in information or evaluate different treatment options. People who lack insight may not recognise that they are unwell and require treatment. The concept of 'capacity' for decision making is important, but there is debate as to how it should be defined (Wong et al., 1999).

In some cases, people may be treated without obtaining their consent. For example, the UK Mental Health Act allows people to be detained and treated without their consent if they pose a serious threat to the health and safety of themselves or other people. Issues of capacity and consent also arise in more common situations.

Although there exist many instruments and tools to aid the assessment of a person's capacity, there is a lack of standardised guidelines to inform the assessment of mental capacity. The results of a research review suggested that a formulaic approach to capacity assessment may not capture the nuances of specific individual cases, and that capacity assessment instruments may support, but cannot replace, clinical judgement (Lamont et al., 2013). Research Box 16.1 illustrates the complexities of the concept of 'consent' in mental health settings. Many of these issues also apply in the neuropsychiatric disorders described in the next section.

RESEARCH BOX 16.1   What does consent mean in practice?

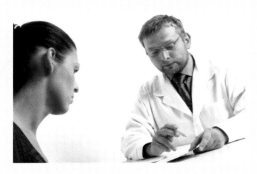

Background

In principle, people with the capacity to make an informed choice about treatment should be appropriately informed and free to give or deny their consent for treatment, without coercion. However, for people detained in psychiatric hospitals, issues of consent are less straightforward.

Method and findings

In-depth interviews were conducted with five Responsible Medical Officers (RMOs) and seven consenting adult patients at a medium-secure psychiatric hospital.

(Continued)

One RMO neatly summed up the paradox of consent with detained patients:

There is no such thing as freely-given consent... even with the patients that are consenting to take the medication, they're not really consenting patients because... they know that taking medication regularly and in a compliant manner is likely to lead to their swift discharge from hospital.

One patient confirmed this:

I've learnt over the years to do as I'm told.

Discussions of consent focused on medication only, and attendance at psychological treatment sessions was presumed to equate to consent. When RMOs talked about being 'cautious' when making decisions about treatment, they actually meant assuming that the person consented to treatment rather than assuming non-consent.

Significance

The concept of 'consent' in mental health settings is not always easy to define. Both patients and RMOs highlighted some of the challenges to the idea that treatment for people with capacity should only be given with the person's informed consent.

Photo © Endostock /Fotolia

Larkin, M., Clifton, E. & de Visser, R. (2009) Making sense of 'consent' in a constrained environment. *International Journal of Law & Psychiatry*, *32*: 176–183.

Summary

- A thorough psychiatric interview involves taking a psychiatric history and conducting a Mental State Examination.
- The Mental State Examination assesses: behaviour and appearance, mood and affect, speech and thought, perception, and insight and cognition.
- Many psychiatric disorders present as syndromes, and symptoms are shared between many of these syndromes. This makes differential diagnosis important.
- When developing a treatment plan, medical, psychological, and social interventions should be considered.
- Transdiagnostic approaches to conceptualising and treating psychiatric disorders can be more effective than disease-specific approaches (Pearl & Norton, 2017).
- There is strong evidence that psychological therapies can be as effective as medication for many psychiatric disorders, in particular mood disorders.

16.3 NEUROLOGICAL DISORDERS

Degeneration or damage within the brain and nervous system can lead to a range of disorders. Their precise nature is determined by the location and extent of the impairment to normal functioning. Altered brain functioning can also be implicated in a range of psychiatric disorders. Because different brain regions have different functions (see Chapter 7), damage or disorders that are localised in specific brain regions tend to have specific outcomes. This section outlines a number of common neurological disorders, their psychological aspects, and their treatment. It is followed by sections on neuropsychological assessment and rehabilitation.

Multiple sclerosis (MS) is characterised by the inflammation and demyelination of the central nervous system. It may result in a loss of sensation or function in the limbs, incontinence, fatigue, pain, cognitive impairments, and mood disorders. In many countries, MS is the most common neurological disorder among young adults. It is believed to be an autoimmune disorder but the exact processes involved are not known and there is no cure. The unpredictable and variable nature of MS affects psychological wellbeing. Depression and anxiety appear to be more common among people with MS than in the general population or among people with similar levels of physical disability due to other causes (Feinstein, 2011; Mohr & Cox, 2001). In addition, learning, attention, and concentration may be impaired. Although there is no effective cure for MS, research suggests that psychological interventions such as CBT can be effective for managing depression and helping people cope with the physical limitations arising from MS (Thomas et al., 2006). However, psychological comorbidities in MS are often under-diagnosed and under-treated (Skokou et al., 2012).

Motor Neurone Disease (also called Amyotrophic Lateral Sclerosis or ALS) is a rare and terminal disorder which involves the progressive degeneration of motor neurons leading to progressive weakness in the skeletal muscles. The cause of the disease is not known and it is also not known why the sensory nerves, which have a similar structure, are not affected. Mood disorders are more common than cognitive impairments (Goldstein & Leigh, 1999). Anxiety and depression also appear to be correlated with the severity of functional impairment and to overall quality of life (van Groenstijn et al., 2016). However, the relationship between functional impairment and overall quality of life appears to be moderated by the degree of social support that is available.

Disorders of the basal ganglia, such as Parkinson's disease and Huntington's disease, cause severe motor deficits (see Chapter 7). However, there are also important cognitive and emotional aspects of these disorders. Indeed, the symptoms of basal ganglia disorders have been referred to as the three Ds: dyskinesia, dementia, and depression (Rosenblatt & Leroi, 2000). **Parkinson's disease** is a severe motor disorder characterised by muscle stiffness, slowness of movement, an unstable posture, and muscle tremors (see Case Study 7.1). It is a progressive degenerative disorder resulting from a severe reduction in dopamine activity in the basal ganglia. There is no cure for Parkinson's disease. Standard pharmacological treatment is the dopamine precursor L-Dopa, but in the last decade the use of deep brain stimulation has progressed, and combined treatment with deep brain stimulation and L-Dopa may be more effective than pharmacotherapy alone (Fang & Tolleson, 2017). Research on the potential of stem-cell therapy is ongoing

(Ali et al., 2014). Cognitive deficits are common and include impairments to memory and information processing. Depression, anxiety, lethargy, sleep disturbances, and pain are more common among people with Parkinson's disease than in the general population (Chaudhuri et al., 2006).

Huntington's disease is characterised by involuntary rapid, ceaseless movements or tics. Other symptoms include a loss of coordination and balance, slurred speech, and difficulties in swallowing. It is a genetically determined disorder caused by the progressive degeneration of neurons with receptors for the neurotransmitters GABA and acetylcholine. There is no cure for Huntington's disease and death usually occurs 15–25 years after symptom onset. Treatment focuses on addressing the symptoms, preventing complications, and providing psychological support. Cognitive deficits are common and include impairments to memory retrieval, attention, and concentration. Compared to the general population, people with Huntington's disease are more likely to experience depression and suicidal behaviour (van Duijn et al., 2014).

Dementia, meaning 'deprived of mind', involves the progressive loss of cognitive function due to damage or disease in the brain. Dementia is not a single disorder but a syndrome, the symptoms of which vary between people, depending on the location and cause of the disorder. Vascular dementias result from multiple small strokes which, in accumulation, produce a sufficient loss of neurons and accompanying changes in behaviour and cognition. The importance of dementia to mortality statistics is increasing in developed countries. In the UK, dementia is now the third most common cause of death (Office for National Statistics, 2015). However, it should also be noted that the 'compression of morbidity' described in Chapter 8 applies to cognitive morbidity: fewer older people are reaching a threshold of significant cognitive impairment, but there is a more rapid decline to death among those who do (Langa et al., 2008).

Dementia of Alzheimer type (DAT or **Alzheimer's disease**) accounts for over half of all dementias. It involves the progressive loss of neurons and synapses in the cerebral cortex and particular subcortical regions. The cause of loss of neurons in DAT is not well understood, but is believed to be due to a combination of genetic factors and environmental influences. DAT is characterised by progressive impairments to memory, cognitive capacities, and social functioning, which are commonly accompanied by confusion, irritability, and mood swings. People with DAT are more likely than the general population to experience anxiety, irritability, depression, and apathy. Anxiety and depression may be predictive of further cognitive decline (Banks et al., 2014). People with DAT may also experience psychosis – including delusions and hallucinations – especially if there is a rapid cognitive decline (Ropacki & Jeste, 2005).

Among older people, it may be difficult to make a differential diagnosis between depression and the early stages of dementia because depressed people often experience impaired concentration and memory. Although depression and dementia often co-occur, it is unclear whether depression is a consequence of neural degeneration in brain structures responsible for mood, a reaction to an awareness of the onset of dementia, or whether both dementia and depression have shared biological pathways (Mendes-Silva et al., 2016). Psychosocial aspects of DAT are addressed in Case Study 16.3.

CASE STUDY 16.3 Identifying the early stages of dementia

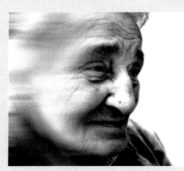

As dementia develops, people may not have full awareness of changes in their behaviour or their own memory problems. Andreas visited his doctor on his own on what was supposed to be a joint visit with his wife Maria. He had become worried about changes in Maria's behaviour. Andreas said that he did not notice the gradual changes occurring day to day, until it was pointed out to him by other people who had less frequent contact with her:

So one example was with my son. He lives overseas, and can only visit a few times a year. He took Maria out shopping for a new coat, and when he came back said 'Why haven't you told me how down she is? She wasn't really interested in any-thing, and when we were having coffee she was just in a world of her own'. When he told me how much she had changed since the summer it really shocked me.

When he said that, it did make me wonder whether she might be depressed. But then there were other things, like forgetting to lock the house when we went out, or not locking the car when she got home, and she didn't like it when I pointed it out. I wasn't sure what was wrong, but it was starting to worry me. That worry must have grown because one time she said 'Why are you always getting annoyed with me?' and I just said 'It's because I'm so worried about you', and that made her really upset. So I suggested that we should go and see the doctor. She reluctantly agreed, but on the day of the appointment, she said she wasn't coming. So I went down on my own.

Andreas recalled how the doctor thought that Maria might be depressed. He called her to ask her to come to the doctor's surgery and she reluctantly agreed. After a productive three-way discussion, the doctor was able to determine that Maria was displaying signs of dementia.

Now that I have spoken to other people, I've found out that a lot of us have been through the same kinds of things. At first, it's hard to notice that there is anything wrong. It's a series of unrelated and apparently insignificant things that you can only make sense of with hindsight. So I think that with hindsight, the changes initially were hard to recognise and hard to interpret because I didn't know there was a problem.

Adapted from accounts at: www.healthtalk.org/peoples-experiences/nerves-brain/carers-people-dementia/suspicions-early-signs-dementia

There is some evidence that drug therapies (cholinesterase inhibitors, memantine, and Ginkgo biloba) have a small but significant impact on cognitive functioning in Alzheimer's disease, and that exercise therapy can also be effective (Ströhle et al., 2015).

Neurological deficits often arise from a cerebrovascular accident or **stroke**: central nervous system neurons die because of disruptions to the blood flow to the brain (see Chapter 12). The reduction of blood flow may be due to a blood vessel blockage (ischaemic stroke) or rupture (haemorrhagic stroke). The outcomes are determined by the size and location of the blood vessels involved. The brain regions affected by the disturbances to blood flow are unable to function properly, and this may result in impairments to voluntary movement, comprehension, and the production of speech or visual impairments. Depression and anxiety are more common, especially in people who have experienced a stroke, than in the general population, and may be more likely among women, younger people, those more functionally disabled from the stroke, and those with less emotional support (Broomfield et al., 2015; Fei et al., 2016). Other common psychological consequences of strokes are increased rates of irritability, agitation, eating disturbances, and apathy (Angelelli et al., 2004). Psychiatric disorders after stroke are important in their own right, but they also hamper physical rehabilitation (Ahn et al., 2015). There is, therefore, a need for physical, cognitive, and psychological rehabilitation (see Research Box 16.2).

RESEARCH BOX 16.2   The influence of social support on quality of life after stroke

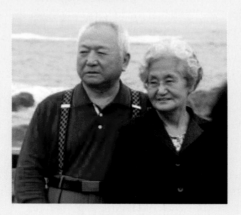

Background

Stroke is a major cause of adult disability and mortality. In addition to its physical impact, stroke is often associated with impairments to quality of life and the development of depression. Depression and impaired quality of life are linked with poorer outcomes after stroke, so it is important to find ways to reduce their impact.

Method and findings

102 adults with their first ischaemic stroke were recruited from a hospital in Taiwan. They took part in structured interviews that assessed social support in four domains – emotional support, affirming support, informational support, and tangible physical support. Depression and quality of life were also assessed.

(Continued)

Half (47%) of the sample had possible depression. Depression was related to significantly lower quality of life, and both were related to greater impairments to daily activities. Statistical modelling revealed that tangible physical support was strongly determined whether impairments to daily activities resulted in depression or impaired quality of life.

Significance

This study shows that enhancing physical support after stroke reduces the likelihood that people will develop depression or have reduced quality of life. Rehabilitation after stroke should give greater attention to how people can develop and use their support networks to reduce negative psychosocial impacts.

Huang, C.Y. et al. (2010) Mediating roles of social support on post stroke depression and quality of life in patients with ischemic stroke. *Journal of Clinical Nursing*, *19*: 2752–2762.

Neurological impairment may be caused by a **traumatic brain injury**. Traumatic brain injuries commonly arise from blunt injuries to the head during 'closed head injuries' such as road traffic accidents, falls, assaults, or sporting injuries (Ponsford, 2004). In contrast, 'open head injuries' occur when a sharp object penetrates the skull and tend to result in more localised damage. Closed head injuries tend to result in a diffuse array of cognitive, behavioural, and emotional symptoms. Contusions occur when the brain is damaged by an impact with the skull (e.g. during car accidents). Such damage is particularly common in the basal forebrain, and frontal and temporal lobes. Shearing strains occur between tissues of different density (e.g. between white matter and grey matter) and can be as a result of rotational forces, such as being punched on one side of the head in boxing. Because multiple mechanisms may be involved in traumatic brain injuries, the resulting neural damage tends to be heterogeneous. Damage to the prefrontal cortex often leads to changes in personality, such as irritability and disinhibition. Rates of depression and anxiety are elevated following traumatic brain injuries, but the prevalence and severity of these psychological outcomes may be influenced more by coping styles and adjustment to the injury than to the extent of the disability (Bowen et al., 1998; Ponsford, 2004). Emotional support and psychological interventions may, therefore, play an important role in rehabilitation (Fandrew et al., 2009).

Summary

- Neurological disorders may arise from progressive degenerative disease processes or acute events such as a stroke or traumatic brain injuries.
- The severity and impact of neurological disorders depends on the location and extent of the neurological damage involved.
- Neurological disorders can cause impairments to physical functioning as well as changes in mood and personality.

16.4 NEUROPSYCHOLOGICAL ASSESSMENT AND REHABILITATION

Neuropsychological rehabilitation focuses on treating the cognitive and emotional deficits arising from neural damage or degeneration. It may form part of a broader approach aimed at improving a person's physical, behavioural, and social functioning. An important part of rehabilitation programmes is a thorough neuropsychological assessment to establish the precise nature of any impairments and to enable the individualisation of rehabilitation programmes (Luria, (1963 [1948]).

16.4.1 NEUROPSYCHOLOGICAL ASSESSMENT

A neuropsychological assessment may be carried out for different purposes, including: (i) describing and measuring cognitive deficits; (ii) a differential diagnosis (e.g. whether the cognitive deficits are part of another psychiatric disorder); and (iii) monitoring the neuropsychological rehabilitation. A complete neuropsychological assessment involves the examination of all modes of sensation as well as memory and problem-solving capacities.

An important part of this process is an evaluation of a person's intellectual capacities. A useful tool is the **Mini-Mental State Examination** (MMSE). The MMSE does not assess all the features assessed by the full Mental State Examination. Instead it provides a brief (10 minute) standardised way of assessing someone's cognitive capacities (Folstein et al., 1975) through:

- Orientation – e.g. the person is asked to give the year, season, day, date, and month.
- Registration – e.g. the person is asked to repeat three unrelated objects named by the healthcare professional.
- Attention and calculation – e.g. the person is asked to count backwards from 100 in 7s.
- Recall – e.g. the person is asked to give the names of the three objects named earlier.
- Language – e.g. the person is shown common objects and asked to name them; asked to repeat the sentence 'No ifs, ands, or buts'; follow some written instructions; and write a sentence.

The Addenbrooke's Cognitive Examination and the Montreal Cognitive Assessment serve similar purposes, and may be easier to use as they do not have the copyright restrictions on the MMSE (Hsieh et al., 2013; Nasreddine et al., 2005; Roalf et al., 2013). It is also possible to use paper and pencil tests of intelligence as part of this process. Recently, the brief self-administered Test Your Memory (TYM) was found to be just as effective as the longer MMSE and Addenbrooke's Cognitive Examination for DAT and other dementias (Brown et al., 2009). Computer-administered tests are also available. For all such tests, standardised scores can be used to classify people as normal or with varying degrees of cognitive impairment.

Physiological or neuroimaging assessments may also be made. Tests of cranial nerve function include assessments of:

- Scent perception, visual acuity, visual fields, and eye movement.
- Colour vision.
- Power of the jaw and facial muscles.
- Hearing.
- Head movements.

Tests of motor nerve function include assessment of the reflexes and observations of any involuntary movements, weakness, or incoordination. Sensation in the limbs can be assessed via the application of appropriate touch and temperature. Further investigation of the nervous system may include computerised tomography (CT), magnetic resonance imaging (MRI), and functional MRI (fMRI). Angiography and venography can provide information about blood flow within the brain. Analysis of cerebrospinal fluid can also give information about infections (e.g. meningitis, encephalitis) and some cancers.

CLINICAL NOTES 16.2

Neuropsychological rehabilitation and goal setting

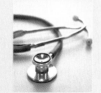

- In designing rehabilitation for people with neuropsychiatric disorders, it is important to set goals and targets that are relevant for each patient. This can increase their motivation and adherence. This general principle can be applied in other medical contexts.
- Goals should be SMART:

  - Specific – stick to specific behaviours.
  - Measurable – behaviour has to be measurable so progress can be recorded.
  - Achievable – within their capabilities. This often means you need to start with very small goals.
  - Realistic – goals need to be easily carried out and attained within the context of the patient's life.
  - Time specific – give a time in which the goal must be achieved.

- An example of a SMART goal for a depressed and withdrawn patient might be to walk to the local shop every day for a week.

16.4.2 NEUROPSYCHOLOGICAL REHABILITATION

The brain exhibits a certain amount of plasticity, and connections between neurons can change in response to experience (see section 7.1.2). The prospects for a recovery from neural damage are influenced by the size and location of any damage, the state of the brain before the injury (influenced by the person's age), and the person's personality and coping styles before the injury (Luria, 1963[1948]; Ponsford, 2004; Prigatano, 1999).

Key tasks for rehabilitation may include the rehabilitation of disorders of language, attention, memory, self-awareness, and behavioural problems. In all cases, it is important to address depression. Prospects for rehabilitation following traumatic brain injury may be hampered if the brain injury means that the person is unaware of the need for rehabilitation, or has experienced changes in attention and personality that make it harder for them to persist with rehabilitation tasks.

Over recent decades, there has been a trend toward community-based neuropsychological rehabilitation. Such programmes are designed to enhance the development of independence (Ponsford, 2004; Wilson et al., 2009). They often involve the provision of appropriate support services in the home and workplace. There has been increased use of technologies to aid memory, decision making, and the organisation of daily activities. Rather than being an exclusive relationship between patients and healthcare professionals, rehabilitation has come to be seen as a partnership involving people's families. All parties in this partnership must work together to achieve optimal cognitive, physical, and social wellbeing.

Rehabilitation should be designed to achieve goals that are relevant to the person's lifestyle. This will make it more likely that the patient and their family will remain involved in goal setting and rehabilitation activities. The general principles of goal setting must apply here. Goals should be agreed with the patient and should be SMART. In other words, they should be:

Specific, Measurable, Achievable, Realistic, and have Timelines for achievement (see Clinical notes 16.2).

Decisions about which approaches to use should be influenced by the nature of the goals to be reached and the capabilities of the patient (Wilson et al., 2009). They may entail learning new ways of performing tasks or interacting with people and coming to terms with limitations. This can be done by employing a range of techniques, including the use of external aids or tools. The techniques chosen should maximise the patient's attention to the immediate tasks (as well as the longer-term goals). This may be particularly important following traumatic brain injury which results in impairments to attention, arousal, self-awareness, and executive function.

There is now much greater recognition of the need to address cognition, emotion, behaviour, and social functioning, and to acknowledge the links between these different aspects of people's lives. This is the basis of the holistic approach to healthcare and treatment. Rehabilitation must aim to improve cognitive functioning but also address any changes in mood and personality associated with the underlying neuropsychological impairment. It is now recognised that rehabilitation requires a broad theoretical base and that no single theoretical approach will be the most appropriate foundation for all people.

Summary

- Neuropsychological rehabilitation focuses on addressing the cognitive and emotional deficits arising from neural damage or degeneration.
- Neuropsychological assessment can be used as part of a diagnosis, for planning rehabilitation, and for monitoring progress. It focuses on cognitive capacity and may also involve physiological or neuroimaging assessments.
- The prospects for rehabilitation in neurological disorders are influenced by the characteristics of the neurological impairment (nature, size, location, etc.) as well as the characteristics of the patient, such as their coping style.
- Neuropsychological rehabilitation should be designed to meet the goals that are important to the patient. In addition to improving physical capacities, it is important to address any changes in mood and personality.

FURTHER READING

Gelder, M. et al. (2012) *Psychiatry* (4th edition). Oxford: Oxford University Press. A comprehensive, clear, and authoritative overview of psychiatry. A major limitation is that it contains no references. More detailed coverage is provided in Cowen, P., Harrison, P. & Burns, T. (2012) *Shorter Oxford Textbook of Psychiatry* (6th edition). Oxford: Oxford University Press.

Stevens, L. & Rodin I. (2010) *Psychiatry: An Illustrated Colour Text* (2nd edition). Edinburgh: Churchill Livingstone. Accessible, brief chapters on a range of topics. Each topic is covered in a two-page spread that gives a good introduction that can be supplemented by further reading.

Wilson, B.A. et al. (eds) (2009) *Neuropsychological Rehabilitation: Theory, Models, Therapy and Outcome*. Cambridge: Cambridge University Press. Provides broad coverage of neuropsychological rehabilitation, including group and individual interventions. It also includes a number of case studies.

REVISION QUESTIONS

1. Describe the 'three Ps' related to the onset and progression of psychiatric disorders.

2. Choose one psychiatric disorder. Outline its key features, causes, and treatment options.

3. What is assessed by the Mental State Examination? How is this done?

4. Briefly describe the applicability of drug therapy, psychotherapy, and electroconvulsive therapy for psychiatric disorders. Discuss the success rates of each.

5. Why are combinations of drug therapy and psychotherapy often more effective than either treatment mode in isolation?

6. Choose one neurological disorder. Outline its causes, physical and psychological symptoms, and prospects for treatment.

7. Why is a thorough neuropsychological assessment for rehabilitation necessary? What procedures are used in this assessment?

8. Outline the purposes and practices of neuropsychological rehabilitation.

SECTION IV

HEALTHCARE PRACTICE

17 EVIDENCE-BASED PRACTICE

Case study

17.1   Barriers to adherence to antiretroviral medication for HIV

Figures

17.1   The cycle of activities in evidence-based practice
17.2   Multidimensional model of barriers to adherence
17.3   How better practitioner–patient communication leads to better adherence

Research box

17.1   How common is shared decision making?

LEARNING OBJECTIVES

This chapter is designed to enable you to:

- Define evidence-based practice.
- Identify the sources of information to be used in evidence-based practice.
- Describe the factors that influence adherence to prescribed treatment.
- Discuss the importance of effective practitioner–patient communication.

Ideally, all decisions about treatment would be based on sound evidence. This ideal lies behind the promotion of evidence-based practice. But what is meant by 'evidence-based practice', and what counts as 'evidence'? This chapter begins with a description of evidence-based practice, the second section focuses on evidence from research on adherence to treatment, and the third section describes research into practitioner–patient communication. Chapter 18 builds on this last section and outlines the communication skills that have been shown to produce better patient outcomes.

17.1 EVIDENCE-BASED PRACTICE

17.1.1 WHAT IS EVIDENCE-BASED PRACTICE?

Evidence-based practice (EBP) is based on the principle of 'integrating individual clinical expertise with the best available external clinical evidence from systematic research' (Sackett et al., 1996: 71). An important aspect of clinical expertise is taking into account the details of particular people's predicaments, rights, and preferences. In their useful guide, Straus et al. (2010) state that to practise EBP we must:

1. Formulate an appropriate question. Questions must be phrased in a way that allows us to determine whether they have been answered. For example, if we want to know which of two possible treatments is better, then we need to define beforehand what we would consider to be a clinically significant difference – we will then have a criterion to apply to our answers.
2. Find the best evidence to answer this question. The different sources of evidence will be discussed in more detail below.
3. Evaluate and appraise the evidence. Medical professionals must know how to distinguish between reliable and unreliable (or good and bad) evidence. Although evidence can aid decision making, the evidence itself does not make decisions.
4. Align our evaluation of the evidence with our own expertise and the details of the particular patient. We must understand how the evidence will apply to particular people. As noted above, this means taking into account people's rights and preferences and any contra-indications for specific treatments.
5. Evaluate steps 1–4 in a process of continual feedback, refinement, and flexibility. It is important to evaluate not only the outcomes (i.e. whether the chosen treatment was successful) but also the processes of integrating the evidence with clinical judgement. Through such self-evaluation the process and practice of EBP should become more effective.

Ideally, steps 1 to 5 will form a feedback loop whereby our evaluation of the processes and outcomes of medical decision making informs the development of more appropriate question formulation, better evidence-gathering, better evaluation, and a better integration of evidence with clinical expertise (see Figure 17.1).

These five steps represent an ideal pattern, which may not be followed by all clinicians all of the time (Straus et al., 2010). Clinicians may shift between different modes of EBP depending on the nature of their work and the presenting condition. Often the third step

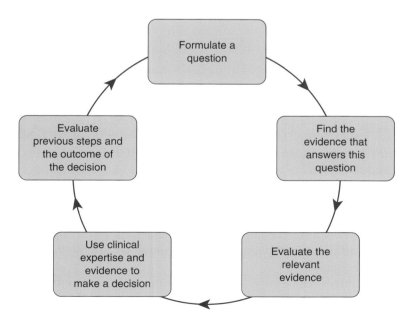

FIGURE 17.1 The cycle of activities in evidence-based practice (based on Strauss et al., 2005)

may be skipped, with practitioners preferring to use others' evaluations. However, all modes of EBP will involve formulating the right questions and integrating evidence with clinical expertise, patient characteristics, and circumstances. It is also important to note that in the domain of psychotherapy, some have identified a need to acknowledge the need for, and value of, practice-based evidence (Margison et al., 2000).

17.1.2 A HIERARCHY OF EVIDENCE

In terms of finding the best evidence to answer appropriate treatment questions, some have identified a **hierarchy of evidence** for EBP (Straus et al., 2010). The components of this hierarchy are systems, synopses, syntheses, and studies. These will be described in an order of decreasing utility for practising EBP.

Systems

These are computerised decision-support systems which contain up-to-date information about different treatments and allow for the input of the details of particular people to aid identification of the most appropriate treatment.

Synopses

These consist of brief, up-to-date summaries of current best practice. Healthcare professionals may benefit from investing in evidence-based practice journals and online resources (see Clinical notes 17.1).

CLINICAL NOTES 17.1

Finding up-to-date research evidence

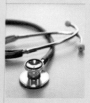

- Use synopses of research such as the Database of Abstracts of Reviews of Effects (DARE), the journal *Evidence Based Medicine*, the American College of Physicians' *ACP Journal Club*, and *BMJ pico*.
- Look for recent meta-analyses or systematic review papers.
- Use the Cochrane database to find up-to-date reviews of different treatments (www.cochrane.org).
- Be sure you know how to find the relevant primary research evidence using databases like PubMed (www.pubmed.gov) and develop the skills required to read such reports critically.
- Access Healthtalk online (www.healthtalkonline.org) for interesting case studies of people's experiences of a range of illnesses and treatments.

Syntheses

Meta-analyses and systematic reviews provide detailed descriptions of research findings through methodical searches of published literature to identify all relevant studies. **Meta-analysis** is used to combine the results of similar studies for statistical data analysis (see Box 17.1). **Systematic reviews** provide summaries of published research, but are not based on the statistical processes of meta-analysis. In both cases there is usually an evaluation of the quality of studies, so that studies with weaker research designs have less influence than studies with more robust methodologies.

BOX 17.1   What is meta-analysis?

- Meta-analysis is a statistical procedure used to combine the samples of several similar studies into one larger analysis. It is particularly useful for evaluating intervention studies because small sample sizes can affect the likelihood of finding statistically significant results.
- The first step in meta-analysis is to identify relevant studies – usually via a systematic search of electronic databases. Once relevant papers have been identified, it is important to determine which studies are of a suitable quality for inclusion. Once suitable studies have been identified, the combined data can be analysed to find the overall 'effect size' – i.e. not only whether a treatment has a statistically significant effect on clinical outcomes, but also the magnitude of that effect.
- Meta-analysis can only be as good as the studies that are entered into it. Furthermore, meta-analysis may be affected by the 'file drawer effect' where studies that do not find significant effects may never be published, and will instead languish in a filing cabinet. The real 'effect size' may therefore never be known. This has led to calls for all clinical trials to be registered before any data are collected so that the extent of the 'file drawer effect' might be estimated (International Committee of Medical Journal Editors, 2017).

The increasing use of qualitative methods in health research (see below) has prompted the development of techniques for **meta-synthesis** of non-numerical data (Melendez-Torres et al., 2015).

Studies

These include individual studies and clinical trials as reported in peer-reviewed journals. One disadvantage of relying on single papers is that no single study will be perfect in terms of its design and execution. Even with good studies, the characteristics of the sample may not be the same as those of the people to whom you are hoping to apply the findings. Thus, you will need to read and evaluate several papers in order to find the appropriate evidence to answer your questions. This is a difficult task: at least half a million English-language records are added to the PubMed database each year. Finding the best and most relevant evidence therefore requires the development of good search skills and devoting a considerable amount of time to this endeavour. The hierarchy of evidence (Straus et al., 2010) suggests that individual research papers found via searches of databases such as PubMed have a low priority for healthcare professionals. However, syntheses, synopses, and systems are all based, one way or another, on original research.

Original research studies may employ one of several study designs. In a **randomised controlled trial** (**RCT**), the efficacy of a treatment or intervention is assessed by comparing clinical outcomes in a group receiving the target treatment with a 'control group' which may receive routine care or a placebo. People are randomly allocated to treatment or control groups and statistical checks are made to ensure that the groups that will be compared at the end of a study do not differ at the start of the study. Methodological rigour is enhanced by ensuring that the people receiving treatment and the researchers measuring clinical outcomes are 'blind' to (unaware of) whether a person received the treatment or a placebo.

Other study designs include **case-control studies**, which compare people with a particular condition (cases) to a group of healthy people (controls), and **cross-sectional surveys**, where standardised questionnaires are used with a group of patients or a sample of the general population.

Qualitative methods are used to examine people's experiences, and typically involve individual interviews or group interviews (focus groups). Qualitative analysis is typically based on the systematic interpretation of oral accounts, rather than statistics. Important information can also be gleaned from case series or **case reports**, but because these are based on small numbers of patients in specific contexts it may be inappropriate to apply their results to other clinical settings.

17.1.3 HOW TO READ A PAPER

It is important to know how to read and critically evaluate individual research papers. Medical research papers usually follow a set structure. The introduction should provide an accurate summary of current knowledge of the topic covered in the paper, give a rationale for the current study, and state clear research aims or hypotheses. The methods section should describe the study methods in sufficient detail that other researchers could replicate the study if they wanted to. The results section should present the results of any statistical or qualitative analyses conducted to address the stated research questions or hypotheses. The discussion should give an accurate description of how the results of the study relate to existing knowledge and the implications for clinical practice.

Box 17.2 outlines several questions to ask when critically reading research papers. These questions cover all four sections of the research papers just described. This list is adapted from Greenhalgh's book, *How to Read a Paper*, which also gives useful tips for reading the different types of papers that appear in medical journals (Greenhhalgh, 2014).

BOX 17.2   How to read a research paper

The following questions may be helpful for guiding critical reading of papers reporting original research. Not all of them will apply to all study designs. You may not be able to answer all of these questions at this stage of your education, but you should aim to be able to.

- Where was the paper published?
  - journal esteem is a good first indicator of the quality of a study
- Was the study original?
  - does the introduction give thorough coverage of existing knowledge of the topic?
  - what does the study offer in terms of new information?
- Who were the participants/patients?
  - how were people selected for the study?
  - who was included/excluded?
  - was it a 'real life' study or an experimental study?
- Was the study design appropriate?
  - what was done and how was it assessed?
- What was done to reduce bias?
  - was it necessary to have a control group (or groups)?
  - were participants randomised to groups?
- Was the treatment/intervention complete?
  - did all participants complete all requirements?
  - was there differential attrition (i.e. did people who dropped out differ from those who completed the study)?
- Was the assessment/analysis blind?
  - did the researchers know who was getting which treatment?
- Were the preliminary statistical issues addressed?
  - was the sample size big enough?
  - was the duration of follow-up long enough to detect effects on key outcomes?
- Were appropriate analyses conducted?
  - were the appropriate statistical or qualitative analyses conducted?
  - where necessary, was there adjustment for differences in the number of participants who dropped out?

(Continued)

- Were the conclusions supported by the analysis?
    - did the authors 'cherry pick' results that supported their argument?
    - were alternative explanations of the results considered?
    - was the influence of unmeasured explanatory factors considered?
- Were all conflicts of interest declared?
    - were all sources of funding and all researcher interests stated clearly?

Summary

- Evidence-based practice (EBP) means integrating the best research evidence with clinical judgement and knowledge of each patient.
- Different sources of information may be more or less useful for the practice of EBP. The availability of research syntheses may facilitate EBP.
- To practise EBP, medical professionals need to be able to assess the quality of individual research papers.

17.2 ADHERENCE TO TREATMENT

One important focus of EBP is an understanding of **adherence** to treatment. Better adherence results in better clinical outcomes (DiMatteo et al., 2002). It is therefore worrying that around 20–30% of patients across a range of medical conditions do not take all of their medication as prescribed (Their et al., 2008). Non-adherence results not only in poorer outcomes for people, but also huge avoidable healthcare costs.

Most adherence research has focused on adherence to medication, but the notion of non-adherence may also apply to other forms of medical treatment or therapy (e.g. exercise or physiotherapy) or behaviour modification (e.g. diet). The terms 'adherence' and 'compliance' are often used interchangeably. However, it has been argued that 'adherence' is preferable because it implies the active involvement of the person in treatment processes, whereas 'compliance' implies that people simply follow doctors' orders.

The relationship between adherence and non-adherence should be thought of not in binary terms but rather in terms of a continuum of 'more or less' adherence. This approach counters the idea that there is a 'non-compliant patient' type and acknowledges that adherence may not be perfect even in those who are strongly motivated to adhere. It also means we need to think of adherence in broad terms and consider the various ways in which people may deviate from a prescribed treatment:

- Taking too little of the prescribed treatment (e.g. too little of recommended exercise).
- Taking too much of the prescribed treatment (e.g. exceeding prescribed drug dosages).
- Not taking the treatment at the prescribed intervals (e.g. exercising too frequently or not as frequently as required).
- Not taking the treatment for the prescribed duration (e.g. ceasing antibiotic medication when one feels better).
- Taking other medication without the knowledge of the prescribing medical professional.

ACTIVITY 17.1

- Think back to the last time you were prescribed medication.
- Did you take all the doses? Did you take all of the doses at the prescribed times?
- If not, why not?

17.2.1 REASONS FOR NON-ADHERENCE: UNINTENTIONAL OR INTENTIONAL?

It is useful to distinguish between intentional and unintentional reasons for non-adherence (Myers & Midence, 1998). There may be various reasons for **unintentional non-adherence**. People may not understand the instructions for treatment or may forget the instructions. Non-adherence may occur because people find it difficult to follow their regimen or simply forget to take doses. To reduce non-adherence we need to consider:

- People's understanding and recall of information (see Chapter 10).
- People's motivation (see Chapter 2).
- The provision of resources to facilitate adherence.

Poor practitioner–patient communication underlies much unintentional non-adherence (see Chapter 18).

Intentional non-adherence occurs when people decide not to follow a treatment regimen. A useful model of behaviour in the domain of adherence is the **self-regulation model** of illness representations (see Chapter 4), which has also been referred to as the common-sense model of self-regulation (Leventhal et al., 2016). This model highlights the need to pay attention to a person's understanding of their illness, including its cause and treatment. According to this model, there are three important aspects of self-regulatory processes. The first is rational planning of responses to illness; the second is emotional responses to illness and its treatment; the third component is the person's monitoring and appraisal of their behaviour and of the progress of treatment. This model therefore emphasises the person's ability to reflect on his/her actions and their consequences. It also highlights the constant interaction between the three components – beliefs, emotions, and appraisal. This model helps explain the various reasons for non-adherence, including defensive coping or denial of the threat posed by the illness, missing medication doses to avoid unpleasant side effects, or stopping treatment early when symptoms subside.

17.2.2 REASONS FOR NON-ADHERENCE: MULTIFACETED MODELS

Although the intentional/unintentional distinction discussed above is helpful, multifaceted models of adherence are probably more useful in prompting clinicians to identify and address a range of barriers to adherence. Recent reviews of research have identified several important characteristics of individuals, medical conditions, and treatment regimens (Beatty & Binnion, 2016; Gellad et al., 2011; Kardas et al., 2013; Zwikker et al., 2014). These are illustrated in Figure 17.2 and Case Study 17.1.

Disease factors

Adherence tends to be better when people experience symptoms of illness. This has clear implications for medical conditions with fluctuating symptoms (e.g. asthma) or no symptoms (e.g. hypertension). For less serious conditions, better adherence is found among people with poorer health. For serious conditions, worse adherence is found among people with poorer health. This difference may arise because people with more serious conditions have more physical, practical, and psychological barriers to adherence.

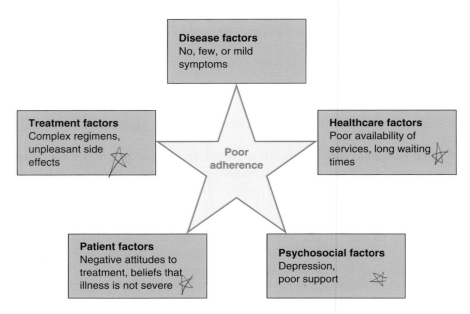

FIGURE 17.2   Multidimensional model of barriers to adherence

CASE STUDY 17.1 Barriers to adherence to antiretroviral medication for HIV

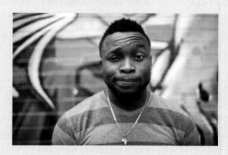

Ben is 40 and was diagnosed with HIV 15 years ago. He has not been diagnosed with AIDS and his health has generally been good. He has been using combination antiretroviral therapy (ART) since his diagnosis. He has changed medication several times to make it easier to manage the timing and number of the doses of drugs. He is currently taking two antiretroviral medications – one of which is a combination of two drugs – in three doses. Ben finds this combination much easier to adhere to than earlier prescriptions:

It's so much easier having the combination pill. Before I started this I had to take three different drugs – one twice a day, one three times a day, and the other one once a day. I also had to try to have some on an empty stomach.

Like many people using ART, Ben has experienced unpleasant side effects such as nausea and headaches. When changing to his current medication, he initially developed a rash and experienced some insomnia. He has also experienced lipodystrophy – a redistribution of body fat caused by a disturbance in the fat metabolism – and his finger and toenails have become discoloured.

Obviously, I haven't been really sick yet, and I want to stay that way. Taking these drugs is probably the best way for me to stay healthy, but the side effects do sometimes make me wonder... I'm also worried about what all these drugs are doing to my liver.

Although Ben tries to maintain his adherence to his medication, and this has been helped by a simpler drug regimen, he does still sometimes miss doses:

Sometimes you go out and you meet someone, and one thing leads to another, and you end up going back to their house, and you don't take your medication. But that's usually only one or two doses. So, I hope that's not going to matter in the long run... it doesn't seem to have so far.

This case study shows how adherence can be affected by a range of factors, including a rational consideration of the potential benefits, concerns about the immediate and long-term side effects, and the difficulties of matching treatment regimens and lifestyles.

Treatment factors

Adherence falls as the complexity or burden of dosing regimens increases. It is generally easier for people to adhere to single daily doses than multiple daily doses and their associated timing schedules. It is also easier to adhere to regimens that do not involve multiple medications, specific times, or dietary requirements. Adherence rates are lower when people experience unpleasant medication side effects.

Patient factors

Adherence is not strongly influenced by demographic factors such as age, sex, or socio-economic status. However, as noted in the discussion of intentional non-adherence, people's beliefs exert an important influence on adherence. As predicted by conceptual frameworks such as the Health Belief Model (see Chapter 5), better adherence is found when:

- People believe their condition is serious.
- People perceive more benefits from adherence.
- There are fewer barriers to adherence.
- People are more motivated.

Barriers to treatment include people not agreeing with their diagnosis or treatment plan. They may also include concerns about side effects or the long-term effects of medication (Horne et al., 2013).

Psychosocial factors

Psychosocial factors are also important. Adherence tends to be poorer in people who are depressed and have lower levels of social support (Grenard et al., 2011). In addition to direct practical or emotional encouragement for treatment adherence, social support may have more general effects. For example, adherence is greater among people in families that are more cohesive and have less conflict.

Healthcare factors

Practical issues, such as accessibility of services and waiting times, may affect adherence. One aspect of healthcare systems that has received much attention is **practitioner–patient communication** and the practitioner–patient relationship. A fuller consideration of the importance of practitioner–patient communication is given in the next section of this chapter but poor communication may be a reason for non-adherence. Adherence tends to be better if people have longer consultations and a trusting relationship with a healthcare practitioner who expresses a genuine interest in their health. Better practitioner–patient relationships lead to better adherence. Figure 17.3 displays the ways in which better practitioner–patient communication can lead to better adherence and better outcomes for patients.

Adherence is also influenced by the provision of information by healthcare professionals and the efficient use of this information. The exchange of information should not just focus on facts about illness and its treatment, but also on the emotional concerns of the patient (see Chapter 18). Good communication skills are required to elicit people's beliefs, to respond to them sensitively, and to include these when developing a treatment plan that will be most likely to be adhered to (see Chapter 18).

Adherence is better when people are satisfied with the amount of information given and when they are able to understand and recall this information (see Clinical notes 10.3). People need information to:

- Help them to be adherent.
- Counter fears or misconceptions about their treatment.
- Counter feelings that they have not received adequate attention.

However, more information is not always a good thing. Too much information can hamper efficient decision making. Information about low treatment efficacy or side effects may lead to lower adherence rates.

CLINICAL NOTES 17.2

Agreeing treatment plans

- Discuss the person's beliefs, concerns, and intentions relating to treatment. Where possible, customise the regimen in accordance with their wishes.
- Simplify the regimen as much as possible.
- Provide simple, clear instructions for taking medication.
- Elicit the person's feelings about her or his ability to follow the regimen and discuss strategies for enhancing adherence.
- Consider the use of medication-taking systems, including electronic reminders.
- Emphasise the value of the prescribed regimen and the important of adherence for producing the best treatment outcomes.
- Obtain any necessary help from family members, friends, etc.

(Osterberg & Blaschke, 2005)

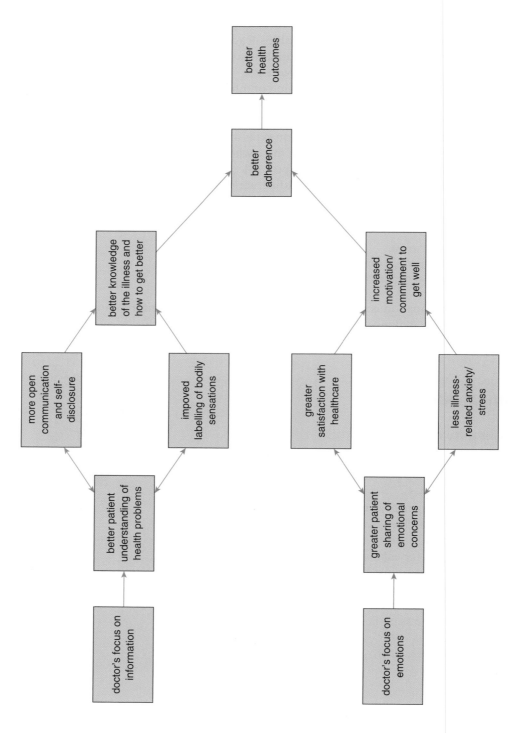

FIGURE 17.3 How better practitioner–patient communication leads to better adherence (adapted from Squier, 1990)

The value of recorded information – in print, digital, or video format – is becoming more widely acknowledged, particularly for complex treatment regimens. Although written information such as instructions or leaflets may help to increase adherence, such information needs to be discussed with people to ensure that they understand the content. Combinations of verbal and written information may be more effective than either verbal or written information in isolation. Combined approaches can repeat and reinforce information, as well as emphasise that the practitioner is interested in the person's understanding of the information and the importance of adherence. The benefits of written information can be further enhanced if that information can be customised or tailored to each patient (as opposed to generic letters, leaflets, or video resources).

17.2.3 STRATEGIES FOR IMPROVING ADHERENCE

Various methods can be used to help people follow through on their intentions to take medication. These include: specific action plans or implementation intentions, clear written or printed information, and the use of electronic reminders, smartphone apps, or monitors of medication use (Hood et al., 2016; Howren et al., 2013; Petrie et al., 2012; Rosen et al., 2002).

A systematic review of interventions found that many are not successful and that many of those which are successful produce only modest improvements in adherence (Nieuwlaat et al., 2014). The fact that many of the interventions are complex and multifaceted means that it is difficult to determine the relative importance of various components. Nevertheless, the evidence suggests that to increase adherence it may be important to: provide information, reminders, counselling, support, and reinforcement; explore the patient's beliefs about their condition and its treatment; discuss the severity of the person's illness; and emphasise the importance of adherence before treatment begins.

Adherence tends to be better when the practitioner and patient are able to talk about it in a non-judgemental way (Noble, 1998; Young et al., 2016). It is preferable that such discussions happen when treatment is being decided on, rather than after the non-adherence has occurred. It is also important to monitor adherence and to give appropriate feedback to people (see Clinical notes 17.3).

CLINICAL NOTES 17.3

Increasing adherence

- Monitor adherence. Watch for the markers of non-adherence, such as missed appointments, missed refills, and a lack of response to medication.

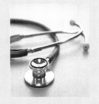

(Continued)

- Express approval of adherence and encourage continued adherence. When appropriate, include objective measures of improvement due to treatment.
- Ask the person about non-adherence and barriers to adherence in an understanding, non-confrontational way.
- If adherence appears unlikely, consider prescribing more 'forgiving' medications – i.e. medications whose efficacy is less affected by missed doses. Options may include: medications with long half-lives, depot (extended-release) medications, or transdermal medication.

(Osterberg & Blaschke, 2005)

Summary

- Many people find it difficult to adhere to treatment regimens.
- Poorer adherence is related to poorer health outcomes.
- A range of factors affect the likelihood of adherence to treatment regimens, including characteristics of the disease, treatment, and patient and healthcare factors.
- Adherence should be discussed at the time treatment is prescribed. Patients should also be given feedback on their adherence.

17.3 PRACTITIONER–PATIENT COMMUNICATION

In addition to helping improve adherence, practitioners who communicate better with their patients are more likely to detect emotional distress in people and respond to it appropriately, make accurate, comprehensive diagnoses, and have patients who are more satisfied with their care and less anxious about their health (Lloyd & Bor, 2009). People often receive less information than they desire from healthcare professionals, and practitioners tend to overestimate the time they spend giving information and answering questions.

Information given to patients should be tailored to their needs and capacities. Practitioners must pay attention to the complexity of their language and the speed of delivery. They should check that a person understands the information they have been given. They should also attend to how a person's emotions may affect their capacity to take in information and recall it after a consultation. (A fuller description of clinical interview skills is given in Chapter 18.)

To understand why practitioner–patient communication is such a powerful phenomenon it is important to consider the purposes of medical communication, the communication behaviours practitioners use, and the influence of communication skills on patient outcomes (Ong et al., 1995). Each of these aspects of communication is described below.

17.3.1 PURPOSES OF MEDICAL COMMUNICATION

Practitioner–patient relationship

One purpose of medical communication is to develop a good practitioner–patient relationship. In psychotherapy, it is understood that a good therapeutic relationship is essential for successful interventions. Although Rogers' (1951) 'client-centred' approach was developed for psychotherapy, several of its principles also apply to practitioner–patient relationships. Practitioners should aim to be non-judgemental, respectful, and empathic by eliciting and responding sensitively to people's concerns. Practitioners should also be aware of the appropriate use of silence and non-verbal behaviour (see Chapter 18). They should also be attentive to what a patient is saying by paraphrasing or reflecting back to the person what they have said. In addition, they need to be aware of what that patient is *un*able to say. Practitioners who employ such techniques are more likely to detect underlying and undeclared emotional concerns (e.g. Del Piccolo et al., 2014; Girón et al., 1998). Practitioners who attend to patients' emotional wellbeing are better able to reduce the anxiety or other heightened emotions which can impair attention being paid to medical information and the later recall of such information (see Chapter 10). Research shows that patients are more satisfied with practitioners who take a partnership approach to treatment that facilitates patient autonomy and involvement through activities such as listening and explanation on the part of the practitioner (see Chapter 18) (Oliveira et al., 2012; Tak et al., 2015).

ACTIVITY 17.2

- Think back to the last time you consulted a healthcare professional.
- How many of the behaviours just mentioned were displayed by the healthcare professional?
- Was the healthcare professional empathic? If so, how did they display their empathy?
- Which undesirable behaviours did they display?
- Reflecting on your own experiences as a patient can be used to improve your own communication skills as a healthcare professional.

Exchanging information

The patient-centred approach emphasises that patients should feel able to express all of their reasons for consulting a healthcare professional, whether these relate to symptoms or emotions. However, clinical interviews cannot be *completely* patient-centred: healthcare professionals do need to gather necessary information from the patient. The ideal medical interview, therefore, will be collaborative, and will integrate patient-centred and practitioner-centred approaches (see Figure 18.2). One pan-European study revealed some differences between countries, but greater similarities in people's preferences for doctors' communication styles (Elnegaard et al., 2015).

Just because a patient is given information there is no guarantee that there will be a transfer of knowledge or skills, or changes in behaviour. Any information given must be understood and used in positive and productive ways. Patients actively process information according to their pre-existing beliefs and understanding. As noted in Chapter 10, memory is an active process with a limited working capacity. Information provided to a person may, therefore, not be remembered:

- if it is not understood in the first place.
- if too much information is given.
- if the information is not stored in memory (i.e. through repetition or rehearsal).

Much of the information given to patients does get forgotten or cannot be recalled accurately (Kessels, 2003). One way to increase the likelihood that information is understood in the first place is to ask patients to put into their own words what they have been told and to then correct any inaccuracies. However, this kind of checking of patients' comprehension is rare (Braddock et al., 1997; Katz et al., 2012).

As noted elsewhere (see Chapter 10), it is also important to consider how strong emotions such as someone's fear and anxiety about their health can affect memory processes by limiting their attentional focus during consultations and thereby reducing the amount of information that they can recall (Kessels, 2003). Recall of information can be improved by developing and using recordings of important information and/or written materials prepared in a patient-friendly style (Watson & McKinstry, 2009). For example, one review of research found that pictures that are relevant to written or verbal information can markedly increase the attention people pay to health information, and their later recall of it (Houts et al., 2006). Another review revealed that audio-visual materials can enhance understanding and recall of information relevant to informed consent procedures for treatment (Schenker et al., 2011).

Medical decision making

In recent decades the paternalistic approach to practitioner–patient relationships – where the practitioner directs the care and makes decisions – has been replaced by a **shared decision making** approach. This term should not be taken to imply a 50/50 share in decision making, because patients may not feel capable of making decisions and may be worried about being responsible if they choose a treatment that is not effective. However, patients should be given as much information as they want about different treatment options before a final decision is made.

Charles et al. (1997) identified four characteristics of shared decision making:

- *Shared decision making involves at least two participants*: The minimum requirement is that a healthcare professional and patient are involved. Other parties may include relatives (e.g. parents), advocates, interpreters, or legal guardians. In some cases, more than one healthcare professional may be involved in decisions about treatment.
- *Both parties must share information*: The minimum requirement is that healthcare professionals give information about a treatment in order to gain informed consent. However, people may bring important information about their circumstances and may have also gathered their own information about treatment options (some of which will be valid, some of which will not). It is important to bear in mind that people may want information for reassurance rather than to become involved in decision making.
- *Both parties must make an effort to be involved*: Although both the healthcare professional and patient should be involved in decision making, different patients may prefer different levels of involvement.
- *A decision must be made and both parties must agree to it*: It is important to consider both the process and outcome of shared decision making. Possible outcomes of shared decision making include no decision, disagreement between the healthcare professional and patient, or agreement about a treatment plan.

Different patients will approach medical encounters in different ways, so healthcare professionals must be adaptable when it comes to decision making. In some situations, shared decision making is not necessarily the 'optimal' mode of decision making (Murray et al., 2006). Patients may not want to share the responsibility for decision making, and will instead prefer an 'informed' model in which they are provided with as much information as they want but can leave the decisions to the healthcare professional. Because patients vary in their desire for involvement in decision making, healthcare professionals must have the necessary skills, patient knowledge, and time to determine when and why patients wish to be involved (McKinstry, 2000). However, the research evidence suggests that the behaviour of many healthcare professionals precludes shared decision making (see Research Box 17.1). To some extent this reflects healthcare professionals' beliefs and behaviour, but structural factors, such as the duration of consultations, may also hamper them.

RESEARCH BOX 17.1   How common is shared decision making?

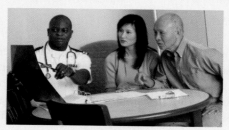

Background

Shared decision making is an important part of patient-centred care. This study was designed to determine how often shared decision making occurs and how it can be encouraged.

Method and findings

The study examined recordings of 62 primary care consultations. Researchers looked at whether criteria for shared decision making had been met in terms of:

1. Both the patient and doctor are involved.
2. Both parties share information.
3. Both parties take steps to reach a consensus about the preferred treatment.
4. An agreement is reached about treatment.

Results showed that the first two criteria (both patient and doctor being involved and sharing information) were not always met. When these first two criteria are not met it is highly unlikely that the last two criteria can be met. For example, dosage and side effects were not always discussed when new medication was prescribed. Furthermore, the fact that many doctors have no idea of their patients' views of medicine makes it harder to decide on the treatment that is most likely to be adhered to.

In interviews, doctors identified several barriers to shared decision making:

*   Time pressures – one suggested it would take an hour to satisfy all four criteria.
*   The assumption that patients merely wanted their problems solved and so doctors gave prescriptions without sharing the decision making.
*   Doubt over people's ability to understand medical terms and information.

Significance

This study shows that more effort is needed to ensure that the sharing of information occurs so as to increase the likelihood of shared decision making about treatment.

Stevenson, F.A., Barry, C.A., Britten, N., Barber, N. & Bradley, C.P. (2000) Doctor–patient communication about drugs: The evidence for shared decision making. *Social Science & Medicine*, 50: 829–840.

17.3.2 COMMUNICATION BEHAVIOURS IN MEDICAL SETTINGS

Analyses of practitioner–patient communication indicate that asking questions is one of the most common practitioner behaviours after giving information and instructions (Bensing et al., 2003; Clayton & Dudley, 2009; Roter et al., 1988). However, such questions are most likely to be closed yes/no questions during the history-taking phase and are more likely to be **instrumental behaviour** (exchanges of facts) rather than **affective behaviour** (sharing emotions) (Mjaaland & Finest, 2009). Time pressures are often cited as a reason for a lack of attention to affective behaviours, as well as a barrier to shared decision making (see Research Box 17.1). However, longer consultations do not necessarily mean greater attention being paid to people's emotions and concerns. One comparative study of US and Dutch physicians identified four different communication patterns which varied in their relative attention to affective and instrumental behaviours (Bensing et al., 2003). There was also variation between countries, suggesting that medical training and professional cultures influence practitioners' attention to affective issues.

Reviews of the research reveal some important sex differences in practitioner–patient communication. Female physicians are more likely to engage in patient-centred behaviours, whether this relates to shared decision making or affective behaviour. In turn, patients speak more in consultations with female physicians (Jefferson et al., 2013; Sandhu et al., 2009). This may mean that fewer consultations are possible. However, not only do patients share more emotional/affective information in longer patient-centred consultations, but they also share more biomedical/instrumental information.

For both male and female practitioners, communication skills can be enhanced by communication skills interventions and training (Berkhof et al., 2011; Rao et al., 2007). Such training should include active, practice-oriented strategies such as role-play, feedback, and small group discussions. There is also evidence that interventions aimed at patients can improve practitioner–patient communication (D'Agostino et al., 2017). Although research has tended to focus on verbal behaviour, nonverbal behaviour is also very important – particularly for communicating emotions (Ong et al., 1995). The full range of communication behaviours employed in medical consultations and their effects is covered in more detail in Chapter 18.

17.3.3 THE INFLUENCE OF COMMUNICATION SKILLS ON PATIENT OUTCOMES

Research reviews confirm that better practitioner–patient communication can result in a range of better patient outcomes, including better emotional wellbeing, the resolution of symptoms, improved functioning, better physiological measures, and better pain control (Boerebach et al., 2014; De Vries et al., 2014). The verbal behaviours that appear to be related to better patient outcomes include patient-centred questioning and empathic responses to patients, along with summarising and clarifying information given to, and received from, patients. Important nonverbal behaviours include adopting an open and direct posture, leaning toward the patient, and nodding where appropriate (Henry et al., 2012). Longer consultations and friendliness and courtesy on the part of practitioners also tend to produce better outcomes.

Better practitioner–patient communication appears to lead to better patient outcomes via several routes (Street et al., 2009). Better communication leads to better proximal outcomes, including mutual understanding, patient satisfaction, trust, decision making, agreement about treatment, and patient motivation (De Vries et al., 2014; Henry et al., 2012). Better intermediate outcomes include better adherence and self-care by patients, both of which lead to improved health outcomes (DiMatteo et al., 2002; Moore et al., 2004). These processes are reflected in Figure 17.3, which was introduced in the section on adherence. It has been suggested that better practitioner–patient relationships may act as a form of social support (Ong et al., 1995). As a result, it has been argued that for the best outcomes clinicians and patients should focus on the proximal and intermediate outcomes of respect, trust, and a commitment to adherence (Street et al., 2009).

17.3.4 COMMUNICATION ABOUT RISK

One important aspect of medical communication is the discussion of risk. However, there are many barriers to people's understanding of risk. As noted earlier, people do not passively receive risk information; rather, they actively process it according to their pre-existing knowledge, beliefs, and preferences (Leventhal et al., 2003; Marteau & Weinman, 2004). Although many models of health behaviour are based on rational decision making (see Chapter 5), it is important to consider the emotional content of medical information. We must also consider whether people can understand risk information in the forms in which it is frequently communicated.

Understanding risk information

One difficulty in communicating risk information is that there are numerous ways to calculate and present risks. Information is often presented in the form of a **relative risk** – e.g. 'Smokers are 10 times more likely than non-smokers to develop lung cancer'. Such information is derived from population-based research which compares the relative likelihood of an outcome (e.g. lung cancer) in people exposed or not exposed to a risk factor such as smoking. Although such data are extremely useful at a population level, it is difficult to convert them into numbers that apply to individuals.

Individuals are more likely to be persuaded by an **absolute risk** – e.g. 'If you continue to smoke there is a 20% chance you will develop lung cancer in the next ten years'. However, absolute risks may be difficult to calculate because you will need to incorporate a range of risk factors. Regardless of whether risk information is presented in relative or absolute terms, risk figures are always estimates which have margins of error – often given as **confidence intervals**. However, providing patients with risk estimates as well as confidence intervals may in fact hinder, rather than aid, comprehension. Simpler numerical information may be preferable because it is easier for people to understand.

Many people have difficulty understanding health statistics and probabilities. The fact that many healthcare professionals also have difficulty understanding probabilities makes it even harder to convey this information accurately to patients (Gigerenzer et al., 2008). This difficulty with medical statistics is a specific aspect of a broader phenomenon. It could be argued that lotteries and the gambling industry rely on the fact that people do not understand probability and statistics! However, patients need to understand risk information so they can participate in shared decision making. To maximise people's comprehension of numerical risk information it is recommended that healthcare professionals use 'real' numbers rather than probabilities (Gigerenzer et al., 2008: see also Table 17.1). Decision aids, such as pictorial representations, may also help people to understand different event likelihoods (Edwards et al., 2002; Garcia-Retamero et al., 2012; Reyna et al., 2009).

Emotional responses to risk information

Even when people understand statistical risks they do not necessarily apply these probabilities to themselves. Affective responses to risk information are an important influence on subsequent behaviour. People can often find exceptions to statistical risk information and apply these to their own preferred patterns of behaviour. For example, a heavy smoker who does not want to follow a recommendation to quit may say 'My grandmother smoked all of her life, and she lived to 94'. A common phenomenon is **unrealistic optimism** about health (Weinstein, 1987): that is, people often feel that they are less likely than other people to experience negative health outcomes and more likely to experience positive outcomes. Unrealistic optimism reduces the likelihood that people will engage in a healthy behaviour change, particularly when they believe they have some control over health outcomes (Klein & Helweg-Larsen, 2002).

To counter unrealistic optimism we must convince patients that the risks are real and serious (Floyd et al., 2000). Some health promotion campaigns use shocking graphic images in order to emphasise the seriousness of health risks and prompt behaviour changes (e.g. images of fatty deposits being squeezed from the arteries of deceased smokers, or graphic images of a motor vehicle accident). In one-to-one medical consultations, techniques based on shock or fear may be employed (e.g. 'If you don't stop smoking you'll die before you're 60'). A paradox of risk communication is that a certain amount of anxiety may be necessary to motivate a behaviour, whereas too much anxiety can lead to inappropriate responses, such as the denial of real risks. If information or images are too shocking or frightening they may cause defensive avoidance of the issue – i.e. people will stop thinking about their behaviour and its associated risks because they do not want to think about the feared outcome. Shocking images that appeal to the sense of fear are most likely to be successful when they are accompanied by clear information about what people can do to avoid undesirable outcomes and programmes are designed to help them carry out healthy behaviours (Ruiter et al., 2014).

TABLE 17.1   Recommendations for communicating risk information (adapted from Gigerenzer et al., 2008)

	What to aim for...	**What to avoid...**
Use frequency statements instead of single-event probabilities	Four out of 10 patients taking this medication will experience insomnia	There is a 40% likelihood of insomnia from taking this medication
Use absolute risks instead of relative risks	Mammograms reduce the risk of dying from breast cancer from five in 1,000 to four in 1,000	Mammograms reduce the risk of dying from breast cancer by 20%
Use mortality rates instead of survival rates	There are three prostate cancer deaths per 1,000 men in the USA, compared to two per 1,000 men in the UK	The five-year survival rate for men with prostate cancer is 98% in the USA and 71% in the UK

Summary

- Practitioner–patient communication serves many purposes and is an important aspect of patient-centred care.
- If people receive the information they need and are able to use this as part of decision making about treatment, they are more likely to be satisfied with consultations, adhere to treatment, and experience positive outcomes.
- Better practitioner–patient communication will result in improved practitioner–patient relationships and exchanges of important information, better medical decision making, and more positive outcomes.
- Communication about risk is an important aspect of medical communication. However, many patients (and healthcare professionals) have difficulty understanding the meaning of risk data. In addition, people's emotional responses to risk information may help or hinder healthy behaviour.

FURTHER READING

Greenhalgh, T. (2014) *How to Read a Paper: The Basics of Evidence-Based Medicine* (5th edition). Oxford: Blackwell. A useful guide on how to approach and make sense of research papers. Includes how to approach different kinds of papers, literature searches, and statistics.

Straus, S.E., Richardson, W.S., Glasziou, P. & Haynes, R.B. (2010) *Evidence-Based Medicine: How to Practice and Teach EBM* (4th edition). London: Elsevier. This book is written mainly for experienced practitioners but does include some useful information that is suitable for students.

Goldacre, B. (2008) *Bad Science*. London: Fourth Estate. Written by a journalist, this book provides an accessible critique of the use and misuse of evidence in mainstream media reporting of health and science issues.

REVISION QUESTIONS

1. Give a definition of evidence-based practice (EBP).

2. Why is it important for medical professionals to practise EBP?

3. What is meant by the hierarchy of evidence in EBP? What distinguishes sources of evidence higher in the hierarchy from those further down?

4. Describe the differences between intentional and unintentional non-adherence.

5. Outline the range of factors which influence adherence to a prescribed treatment.

6. Describe the different purposes of practitioner–patient communication.

7. Describe the characteristics of shared decision making as identified by Charles et al. (1997).

8. Better practitioner–patient communication leads to better patient outcomes. Outline the mechanisms that explain this link.

18 CLINICAL INTERVIEWING

(Continued)

Figures

Research box

LEARNING OBJECTIVES

This chapter is designed to enable you to:

- Describe different ways we communicate.
- Recognise the importance of the person's agenda in clinical interviews.
- Outline communication skills for different stages of the clinical interview.
- Describe effective ways to deal with strong emotions in the clinical interview, such as anger, anxiety, and distress.
- Consider important factors when giving bad news.

Most clinicians do between 140,000 and 160,000 clinical interviews during their career (Frankel & Sherman, 2015). As we have seen in the previous chapter, how we communicate in clinical consultations is an important part of good medical practice. Good communication is associated with more accurate diagnoses, enhanced understanding, better adherence to treatment, greater satisfaction, and improved physical and emotional outcomes for patients. Good communication is also associated with less iatrogenesis (i.e. adverse effects or complications), fewer complaints, and less litigation.

Communication in clinical settings requires particular skills. Communication skills training may involve mock clinical interviews, role-play, video recording, and feedback. Some students find this kind of training artificial but evidence shows it is an effective way to learn these skills. For example, one study evaluated third-year medical students' performance in clinical exams (OSCEs) before and after communication skills training was introduced. Students who had communication skills training did better in their OSCEs. They were rated as more competent, having a better relationship with the patient, and being better at clinical assessment, negotiation, and decision making. They also showed better organisation and time management during the consultation (Yedidia et al., 2003).

In this chapter we shall start by examining how we communicate through verbal and nonverbal behaviour. The second section looks at clinical interviewing, including different models of clinical interviews as well as specific skills and techniques to use in clinical interviews. The final section considers the communication skills required in difficult encounters, such as how to cope with angry or upset people, or when giving bad news.

18.1 HOW WE COMMUNICATE

Communication is the process through which people provide and exchange information through a common system of signs, symbols, or behaviour. Communication in healthcare is frequently thought of in terms of verbal and nonverbal behaviour in one-to-one consultations. However, the increase in e-health and tele-health means care is increasingly provided through technology such as text or in-app messaging, email, video, or telephone consultations. This raises further challenges in terms of communication in clinical consultations.

18.1.1 VERBAL COMMUNICATION

Verbal communication includes both *what* we say and *how* we say it. Speech is often surprisingly disjointed, but we are still able to understand the message being conveyed. The example below is a man talking about his sexual activity.

> Question: 'How important is it to be sexually active?'
>
> 'Sexually active is important. It is just now. Well... I've got – I don't treat women very well, I suppose. My mum always gets on my back for this, but I don't – I mean I cheat on them, and I deceive them, which is wrong, and I know it's wrong, but I think I'm kind of insecure in myself in that respect. Which is... I don't know why, but I just am. Yeah... I like to have sex quite a lot.'

In day-to-day interaction many factors are used to interpret the meaning of what is said – including nonverbal behaviour and the social context. Consequently, even if *what* we say is very clear, people may still misinterpret it because of their expectations, beliefs, social context, the speech characteristics (e.g. our tone of voice), and nonverbal behaviour.

At a simple level, communication can be conceptualised as a messaging process where a message is encoded, transmitted, and received. It is possible for communication to break down at each of these stages. The message might be ambiguous, that is, difficulty may result from the way we write or say the message (*encoding*), the message might not transmit properly through faulty technology, delivery or noise (*message transmission*), or the other person might misinterpret the message (difficulty *decoding*).

In medical practice, the words we use and the way we say things are both important. The way in which questions are asked can also influence how people respond. **Closed questions**, which tend to start with words like *did*, *is*, *have*, *can*, require people to respond in fixed ways (typically, by saying *yes* or *no*). Such questions are useful for obtaining specific information or clarifying points, such as '*Have you taken any medication for this?*' or

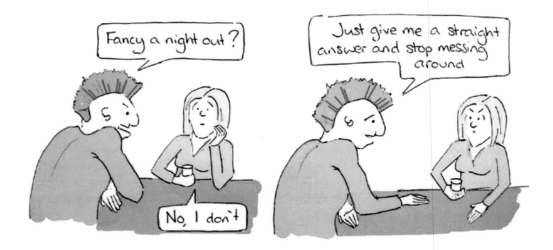

'*Is the pain sharp or dull?*' The disadvantage of closed questions is that very limited amounts of information are obtained. **Open questions**, on the other hand, encourage respondents to talk freely and tend to start with *what, how, when, why*, etc. Such questions are useful because they encourage the patient to express what is important in their own words, for example '*What have you come to see me about today?*' or '*What does the pain feel like?*' The disadvantage is that they are less well suited for reaching definite goals or clarifying points.

Open and closed questions are both useful in clinical interviews. A common approach is the '**open-to-closed cone**' or '**funnel approach**', in which open questions predominate at the start of an interview and closed questions are used later. Open questions may be used first to obtain a broad picture of the problem from the person's perspective. This provides an opportunity for the healthcare professional to listen to the person and consider what other information might be important. The use of open questions at the beginning of an interview is extremely helpful in the exploration of problems: their power as an information-gathering tool cannot be over-emphasised. A common mistake in clinical interviews is to move to closed questions too quickly. As the interview moves on, however, using more specific open questions, probes, and closed questions can clarify information and find out more details that the person might not mention otherwise.

There are some types of questions that need to be avoided. These include multiple and leading questions. **Multiple questions** are those in which two or more questions are asked together – e.g. '*Have you seen a doctor for this and what treatment did you have?*' Such questions often result in people answering only one part of the question. **Leading questions** are those that imply a right answer – e.g. '*You don't have any pain then?*' or '*No history of heart problems?*' Questions of this type impose our own assumptions on the person and make it difficult for them to disagree. Research on forensic interviews has shown that even slight variations in wording can influence people's judgements. For example, assessing how fast a car was going when it hit a lorry will be influenced by the choice of verb used in the question (e.g. 'smash' or 'hit'): people will say the car was going faster if the word *smashed* is used (Wright & Loftus, 2008). Therefore leading questions, or questions using words that imply extent, can influence a person's responses and should be avoided.

Characteristics of speech also influence the interpretation of meaning. Features such as tone, pitch, pauses, sighs, and speed influence how speech is interpreted. These features may completely change the meaning of a sentence. For example, a sarcastic tone of voice may indicate that a person means the opposite of what they are actually saying. Speech characteristics may also be used as a guide to a person's mood. Fast, high-pitched speech usually indicates arousal, such as excitement or anxiety, whereas very slow speech can be characteristic of depression. This can be used in clinical practice to gauge and influence a person's mood. For example, if you are talking to a person who is angry or anxious, deliberately slowing your speech and using a lower pitch may help calm them.

In healthcare practice, the characteristics of our speech can influence the relationship with the person and the confidence they have in us. A study of 1,411 patients or carers in Japan found that speech (way of speaking, volume, tone, pitch, etc.) was more important than a doctor's reputation, title, attire, age, or gender in determining people's confidence in the doctor (Kurihara et al., 2014). Similarly, a study in the USA which audiotaped surgeons' consultations and rated their speech for warmth, hostility, dominance, concern, and anxiety found that surgeons who were high on dominance and low on concern or anxiety were almost three times more likely to have been sued by patients (Ambady et al., 2002).

18.1.2 NONVERBAL COMMUNICATION

Nonverbal communication plays a crucial part in communication. It includes facial expression, eye movements, spatial behaviour, posture, gestures, touch, and bodily contact. **Facial expression** is important in indicating mood or emotions, as shown in Chapter 2 (see Figure 2.2). **Eye movements** and eye contact help establish a rapport with another person. People look more at people they like, and frequent or sustained eye contact is usually a sign of attentiveness. Conversely, reduced eye contact may signal avoidance or emotional problems, such as depression. It is important to get the balance of eye contact right.

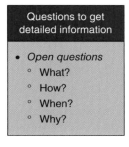
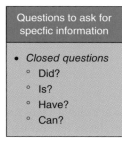
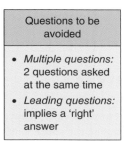

FIGURE 18.1   Different types of questions

On the one hand, we want to appear attentive, so we need to have plenty of eye contact, especially at the beginning of a consultation. On the other hand, prolonged eye contact can be interpreted as too intimate or aggressive: after all, long, and direct eye contact can be observed in courting couples, and boxers may try to intimidate their opponents by 'staring them down' before a fight.

Spatial behaviour is a form of nonverbal behaviour that may be either supportive or intimidating (see Chapter 9 for information on social roles). It has been suggested that personal space can be divided into four zones (Hall, 1966):

1. Intimate zone (0–45cm) – only lovers, close relatives, and very close friends are normally allowed into this zone.
2. Personal zone ranges (45–120cm) – friends and family members are allowed into this zone.
3. Social zone (120–360cm) – conversations with acquaintances and work colleagues usually take place in this zone.
4. Public zone (360–760cm) – this is the zone that is often used when someone is giving a talk to an audience.

These distances apply to North American and Northern European cultures. However, there are large cultural differences in the demarcation of zones. For example, many Middle Eastern, Latin American, and Mediterranean cultures favour smaller distances in ordinary conversations. This variation in norms can create problems when people from different cultures meet because the person who is used to more space may feel uncomfortable, or that the other person is assuming a closer relationship than they have. There can also be differences between certain patient groups, or under particular circumstances. For example, feeling threatened is associated with a need for greater personal space in most people (Stamps, 2011). There is evidence that people with schizophrenia often need a larger personal space zone around them, which may be due to symptoms of paranoia (Schoretsanatis et al., 2016). In contrast, people with autism spectrum disorder have a reduced personal space zone (Asada et al., 2016).

Cultures have implicit rules about the use of space which affect everything from which seat we take in a lecture to where we put our towels on a beach. If someone's personal space is invaded they will usually withdraw. If this is not possible, people may use other nonverbal behaviour to diffuse the situation. For example, if we are forced to stand close to strangers we are able to tolerate it better if eye contact is reduced (Yoshida & Hori, 1989). This probably explains why commuters on very crowded trains do not look at each other!

ACTIVITY 18.1

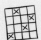

- Next time you are on a train or in a cinema, pay attention to where people sit. Usually, as long as the space is not completely full, people will try to keep a certain distance from people they do not know.

Spatial behaviour has a number of implications for clinical practice. First, we must be careful how we position ourselves in relation to the person. We must not be so close that we invade their personal space, or so far away that we signal this is a formal 'public zone' encounter. The traditional consultation room set-up, where the healthcare professional sits behind a desk, is not conducive to a good rapport. If a desk is necessary, it is far better to position ourselves at the corner so that there is no barrier between us and the person.

Second, physical examinations and procedures need to be performed with a lot of care because we are entering a person's intimate zone. Uncaring remarks or even a lack of acknowledgement of the person during this time can have a particularly negative impact because they have allowed us into their intimate space. Finally, personal space varies between individuals, so we should not assume we know what is appropriate. Instead, we should watch for nonverbal cues that a person might not be comfortable with our proximity.

Posture is an indicator of attentiveness, interest, a social relationship, and someone's attitude toward us. Closed postures, where people have their arms and legs crossed and/or are hunched, indicate a lack of engagement or defensiveness. Good postures for clinical interviewing include:

- An open posture (nothing crossed).
- Body facing toward the person.
- Attentive (leaning forward).
- Relaxed (sends the message 'I am relaxed; I have time for you').

People rate clinicians who use such postures as having more empathy and better rapport. For example, research shows that something as simple as sitting by a person's bedside rather than standing is associated with better ratings of doctors' communication, the interaction, and understanding of the person's condition, despite there being no difference in the amount of time spent with the person (Merel et al., 2016; Swayden et al., 2012).

In social situations, posture also indicates personal alliances. When people like each other they often mirror each other's posture. Research shows that mirroring strengthens the rapport with patients in clinical interviews (Sharpley et al., 2001), though it needs to be used judiciously. It is obviously not appropriate to mirror the posture of a highly anxious person who has crossed their arms and legs or is fidgeting. Mirroring is best used after the initial session, as there is some evidence it can have a negative effect if used in the first encounter (LaFrance & Ickes, 1981).

Finally, **touch** can be a very powerful, human response, particularly when someone is distressed. Touch must always be used appropriately, with due regard to the sensitivities of the person and professional codes of conduct. People vary greatly on what they consider to be acceptable touch and there are strong cultural differences.

Clinical examinations involve touch – sometimes of very intimate areas. This will be accepted by most people because of the social roles of patient and doctor or other healthcare professional. A professional intimate examination is associated with improved patient outcomes (Field et al., 2007; Kiernan, 2002). Four factors are important if we are to use touch positively (Gelb, 1982):

1. The therapeutic encounter must have clear boundaries.
2. The touch must be appropriate to the circumstances.
3. The person should feel they have control over physical contact.
4. The touch must be for the person's benefit not the therapist's.

Guidelines for physical examinations are given in the Clinical notes 18.1.

CLINICAL NOTES 18.1

Physical examinations

When carrying out clinical examinations it is basic good practice to:

*   Explain what you are going to do.
*   Ask the person's permission.
*   Ask if they have any concerns.
*   Respect their modesty.
*   Never comment on their anatomy or state while carrying out the examination.
*   Watch the person's body language for any signs of discomfort.

Summary

*   We communicate through verbal and nonverbal behaviour.
*   Verbal communication includes both what we say and how we say it.
*   Communication can break down at the stages of (a) encoding, (b) message transmission, or (c) decoding.
*   The way in which we say things (e.g. tone of voice) can override the meaning of what we say, such as when using sarcasm. Paralinguistic cues are often good indicators of emotional state.
*   Nonverbal behaviours include facial expression, eye movements, spatial behaviour, posture, and touch.
*   Good clinical interview skills include a relaxed, open posture, good eye contact, and appropriate use of space and touch.

18.2 CLINICAL INTERVIEWING

Models of the clinical interview have been developed to help healthcare professionals understand the processes involved and improve their communication and interview skills. Many models have been proposed and in this section we concentrate on two that are relevant to general consultations. The first outlines the different perspectives of clinicians and patients and encourages a more patient-centred approach to interviewing (the Patient-Centred Clinical Method; Stewart et al., 1995). The second outlines the various stages of a clinical interview and considers which communication skills and techniques may be useful for each stage (the Calgary-Cambridge model; see Silverman et al., 2013). Models that are not outlined here include the Healthcare communication E4 model (Keller & Caroll, 1994), the Three-function model (Cole & Bird, 2000), the Four habits model (Frankel & Stein, 1999), or the SEGUE Framework for teaching and assessing communication skills (Makoul, 2001).

18.2.1 THE PATIENT-CENTRED CLINICAL METHOD

The patient-centred clinical method is shown in Figure 18.2. This model highlights the importance of considering different agendas during the clinical interview. The first is the **clinician's agenda**: the clinician needs to explore and identify any underlying disease. For this reason, they need to ask about symptoms, carry out investigations, and consider differential diagnoses. The second is the **person's agenda**: this arises from the person's concern with their illness (e.g. their experience of sickness). As we have already seen in Chapter 4, people come to consultations with ideas and beliefs about what is wrong and they may have concerns about the illness and the impact it will have on them.

One strength of this model is the equal emphasis placed on the two agendas. Substantial evidence confirms the importance of considering the person's agenda and using patient-centred clinical interviews. For example, consideration of a person's beliefs and concerns in a consultation has been shown to lead to more positive perceptions of the consultation, fewer follow-up appointments, investigations, referrals (Stewart et al., 2000), complaints, and malpractice claims. People are also more likely to discuss difficult issues like a prognosis in cancer and report more satisfaction (Shields et al., 2009).

Another strength of this model is the focus on collaboration between the clinician and patient. The model specifies that, after considering the different agendas, there should be an integration of agendas and shared planning and decision making about the treatment. Evidence confirms that collaborative approaches to treatment are more effective. For example, a review of 48 studies found that consultations with a collaborative relationship where the person's perspective was considered led to better adherence in paediatric and adult samples, as well as in primary and secondary care (Arbuthnott & Sharpe, 2009). Similarly, a review of 55 studies of patient experience across a wide range of services found a good patient experience is associated with better health outcomes, adherence to treatment, preventative care, resource use, and possibly fewer adverse events (Doyle et al., 2013).

However, consideration of the person's perspective is not always carried out in practice. A review of surgeons' communication found that, although surgeons were good at providing information about surgical conditions and treatment, they rarely explored the person's concerns or feelings (Levinson et al., 2013).

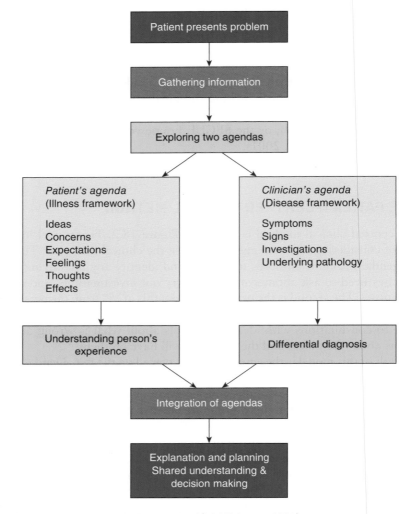

FIGURE 18.2   Patient-centred clinical method (McWhinney, 1989)

18.2.2 THE CALGARY-CAMBRIDGE MODEL

The Calgary-Cambridge model of clinical interviewing is shown in Figure 18.3. This model is different from the previous one in that it focuses on the structure of the interview and indicates what skills may be relevant to each stage of the clinical interview. It provides a clear structure that is useful for medical education because it helps us to concentrate on the learning skills that are relevant to each stage. Students can thus build up their skills as they become competent at each stage.

Initiating the session involves starting to establish a rapport with the person and identifying the reason for the consultation. The skills that the Calgary-Cambridge guide lists as important at this stage are shown in Box 18.1. It is vital, especially in hospital settings, to get your introduction right and not to assume the person knows either who you are or what the interview will involve. Getting the introduction right is not as easy as you might think. A study in the USA observed medical students' consultations in emergency medicine to see whether students acknowledged the patient, introduced themselves, identified they were a student, explained the care plan, that other providers would be involved in their care, and the duration of care. This study showed that students were good at introducing themselves in consultations (91%), but didn't always remember to identify themselves as a student (58%), or acknowledge the patient (61%). Only one consultation out of 246 managed to cover all these elements (Turner et al., 2016).

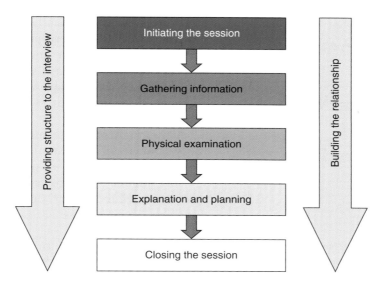

FIGURE 18.3   Calgary-Cambridge model of clinical interviewing

---

BOX 18.1   Initiating the clinical interview

Establish an initial rapport

- Greet the person and ask for or check their name.
- Introduce yourself and tell the person what your role is in their care.
- Show interest and respect for the person.
- Maintain good eye contact and body posture.

Identify the reasons for the consultation

- Use open questions to find out about the problems the person would like to discuss.
- Listen carefully to what the person says and do not interrupt.
- Check whether there is anything else the person wants to discuss (e.g. 'so you've come about these headaches, is there anything else you'd like to discuss today?')

Adapted from Silverman et al. (2013)

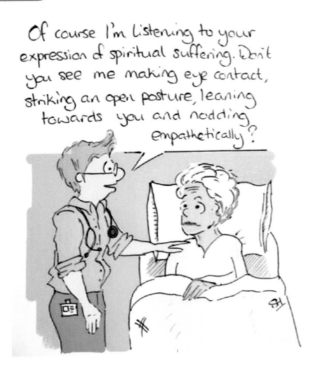

Of course I'm listening to your expression of spiritual suffering. Don't you see me making eye contact, striking an open posture, leaning towards you and nodding empathetically?

Using open questions at the beginning of the consultation is a very good way to obtain maximum information from the person – providing we then listen to what they say! A classic research study in the 1980s found that doctors interrupted a person an average of 18 seconds after they started talking (Beckman & Frankel, 1984). Yet contrary to popular belief, the more a doctor interrupts, the longer a clinical interview will typically take (Menz & Al-Roubaie, 2008). Interruptions disrupt the person's concentration and lead them to expect they will only have a few seconds to say what they want to say. Attentive listening is therefore as important as asking the right kind of questions.

Active or attentive listening is a skilled process that involves listening, facilitating responses, and picking up on cues from the person. A number of skills can be used to help the person tell their 'story' or expand on their situation. These include:

- **Encouragement:** Nonverbal and verbal encouragement, such as 'uh-huh', 'go on', or 'I see', signal that the person should go on with their story. This involves only minimal interruption and gives the person the necessary confidence to keep going. Facilitative comments should be **neutral** – e.g. not using words like 'right' or 'good' which can be misinterpreted as meaning that what the person is saying is correct.
- **Silence:** Verbal facilitation is ineffective unless it is followed by an attentive silence, yet many of us find silences uncomfortable and tend to leap in quickly if a response is not forthcoming. A useful skill therefore is to leave a slightly longer pause after the person has finished speaking before you start speaking – try counting to three in your head.
- **Reflection (echoing):** Reflecting back or echoing the last few words the person has said may encourage them to expand or continue talking. Students sometimes worry that echoing will sound unnatural but it is remarkably well accepted by people. Repetition encourages the person to continue with their last phrase so is more directive than encouragement or silence.
- **Paraphrasing:** Paraphrasing involves restating in your own words the content or feelings behind the person's message. It is not quite the same as summarising or checking because it is intended to sharpen rather than just confirm your understanding. Paraphrasing checks whether your *interpretation* of what the person said is correct.

Gathering information is the second stage of the clinical interview and involves exploring the problem further, understanding the person's perspective, and providing structure to the consultation. The communication skills that the Calgary-Cambridge guide identifies as important for this stage are shown in Box 18.2.

BOX 18.2   Gathering information

Explore the problem further

- Facilitate and clarify the person's story of the problem.
- Use open and closed questions.
- Use active listening.
- Summarise the person's points from time to time to check your understanding.
- Use clear, concise questions or comments and avoid jargon.

Understand the person's perspective

- Explore and acknowledge the person's ideas and concerns about the problem.
- Determine how it affects the person's life.
- Explore the person's goals and expectations.
- Encourage the person to express feelings and thoughts.
- Pick up on the person's verbal and nonverbal cues and check and acknowledge as appropriate.

Provide a structure to the consultation

- Summarise the person's points at the end of a line of enquiry to check for understanding before progressing.
- Signpost moving from one section to another (e.g. *'We'll come back to that in a minute, but first I would like to ask you a few questions about your family history'*).
- Sequence the interview logically.
- Use appropriate timing to keep the interview on task.

Adapted from Silverman et al. (2013)

Explanation and planning involves the aspects covered in Chapter 17. These include: providing the correct amount and type of information; aiding accurate recall and understanding; achieving a shared understanding that incorporates the person's perspective; and shared decision making. The communication skills that the Calgary-Cambridge guide lists as important for this stage are shown in Box 18.3.

The final stage of the interview consists of **closing the interview**. This stage can have a disproportionate effect on what people take away from the interview (see 'primacy and recency effect' in Chapter 10). Providing a summary of what has been discussed and agreed gives an opportunity to check that understanding has been shared and that the person is happy with the agreed treatment. In addition, **safety netting** – where we tell the person what to do if the treatment plan does not work or if other symptoms arise – may prevent future difficulties. Simple things such as asking whether there is anything else the person wants to discuss and saying goodbye properly can make a big difference to the person's experience of the consultation. The communication skills that the Calgary-Cambridge guide identifies as important for this stage are shown in Box 18.4.

BOX 18.3   Explanation and planning

Provide the correct amount and type of information

- Establish what the person knows already.
- Give information in manageable chunks.
- Check for understanding.
- Ask what other information might be helpful.
- Make sure information is given at appropriate times.

Aid accurate recall and understanding

- Organise information into logical, discrete sections.
- Use explicit categorisation or chunks (e.g. *'There are three things that are important…'*).
- Repeat and summarise information.
- Use concise statements that are easily understood and avoid jargon.
- Check their understanding at the end and clarify where necessary.

Achieve a shared understanding

- Link explanations to the person's agenda.
- Encourage the person to contribute.
- Pick up on verbal and nonverbal cues.
- Elicit the person's beliefs, reactions, and feelings about the information given.

Shared planning and decision making

- Share your own thoughts, ideas, and dilemmas as appropriate.
- Involve the person by offering suggestions rather than orders and giving the person a choice.
- Negotiate a mutually acceptable plan.
- Check with the person if the plan is acceptable and whether they have any concerns.

Adapted from Silverman et al. (2013)

In approximately one in five consultations people raise a new problem in the final stage of the interview (White et al., 1994). Often this will be the problem the person is most worried about. One way to avoid the problem being raised only at the end of the interview is to gather information as skilfully as possible earlier on. Research confirms that healthcare professionals who ask about people's beliefs, who are responsive to people, give plentiful information, and discuss treatments with people are less likely to find such new problems being raised during the closing stage of interviews (White et al., 1994).

The Calgary-Cambridge model provides a useful and detailed framework of strategies that healthcare professionals can use during different stages of a consultation.

BOX 18.4 Closing the clinical interview

- Briefly summarise the session and agreed treatment plan.
- Lay out and agree with the person the next steps both for you and them.
- Provide a safety net: explain any possible unexpected outcomes and what to do if the plan doesn't work – as well as how and when to seek help.
- Make a final check that the person agrees and is comfortable with the plan.
- Ask if there are any questions or other items to discuss.

Adapted from Silverman et al. (2013)

Since it was proposed it has formed the basis for training programmes in many countries, as well as rating scales that can be used for self-evaluation, peer evaluation, and examination of communication skills (e.g. Axboe et al., 2016; Burt et al., 2014; Edgcumbe et al., 2012; Sommer et al., 2016). Researchers have also expanded the number of strategies that can be included. For example, Lefroy et al. (2014) identified 249 different strategies students can use to improve their consultation skills either alongside or separately to the Calgary-Cambridge model. Although originally developed for medical students, the Calgary-Cambridge and Patient-centred approaches have since been used to train healthcare professionals from many disciplines, including dentistry, pharmacy, and veterinary medicine (Englar et al., 2016; Greenhill et al., 2011; Rosenzweig et al., 2016).

However, a criticism of this model is that it does not explicitly include relationship factors that are highly important, such as the quality of the therapeutic relationship, trust, and empathy. For example, a study of communication between healthcare providers and people with HIV found that when healthcare providers had greater respect for patients it was associated with consultations having a more positive emotional tone, being more patient-centred, and healthcare providers using less verbal dominance (Flickinger et al., 2016). Non-specific factors are also rated highly by lay people. Research Box 18.1 describes an international study of medical student consultations where students' affective communication skills (attitude, empathy, and listening) were more highly valued by lay people than process- or task-orientated skills (Mazzi et al., 2015).

These models of clinical communication are therefore useful aides for developing communication skills and conducting consultations that are in line with good practice and consider the person's agenda. However, non-specific factors such as the attitude of healthcare providers, respect, and empathy are also critical and need to be maintained – especially because research shows there is a common decline in factors such as empathy during clinical training (Neumann et al., 2011).

RESEARCH BOX 18.1   What do people appreciate in healthcare students' communication?

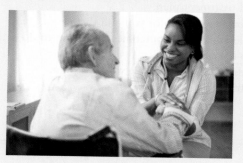

Background

Although evidence shows good communication is important and leads to better patient outcomes, what constitutes good communication is usually determined from the healthcare professionals' perspective. This study examined what communication skills are valued by patients.

Method and findings

Focus groups were conducted with 259 lay people from The Netherlands, Italy, the UK, and Belgium. Each group watched the same videos of medical students conducting consultations with patients. Participants rated the communication in each consultation and then discussed their reasons for positive or negative ratings. Discussions were recorded and analysed for people's preferences.

Participants' comments on medical students' behaviours fell into four categories:

- Affective-orientated/emotional expressions (e.g. attitude, empathy, listening).
- Task-orientated expressions (e.g. competency, self-confident, providing solutions).
- Process-oriented expressions (e.g. structure of the interview, flexibility, summarising, verifying).
- Nonverbal communication (e.g. eye contact).

People most appreciated **affective-orientated** behaviours, which were positively rated by 93% of participants. These behaviours included being facilitating, having an inviting attitude, reassurance/trust, showing interest in the patient, listening, having a pleasant attitude, and being empathic. The next most appreciated behaviours were **task orientated**, which were rated positively by 85%. These behaviours included clarity of the interview, self-confidence, getting a complete picture, competency, and being business like.

Most negative statements were about difficulty understanding students' speech, poor nonverbal behaviours (e.g. lack of eye contact, reading, or writing), not involving the patient, and not collecting enough information.

(Continued)

Significance

This study and other studies demonstrate quite clearly that good communication skills are important – particularly affective communication, which is highly valued by nearly everybody. It also demonstrates the significance of para-verbal and nonverbal communication, which can result in negative evaluations if not done well.

Mazzi, M.A., Rimondini, M., Deveugele, M., Zimmermann, C., Moretti, F., van Vliet, L., Deledda, G., Fletcher, I. & Bensing, J. (2015) What do people appreciate in physicians' communication? An international study with focus groups using videotaped medical consultations. *Health Expectations*, *18*(5): 1215–1226.

Summary

- The patient-centred clinical method indicates the importance of considering the person's agenda.
- The Calgary-Cambridge model is a useful guide to the communication skills that are important at different stages of the clinical interview.
- Good clinical skills include thorough introductions that encompass an explanation of who you are, what the interview is about, and consent.
- Gathering information is best achieved using a funnel of open-to-closed questions.
- Physical examinations should involve an explanation, respect, and sensitivity to a person's cues.
- Explanation and planning involves providing the right amount and type of information in a way that achieves a shared understanding and a treatment plan.
- Closing the interview should include a summary, a check of understanding and agreement, and safety netting.
- Relational factors, such as the attitude of the clinician and empathy, are also critical and need to be developed and/or maintained during training.

18.3 DIFFICULT INTERVIEWS

In healthcare we work with people from cradle to grave. Care, therefore, often involves extreme emotions in response to birth, challenging events or illnesses, life-threatening events, and death. Some of the most difficult interviews for healthcare professionals are those that involve high levels of negative emotions, such as anger, distress, grief, anxiety, or fear, or those that are hard because people have difficulty with communicating, such as with language or hearing difficulties. These raise challenges for healthcare professionals in that it is hard to discuss and make decisions about treatment with a person who is highly emotional or has difficulty communicating.

In this section we focus on the communication skills healthcare professionals need to help people who are angry, anxious, distressed, or those with communication difficulties. Then, in the final section of the chapter, we look at how to give sad or bad news.

18.3.1 COMMUNICATING WITH ANGRY PEOPLE

Though anger and aggression are linked, they are not the same. Anger is an emotion, whereas aggression is a behavioural response involving some form of attack on an object or person. The link between anger and aggression means that when we are confronted with an angry person it is normal to feel under attack, particularly if the anger is directed at us. However, the true cause of the anger may be something completely different, such as illness, a disability, or frustration.

When confronted with an angry person it has been suggested that healthcare professionals typically respond in one of three ways (Lipp, 1986): they may try to ignore the anger and keep going with the interview as 'normal'; they may get angry back; or they may try to pacify the person. Each of these strategies may make the anger worse. Ignoring someone's anger rarely diffuses it and consequently the consultation is likely to go badly. Although getting angry in return is an understandable human response, it merely escalates the situation. In addition, trying to pacify the person (e.g. by telling them to calm down) may potentially inflame the situation.

As we saw in Chapter 2, anger has a range of effects on us. It is associated with strong physiological arousal and a narrowed focus on what provoked the anger. Until the anger has dissipated, it will be hard for the person to think about or deal with anything else. Common underlying reasons for anger can include:

- Feeling hurt or let down: If people are emotionally hurt they will often protect themselves by getting angry about it. In this case the anger will usually be directed at a particular person or group. Expressing this type of anger may lead to crying.
- Perceived injustice or broken rules: Perceived injustice can lead to anger and can arise in situations where a particular treatment is given to some people but not others. Cognitive theory suggests that we all have our own 'rules' about how both we and other people should behave (see Chapter 19). If people break our rules we may get angry. For example, I might have a rule that 'I must always be there for people when they need me'. If a healthcare professional is then not there for me when I need them (e.g. cancels an appointment or keeps me waiting for a long time), I might get angry.
- Goal frustration: If we are prevented from doing things or reaching goals that are important to us, then it is common to feel frustration and anger (see Chapter 9). Injury and illness often prevent people from attaining their goals so anger and frustration may be common.

ACTIVITY 18.2

- Think back to the last time you were really angry with someone.
- Why was this?
- Were you hurt, frustrated or had they broken one of your rules?
- What could they have done that would have stopped you feeling angry?

Like all strong emotions, anger needs to be expressed and diffused before a clinical consultation can continue. The following points can be helpful when trying to achieve this:

- **Check your own emotional response**: If you feel angry, anxious, or upset it will be harder for you to calm the person. Remind yourself that anger is an emotion and not necessarily an attack and that the source of their anger can be the illness or hurt and so is not necessarily about you.
- **Acknowledge the anger**: Recognise that the person is angry and that it is important to deal with this. For example, you may say, '*I can see you're angry and I think it's important we talk about this first*'.
- **Find out the source of the anger**: Let the person talk. Giving them space to verbalise and vent what they are angry about is the first step toward diffusing that anger. People cannot remain angry forever – especially when they are with a sympathetic person.
- **Empathise**: The most effective way to tackle anger is to sympathise or understand. You do not have to agree with the person to be able to understand why they might be angry. Simple statements such as '*I can see why you're angry*' may prove very effective.
- **Disarm**: Many people who are angry say all they want is for the other person to understand and apologise. Some healthcare professionals worry that an apology means they are admitting fault or liability, but it is possible to express regret without agreeing that the person is right by saying something like '*I'm sorry if that upset you*'. In some circumstances it may be appropriate to give a clear apology.

18.3.2 COMMUNICATING WITH ANXIOUS PEOPLE

Anxiety and fear are a normal response to the perceived threat of illness or injury and thus are common in healthcare settings. People differ in their anxiety levels and responses. Those with the personality trait of neuroticism will have higher levels of anxiety (see Chapter 2).

Anxiety makes people hypervigilant for signs of threat. Consequently, they are likely to react strongly to unexpected events, symptoms, or negative news. Anxiety also makes people less flexible in their coping strategies, so specific strategies become more rigidly applied. For example, anxious people may need to know exactly what will happen next so that the additional threat of unexpected events is reduced. Mere reassurance rarely works with anxious people – in fact it can backfire because they may feel that you do not understand. In dealing with an anxious person the following may help:

- **Use your body language and speech**: As we saw at the beginning of this chapter, characteristics of speech and nonverbal communication can help someone calm down. Adopt a relaxed and open body posture (non-threatening), lower the tone of your voice slightly, and slow your speech down.
- **Acknowledge the anxiety**: As with anger, recognise the person's anxiety (e.g. '*You seem quite worried*').
- **Find out the main source of the anxiety**: Anxiety can become generalised, so asking someone why they are anxious may elicit only a general or defensive response. Use a more focused question such as '*Are you worried about anything in particular?*', '*What is it you are particularly worried/anxious about?*', or '*What was it that brought this anxiety on?*'
- **Empathise**: As with anger, empathy and understanding can be very helpful responses to strong emotion. In cases of terminal illness, where the threat of death is inevitable, empathy is crucial. In these cases, we cannot 'fix' anxiety or any other strong emotion – we can only empathise and provide support.
- **Minimise the threat**: Anxiety is based on a perceived threat. Therefore, one way to lower anxiety is to reduce or remove that threat. This is best done by providing information as opposed to mere reassurance. For example, a pregnant woman might be anxious about her baby dying. In this instance, finding out why she believes this will happen and giving her information about the actual risk of it happening (or not) will be more effective than telling her not to worry. If there is a high risk, then involve her in planning screening or treatment so that the risk of adverse consequences is minimised.
- **Increase feelings of safety**: A related technique is to increase feelings of safety through information. For example, you might tell the person about self-monitoring or other things they can do to prevent complications developing, or about medical tests that can be done to check whether the perceived threat is real or likely.

Fear and panic are extreme forms of anxiety and require a different approach. They invoke very strong physical and behavioural responses, such as fight, flight, freezing, or turning to the group (see Chapter 4). Soothing responses in these circumstances are similar to those we might use with a frightened animal. Our body language and voice can be used to calm the person. Offer support and empathy and, if something triggered their fear or panic, remove them from that situation or stop the procedure. Strong fear or panic rarely lasts long so this should subside after a few minutes at most. Be prepared to stay with the person and remain calm while their fear or panic reduces. Distraction can be useful, when it is sensitively timed, because this can help the person refocus away from the threat.

18.3.3 PEOPLE WITH COMMUNICATION DIFFICULTIES

People can have difficulty communicating for a wide range of reasons. Common difficulties are communicating with people who have hearing, speech, or language difficulties. This means consultations might involve interpreters or a family member to facilitate communication. These consultations raise specific challenges but do not need to be difficult if you are patient and take time to communicate in the best way possible for that person. Remember that difficulties communicating do not mean the person is not intellectually capable.

Guidance for communicating with various groups, such as people with hearing loss or speech and language difficulties, has a few core things in common:

- **Find out about the person's communication difficulties** so you know how to best adapt your communication style to help them. For example, if someone is hearing impaired, you might ask if they need to lip read.
- **Check whether the person would prefer to be seen alone or with a companion** for part or all of the consultation.
- **Get the person's attention before you start talking to them**: For example, by addressing them by name, or waving, or tapping them on the arm.
- **Address the person directly**: It is important to address the person directly and treat them with respect in the same way you would with someone without communication difficulties. Talk directly to them, not to the interpreter or a family member. For people with hearing impairments, face-to-face contact is important for lip reading so look at them directly when you talk and do not cover your mouth with your hand or clothing.
- **Speak clearly but naturally**: Do not excessively slow down, shout or exaggerate your words or movements. Although it can help to slow your speech slightly to make words clearer do not overdo it because this can appear patronising. Shouting might appear aggressive and is uncomfortable for people wearing hearing aids. Natural facial expressions and gestures are easier for people to understand and interpret so do not exaggerate them.
- **Listen to the response**: Give the person enough time to respond and do not try to finish their sentences or words for them, or cut them off. Be patient and if you do not understand something it's fine to ask them to repeat it. If the person has a speech problem, such as a stammer, do not tell them to slow down or start again as this can increase stress.
- **Pay attention to nonverbal communication**: You can pick up a lot from the person's facial expressions, gestures, and other responses that they may not be able to verbalise.
- **Check that the person understands**: Use plain language and don't over-elaborate or repeat things. If the person doesn't understand, try saying it in a different way.

In addition, there are specific aspects that need to be considered. For example, if someone has a hearing impairment it helps if there is no background noise and the room is well lit so they can clearly see your face. When working with interpreters it is important to focus and talk to the person, not to the interpreter.

18.3.4 DEALING WITH DISTRESS

Distress is a very general term. It is used here to describe situations where people break down and cannot stop crying. Distress can result from anger, anxiety, or fear and so dealing with this draws on similar principles to dealing with those emotions. Two particular points should be borne in mind:

- Though it is natural to want to stop someone crying, it is not helpful to tell the person to stop. Even if you say this empathically, the underlying message is that you think they should not be upset or crying.

- Though empathy and understanding are important, too much empathy can *increase* someone's distress. If they are really distressed they will be consumed by their feelings so in these circumstances too much empathy can keep them focused on these feelings and feel overwhelmed. In such cases it is more useful to try to get them to focus on specific events or facts which will lower their distress. This is not to say you need to be completely unempathic, only that you need to help them focus. For example, you might say '*I can see it's really upsetting – can you tell me exactly what happened?*' or '*Is there anyone I can call at home who can come and be with you?*'

ACTIVITY 18.3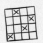

- Think about a time when you were really upset about something important.
- When someone was sympathetic did it make you more or less upset?

CLINICAL NOTES 18.2

Dealing with strong emotions

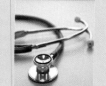

- If strong emotions are ignored the consultation will be difficult and ineffective.
- Anger is associated with aggression/attack but people can express anger safely if helped to do so.
- Useful techniques include acknowledging the emotion, identifying the reason for the emotion, empathising/understanding, and disarming.
- Anxiety is the result of a perceived threat and is associated with hypervigilance and inflexible coping.
- Anxiety can be helped by reducing the perceived threat and increasing feelings of safety.
- Consultations with people with communication difficulties, such as hearing, speech, and language difficulties, do not need to be difficult if you adapt your communication style accordingly.
- High levels of distress will reduce if the person has to focus on specific events or facts.

18.4 GIVING BAD NEWS

One of the hardest tasks in healthcare is to give bad news to people. This can range from diagnosing a chronic or terminal illness to giving news about death or disability. However, any news that brings with it some restriction or potential loss can be sad or bad news.

A useful definition of bad news is that it is 'any information that produces a negative alteration to the person's expectations about their present and future' (Fallowfield & Jenkins, 2004: p312). This recognises the subjective nature of bad news and the importance of each individual's perception of what the news means for them. Thus, a sprained ankle can be bad news for someone who has a job that requires them to be on their feet all day; an infectious illness can be bad news if diagnosed the day before someone planned to go away on the holiday of a lifetime.

Reviews of research in this area have identified three important factors when giving bad news. First, people appreciate it if the clinican is kind, confident, sensitive, and caring. People also prefer clinicians to show concern and distress rather than being aloof and detached. Second, people appreciate it more if the news is given clearly, using simple terms, and if they have time to talk about it with the clinician and ask questions. Third, people appreciate a quiet and private setting (Joekes, 2018).

A number of things can affect a healthcare professional's ability to give bad news sensitively. These include burnout, fatigue, stress, and if the healthcare professional has a fear of death (Brown et al., 2009; Cialkowska-Rysz & Dzierzanowski, 2013). Training for healthcare professionals in giving bad news is increasingly available, with some evidence that it improves clinicians' competency at giving bad news (Alelwani & Ahmed, 2014).

Many guidelines for how to give bad news have been proposed, although these have been based more on consensus than research evidence. The principles in these guidelines overlap a good deal. Here, a six-step approach (or SPIKES) is outlined (Baile et al., 2000; Buckman, 1992).

1. **Setting up:** Prepare thoroughly for the interview. Make sure you have all the relevant information. Locate the interview somewhere private, where you will not be interrupted. Allow yourself the time to give the news and then deal with people's responses and questions.
2. **Person's perception:** Start by checking how much the person already knows and understands so you can tailor the bad news appropriately. Use an open question here such as, '*What have you been told so far?*'
3. **Information needed:** Ask the person how much they want to know about the diagnosis, prognosis, and treatment. This helps tailor the type and amount of information you give in this session to what the person wants and is able to cope with.
4. **Knowledge given:** Impart knowledge of the bad news. It can help to pre-warn the person by saying something like, '*It's not the good news we hoped for*', and then pausing. This allows the person a short time to prepare for the bad news. Give the bad news clearly and in simple language. Ambiguous statements should be avoided (e.g. saying a test was '*positive*', which means the opposite in pathology to lay language). Give the information in small, manageable chunks.
5. **Emotional response:** A range of emotional responses may arise when giving bad news, including shock, disbelief, fear, anxiety, distress, grief, and anger. As discussed in the previous section, the best way to deal with strong emotions is to recognise them and sympathise. With very bad news there is little you can do but offer sympathy and support. Evidence suggests that people will appreciate this.
6. **Summarising and strategy:** Toward the end of the interview the clinician should summarise the main points or outcomes of the interview and consider or agree a future strategy, such as curative or palliative treatment. This helps focus the person on the next steps, gives some certainty, provides a known support structure, and provides hope where possible.

CASE STUDY 18.1   Giving bad news

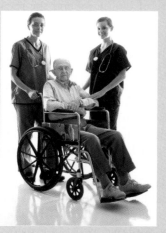

Jack is a 70-year-old man who has been diagnosed with secondary progressive multiple sclerosis.

> When I was first diagnosed in the hospital, a consultant, who I'm glad to say has now retired, said to me, 'Oh, we've got your diagnosis. I'm sorry, you've got an incurable disease and we can't treat it'.

> Now that was true, but I think the [other] doctor, the ward doctor, came back to me and when he explained it to me in detail and in drawings, I felt much happier.

Interviewer: Can you tell me how you would have preferred to have been told?

As the [other] doctor did, he sat on the side of the bed, he had a pad of plain paper and a pencil and he drew the spinal column, right, and he showed the scarring as much, as near as he could, my particular scarring.

He explained how messages travelled and he said, 'The trouble is when they hit a scar they're delayed, they go to the next scar and they're delayed a bit further, and further and further and further.' If you've only got slight scarring or very little scarring that's when it's MS. But unfortunately I've got quite severe scarring, and so the messages are delayed quite a bit.

Interviewer: How do you think that information should be given?

Well, I think it should be given in the way that my present consultant has given me other news. He sits you down and he smiles at you and first of all you realise that he's on your side, he's with you and he understands you as a person, and when he tells you or gives you news – like when he gave me the final diagnosis – it was done in a way that, in fact he held my hand, you know, and he told me first of all, he built up to it, he didn't just blurt it out.

Interviewer: You were talking about how you feel information like that should be given?

Gently, but factually, I mean when, certainly people like to know the facts and I'm one of them, but if they're going to be pretty dramatic then I think it's only right that they should be given to you in a very sympathetic, that's the word I think, in a sympathetic way and that you realise, as the patient, that the person giving you that

(Continued)

information understands that you're going to have to take that, take it on board and, and come to terms with that, which for me has been very difficult because of other reasons, not that, I think it's very important the way that these things are broken.

It doesn't really matter how brave you are or how not brave you are, if you're going to have bad news of any sort, any sort of bad news, I'm sure there must be a way of, of easing it so that you can make it as gentle as you can to the person that's going to have to receive it.

(Adapted from www.healthtalkonline.org.uk © DIPEx. Photo © iofoto/Fotolia)

CLINICAL NOTES 18.3

Giving bad new

- Give bad news in a private setting.
- Give the news clearly and make sure there is enough time to talk about it.
- Be kind and caring.
- **SPIKES** is a useful mnemonic to remember the Setting, Person's perception (what do they know), Information needed (what do they want to know), Knowledge giving, Emotional response, Summarising and strategy.

CONCLUSION

In this chapter we have looked at the different ways in which we communicate and how these may be used in clinical practice to be more effective. The Patient-centred clinical method reminds us that the person's agenda is as important as the clinician's agenda and that the relationship should be collaborative. The Calgary-Cambridge model provides a useful framework to think about the different stages of a clinical interview and which skills are relevant to each. Both these approaches have been used in training and assessment of clinical communication in a range of disciplines. However, neither approach explicitly considers relationship factors, which are also important, such as the clinician's attitude and empathy.

This chapter has covered a variety of techniques and skills that can be useful in both routine and difficult clinical interviews. However, skills need to be practised in order to learn them. They may feel awkward and demanding initially, but with practice they will feel more easy and natural. Usually, with learning skills we move from (a) unconscious incompetence to (b) conscious incompetence to (c) conscious competence to (d) unconscious competence. Clinical skills are a good example of this, so the more you practise the more quickly you will reach unconscious competence.

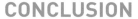

FURTHER READING

Llewellyn, C.D. et al. (eds) (2018) *The Cambridge Handbook of Psychology, Health and Medicine* (3rd edition). Cambridge: Cambridge University Press. Includes short chapters on communicating risk, healthcare professional–patient communication, breaking bad news, medical interviewing, and communicating health information.

Coulehan, J.L. et al. (2001) 'Let me see if I have this right…': Words that help build empathy. *Annals of Internal Medicine, 135:* 221–227. This is a useful article on how to be empathic in clinical situations.

Platt, F.W. & Gordon, G.A. (2004) *Field Guide to the Difficult Patient Interview* (2nd edition). Philadelphia, USA: Lippincott Williams & Wilkins. A pocket guide to communication skills for difficult clinical interviews. An easy, accessible book with useful tips.

Silverman, J., Kurtz, S. & Draper, J. (2013) *Skills for Communicating with Patients* (3rd edition). Oxford: Radcliff Medical Press. Describes the Calgary-Cambridge approach to communication skills in detail and is written in an accessible style.

REVISION QUESTIONS

1. Describe three types of nonverbal behaviour and discuss how these are relevant to clinical practice.

2. How do our characteristics of speech influence communication?

3. Describe the patient-centred clinical method for clinical interviews.

4. Discuss the evidence that clinicians' communication affects patient outcomes.

5. Outline the Calgary-Cambridge model of clinical interviewing and illustrate it with the communication skills that are relevant to the different stages of the interview.

6. Describe the key communication skills for effective information gathering in clinical interviews.

7. Outline the six main points for good clinical practice when conducting a physical examination.

8. What communication skills are useful for diffusing anger in clinical settings?

9. Discuss the key communication skills for closing a clinical interview.

10. Outline the SPIKES model for giving bad news.

19 PSYCHOLOGICAL INTERVENTION

CHAPTER CONTENTS

(Continued)

Case studies

19.1   CBT for postnatal PTSD
19.2   Psychodynamic therapy for sexual dysfunction

Figures

19.1   Main approaches to psychotherapy
19.2   Case formulation of woman with PTSD after a difficult birth
19.3   Targeted health promotion: anti-smoking campaign

Research box

19.1   Effects of mindfulness-based interventions on biomarkers in people who are healthy or have cancer

LEARNING OBJECTIVES

This chapter is designed to enable you to:

- Outline different psychological specialties and their applications to medical settings.
- Understand the theoretical basis of psychological therapies.
- Describe cognitive behaviour therapy, third wave therapies, psychodynamic therapy, and counselling.
- Understand the use of psychotherapeutic techniques in clinical practice.

Mental illness is surprisingly common. It is estimated that 322 million people worldwide suffer from depressive disorders and 264 million from anxiety disorders – each of these figures represent about 4% of the global population (World Health Organisation, 2015). Less severe problems, such as mild or moderate symptoms of depression or anxiety, will be experienced by many more people at some point in their lives.

Psychological interventions have the potential to make a huge difference to individuals and society and are likely to play an increasing role in clinical practice. However, the range of psychological professionals and interventions can be confusing. Many professions are involved in psychotherapy, such as psychiatrists, psychologists, counsellors, mental health nurses, and psychotherapists. It is not always clear who does what. As with medicine, psychology includes many specialisms. These include: health psychology, clinical psychology, counselling psychology, occupational psychology, neuropsychology, and research. Table 19.1 summarises a range of psychological specialties. In practice, an individual's work may span two or three specialisms: for example, a clinical psychologist may also work in a forensic setting.

TABLE 19.1 Psychology specialities

Specialty	What do they do?	Where do they work?	Typical training
Clinical psychologist	Assess and treat mental health problems such as depression, schizophrenia, and personality disorders	Health and social care settings like hospitals, community mental health teams, and health centres	Clinical doctorate degree, including work placements in mental health settings
Counselling psychologist	Assess and treat moderate mental health problems such as depression and anxiety	Wide variety of places such as hospitals, prison services, education, and industry	Undergraduate degree plus specialist diploma and sometimes a doctoral degree
Health psychologist	Health promotion, health services research, treats health problems such as obesity, smoking cessation, and pain management	Health and social care settings like hospitals, health centres, and other health-related organisations	Health psychology Master's degree and often a doctoral degree
Forensic psychologist	Work in legal processes, criminal behaviour, and investigations, including rehabilitation work with offenders	Prison services, secure hospitals and rehabilitation, police and probation services	Forensic psychology Master's degree and diploma, including work placements in forensic settings
Educational psychologist	Assess and provide remedial work for children with behavioural or learning difficulties	Schools, education departments, and local authorities	Educational doctoral or Master's degree plus work placements in educational settings
Occupational psychologist	Work with individuals and organisations to increase the effectiveness of employees and organisations	Industry, commerce, and other large organisations	Occupational psychology Master's degree plus work placements in occupational settings
Neuropsychologist	Assess and rehabilitate people with brain injury or disorders	Healthcare settings such as hospitals and neurological and community rehabilitation services	Doctoral degree (usually clinical, educational or health) plus diploma in neuropsychology
Sport and exercise psychologist	Work with athletes, sports people, and teams to enhance performance	Health services, professional sports teams and national governing bodies	Three-year training, including sport and exercise Master's or doctoral degree, plus work placements in sport and exercise settings

In most countries psychology is regulated by organisations such as the European Federation of Psychologists' Associations, or the American Psychological Association. These organisations monitor and regulate the content of psychological degrees and training in the same way that medicine is regulated by organisations such as the General

Medical Council (UK) or the Liaison Committee on Medical Education (USA). Psychologists need to be registered with the relevant organisation and apply for professional status in order to practice.

This chapter focuses on the use of psychotherapy in healthcare settings. First, it explains the main types of psychotherapy used to treat mental health problems. Then it looks more specifically at interventions for physical health problems, such as motivational interviewing to help people change their behaviour and the provision of support groups for people with cancer.

19.1 DIFFERENT APPROACHES TO PSYCHOTHERAPY

Here we shall use the term 'psychotherapy' very broadly to mean any form of therapy that involves talking and exploring psychological issues. The aim of **psychotherapy** is to resolve mental health problems and help a person thrive. Psychotherapy usually involves one-to-one sessions in which people talk through their problems. However, there are different types of psychotherapy, each with its own theoretical foundations. As a consequence, the content of psychotherapy can differ hugely and in addition to talking therapies may involve writing, drawing, imagery work, role-play, or homework.

The main theories on which psychotherapies are based include psychodynamic (Freudian) theory, humanistic and existential theory, behaviourism, and cognitive theory. Figure 19.1 shows how these theories have resulted in different approaches to psychotherapy, each with their own philosophical assumptions and techniques. For example, **humanism** assumes (i) that humans are essentially good, (ii) that we strive for personal growth and development, and (iii) that we have free will and can therefore make choices. The humanistic approach to therapy, which was very popular in the 1960s and 1970s, is founded on the principle that the therapist provides an **unconditional positive regard**: in other words, whatever a person has done will be understandable given that person's experience. The focus in humanistic therapy is on the person's unique experience, needs, and personal growth. The humanistic approach continues to be used in therapy today and is also evident in patient-centred medicine.

Modern psychotherapy draws on a range of theoretical approaches, including cognitive behaviour therapy (CBT), third wave CBT therapies, psychodynamic therapies, and counselling.

Psychotherapies often overlap with each other and thus are not always easy to classify. For example, cognitive analytic therapy (CAT) combines CBT and psychoanalytic principles in therapy. Interpersonal therapy focuses on relationship processes in depression and draws on psychodynamic principles, CBT techniques, and brief crisis intervention. Eye-movement desensitisation and reprocessing is a specific therapy used to treat post-traumatic stress disorder (PTSD): it is referred to as integrative but incorporates a lot of CBT principles. The next section will look in more detail at the most widely used psychotherapies in healthcare settings, namely CBT, psychodynamic therapy, and counselling.

19.1.1 COGNITIVE BEHAVIOUR THERAPY (CBT)

CBT is founded on behaviourism and cognitivism. CBT is not a single therapy but rather a group of therapies that are founded on shared core principles. Consequently, some argue that the term 'cognitive and behaviour therapies' is a more accurate label (Eagle & Worrell, 2018). These therapies have developed in three waves (Hayes, 2004). The first wave derived from **behaviourism**, which focuses on people's behaviour and how it is learned and shaped by events. Behaviourism describes the processes through which people's behaviour is shaped, including classical conditioning, operant conditioning, and modelling (outlined in Chapter 10). Behavioural therapy uses these processes to change maladaptive behavioural responses and substitute them with new adaptive behaviours. For example, phobias are often conditioned responses to an object that is associated with fear because of a negative or traumatic experience in the past. Behaviour therapy would involve trying to counter-condition this response through techniques like exposure to the feared object, systematic desensitisation to the object, relaxation training, modelling of adaptive behaviour, and reinforcement of adaptive behaviour. A well-known example of positive reinforcement is the use of reward charts and stickers with children to encourage good behaviours. Wearable technology that monitors health behaviours, such as exercise, can encourage behaviour modification using principles of behavioural monitoring and reinforcing healthy behaviour (Davision & Garcia, 2017).

Behaviourism emphasises scientific, or empirical, testing. Behavioural therapy therefore includes carrying out **behavioural experiments** in which people test their views of what will happen under certain circumstances. Consider, for example, the case of a person who has social phobia and avoids social situations because they get highly anxious, assume that everyone notices and thinks they are odd. This can lead to a vicious cycle where social situations are avoided. The more these situations are avoided the more anxious the person will become about attending them. The person's assumptions are not challenged or disproved because there is no opportunity for them to have a good experience of a social situation. This combination of negative assumptions and avoiding social events (avoidance behaviour) creates a negative cycle that perpetuates the phobia. In these circumstances, a behavioural experiment might be for the person to attend a social situation, monitor their anxiety (which should reduce over time), monitor how they act, and also notice how other people respond to them – whether positively or negatively. Another possibility might be to ask other people how they feel in social situations and whether they ever get anxious. This can normalise a certain degree of social anxiety. Behavioural experiments can reduce anxiety in many ways: the increased exposure to social situations can reduce anxiety through habituation, challenge negative beliefs, and break the negative cycle. We once heard of a therapist who went out and acted in bizarre ways in an attempt to show a person how *little* other people would notice!

It can be seen that behavioural experiments affect a person's thoughts as well as their behaviour. From a cognitive viewpoint, behavioural experiments encourage people to become aware of underlying assumptions, specify and test them, and then revise their thoughts and behaviour accordingly. There is ongoing debate about whether behavioural

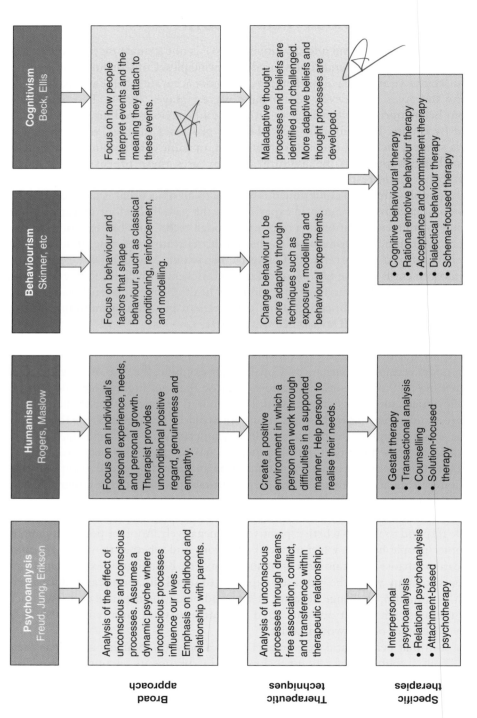

FIGURE 19.1 Main approaches to psychotherapy

experiments work mainly through behavioural or cognitive means (Ougrin, 2011; Salkovskis et al., 2006). Regardless of how they work, however, behavioural experiments can be powerful tools of change and are particularly effective for anxiety disorders. They are also useful when treating people with less cognitive ability, such as young children or people with learning difficulties. Case Study 19.1 gives an example of how cognitive and behavioural methods were used to treat a woman with PTSD after a difficult birth.

CASE STUDY 19.1   CBT for postnatal PTSD

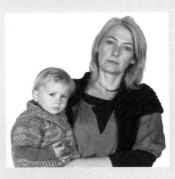

Sarah is 35 years old, married, and has a 14-month-old daughter. Sarah had a termination of a pregnancy when she was 19 years old, which she kept a secret for 16 years because she thought people would judge her negatively.

Sarah's labour was induced and there was confusion over when it would happen. Sarah panicked because she was unprepared and her husband was not there. The midwife was not sympathetic to Sarah's high levels of anxiety. After a painful internal examination during which Sarah cried and asked the midwife to stop, the midwife said 'If you think that's painful, what are you going to be like giving birth?' From this point onwards Sarah's labour and delivery were characterised by pain, extreme distress, and fear of the midwife.

Sarah's daughter was delivered by emergency caesarean section after a long labour during which Sarah thought she might die. Sarah started to feel the surgery half way through and was given morphine. She reported dissociating (feeling detached from herself and like the labour was unreal) and cannot remember anything for 12 hours after the delivery. She said the first few months after the birth 'are a blur' and it took her a year to bond with her daughter. The main themes of Sarah's birth seemed to be feeling terrified, vulnerable, and out of control; high levels of confusion and dissociation; and confirmation of her belief that others will judge her and hurt her through her experience with the midwife.

After the birth Sarah suffered from postnatal depression, was prescribed antidepressants, and attended a support group. Sarah first attended CBT 14 months after giving birth. She was highly distressed, appeared to be reliving the birth experience, was crying and shaking. She had the full range of PTSD symptoms, including flashbacks, nightmares, and strong physical and emotional reactions to reminders of birth, feeling emotionally numb yet crying all the time. Her flashbacks were of seeing herself lying in the delivery room feeling helpless and terrified as the midwife came into the room.

Therapy consisted of various cognitive and behavioural techniques. Techniques used in treatment included:

(Continued)

1. *A behavioural experiment* where an anonymous survey was carried out of people's opinions of Sarah's abortion to challenge her belief that others would judge her. The survey described the circumstances in which Sarah fell pregnant and had the abortion and asked people what they would think of her. People who did not know Sarah completed the survey and responses included pro-life and pro-abortion views. This dramatically changed Sarah's beliefs about herself, the abortion, what others would think of her, and the importance she placed on others' views.

2. *Mild exposure in the form of reliving exercises.* Sarah was asked to imagine the birth as if it were currently happening and talk through the events in detail.

3. *Stronger exposure* through visiting the labour ward with the therapist to help Sarah overcome her fear and avoidance.

4. *Cognitive exercises* to change Sarah's appraisals of difficult events in the birth, such as using a role-play to act out confronting the midwife and reducing Sarah's fear.

5. *Visualisation exercises* to rewrite her flashbacks. For example, she imagined the anaesthetist in the delivery room whom she felt comfortable and safe with, as opposed to the frightening midwife.

6. *Positive reformulation* to consolidate these changes in Sarah's beliefs.

7. After ten sessions of CBT, Sarah's PTSD symptoms had gone and her maladaptive beliefs about herself and others changed.

(Ayers et al., 2007)

The second wave of CBT derived from cognitivism, which views thoughts as being central to how we feel and behave. Cognitivism was the dominant paradigm in psychology for many years and the importance of cognition is apparent in many of the theories and research outlined in this book. The main cognitive theory of mental illness was proposed by Aaron Beck (1967), who argued that appraisal and the personal meaning of events are central in the development and maintenance of psychopathology. According to Beck, early experiences lead to sets of **core beliefs** or **schema** about ourselves, the world, and others. These beliefs are not necessarily rational because most of them are formed in childhood without the benefit of adult logic. Core beliefs can lead to **maladaptive assumptions** – sometimes referred to as 'rules for living'.

Beck was particularly interested in depression. He argued that people become depressed when they have a depressogenic triad of negative beliefs about themselves (e.g. they are deficient in some way), others and the world (e.g. others don't like them or treat them badly), and the future (e.g. negative expectations or hopelessness).

Evidence supports the existence of this depressogenic style of thinking: it has been observed in adults and children during depression (Beck & Perkins 2001; Braet et al., 2015). It has led to the cognitive content-specificity model which proposes that, although anxious and depressed people have maladaptive cognitions, the content of these differ for each disorder. Following on from Beck's work, it has been hypothesised that depressive cognitions are largely focused on negative beliefs about the self, the future, and loss, whereas anxious cognitions are largely focused on perceived danger or threat. There is some evidence to support this. For example, a study of anxiety and depression from childhood to early adulthood in over 1,600 pairs of twins found that anxiety sensitivity (fear of bodily sensations) was associated with anxiety but not depression (Brown et al., 2014). However, the same study found that social concerns (fear of publicly observable symptoms) were associated with both anxiety and depression, and so were not disorder-specific. The authors therefore concluded that there are both specific and shared thought patterns in anxiety and depression (Brown et al., 2014).

CBT is used to treat a wide range of psychological problems, not only depression. Cognitive theories have been developed for different psychological disorders such as depression (Beck, 1967), panic (Clark, 1986), anxiety (Wells, 1997, 2010), PTSD (Brewin & Holmes, 2003), and personality disorders (Young et al., 2004). These theories and the evidence for content-specificity have informed the development of cognitive therapy protocols for different psychological disorders. The defining features of CBT are given in Box 19.1. CBT is now being applied to an increasing range of mental and physical disorders and is also developing to incorporate different techniques based on mindfulness meditation, and acceptance. These are collectively referred to as the third wave therapies and are outlined in the next section.

However, the underlying theory can be applied to most of us, even when we are functioning well. Consider, for example, a person whose core beliefs include that they are unlovable and that other people will judge them, which could stem from having overly judgemental or unloving parents. This person might compensate for these core beliefs by having rules for living such as:

'If I do everything perfectly then people will love me.'

'If I do what people want they will not criticise me.'

'I must not show negative emotions or people will judge me.'

These rules can help the person to function well and feel good about themselves as long as they adhere to these high standards. However, keeping up these standards will put them under considerable strain and make them vulnerable if something happens to make them think they've failed, such as not doing well in an exam or being made redundant from work. Under these circumstances it is possible they will develop depression because they have violated their rules and so activated their underlying belief that they are unlovable.

One difficulty in cognitive therapy is that people are not consciously aware of their own core beliefs and rules for living. However, these beliefs are usually reflected in the moment-to-moment **automatic thoughts** they have, especially in difficult situations. Thus CBT involves monitoring automatic thoughts

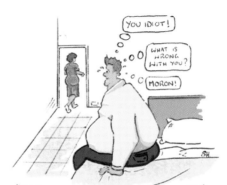

"I'll leave you alone with your thoughts," she said. How cruel.

to help uncover a person's rules and core beliefs. These are put together in a formulation, which can be written or diagrammatic. The formulation is then used as a guide for the therapist and person to understand the problem and work out ways to test and challenge existing beliefs and build new, more adaptive beliefs. Testing beliefs can be done using cognitive and behavioural methods. Cognitive methods include guided discovery or Socratic questioning, where the therapist helps the person examine and question their existing beliefs by considering evidence of whether or not they are correct. Case Study 19.1 illustrates the testing of beliefs using cognitive and behavioural methods. The formulation for the woman featured in this case study is shown in Figure 19.2.

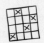

ACTIVITY 19.1

- Think about the last time you felt upset or angry and write down the following:

  o   What was the situation or trigger?
  o   What thoughts went through your mind (automatic thoughts)?
  o   How did these thoughts influence how you felt?
  o   Can you identify any of your rules (assumptions) that might have been broken?

BOX 19.1   Core features of CBT

1. It is a collaborative relationship between the therapist and the client.
2. The client is educated about the CBT approach so that they can become their own 'therapist'.
3. The focus is on the present problem – 'here and now'.
4. Structured sessions with content (an agenda) are agreed between the therapist and the client at the beginning of each session.
5. It is goal directed, with aims for therapy being stated at the beginning and work in therapy is directed toward achieving these aims.
6. It is short-term therapy, typically between six and 24 sessions.
7. It is an examination of maladaptive beliefs.
8. Maladaptive beliefs are cognitively challenged through Socratic questioning.
9. Behavioural experiments are used to test maladaptive beliefs (empirical approach).
10. General and specific formulations are used to guide understanding and change.

There is little doubt that CBT is a popular and effective treatment for a variety of conditions. It is now the recommended treatment for many psychological disorders, including depression, PTSD, generalised anxiety disorder, panic, and obsessive compulsive disorder (National Institute for Health and Care Excellence (NICE), 2011). The widespread use of CBT is based on evidence that it is an effective treatment for these disorders. Reviews of

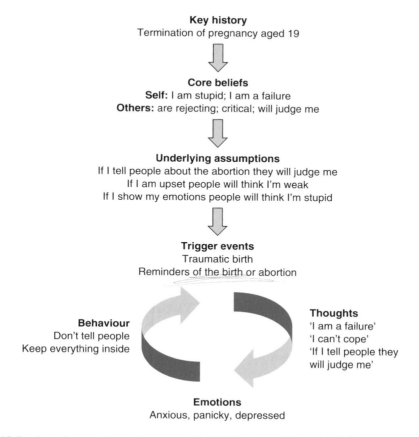

FIGURE 19.2 Case formulation of woman with PTSD after a difficult birth (Ayers et al., 2007)

CBT for anxiety disorders show that it is better than wait-list or placebo controls and as effective as pharmacological treatment in reducing anxiety, depression, and increasing quality of life (Mitte, 2005; Olatunji et al., 2010). In addition, CBT has lower dropout rates than pharmacological treatment (Mitte, 2005).

CBT is also increasingly used as an adjunct to treatments of chronic illnesses. Reviews of randomised controlled trials have generally found positive effects of CBT treatment for illnesses as diverse as chronic fatigue (Price et al., 2008), fibromyalgia (Bernardy et al., 2013), traumatic brain injury (Soo & Tate, 2007), sleep problems (Montgomery & Dennis, 2003), and asthma (Kew et al., 2016). However, the assessment of the effects of CBT is often limited to psychological outcomes, such as quality of life and measures of distress, rather than to physical functioning.

The popularity of CBT means it is now in danger of being applied in a blanket fashion to areas where there is inconsistent evidence of its efficacy. For example, there are instances where CBT appears helpful but does not result in clinically significant change, such as with child sexual abuse (MacDonald et al., 2012) or domestically abusive men

(Smedslund et al., 2007). There is also evidence that other therapies can be just as effective as CBT, or more so (Stoffers et al., 2012). A more considered view might be to recognise that CBT works very well for *some* disorders where it can lead to an improvement in *some* outcomes, but that it is by no means a panacea.

19.1.2 THIRD WAVE CBT THERAPIES

The most recent developments in CBT have been referred to, collectively, as third wave cognitive and behavioural therapies (Hayes, 2004). These therapies focus less on challenging the *content* of thoughts and more on the *relationship* that an individual has with their thoughts and emotions. Techniques such as acceptance, mindfulness, and cognitive defusion help a person to accept their thoughts and emotional responses and not see them as all-defining or permanent. This prevents psychological symptoms being made worse by negative appraisals of thoughts and emotions. There is also a focus on life values and spirituality in many third wave therapies.

Various third wave therapies have been developed. A review identified 17 therapies classified in the literature as 'third wave' (Dimidjian et al., 2016). Those most widely cited were Acceptance and Commitment Therapy (ACT), Dialectical Behaviour Therapy (DBT), and mindfulness, which are described below. Other third wave therapies include functional analytic psychotherapy, behavioural activation, compassion-focused therapy, metacognitive therapy, and integrative behavioural couples therapy.

Mindfulness is based on meditative practices which have been used for centuries. In its contemporary form, mindfulness has been defined as bringing non-judgemental awareness to an object of attention, being receptive, and in the present moment (Kristeller, 2018). Mindfulness interventions involve regular meditation to practise raising awareness of factors such as breathing, bodily sensations, or thoughts and emotions. Specific techniques, such as guided meditation, walking meditation, body scan meditation, or mindful eating, can be incorporated into a range of different psychotherapeutic approaches. These techniques involve focusing on a particular task (e.g. walking or eating meditation) or different parts of the body (e.g. body scan meditation) in order to be in the present moment, to notice and pay attention to what we are doing or feeling.

There are also stand-alone mindfulness therapies which have been widely applied and evaluated. The most commonly known are Mindfulness-Based Stress Reduction (MBSR) (Kabat-Zinn, 1990) and Mindfulness-Based Cognitive Therapy (MBCT) (Segal et al., 2002). Both these therapies consist of eight weekly sessions of mindfulness meditation with daily mindfulness practice in between to teach people mindfulness skills with the goal of reducing stress or depression. The therapist or instructor provides psychoeducation about mindfulness and emotions, guides mindfulness practice in person or via audio-recordings, and provides specific content relevant to the intervention (e.g. risk factors for stress or depression).

Many mindfulness interventions have been developed for specific health problems or illnesses with mixed evidence for efficacy. Interventions have been developed for changing health behaviours such as smoking (Maglione et al., 2017) or obesity (Ruffault et al., 2016); for symptoms such as chronic pain (Hilton et al., 2016); for psychological disorders such as attention deficit/hyperactivity disorder (Mitchell et al., 2015) or psychosis (Aust & Bradshaw, 2017); for physical illnesses such as breast cancer (Zhang et al., 2016) and respiratory disorders (Harrison et al., 2016); and for groups of people such as carers (e.g. Rayan & Ahmad, 2017) and healthcare professionals (Burton et al., 2017).

Mindfulness interventions have been widely evaluated with evidence that they are effective compared to wait-list controls or treatment as usual. A review of 47 randomised controlled trials found that mindfulness meditation programmes, such as MBSR and MBCT, result in small to moderate improvements in anxiety, depression, and pain (Goyal et al., 2014) but there was poor or insufficient evidence of effects on positive mood or stress-related behaviours, such as substance use, eating habits, sleep, or weight. Mindfulness interventions are not more effective than other active treatments, such as behavioural therapies or exercise (Goyal et al., 2014). However, there is interesting evidence emerging about physiological responses to mindfulness interventions (see Research Box 19.1).

Acceptance and Commitment Therapy (**ACT**) (Hayes et al., 1999) incorporates mindfulness and other techniques to help people accept events, thoughts, and feelings that are outside our control and instead identify personal values and commit to acting on these. ACT rests on the assumption that trying to avoid or get rid of symptoms perpetuates negative emotions and suffering – hence the focus on accepting these symptoms and commitment to living a valued life. The core principles of ACT are shown in Box 19.2. The evidence for ACT is similar to that for mindfulness in that it appears to be an effective treatment but no more effective than standard CBT. A meta-analysis of 60 randomised controlled trials of ACT for stress, physical, and psychological disorders found a small effect of ACT compared to wait-list controls or treatment as usual (Ost, 2014). The evidence suggested ACT was most effective for chronic pain and tinnitus, and possibly effective for psychological disorders and stress. However, ACT was not significantly better than other forms of cognitive or behavioural therapy (Ost, 2014).

Dialectical Behaviour Therapy (**DBT**) (Linehan, 2014) was originally developed as a treatment for suicidal people and then tailored for people with borderline personality disorder. Since then, it has been used as a treatment for a range of psychological and behavioural problems. DBT uses standard CBT techniques for emotion regulation along with mindfulness and acceptance. DBT has four components: (i) individual therapy to address problem behaviours, set goals for quality of life, and work toward them; (ii) group sessions to teach core skills of mindfulness, emotion regulation, tolerance of distress, and interpersonal skills; (iii) a therapist consultation team to support therapists providing DBT; and (iv) telephone coaching to help people apply skills in their daily life. As with other third wave therapies, reviews of the evidence suggest DBT is more effective than usual treatment for borderline personality disorder and suicidality (Stoffers et al., 2012), and eating disorders (Lenz et al., 2014). However, DBT is not necessarily more effective than other psychotherapies. Although DBT has been used to treat other conditions, such as depression, anxiety, and intellectual disabilities, there is not yet enough evidence on which to draw conclusions (McNair et al., 2016).

RESEARCH BOX 19.1   Effects of mindfulness-based interventions on biomarkers in people who are healthy or have cancer

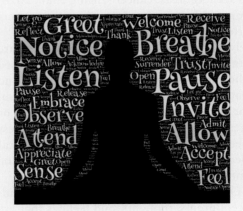

Background

A previous review and meta-analysis found that mindfulness-based interventions have a small beneficial effect on cortisol levels in healthy adults (Sanada et al., 2016). This systematic review looked at the effect of mindfulness-based interventions on biomarkers (cytokines, neuropeptides, and C-reactive protein (CRP)) in healthy people and people with cancer.

Method and findings

A search of the literature between 1980 and 2016 found 13 research studies with a total of 1,110 participants: seven studies with healthy subjects (n=750) and six studies of people with various types of cancer (n=360). Results showed mindfulness-based interventions had no effect on cytokines in healthy people but were associated with a reduction in pro-inflammatory cytokines and possibly an increase in anti-inflammatory cytokines in people with cancer. In healthy people, mindfulness interventions were associated with increased levels of the neuropeptide insulin-like growth factor (IGF-1) as well as short-term increases in neuropeptide Y, which is associated with more beneficial responses to acute stress.

Significance

The authors suggest that the changes in biomarkers observed in healthy adults after mindfulness interventions might offer protection against acute stress. Changes observed in cancer patients might indicate a change from a depressive/carcinogenic profile to a more normal one. However, given the complexity and different contexts of the immune system, additional evidence is necessary to confirm the impact of mindfulness interventions on biomarkers.

Sanada, K., Alda Díez, M., Salas Valero, M., Pérez-Yus, M.C., Demarzo, M.M., Montero-Marín, J., García-Toro, M. & García-Campayo, J. (2017) Effects of mindfulness-based interventions on biomarkers in healthy and cancer populations: A systematic review. *BMC Complementary and Alternative Medicine*, *17*(1): 125.

Third wave therapies such as mindfulness, ACT and DBT share a number of similarities. Common characteristics are the focus on mindfulness, acceptance, and cognitive defusion. There is substantial evidence that these third wave therapies are effective. A review of meta-analyses conducted for common third wave therapies (including those described here) concluded they have 'at least moderate to large effects' for treatment of anxiety, depression, eating disorders, borderline personality disorder, and suicidal behaviours compared to wait-list controls or treatment as usual (Dimidjian et al., 2016). For example, a review of psychological therapies for depression found that third wave therapies and standard CBT approaches were equally effective and acceptable treatments (Hunot et al., 2013). Third wave therapies therefore provide a useful extension of cognitive and behavioural therapies to include new techniques and approaches that are as effective as standard CBT, but not necessarily more effective.

BOX 19.2 Core features of ACT

ACT frequently uses six core principles to help people develop psychological flexibility:

1. **Cognitive defusion**: helping people to realise that their thoughts, emotions, and memories are not necessarily true or define them.
2. **Acceptance**: helping people to allow their thoughts and feelings to come and go rather than struggling with them.
3. **Present moment**: helping people to be aware of the here and now, and to experience it with openness, interest, and receptiveness.
4. **Observing the self**: helping people to develop a transcendent sense of self and a continuity of consciousness that is unchanging.
5. **Values**: helping people to discover what is most important to them.
6. **Committed action**: helping people to set goals according to their core values and acting on them.

19.1.3 PSYCHODYNAMIC THERAPY

Psychodynamic therapy is based on Freud's theory of the psyche and psychopathology. The central idea is that we have a dynamic unconscious – hence the term psycho*dynamic* therapy. This dynamic unconscious involves a continuous conflict between drives and impulses on the one hand, and our ego and social constraints on the other hand. Conflict, suppression, and a building up of psychological defences then influence our behaviour, thoughts, and feelings which can lead to psychopathology.

Psychodynamic theory has been extensively developed and refined and there are now many different types of psychodynamic therapy. These include interpersonal psychoanalysis, relational psychoanalysis, and attachment-based psychotherapy. Carlyle (2007) outlines three common principles in psychodynamic therapies. The first is the importance of early childhood experience. Modern psychodynamic theory incorporates work on **early attachments** (Bowlby, 1958), which indicates that the relationship a child has with their primary caregiver between the ages of six months and 3 years of age is fundamental in forming a person's early experience and their expectations of social relationships (see Chapter 8). Attachment is not the only important early experience. Research suggests that playing helps children to learn about the rules for appropriate behaviour and social roles. It also helps them to test their own abilities and regulate their emotions. For example, a child play-fighting with a parent will learn about acceptable and unacceptable levels of aggression.

Psychodynamic theory puts forward two processes by which early experiences affect development. These are introjection, where the child internalises aspects of their parents or other significant people into themselves. The other process is projection, where people project aspects of their own internal world onto others. The most well-known example of projection is when you view another person negatively because they do something or represent something you dislike about yourself. For example, a father may react angrily when his son does not achieve top grades at school because the father is frustrated by his own lack of achievement and success. The father is therefore projecting a part of himself that he dislikes onto his son and reacting strongly because of this.

Psychopathology in adults is therefore thought to result from early experiences being negative in some way, such as having neglectful or over-intrusive parents or a childhood that involved trauma, loss, or separation. The negative experience then results in adults who have difficulties coping with life or relationships. As a result, the second common principle in psychodynamic therapies is the importance of relationships, particularly the **therapeutic relationship**. The therapeutic relationship is thought of as a regular, contained space for people to work through and understand their difficulties. This means psychodynamic therapy is regular and intensive – often happening more than once a week for more than a year – to provide the patient with a frequent and predictable time in their life to deal with their difficulties.

Through regular contact, the therapist starts to symbolise a parent for the patient. The therapeutic relationship therefore becomes a 'stage' on which interpersonal difficulties are played out. This is known as **transference**, where the way the patient views and relates to the therapist is thought to represent their underlying issues or interpersonal difficulties with parents or other significant people. A psychodynamic therapist therefore remains as neutral as possible and is not supposed to bring their own characteristics or feelings into therapy. This aspect of psychodynamic therapy is summed up by the (often untrue) stereotype of the therapist who says nothing while the person lies on the couch and talks.

The third common principle in psychodynamic therapies is the importance of **personal defences**, which are the ways in which people avoid difficult or painful thoughts. There are many different types of defences, including denial, repression, humour, rationalisation, escapism, and regression. Like coping strategies, defences are not necessarily maladaptive. For example, a person who has to have complicated surgery may well deny or repress thoughts of possible complications or a painful recovery, which will minimise the threat of surgery and reduce their anxiety beforehand. The defining features of psychodynamic therapy are given in Box 19.3. Case Study 19.2 illustrates the psychodynamic treatment of sexual dysfunction.

The emphasis on unconscious processes means psychodynamic theory is difficult to test scientifically and it has been criticised for this. However, advances in neuroscience and research using imaging, such as fMRI, have demonstrated that unconscious neural activity in the brain often pre-empts our voluntary action (Bonn, 2013). Because of various criticisms and the lack of consistent evidence, psychodynamic therapy is not as commonly recommended in guidelines for the treatment of mental health disorders as CBT. Proponents of the psychodynamic approach argue that this dismissal of psychoanalysis by treatment guidelines is premature and unjustified (Smith, 2007). Reviews of the research into the effectiveness of psychoanalysis for disorders such as personality disorders, anxiety, and depression have reached different conclusions. Some find that psychodynamic therapy is ineffective (Roth & Fonagy, 2004), but others conclude it is effective (Driessen et al., 2015; Leichsenring, 2005). However, this might reflect the variability of disorders and contexts in which it has been applied. Two notable reviews concluded that psychodynamic psychotherapy is effective. A Cochrane review of randomised controlled trials of short-term psychodynamic psychotherapy concluded that there is evidence for 'modest to large gains' for common disorders such as anxiety, depression, and interpersonal problems (Abbass et al., 2014). Another review and meta-analysis of the effect of psychodynamic therapy over time concluded that psychodynamic therapy is as effective as other types of psychotherapy for a range of outcomes (Kivlighan et al., 2015).

BOX 19.3   Core features of psychodynamic therapy

1. It is based on the assumption that we have a dynamic unconscious.
2. It is focused on the past, particularly early childhood experience and conflict, and on the suppression or psychological defences that have resulted.
3. The therapist remains neutral so transference can occur and the underlying issues can be explored.
4. The focus is on interpersonal relationships and how these are influenced by childhood experience, subsequent defences, projection, etc.
5. Maladaptive personal defences are explored.
6. It is an intensive therapy, typically comprising one or more sessions a week for at least a year.

CASE STUDY 19.2   Psychodynamic therapy for sexual dysfunction

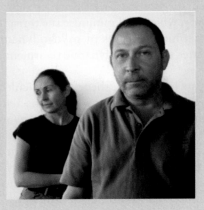

Laura is 38 and suffers from dyspareunia (pain on intercourse) and an inability to have sexual intercourse. Dan suffers from dyspepsia (indigestion) and backache. His mother died when he was five.

Laura and Dan had a son who died of a hereditary brain disorder at 15 months. When he died Laura was pregnant and this baby also died of the same disorder when 10 months old. The following year Laura had an ectopic pregnancy and chose to be sterilised.

At the funeral of their first child Laura said she felt 'numb' and her family sent her shopping to distract her. Laura and Dan went on to foster and adopt two children. Their sexual dysfunction started after the death of their first child.

Psychodynamic therapy

Laura and Dan's symptoms were interpreted as physical manifestations of the distress caused by the loss of their children and fertility. Their problems were therefore thought to be due to unresolved loss and bereavement. Dan and Laura were seen individually and as a couple by the same therapist for a year.

The therapist described Laura as 'wooden and lifeless' when discussing her experiences. This was interpreted as a defence mechanism where Laura was no longer in touch with her feelings but projected them onto others so that they felt distress. The fostering, adoption, and work with disabled children was her way of escaping from the pain of bereavement.

The therapist explored Dan's relationship with his mother, who died when he was 5 years old. The therapist suggested his marriage was an attempt to replace the relationship he had with his mother. Dan therefore felt rivalry with his own children while they were alive because they took away Laura's attention. When the babies died he felt responsible and guilty so reacted very negatively to Laura's distress because it reminded him of this. Laura's dyspareunia and inability to have intercourse may therefore have been an angry attempt at retribution because he did not allow her to grieve.

Following this insight the couple was able to have intercourse again. After Laura had an orgasm she broke down and said it was as if she was 'crying from the deepest depths of herself'. She reported recovering mental images of her babies when they were dead, whereas previously she could only picture them alive. By the end of therapy Dan's symptoms had disappeared and Laura's dyspareunia was intermittent but tolerable. The couple was sexually active and reported that their marriage had improved greatly.

(Adapted from Lewis & Casement, 1986)

19.1.4 COUNSELLING

Counselling is an integrative approach that draws on various psychotherapeutic techniques so there is considerable variety, which makes counselling difficult to summarise. However, there are three core principles. The first is that it is **client-focused**. The needs of the client are put first and the aim of counselling is to increase or protect the person's psychological well-being (Farsides, 2009).

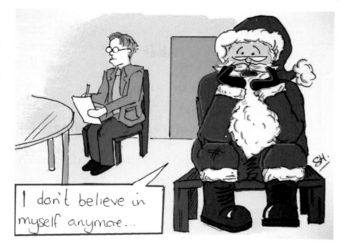

The second principle is that counselling is **non-directive** and the emphasis is on the person exploring, clarifying, and solving their problems. The role of the counsellor is to facilitate this process (Bor & Allen, 2007). The third core principle is that counselling aims to provide a safe and accepting environment in which the person can explore and reflect on their difficulties. This is partly based on the principle of providing people with **unconditional positive regard** to facilitate self-acceptance and feelings of self-worth. For example, parents and society place expectations on us about performance, achievement, and what is seen as successful or worthwhile. This means many people might only feel worthwhile if they reach expectations and perform well in these areas. A counsellor might explore this with a person while at the same time accepting them regardless of their achievements or failures. This provides the person with an insight into their behaviour and feelings at the same time as allowing them to experience a relationship where they are liked and accepted for who they are.

Counselling tends to be used with mild or moderate anxiety and depression, or with people who are in difficult circumstances, or crises. Counselling is also increasingly used in healthcare settings to help people adjust and cope with difficult events, such as a diagnosis of HIV, coronary heart disease, a late miscarriage or stillbirth, or to help people make difficult decisions, such as during infertility treatment or genetic testing (Bor & Eriksen, 2018). For example, in the UK, counsellors are often employed in primary care settings so that doctors can refer people to them immediately, without having to refer to secondary care teams in hospitals or community mental health teams. The defining features of counselling are given in Box 19.4.

Currently, evidence for the efficacy of counselling is limited. This is partly because it is difficult to define a 'standard' approach to counselling so research has focused on evaluating more clearly outlined therapies like CBT. Research into counselling is often methodologically limited by factors such as counselling being poorly defined or not compared to other forms of therapy. However, where evidence is available it suggests that counselling is evaluated positively by participants and can improve some outcomes in the short term. For example, a review of counselling in primary care settings for psychological and psychosocial problems concluded that this was more effective than usual care in the short term. However, over the long term counselling was no more effective than usual care (Bower et al., 2011). Similarly, a review of telephone counselling for carers of people with dementia concluded that it led to reduced symptoms of depression in carers but that the evidence for other outcomes was limited (Lins et al., 2014).

BOX 19.4   Core features of counselling

1. The therapist provides unconditional positive regard and accepts the person for who they are.
2. The therapist is non-judgemental and provides a safe space in which the person can work through their problems.
3. The needs of the client are primary.
4. The person explores their problems and solutions and the therapist facilitates this.
5. Sessions are directed toward the overall aim of improving a person's psychological wellbeing.
6. An integrative or eclectic approach is taken toward therapeutic techniques. These are drawn from various psychotherapeutic approaches, such as CBT and psychodynamic therapy.
7. It is a short-term therapy, typically consisting of between six and 16 sessions.

19.2 WHICH THERAPY IS BEST?

The issue of whether one type of therapy is better than another is contentious. There is evidence to suggest that various different psychotherapies are effective treatments for depression and anxiety disorders. Richardson (2006) argues that 'where one therapy appears to have an advantage over others in terms of empirical research this is usually because the others have failed to accumulate the relevant evidence'. It may be that different therapies are equally effective for some disorders and there is emerging evidence that this may be the case. For example, a review of 257 meta-analyses of the effect of psychotherapy on a range of outcomes showed that the majority (80%) reported a significant effect on outcomes. The authors concluded that the most convincing evidence for the efficacy of psychotherapy were for: CBT, meditation, cognitive remediation, counselling, and mixed psychotherapy (Dragioti et al., 2017). Similarly, a study of more than 5,600 people who had had CBT, person-centred therapy, or psychodynamic therapy found that all three therapies resulted in an improvement and were equally effective (Stiles et al., 2008).

This suggests that non-specific factors, such as the therapeutic relationship or placebo effect, may play an important role in the effectiveness of psychotherapy. The importance of a good relationship between the person and therapist is well established, and evidence shows that it leads to better outcomes, regardless of the type of psychotherapy (Department of Health, 2001). Whether therapy also works through a placebo effect is less widely considered, though Kirsch (2007) has suggested that this is the case because psychotherapy involves no active physiological substances and instead relies on a person's expectations, experience of therapy, and beliefs about therapy to treat illness.

So what can we conclude from this? There is little doubt that psychotherapy is effective in the treatment of mental health. Which type of psychotherapy is best is likely to vary for different psychological problems and individuals. Although the current guidelines favour CBT and third wave therapies, this position may change as the evidence accumulates for counselling and psychodynamic approaches. It would be nice to think that in the future psychotherapy will move away from a 'winner takes all' mentality where one type of therapy has to prove itself as being better than all the others and will integrate those approaches and techniques that are shown to be effective under different circumstances. This is already evident in counselling, which draws on techniques from many different approaches to therapy.

Summary

- There are many different types of psychotherapy.
- Therapies have developed from theories of psychoanalysis, humanism, behaviourism, and cognitivism.
- Dominant approaches to therapy at present are CBT, third wave cognitive therapies, psychodynamic therapy, and counselling.
- CBT is a structured, short-term therapy that focuses on the present problem and changes maladaptive beliefs and behaviour.
- Third wave cognitive therapies focus on the relationship people have with their thoughts and changing this through techniques such as mindfulness meditation, acceptance, and cognitive defusion.
- Psychodynamic therapy is an intensive, long-term therapy that focuses on a person's early childhood experience, interpersonal relationships, and unconscious conflicts.
- Counselling is a short-term therapy that can consist of one approach to therapy, such as psychoanalysis, but is often more integrative or eclectic.
- There is some indication that different types of therapy may be equally effective for some disorders. This may be due to the importance of non-specific factors such as the therapeutic relationship or a placebo effect.

19.3 PSYCHOLOGICAL INTERVENTIONS IN MEDICAL SETTINGS

Psychological interventions in medical settings extend beyond psychotherapy. They do not purely aim to resolve mental health problems but also include any intervention to promote physical or mental health in medical settings. This includes health promotion, pain management, self-management in chronic illnesses, crisis intervention, stress management, and support groups. Descriptions of some of these interventions are given in Table 19.2. Examples and case studies of these interventions can be found throughout the chapters in this book.

There is general support for the effectiveness of psychological interventions for promoting health and wellbeing, although this varies according to the type of intervention and target group. Interventions can be broadly grouped into:

• Those that aim to change health behaviours.
• Those that aim to help people cope with difficult or stressful circumstances.
• Those that target particular symptoms or illnesses, such as pain management.

TABLE 19.2 Psychological interventions in medical settings

Psychological intervention	Aims	What it consists of	Use	See example
Assessment	Assess an individual's psychosocial needs	Interview and questionnaires to assess people's needs and mental state	For severe or chronic illnesses that require multidisciplinary management	
Pain management	Help people manage their pain to increase activity levels and wellbeing	Education about pain, CBT techniques such as monitoring activity and pain, setting goals, empowering people	For chronic pain of any kind, e.g. back pain, pelvic pain, arthritis, etc.	Chapter 4
Motivational interviewing	Help people to change risky health behaviours	Exploring and understanding a person's current beliefs and behaviour, facilitating change through developing the discrepancy between a person's values and current behaviour, and building confidence that change is possible	For smoking, alcohol use, other drug addictions, eating disorders and depression	Chapter 2
Self-management	Help people manage their illness or recovery, including adherence to medication, rehabilitation and facilitating psychological wellbeing	Examining beliefs about illness, illness behaviour, and emotions, and facilitating change to promote good self-management of illness	For chronic illnesses, e.g. multiple sclerosis, diabetes, heart disease, asthma, irritable bowel syndrome, arthritis, etc.	Chapter 4

Psychological intervention	Aims	What it consists of	Use	See example
Health promotion	Promote health and positive health behaviours and reduce risky health behaviours	Education and promotion of health through information and interventions to reduce risky behaviours	With the normal population, e.g. people attending primary care, antenatal clinics, sexual health clinics, and smoking cessation	Chapter 5
Crisis intervention	Support people in times of crisis and help them adjust and cope	Supporting people to work through what has happened and encourage positive adjustment	After a diagnosis of a serious illness such as cancer, heart disease, multiple sclerosis, etc., and in palliative care	Chapters 6, 11 & 12
Stress management	Help people to manage stress effectively	Education about stress: understanding and breaking down stress, appraisal processes and responses, and exploring more adaptive ways to cope	When stress may exacerbate conditions such as heart disease, premenstrual tension, and for healthcare professionals in high stress jobs	Chapter 3
Support groups	Encourage contact with, and support from, other people in similar circumstances	Small groups of people with similar problems, which are usually facilitated by a healthcare professional	With groups such as people with cancer, heart disease, or following stillbirth	Chapter 11
Bereavement counselling	Help people cope with and come to terms with their loss	Individual or couple counselling to help people mourn their loss and find ways to cope	For the loss or bereavement of a significant other, e.g. a stillbirth, relatives of people who are dying	Chapter 6
Neuropsychological rehabilitation	Assess, treat and rehabilitate people with a brain injury to reduce disability and increase quality of life	Examination of cognitive, behavioural, emotional, and social function, and rehabilitation through various techniques, e.g. goal setting, skill training, and increasing awareness	Following brain injury or neurodegenerative diseases such as dementia	Chapter 16

19.3.1 INTERVENTIONS FOR CHANGING BEHAVIOUR

Interventions to change health behaviours include health education, health promotion, and motivational interviewing. **Health promotion** is a broad area, ranging from national advertising campaigns to group interventions with people who have a particular illness. Its effectiveness varies according to the method chosen and the people targeted. Providing blanket information to everyone is less effective than targeting information. Evidence has clearly shown that educational interventions are more effective if they are relevant to the people they target, are individualised, can provide feedback on people's learning, facilitate change by explaining how people can take action, can help people to develop the required skills to change, and can reinforce the desired behaviour (Kok, 2007). This has informed health promotion and there are many advertising campaigns targeting specific groups, such as those in Figure 19.3.

Motivational interviewing is used to change risky behaviour and promote healthy behaviour. Motivational interviewing was developed as a treatment for substance misuse, where people often have positive and negative attitudes toward the problem behaviour. It is a form of directive counselling that helps patients to explore their reasons for a behaviour and their ambivalence toward a problem behaviour and to try to resolve it. Motivational interviewing is more focused and goal-directed than normal counselling, although the emphasis here is not on *persuading* someone to change but on *helping* them to develop their own motivation to change. This is done through (i) empathising with the situation the person is in, (ii) avoiding argumentation or persuasion, (iii) examining the discrepancy between what the person wants to do and what they are actually doing, (iv) examining resistance, and (v) bolstering the person's self-efficacy (Miller, 1995). An example of motivational interviewing is given in Chapter 2 (see Case Study 2.2).

Evidence shows that motivational interviewing can be highly effective. A review of 72 clinical trials of using motivational interviewing across a wide range of behaviours showed it is very effective in the short term. In the long term, change was most likely when motivational interviewing was used in addition to a standard treatment (Hettema et al., 2005). It is therefore a useful approach for healthcare practitioners to use to help people change behaviours, such as substance abuse and non-adherence to treatments.

19.3.2 INTERVENTIONS FOR STRESSFUL OR DIFFICULT CIRCUMSTANCES

Interventions to help people cope with stressful or difficult circumstances include stress management, critical incident debriefing, crisis intervention, bereavement counselling, and support groups. **Stress management** has been used with occupational groups, patient groups, and health professionals. It is based on our understanding of the processes of stress and coping (see Chapter 3) and helps people identify the factors contributing to their

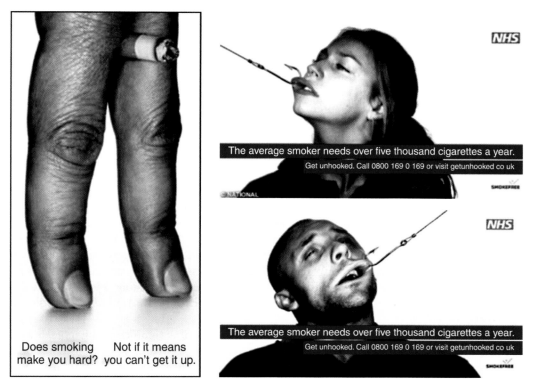

FIGURE 19.3   Targeted health promotion: anti-smoking campaign. © Nick Georghiou

stress and to find more adaptive ways to cope. In healthcare settings, stress management has most often been provided for people with cancer or heart disease. In this context, stress management reduces anxiety, depression, perceived pain, and increases quality of life for people. However, it may have no effect on the course of illness or morbidity (Kenny, 2007).

   Critical incident debriefing was initially developed to help emergency service workers cope with the traumatic events they attended, such as disasters, homicide, or road traffic accidents. Debriefing was carried out in groups and this approach was rapidly applied to a range of traumatic situations. However, evidence has shown that debriefing is *not* effective and in some cases can make people worse. As a result, many guidelines recommend against using it. Despite this, debriefing is still used in some settings in varying forms. For example, 78% of hospitals in the UK offer some form of midwife-led debriefing to women after difficult or traumatic birth experiences (Ayers et al., 2006). However, the content of midwife-led debriefing is different from critical incident debriefing so these services are usually referred to by other names, such as 'birth afterthoughts'.

ACTIVITY 19.2

- Think of a time you found really stressful or difficult.
- How did you cope with it?
- What did you find most helpful?

Debriefing shares some similarities with **crisis intervention** and bereavement intervention in that all of these try to ameliorate a situation rather than prevent it happening in the first place. Crisis intervention is used in situations where there has been threat of harm or violence, such as terrorist attacks, violent crime, domestic violence, or suicide attempts. It draws on a range of psychological theories and techniques to support people through a critical period (Roberts, 2005). Evidence for crisis intervention in medical settings suggests it reduces anxiety and PTSD, but is less effective for reducing depression (Stapleton et al., 2006). In addition, crisis intervention is more effective when it involves more than one session and is carried out by an experienced therapist (Stapleton et al., 2006).

Bereavement intervention is used following the death of a significant other, such as a spouse, parent, or child. Bereavement interventions vary according to which theoretical view is taken of bereavement. The psychodynamic view focuses on unresolved conflicts or issues with the deceased. Stage theories of bereavement emphasise the different stages a person needs to go through, such as numbness, yearning, despair, and recovery (Payne et al., 1999). Stress theories of bereavement emphasise the stress of bereavement and the loss of resources to cope. Support theories emphasise the loss of social support and the disruption of support networks.

A review of bereavement intervention considered the different theoretical viewpoints and whether these can account for the evidence that (i) men are more affected by the death of a spouse than women; and (ii) that how the person dies affects the nature of grief – for example, an unexpected death is likely to result in more severe grief than an expected death. The review concluded that these facts were best accounted for by stress or support theories of bereavement (Kato & Mann, 1999). However, this and other reviews of the evidence suggest that bereavement interventions as a whole may be limited in their impact. Although they improve short-term outcomes compared to no treatment, these differences are not observed in the longer term, which might be because grief tends to reduce naturally over time in those who have no treatment (Currier et al., 2008). There is also evidence that suggests bereavement interventions are only really effective for high-risk individuals – for example, in cases where the death was unexpected, where there was a high level of dependency in the relationship, or where the person had a history of psychological problems (Currier et al., 2008; Jordan & Neimeyer, 2003).

CLINICAL NOTES 19.1

Psychotherapy techniques and clinical practice

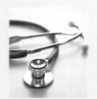

- Recognise that individuals come to you with their own emotional baggage, core beliefs, past experience, and relationship history.
- Do not underestimate the effects of a good practitioner–patient relationship and placebo.
- Give people unconditional positive regard to improve the practitioner–patient relationship and the person's psychological wellbeing.
- Be on the person's side, understand their experience, and work with them to encourage change.
- Remember that helping people to 'face their fear' is essentially a form of exposure and so can be an effective treatment for anxiety.
- Help people to distance themselves from negative thoughts – e.g. to accept the thoughts and think of them as a wave that will just wash over them and recede.

19.3.3 INTERVENTIONS FOR SPECIFIC ILLNESSES OR SYMPTOMS

Interventions targeted at specific illnesses or symptoms are wide-ranging and include self-management interventions, support groups for people with particular problems or illnesses, pain management, and neuropsychological rehabilitation.

Self-management interventions draw on the theories outlined in Chapters 4 and 5 to help people manage their illness or rehabilitation effectively, with the aim of improving their psychological and physical wellbeing. Specific self-management interventions have been designed for many illnesses, such as arthritis, asthma, diabetes, hypertension, chronic obstructive pulmonary disease (COPD), headache, and back pain (Mulligan & Newman, 2018). Generic self-management programmes for chronic disease have also been developed (Lorig et al., 2001). Most self-management programmes involve five core components to increase people's skills at managing their illness. These are: problem solving, decision making, how to find and use resources, forming partnerships with healthcare professionals, and taking action (Lorig & Holman, 2003).

Evidence shows self-management interventions are effective in the short term and can improve health behaviours and the management of an illness, such as adherence to medication. Self-management interventions can also lead to improved physical and emotional wellbeing. For example, a review of 969 randomised controlled trials of self-management interventions for different conditions found strong evidence that self-management interventions for diabetes improve blood glucose control; self-management interventions for rheumatoid arthritis lead to improved disability and psychological wellbeing; and self-management interventions for asthma reduce hospital admissions and emergency healthcare services (Taylor et al., 2014). However, these effects are not always maintained over the long term (Mulligan & Newman, 2018).

Support group interventions are based on substantial evidence that social support is associated with better health and wellbeing and that, conversely, social isolation is a risk for many illnesses. Support interventions usually consist of a group of up to 12 people with similar problems or circumstances who meet eight to ten times. Groups can be facilitated by a health professional or be patient-led. Support groups aim to increase the support available to people, increase education and the sharing of knowledge about relevant circumstances, and increase the sharing and modelling of positive coping strategies.

The popularity of support groups in medical settings was boosted by a study that showed that women with breast cancer who attended a support group lived on average 18 months longer than those who did not attend a support group (Spiegel et al., 1989). Since then the evidence has been less consistent: although support groups usually improve psychological wellbeing and quality of life, they do not have a consistent impact on morbidity or mortality (Gottlieb, 2007). It is possible this is because they work better for some people than others. For example, if a person has a poor social network and does not express their emotions or cope particularly well, then a support group can be very helpful by increasing their social network, helping them talk about their feelings, and letting them see other group members modelling better ways of coping. Conversely, a person with many close friends and family members supporting them may not benefit from a support group.

There are many other interventions for specific illnesses. Evidence shows that **pain management** programmes based on CBT can lead to short-term reductions in pain, disability, negative mood, and catastrophising compared to usual treatment (Williams et al., 2012; see also Chapter 4). **Neuropsychological rehabilitation** uses a wide range of psychological theory to treat and rehabilitate people with neuropsychological problems, such as brain injury (see Chapter 16). Families are usually highly involved in this process. Technologies, such as computer programs, virtual reality training, electronic reminders, and memory aids, are rapidly being developed to help people adapt and function in the community (Wilson, 2007). Research into the effectiveness of neuropsychological rehabilitation has focused on specific techniques. For example, there is evidence that memory rehabilitation and specific attention skills training can be effective, but that general attention training is not (Rohling et al., 2009).

Summary

- Psychological interventions in medical settings include health promotion, interventions for stressful or difficult circumstances, and interventions for specific illnesses or groups of people.
- These interventions are wide-ranging and draw on a range of psychological theories and techniques.

(Continued)

- Evidence shows that health promotion, motivational interviewing, self-management, pain management, and neuropsychological rehabilitation are effective.
- However, the beneficial effect of many psychological interventions in healthcare settings can be short term and limited to psychosocial outcomes.
- Critical incident stress debriefing is the only intervention where there is evidence that it should not be used.
- Bereavement interventions only appear to be effective with high-risk individuals.

19.4 TECHNOLOGY AND PSYCHOLOGICAL INTERVENTION

The cost and limited availability of psychological services in many countries means there is increasing use of technology to support or deliver psychological interventions. The advantages to this are that treatment is accessible, convenient, and can be provided over a wide geographical area. People sometimes refer to the three 'A's of the internet: availability, accessibility, and affordability. Online interventions may also provide a fourth 'A', anonymity, which can reduce barriers to accessing treatment, such as the stigma associated with various illnesses.

Tailored psychological interventions are increasingly accessible through the web, smartphones, and tablets. Online resources are available to treat illnesses, such as computerised therapy for anxiety and depression. Technology can also be used to facilitate support groups through online forums, email discussion groups, and social media. People generally rate online groups positively but there is a lack of high-quality evidence for the effectiveness of online groups (Griffiths et al., 2009). Technology-assisted programs are also available to assist people in lifestyle change or therapy, such as exercise trackers, mood trackers, and meditation apps.

Technology-mediated psychotherapy programmes are usually self-directed, where people work through a series of modules in their own time. Some are supported by a healthcare professional who oversees people's progress via telephone, email, or messaging. Programmes are available for a range of common psychological problems, such as insomnia, stress, depression, anxiety, phobias, etc. (see Clinical notes 19.2). Most are based on CBT or third wave cognitive therapy techniques, which are relatively easily adapted for this medium. There is now substantial evidence that online and computerised programs can be an effective treatment for less severe affective disorders. Reviews and meta-analyses show that web-based treatments for stress, depression, and anxiety disorders are more effective than no treatment or placebo controls, and in some cases are as effective as face-to-face psychotherapy treatment (Andrews et al., 2010; Heber et al., 2017; Mayo-Wilson & Montgomery, 2013; Olthuis et al., 2016).

For example, *Beating the Blues* is a therapy programme developed for moderate depression. It has been used in primary care settings and is also available online. The programme involves individuals watching an introductory videotape and then carrying out eight sessions of one hour each with homework between each session. At the end of each session a printed summary of the session is provided for the person and can be shared with the healthcare professional supporting the programme. People can then meet with their healthcare professional to check on their progress and medication if this is needed. Evidence suggests that this programme is more effective than GP treatment alone at reducing moderate anxiety and depression, facilitating social adjustment and a return to work (Proudfoot et al., 2003, 2004).

The advantages and potential efficacy of programmes delivered through technology means this is a rapidly expanding area. However, not all programmes have evidence of efficacy from methodologically rigorous trials (Ashford et al., 2016). Web-based interventions have also been developed to help people manage long-term physical health conditions such as diabetes (Hofmann et al., 2016), and to encourage more healthy behaviours. However, programmes available via the web vary in quality and content. It is clear from reviews that some web-based programmes are more effective than others, and that not all of them are founded on validated theories of psychological disorder or behaviour change (Murray, 2012). Similarly, there are huge numbers of health apps available, but many of them do not have a theoretical basis or evidence of efficacy. Apps that do have a theoretical basis, such as self-monitoring for behaviour change, have been positively evaluated but the evidence is currently limited to feasibility and pilot studies (Payne et al., 2015). It is therefore important that people are directed to programmes with some evidence of effectiveness.

More recent developments include the use of games and virtual reality to monitor or improve health. Games such as *Wii Fit* promote physical activity and have been used as a part of neuropsychological rehabilitation, e.g. with people who have had a stroke as part of rehabilitation to regain mobility. Although improvements are similar to those observed after conventional rehabilitation, people were less likely to drop out from the *Wii Fit* programme (Cheok et al., 2015). Games have also been developed for specific health issues. These can be to help patients, such as *Bobby got a Burn*, which prepares children for standard medical procedures, or *iSpectrum*, which aims to improve social interaction skills in people with autism or Asperger's syndrome. Games have also been developed to help healthcare students. A scoping review in 2014 identified a wide range of games to help students learn procedures in surgery, radiology, dentistry, nursing, cardiology, dietitians, and first aid (Ricciardi & Tommaso de Paolis, 2014).

Virtual reality programs enable various situations to be simulated and therefore have potential applications in psychological interventions such as neuropsychological rehabilitation and psychotherapy for anxiety disorders. Virtual reality has been used in rehabilitation for conditions such as Parkinson's (Dockx et al., 2016), stroke (Laver et al., 2015), brain injury (Shin & Kim, 2015) and cerebral palsy (Ravi et al., 2016), with some evidence that it is a promising method in terms of increasing mobility and motor skills. Virtual reality programs are also used as part of exposure treatment for anxiety disorders. As mentioned earlier, an effective behavioural treatment for fears and phobias is to expose people to the feared object until their anxiety reduces. Obviously, being exposed to fearful situations can be very challenging for people, so virtual reality is a useful medium through which to 'expose' someone to their feared object or situation but where the person knows it is not real. Virtual exposure has been used as part of treatment for a range of problems, including fear of flying, dental phobia, spider phobia, social anxiety, and PTSD. Several reviews show that virtual reality exposure is an acceptable and effective treatment for phobias and anxiety disorders (Botella et al., 2015). For example, a review of 14 randomised controlled trials of virtual reality exposure for phobias found it resulted in improved outcomes and that improvements are similar to those observed after real-life exposure (Morina et al., 2015).

CLINICAL NOTES 19.2

Computerised and online psychotherapy

- *Beating the Blues* (for depression), www.beatingtheblues.co.uk
- *Fear fighter* (for anxiety and panic), www.fearfighter.com
- *Headspace*: a mindfulness app
- *Big White Wall*: an online community for people with depression and anxiety, www.bigwhitewall.com
- *Sleepio*: an insomnia app, www.sleepio.com
- For a wide range of free self-help resources, see the Centre for Clinical Interventions resources: www.cci.health.wa.gov.au

CONCLUSION

In this chapter we have looked at different types of psychotherapy and the theories underlying them. First we looked at cognitive behaviour therapy and third wave therapies such as mindfulness, ACT and DBT. Then we looked at different approaches of psychodynamic therapy and counselling. There is now extensive evidence that psychotherapy is more effective than no treatment for common affective disorders. However, at this stage there is little conclusive evidence that one therapy is more effective than another. Nonspecific factors, such as the relationship between the therapist and client, are likely to be important in the efficacy of psychotherapy. In the future psychotherapies may therefore move away from focusing on one particular approach to using techniques that are shown to be effective under different circumstances.

Psychological interventions in medical settings draw on psychotherapy and health behaviour change techniques to promote physical and mental health. These interventions may aim to (i) reduce negative health behaviours, such as health promotion and motivational interviewing; (ii) help people cope with stressful circumstances, such as stress management, debriefing, crisis intervention and bereavement interventions; or

(iii) target specific illnesses or symptoms, such as pain, self-management of chronic illnesses, or neurological rehabilitation. The evidence for the effectiveness of such interventions is mixed – probably due to the wide range of interventions and target populations. For example, there is good evidence that motivational interviewing and self-management programmes are effective, but little evidence bereavement interventions are effective unless targeted at high-risk individuals.

Technology is increasingly used to deliver computerised or app-based psychotherapy. These are usually based on CBT and third wave cognitive therapy techniques, which lend themselves well to self-directed psychotherapy. There is substantial evidence computerised psychotherapy is effective for less severe affective disorders, such as depression and anxiety. Recent developments also include use of games and virtual reality to improve psychological and physical health in specific groups, such as people with phobias or neurological disorders.

FURTHER READING

Llewellyn, C.D. et al. (eds) (2018) *The Cambridge Handbook of Psychology, Health and Medicine* (3rd edition). Cambridge: Cambridge University Press. Includes short chapters on behaviour therapy, cognitive behaviour therapy, behavioural couples therapy, biofeedback, counselling, group therapy, technology-assisted interventions, hypnosis, mindfulness, motivational interviewing, pain management, peer support interventions, psychodynamic therapy, self-help interventions, stress and crisis management, and worksite interventions.

Bramber, M.R. (2006) *CBT for Occupational Stress in Health Professionals*. Hove: Routledge. Outlines the use of CBT to help cope with problems like performance anxiety, health anxiety, perfectionism, and burnout.

Rollnick, S., Miller, W.R. & Butler, C.C. (2008) *Motivational Interviewing in Health Care: Helping Patients Change Behavior*. New York: Guilford Press. Outlines the basic principles and core skills required for motivational interviewing.

White, C.A. (2001) *Cognitive Behaviour Therapy for Chronic Medical Problems*. Chichester: Wiley. Provides an introduction to using CBT with a wide range of medical problems, including surgical, cardiac, dermatological, cancer, pain, and diabetes.

REVISION QUESTIONS

1. Describe third wave cognitive therapies and illustrate this with an example.

2. Describe the core features of cognitive behaviour therapy (CBT).

3. Outline the cognitive theory of depression and discuss the role of the depressogenic triad of negative beliefs.

4. Briefly compare and contrast behavioural and cognitive techniques for treating psychological problems.

5. What is a formulation and what is its role in psychotherapy?

6. Briefly outline the three core principles of psychodynamic therapy.

7. Describe the five core features of counselling.

8. Outline three psychological interventions used in medical settings and discuss whether these are effective.

9. What is unconditional positive regard and from which theory or theories does it originate?

10. Outline three psychological specialties and discuss their potential application to healthcare.

BIBLIOGRAPHY

Abbass, A.A., Hancock, J.T., Henderson, J. & Kisely, S. (2006) Short-term psychodynamic psychotherapies for common mental disorders. *Cochrane Database of Systematic Reviews*, *4* (Art. CD004687).

Abbass, A.A., Kisely, S.R., Town, J.M., Leichsenring, F., Driessen, E., De Maat, S., Gerber, A., Dekker, J., Rabung, S., Rusalovska, S. & Crowe, E. (2014) Short-term psychodynamic psychotherapies for common mental disorders. *Cochrane Database Systematic Reviews*, July, *1*(7): (Art. CD004687).

Abbey, G. et al. (2015) A meta-analysis of prevalence rates and moderating factors for cancer-related post-traumatic stress disorder. *Psycho-Oncology*, *24*: 371–381.

Abraham, C. & Michie, S. (2008) A taxonomy of behavior change techniques used in interventions. *Health Psychology*, *27*: 379–387.

Abraham, C. & Sheeran, P. (2007) The health belief model, in S. Ayers et al. (eds), *Cambridge Handbook of Psychology, Health and Medicine* (2nd edition). Cambridge: Cambridge University Press. pp. 97–102.

Abrahams, H.J. et al. (2015) A randomized controlled trial of web-based cognitive behavioral therapy for severely fatigued breast cancer survivors (CHANGE-study): Study protocol. *BMC Cancer*, *15*: 765.

Ackermann, S. & Rasch, B. (2014) Differential effects of non-REM and REM sleep on memory consolidation? *Current Neurology and Neuroscience Reports*, *14*: 430.

Adams, J.A. (1971) A closed loop theory of motor control. *Journal of Motor Behaviour*, *3*: 111–150.

Adamson, S.J., Sellman, J.D. & Frampton, C.M.A. (2009) Patient predictors of alcohol treatment outcome: A systematic review. *Journal of Substance Abuse Treatment*, *36*: 75–86.

Addis, M.E. & Mahalik, J.R. (2003) Men, masculinity, and the contexts of help seeking. *American Psychology*, *58*: 5–14.

Ader, R. (2003) Conditioned immunomodulation: Research needs and directions. *Brain, Behavior and Immunity*, *17* (suppl. 1): s51–s57.

Ahmad, A.S., Ormiston-Smith, N. & Sasieni, P.D. (2015) Trends in the lifetime risk of developing cancer in Great Britain: Comparison of risk for those born from 1930 to 1960. *British Journal of Cancer*, *112*: 943–947.

Ahmid, M. et al. (2016) Growth hormone deficiency during young adulthood and the benefits of growth hormone replacement. *Endocrine Connections*, *2*(5): R1–R11.

Ahn, D.H. et al. (2015) The effect of post-stroke depression on rehabilitation outcome and the impact of caregiver type as a factor of post-stroke depression. *Annals of Rehabilitation Medicine*, *39*: 74–80.

Ainsworth, M.D.S., Blehar, M.C., Waters, E. & Wall, S. (1978) *Patterns of Attachment: A Psychological Study of the Strange Situation*. Hillsdale, NJ: Erlbaum.

Ajzen, I. (1988) *Attitudes, Personality, and Behaviour*. Buckingham: Open University Press.

Akbar, H., Anderson, D. & Gallegos, D. (2015) Predicting intentions and behaviours in populations with or at-risk of diabetes: A systematic review. *Preventative Medicine Reports, 2*: 270–282.

Akobeng, A.K., Ramanan, A.V., Buchan, I. & Heller, R.F. (2006) Effect of breast feeding on risk of coeliac disease: A systematic review and meta-analysis of observational studies. *Archives of Disease in Childhood, 91*: 39–43.

Albarracín, D. et al. (2001) Theories of reasoned action and planned behavior as models of condom use. *Psychological Bulletin, 127*: 142–161.

Albarracín, D. et al. (2003) Persuasive communications to change actions: An analysis of behavioral and cognitive impact in HIV prevention. *Health Psychology, 22*: 166–177.

Alder, J., Fink, N., Bitzer, J., Hösli, I. & Holzgreve, W. (2007) Depression and anxiety during pregnancy: A risk factor for obstetric, fetal and neonatal outcome? A critical review of the literature. *Journal of Maternal-Fetal and Neonatal Medicine, 20*: 189–209.

Alelwani, S.M. & Ahmed, Y.A. (2014) Medical training for communication of bad news: A literature review. *Journal of Education and Health Promotion, 3*: 51.

Alexandrova-Karamanova, A., Todorova, I., Montgomery, A., Panagopoulou, E., Costa, P., Baban, A., Davas, A., Milosevic, M. & Mijakoski, D. (2016) Burnout and health behaviors in health professionals from seven European countries. *International Archive of Occupational and Environmental Health, 89*(7): 1059–1075.

Ali, F. et al. (2014) Stem cells and the treatment of Parkinson's disease. *Experimental Neurology, 260*: 3–11.

Allen, K., Blascovich, J. & Mendes, W.B. (2002) Cardiovascular reactivity and the presence of pets, friends, and spouses: The truth about cats and dogs. *Psychosomatic Medicine, 64*: 727–739.

Alsaker, F.D. (1992) Pubertal timing, overweight, and psychological adjustment. *Journal of Early Adolescence, 12*: 396–419.

Althaus, D., Stefanek, J., Hasford, J. & Hegerl, U. (2002) Knowledge and attitude of the general public regarding symptoms, etiology and possible treatments of depressive illnesses. *Nervenarzt. 73*(7): 659–664.

Alvarez, G.G. & Ayas, N.T. (2004) The impact of daily sleep duration on health: A review of the literature. *Progress in Cardiovascular Nursing, 19*: 56–59.

Ambady, N., LaPlante, D., Nguyen, T., Rosenthal, R., Chaumeton, N. & Levinson, W. (2002) Surgeons' tone of voice: A clue to malpractice history. *Surgery, 132*: 5–9.

American Psychiatric Association (1994) *Diagnostic and Statistical Manual of Mental Disorders* (3rd edition). Washington, DC: APA.

American Psychiatric Association (2004) *Diagnostic and Statistical Manual of Mental Disorders* (4th edition). Washington, DC: APA.

American Psychiatric Association (2013) *Diagnostic and Statistical Manual of Mental Disorders* (5th edition). Washington, DC: APA.

Amieva, M. & Peek, R.M. (2016) Pathobiology of helicobacter pylori-induced gastric cancer. *Gastroenterology, 150*: 64–78.

Amsel, E. & Renninger, K.A. (eds) (1997) *Change and Development: Issues of Theory, Method and Application*. Mahwah, NJ: Lawrence Erlbaum.

Anderson, C.A. (2004) An update on the effects of playing violent video games. *Journal of Adolescence, 27*: 113–122.

Anderson, E.M. & Lambert, M.J. (1995) Short-term dynamically oriented psychotherapy: A review and meta-analysis. *Clinical Psychology Review, 15*: 503–14.

Anderson, L. & Taylor, R.S. (2014) Cardiac rehabilitation for people with heart disease: An overview of Cochrane systematic reviews. *Cochrane Database Systematic Reviews, 12*(12): CD011273.

Andrade, J., Deeprose, C. & Barker, I. (2008) Awareness and memory function during paediatric anaesthesia. *British Journal of Anaesthesia, 100*(3): 389–396.

Andrews, G., Cuijpers, P., Craske, M.G., McEvoy, P. & Titov, N. (2010) Computer therapy for the anxiety and depressive disorders is effective, acceptable and practical health care: A meta-analysis. *PLoS One, 5*(10), e13196.

Anestis, M.D., Smith A.R., Fink, L.E. & Joiner, T.E. (2009) Dysregulated eating and distress: Examining the specific role of negative urgency in a clinical sample. *Cognitive Therapy Research, 33*: 390–397.

Angelelli, P. et al. (2004) Development of neuropsychiatric symptoms in poststroke patients: A cross-sectional study. *Acta Psychiatrica Scandinavica, 110*: 55–63.

Angevaren, M., Aufdemkampe, G., Verhaar, H.J., Aleman, A. & Vanhees, L. (2008) Physical activity and enhanced fitness to improve cognitive function in older people without known cognitive impairment. *Cochrane Database of Systematic Reviews, 3* (Art. CD005381).

Anstey, K.J. & Luszcz, M.A. (2002) Mortality risk varies according to gender and change in depressive status in very old adults. *Psychosomatic Medicine, 64*: 880–888.

Antoni, M.H. (2013) Psychosocial intervention effects on adaptation, disease course and biobehavioral processes in cancer. *Brain, Behavior and Immunity*, 30 (Suppl.): s88–s98.

Antoni, M.H. et al. (2006) Randomized clinical trial of cognitive behavioral stress management on Human Immunodeficiency Virus viral load in gay men treated with highly active antiretroviral therapy. *Psychosomatic Medicine, 68*: 143–151.

Antonovsky, A. (1987) *Unraveling the Mystery of Health: How People Manage Stress and Stay Well*. San Francisco, CA: Jossey-Bass.

Arbuthnott, A. & Sharpe, D. (2009) The effect of physician–patient collaboration on patient adherence in non-psychiatric medicine. *Patient Education and Counseling, 77*: 60–67.

Arden-Close, E., Gidron, Y. & Moss-Morris, R. (2008) Psychological distress and its correlates in ovarian cancer: A systematic review. *Psycho-Oncology, 17*: 1061–1072.

Armfield, J.M. & Heaton, L.J. (2013) Management of fear and anxiety in the dental clinic: A review. *Australian Dental Journal, 58*: 390–407.

Arminjon, M., Preissmann, D., Chmetz, F., Duraku, A., Ansermet, F. & Magistretti, P.J. (2015) Embodied memory: Unconscious smiling modulates emotional evaluation of episodic memories. *Frontiers in Psychology, 26*(6): 650.

Arnett, J.J. (2004) *Emerging Adulthood: The Winding Road from Late Teens through the Twenties*. Oxford: Oxford University Press.

Arnold, R., Ranchor, A., Sanderman, R., Kempen, G., Ormel, J. & Suurmeijer, T. (2004) The relative contribution of domains of quality of life to overall quality of life for different chronic diseases. *Quality of Life Research*, 13: 883–896.

Arseneault, L., Cannon, M., Witton, J. & Murray, R.M. (2004) Causal association between cannabis and psychosis: Examination of the evidence. *British Journal of Psychiatry*, 184: 110–117.

Arseniou, S., Arvaniti, A. & Samakouri, M. (2014) HIV infection and depression. *Psychiatry and Clinical Neurosciences*, 68(2): 96–109.

Asada, K., Tojo, Y., Osanai, H., Saito, A., Hasegawa, T. & Kumagaya, S. (2016) Reduced personal space in individuals with Autism Spectrum Disorder. *PLoS One*, 11(1): e0146306.

Asch, S.E. (1956) Studies of independence and conformity: A minority of one against a unanimous majority. *Psychological Monographs: General and Applied*, 70: 1–70.

Asher, R. (1949) Myxoedematous madness. *British Medical Journal*, 2: 555–562.

Ashford, M.T., Olander, E.K. & Ayers, S. (2016) Finding web-based anxiety interventions on the World Wide Web: A scoping review. *JMIR Mental Health*, 3(2): e14.

Ashley, W.R., Harper, R.S. & Runyon, D.L. (1951) The perceived size of coins in normal and hypnotically induced economic states. *American Journal of Psychology*, 64: 564–572.

Ashworth, M., Godfrey, E., Harvey, K. & Darbishire, L. (2003) Perceptions of psychological content in the GP consultation: The role of practice, personal and prescribing attributes. *Family Practice*, 20: 373–375.

Aspen, V., Darcy, A.M. & Lock, J. (2013) A review of attention biases in women with eating disorders. *Cognition and Emotion*, 27: 820–838.

Astin, F., Horrocks, J. & Closs, S.J. (2014) Managing lifestyle change to reduce coronary risk: A synthesis of qualitative research on people's experiences. *BMC Cardiovascular Disorders*, 14: 96.

Astramskaitė, I., Poškevičius, L. & Juodžbalys, G. (2016) Factors determining tooth extraction anxiety and fear in adult dental patients: A systematic review. *International Journal of Oral Maxillofacial Surgery*, 45(12): 1630–1643.

Atlas, L.Y. & Wager, T.D. (2012) How expectations shape pain. *Neuroscience Letter*, 520: 40–48.

Atlas, L.Y. & Wager, T.D. (2014) A meta-analysis of brain mechanisms of placebo analgesia: Consistent findings and unanswered questions. *Handbook of Experimental Pharmacology*, 225: 37–69.

Aust, J. & Bradshaw, T. (2017) Mindfulness interventions for psychosis: A systematic review of the literature. *Journal of Psychiatric and Mental Health Nursing*, 24(1): 69–83.

Axboe, M.K., Christensen, K.S., Kofoed, P.E. & Ammentorp, J. (2016) Development and validation of a self-efficacy questionnaire (SE-12) measuring the clinical communication skills of health care professionals. *BMC Medical Education*, 16(1): 272.

Ayers, S., Bond, R., Bertullies, S. & Wijma, K. (2016) The aetiology of post-traumatic stress following childbirth: A meta-analysis and theoretical framework. *Psychological Medicine*, 46(6): 1121–1134.

Ayers, S., Claypool, J. & Eagle, A. (2006) What happens after a difficult birth? Postnatal debriefing services. *British Journal of Midwifery*, 14: 157–161.

Ayers, S., Copland, C. & Dunmore, E. (2009) A preliminary study of negative appraisals and dysfunctional coping associated with post-traumatic stress disorder symptoms following myocardial infarction. *British Journal of Health Psychology*, 14: 459–471.

Ayers, S. & Ford, E. (2015) Posttraumatic stress in pregnancy and the postpartum period, in A. Wenzel & S. Scott (eds.), *Oxford Handbook of Perinatal Psychology*. Oxford: Oxford University Press.

Ayers, S., Joseph, S., McKenzie-McHarg, K., Slade, P. & Wijma, K. (2008) Post-traumatic stress disorder following childbirth: Current issues and recommendations for research. *Journal of Psychosomatic Obstetrics & Gynaecology*, 29: 240–250.

Ayers, S., McKenzie-McHarg, K. & Eagle, A. (2007) Cognitive behaviour therapy for postnatal post-traumatic stress disorder: Case studies. *Journal of Psychosomatic Obstetrics & Gynaecology*, 28: 177–184.

Ayers, S. & Olander, E.K. (2013) What are we measuring and why? Using theory to guide perinatal research and measurement. *Journal of Reproductive and Infant Psychology*, 31(5): 439–448.

Ayers, S. & Pickering, A.D. (2005) Women's expectations and experience of birth. *Psychological Health*, 20(1): 79–92.

Ayorinde, A.A. et al. (2017) Chronic pelvic pain in women of reproductive and post-reproductive age: A population-based study. *European Journal of Pain*, 21: 445–455.

Aziz, R. & Steffens, D.C. (2013) What are the causes of late-life depression? *Psychiatric Clinics of North America*, 36: 497–516.

Babor, T.F., Higgins-Biddle, J.C., Saunders, J.B. & Monteiro, M.G. (2007) *AUDIT: The Alcohol Use Disorders Identification Test: Guidelines for Use in Primary Care* (2nd edition). Geneva: World Health Organisation. Available at: http://whqlibdoc.who.int/hq/2001/WHO_MSD_MSB_01.6a.pdf.

Bachen, E., Cohen, S. & Marsland, A.L. (2007) Psychoneuroimmunology, in S. Ayers et al. (eds), *Cambridge Handbook of Psychology, Health and Medicine* (2nd edition). Cambridge: Cambridge University Press. pp. 167–172.

Bae, J.-M., Lee, E.J. & Guyatt, G. (2008) Citrus fruit intake and stomach cancer risk: A quantitative systematic review. *Gastric Cancer*, 11: 23–32.

Bagnardi, V., Zatonski, W., Scotti, L., La Vecchia, C. & Corrao, G. (2008) Does drinking pattern modify the effect of alcohol on the risk of coronary heart disease? Evidence from a meta-analysis. *Journal of Epidemiology and Community Health*, 62: 615–619.

Bahrke, M.S., Yesalis, C.E. & Brower, K.J. (1998) Anabolic-androgenic steroid abuse and performance-enhancing drugs among adolescents. *Child & Adolescent Psychiatric Clinics of North America*, 7: 821–838.

Baile, W.F. et al. (2000) SPIKES – a six-step protocol for delivering bad news: Application to the patient with cancer. *The Oncologist*, 5: 302–311.

Baker, F.C. & Driver, H.S. (2004) Self-reported sleep across the menstrual cycle in young, healthy women. *Journal of Psychosomatic Research*, 56: 239–243.

Baker, F.C. & Driver, H.S. (2007) Circadian rhythms, sleep, and the menstrual cycle. *Sleep Medicine*, 6: 613–622.

Balsa, A.I. & McGuire, T.G. (2003) Prejudice, clinical uncertainty and stereotyping as sources of health disparities. *Journal of Health Economics*, 22: 89–116.

Bambra, C., Pope, D., Swami, V., Stanistreet, D., Roskam, A., Kunst, A. & Scott-Samuel, A. (2009) Gender, health inequalities and welfare state regimes: A cross-national study of 13 European countries. *Journal of Epidemiology and Community Health*, 63(1): 38–44.

Bandelow, B. & Michaelis, S. (2015) Epidemiology of anxiety disorders in the 21st century. *Dialogues in Clinical Neuroscience*, 17: 327–335.

Bandura, A., Ross, D. & Ross, S.A. (1961) Transmission of aggression through imitation of aggressive models. *Journal of Abnormal and Social Psychology*, 63: 575–582.

Banks, S.J. et al. (2014) The Alzheimer's disease cooperative study prevention instrument project: Longitudinal outcome of behavioral measures as predictors of cognitive decline. *Dementis and Geriatric Cognitive Disorders Extra*, 4: 509–516.

Bar-Haim, Y., Lamy, D., Pergamin, L., Bakerman-Kranenburg, M.J. & van Ijzendoorn, M.H. (2007) Threat-related attentional bias in anxious and non-anxious individuals: A meta-analytic study. *Psychological Bulletin, 133*: 1–24.

Barak, Y. (2006) The immune system and happiness. *Autoimmunity Reviews, 5*: 523–527.

Barskova, T. & Oesterreich R. (2009) Post-traumatic growth in people living with a serious medical condition and its relations to physical and mental health: A systematic review. *Disability and Rehabilitation, 31*(21): 1709–1733.

Barth, J., Schneider, S. & von Känel, R. (2010) Lack of social support in the etiology and the prognosis of coronary heart disease: A systematic review and meta-analysis. *Psychosomatic Medicine*, 72: 229–238.

Barton, J.L. et al. (2010) Patient–physician discordance in assessments of global disease severity in rheumatoid arthritis. *Arthritis Care and Research*, 62: 857–864.

Batson, C.D., Duncan, B., Ackerman, P., Buckley, T. & Birch, K. (1981) Is empathic emotion a source of altruistic motivation? *Journal of Personality & Social Psychology, 40*: 290–302.

Bauer, A., Parsonage, M., Knapp, M., Iemmi, V. & Adelaja B. (2014) *Costs of Perinatal Mental Health Problems: The Costs of Perinatal Mental Health Problems*. London: Centre for Mental Health.

Baumeister, H., Haschke, A., Munzinger, M., Hutter, N. & Tully, P.J. (2015) Inpatient and outpatient costs in patients with coronary artery disease and mental disorders: A systematic review. *Biopsychosocial Medicine*, 9: 11. (doi: 10.1186/s13030-015-0039-z)

Baumeister, R.F., Campbell, J.D., Krueger, J.I. & Vohs, K.D. (2003) Does high self-esteem cause better performance, interpersonal success, happiness, or healthier lifestyles? *Psychological Science in the Public Interest*, 4: 1–44.

Beatty, L. & Binnion, C. (2016) A systematic review of predictors of, and reasons for, adherence to online psychological interventions. *International Journal of Behavioral Medicine*, 23: 776–794.

Beck, A.T. (1967) *Depression: Clinical, Experimental and Theoretical Aspects*. New York: Harper & Row.

Beck, R. & Perkins, T.S. (2001) Cognitive content-specificity for anxiety and depression: A meta-analysis. *Cognitive Therapy and Research, 25*(6): 651–663.

Beck, R.S., Daughtridge, R. & Sloane, P.D. (2002) Physician–patient communication in the primary care office: A systematic review. *Journal of the American Board of Family Practice*, 15: 25–38.

Beckie, T.M. (2012) A systematic review of allostatic load, health, and health disparities. *Biological Research for Nursing, 14*(4): 311–346.

Beckman, H.B. & Frankel, R.M. (1984) The effect of physician behaviour on the collection of data. *Annals of Internal Medicine*, *101*: 692–696.

Beer, J.S. & Lombardo, M.V. (2007) Insights into emotion regulation from neuropsychology, in J.J. Gross (ed.), *Handbook of Emotion Regulation*. New York: Guilford Press. pp. 69–86.

Beer-Borst, S. et al. (2000) Dietary patterns in six European populations: Results from EURALIM, a collaborative European data harmonization and information campaign. *European Journal of Clinical Nutrition*, *54*: 253–262.

Bellisle, F., Monneuse, M.O., Steptoe, A. & Wardle, J. (1995) Weight concerns and eating patterns: A survey of university students in Europe. *International Journal of Obesity and Related Metabolic Disorders*, *19*: 723–730.

Belloc, N.B. (1973) Relationship of health practices and mortality. *Preventative Medicine*, *2*: 67–81.

Benarroch, E.E. (2007) Enteric nervous system: Functional organization and neurologic implications. *Neurology*, *69*: 1953–1957.

Benedetti, F., Maggi, G., Lopiano, L., Lanotte, M., Rainero, I., Vighetti, S.& Pollo A. (2003) Open versus hidden medical treatments: The patient's knowledge about a therapy affects the therapy outcome. *Prevention & Treatment*, 6, Article 1.

Benjamin, E.J., Blaha, M.J., Chiuve, S.E., Cushman, M., Das, S.R., Deo, R., de Ferranti, S.D. et al. (2017) Heart disease and stroke statistics – 2017 update: A report from the American Heart Association. *Circulation*, 135.

Bennett, D.S. (1994) Depression among children with chronic medical problems: A meta-analysis. *Journal of Pediatric Psychology*, *19*: 149–169.

Bensing, J.M., Roter, D.L. & Hulsman, R.L. (2003) Communication patterns of primary care physicians in the United States and the Netherlands. *Journal of General Internal Medicine*, *18*: 335–342.

Berk, L.S., Felten, D.L., Tan, S.A., Bittman, B.B. & Westengard, J. (2001) Modulation of neuro-immune parameters during the eustress of humor-associated mirthful laughter. *Alternative Therapies in Health & Medicine*, *7*: 62–76.

Berkhof, M. et al. (2011) Effective training strategies for teaching communication skills to physicians: An overview of systematic reviews. *Patient Education and Counselling*, *84*(2): 152–162.

Berkman, L.F. et al. (2003) Effects of treating depression and low perceived social support on clinical events after myocardial infarction. *Journal of the American Medical Association*, *289*: 3106–3116.

Berkowitz, L. (1989) Frustration-aggression hypothesis: Examination and reformulation. *Psychological Bulletin*, *106*: 59–73.

Berlan, E.D. & Bravender, T. (2009) Confidentiality, consent, and caring for the adolescent patient. *Current Opinion in Pediatrics*, *21*: 450–456

Bernal, M. et al. (2007) Risk factors for suicidality in Europe: Results from the ESEMED study. *Journal of Affective Disorders*, *101*: 27–34.

Bernardy, K., Klose, P., Busch, A.J., Choy, E.H. & Häuser, W. (2013) Cognitive behavioural therapies for fibromyalgia. *Cochrane Database of Systematic Reviews*, *9*: CD009796.

Berry, L.M., Andrade, J. & May, J. (2007) Hunger-related intrusive thoughts reflect increased accessibility of food items. *Cognition and Emotion*, *21*: 865–878.

Beswick, A.D. et al. (2004) Provision, uptake and cost of cardiac rehabilitation programmes: Improving services to under-represented groups. *Health Technology Assessment*, 8(41).

Betrán, A.P., Ye, J., Moller, A.B., Zhang, J., Gülmezoglu, A.M. & Torloni, M.R. (2016) The increasing trend in caesarean section rates: Global, regional and national estimates: 1990–2014. *PLoS One*, 11(2): e0148343.

Bibace, R. & Walsh, M.E. (1980) Development of children's concepts of illness. *Pediatrics*, 66: 912–917.

Binmoammar, T.A. et al. (2016) The impact of poor glycaemic control on the prevalence of erectile dysfunction in men with Type 2 diabetes mellitus: A systematic review. *Journal of the Royal Society of Medicine Open*, 7.

Birthplace in England Collaborative Group, Brocklehurst, P., Hardy, P., Hollowell, J., Linsell, L., Macfarlane, A., McCourt, C., Marlow, N., Miller, A., Newburn, M., Petrou, S., Puddicombe, D., Redshaw, M., Rowe, R., Sandall, J., Silverton, L. & Stewart, M. (2011) Perinatal and maternal outcomes by planned place of birth for healthy women with low risk pregnancies: the Birthplace in England national prospective cohort study. *British Medical Journal*, 343: d7400.

Bischofberger, J. (2007) Young and excitable: New neurons in memory networks. *Nature Neuroscience*, 10: 273–275.

Bisson, J.I., Jenkins, P.L., Alexander, J. & Bannister, C. (1997) Randomised controlled trial of psychological debriefing for victims of acute burn trauma. *British Journal of Psychiatry*, 171: 78–81.

Blaxter, M. (1990) *Health and Lifestyles*. London: Routledge.

Bleich, S.N. et al. (2012) Health inequalities: Trends, progress, and policy. *Annual Review of Public Health*, 33: 7–40

Blyth, F.M., March, L.M., Brnabic, A.J., Jorm, L.R., Williamson, M. & Cousins, M.J. (2001) Chronic pain in Australia: A prevalence study. *Pain*, 89: 127–134.

Bodley-Tickell, A.T. et al. (2008) Trends in sexually transmitted infections (other than HIV) in older people: Analysis of data from an enhanced surveillance system. *Sexually Transmitted Infections*, 84: 312–317.

Boerebach, B.C. et al. (2014) The impact of clinicians' personality and their interpersonal behaviors on the quality of patient care: A systematic review. *International Journal for Quality in Health Care*, 26: 426–81.

Boeschoten, R.E., Braamse, A.M., Beekman, A.T., Cuijpers, P., van Oppen, P., Dekker, J. & Uitdehaag, B.M. (2017) Prevalence of depression and anxiety in multiple sclerosis: A systematic review and meta-analysis. *Journal of the Neurologial Sciences*, 15(372): 331–341.

Bogart, L.M., Bird, S.T., Walt, L.C., Delahanty, D.L. & Figler, J.L. (2004) Association of stereotypes about physicians to health care satisfaction, help-seeking behavior, and adherence to treatment. *Social Science & Medicine*, 58: 1049–1058.

Bolling, K., Grant, C., Hamlyn, B. & Thornton, A. (2007) *Infant Feeding Survey, 2005*. London: The Information Centre.

Bonanno, G.A. & Kaltman, S. (2001) The varieties of grief experience. *Clinical Psychology Review*, 21: 1–30.

Bonn, G.B. (2013) Re-conceptualizing free will for the 21st century: Acting independently with a limited role for consciousness. *Frontier in Psychology*, 4: 920.

Boots Family Trust Alliance (2013) *Perinatal mental health: Experiences of women and health professionals*. London: Boots Family Trust. www.tommys.org/sites/default/files/Perinatal_Mental_Health_Experiences%20of%20women.pdf

Bor, R. & Allen, J. (2007) Counselling, in S. Ayers et al. (eds), *Cambridge Handbook of Psychology, Health and Medicine* (2nd edition). Cambridge: Cambridge University Press. pp. 348–351.

Bor, R. & Eriksen, C. (2018) Counselling, in C.D. Llewellyn et al. (eds), *The Cambridge Handbook of Psychology, Health and Medicine* (3rd edition). Cambridge: Cambridge University Press.

Borg, V. & Kristensen, T.S. (2000) Social class and self-rated health: Can the gradient be explained by differences in life style or work environment? *Social Science & Medicine, 51*: 1019–1030.

Borrell-Carrio, F., Suchman, A.L. & Epstein, R.M. (2004) The biopsychosocial model 25 years later: Principles, practice and scientific enquiry, *Annals of Family Medicine, 2*: 576–582.

Bosque-Prous, M., Espelt, A., Borrell, C., Bartroli, M., Guitart, A.M., Villalbí, J.R. & Brugal, M.T. (2015) Gender differences in hazardous drinking among middle-aged in Europe: The role of social context and women's empowerment. *European Journal of Public Health, 25*(4): 698–705.

Botella, C., Serrano, B., Baños, R.M. & Garcia-Palacios, A. (2015) Virtual reality exposure-based therapy for the treatment of post-traumatic stress disorder: A review of its efficacy, the adequacy of the treatment protocol, and its acceptability. *Neuropsychiatric Disease and Treatment, 11*: 2533–2545.

Boudreau, F. & Godin, G. (2007) Using the theory of planned behaviour to predict exercise intention in obese adults. *Canadian Journal of Nursing Research, 39*: 112–125.

Bowen, A., Neumann, V., Conner, M. & Tennant, A. (1998) Mood disorders following traumatic brain injury: Identifying the extent of the problem and the people at risk. *Brain Injury, 12*: 177–190.

Bower, P., Knowles, S., Coventry, P.A. & Rowland, N. (2011) Counselling for mental health and psychosocial problems in primary care. *Cochrane Database of Systematic Reviews, 9*: CD001025.

Bower, P. & Rowland, N. (2006) Effectiveness and cost effectiveness of counselling in primary care. *Cochrane Database of Systematic Reviews, 3* (Art. CD001025).

Bowlby, J. (1958) The nature of the child's tie to his mother. *The International Journal of Psycho-Analysis, 39*: 350–371.

Bowlby, J. (1969) *Attachment and Loss: Vol. 1. Attachment*. New York: Basic Books.

Bowlby, J. (1973) *Attachment and Loss: Vol. 2. Separation: Anxiety and Anger*. New York: Basic Books.

Boyce, W.T., Chesney, M., Alkon, A., Tschann, J.M., Adams, S., Chesterman, B., Cohen, F., Kaiser, P., Folkman, S. & Wara, D. (1995) Psychobiologic reactivity to stress and childhood respiratory illnesses: Results of two prospective studies. *Psychosomatic Medine, 57*(5): 411–422.

Braddock, C.H., Fihn, S.D., Levinson, W., Jonsen, A.R. & Pearlman, R.A. (1997) How doctors and patients discuss routine clinical decisions. Informed decision-making in the outpatient setting. *Journal of General Internal Medicine, 12*: 339–345.

Bradt, J., Dileo, C., Grocke, D. & Magill, L. (2011) Music interventions for improving psychological and physical outcomes in cancer patients. *Cochrane Database of Systematic Reviews, 10*(8): CD006911.

Braet, C., Wante, L., Van Beveren, M.L. & Theuwis, L. (2015) Is the cognitive triad a clear marker of depressive symptoms in youngsters? *European Child & Adolescent Psychiatry*, 24(10): 1261–1268.

Bramley, N. & Eatough, V. (2005) The experience of living with Parkinson's disease: An interpretative phenomenological analysis case study. *Psychology & Health*, 20: 223–235.

Brandt, C.P. et al. (2017) Main and interactive effects of emotion dysregulation and HIV symptom severity on quality of life among persons living with HIV/AIDS. *AIDS Care*, 29: 498–506.

Bräscher, A.K., Raymaekers, K., Van den Bergh, O. & Witthöft, M. (2017) Are media reports able to cause somatic symptoms attributed to WiFi radiation? An experimental test of the negative expectation hypothesis. *Environmental Research*, 31(156): 265–271.

Braveman, P. & Gottlieb, L. (2014) The social determinants of health: It's time to consider the causes of the causes. *Public Health Reports*, 29(Suppl 2): 19–31.

Bray, G.A. (2000) Reciprocal relation of food intake and sympathetic activity: Experimental observations and clinical implications. *International Journal of Obesity Related Metabolic Disorders*, 24: s8–s17.

Breiding, M.J., Smith, S.G., Basile, K.C., Walters, M.L., Chen, J. & Merrick, M.T. (2014) Prevalence and characteristics of sexual violence, stalking, and intimate partner violence victimization – National Intimate Partner and Sexual Violence Survey, United States, 2011. *Morbidity and Mortality Weekly Report: Surveillance Summary 5*, 63(8): 1–18.

Brewin, C.R., Andrews, B. & Valentine, J.D. (2000) Meta-analysis of risk factors for posttraumatic stress disorder in trauma-exposed adults. *Journal of Consulting and Clinical Psychology*, 68: 748–766.

Brewin, C.R. & Holmes, E.A. (2003) Psychological theories of posttraumatic stress disorder. *Clinical Psychology Review*, 23(3): 339–376.

Brewster, K.L. & Rindfuss, R.R. (2000) Fertility and women's employment in industrialized nations. *Annual Review of Sociology*, 26: 271–296.

Briggs, G.F., Hole, G.J. & Land, M.F. (2016) Imagery-inducing distraction leads to cognitive tunnelling and deteriorated driving performance. Transportation Research Part F: *Traffic Psychology and Behaviour*, 38: 106–117.

Broadbent, E. & Petrie, K.J. (2018) Symptom perception, in C.D. Llewellyn et al. (eds), *The Cambridge Handbook of Psychology, Health and Medicine* (3rd edition). Cambridge: Cambridge University Press.

Brocklehurst, P., et al. (2011) Perinatal and maternal outcomes by planned place of birth for healthy women with low risk pregnancies: The Birthplace in England National Prospective Cohort Study. *British Medical Journal*, 343: d7400.

Brod, S., et al. (2014) 'As above, so below' examining the interplay between emotion and the immune system. *Immunology*, 143: 311–318.

Brooks-Gunn, J. & Paikoff, R.L. (1992) Changes in self feelings during the transition toward adolescence, in H. McGurk (ed.), *Childhood Social Development*. Hove: Laurence Erlbaum. pp. 63–97.

Broom, A. & Tovey, P. (eds) (2009) *Men's Health*. New York: Wiley.

Broomfield, N.M. et al. (2015) Poststroke anxiety is prevalent at the population level, especially among socially deprived and younger age community stroke survivors. *International Journal of Stroke*, 10: 897–902.

Brown, H. & Randle, J. (2005) Living with a stoma: A review of the literature. *Journal of Clinical Nursing*, *14*: 74–81.

Brown, H.M., Waszczuk, M.A., Zavos, H.M., Trzaskowski, M., Gregory, A.M. & Eley, T.C. (2014) Cognitive content specificity in anxiety and depressive disorder symptoms: A twin study of cross-sectional associations with anxiety sensitivity dimensions across development. *Psychological Medicine*, *44*(16): 3469–3480.

Brown, J., Pengas, G., Dawson, K., Brown, L.A. & Clatworthy, P. (2009) Self administered cognitive screening test (TYM) for detection of Alzheimer's disease. *British Medical Journal*, *338*: 1423–1430.

Brown, J.L. & Vanable, P.A. (2008) Cognitive-behavioral stress management interventions for persons living with HIV: A review and critique of the literature. *Annals of Behavioral Medicine*, *35*: 26–40.

Brown, R., Dunn, S., Byrnes, K., Morris, R., Heinrich, P. & Shaw, J. (2009) Doctors' stress responses and poor communication performance in simulated bad-news consultations. *Academic Medicine*, 84(11): 1595–602.

Brown, R.J. (2007) Introduction to the special issue on medically unexplained symptoms: Background and future directions. *Clinical Psychology Review*, 27(7): 769–780.

Bruinsma, F. et al. (2006) Concern about tall stature during adolescence and depression in later life. *Journal of Affective Disorders*, *91*: 145–152.

Brumariu, L.E. & Kerns, K.A. (2010) Parent–child attachment and internalizing symptoms in childhood and adolescence: A review of empirical findings and future directions. *Development and Psychopathology*, *22*: 177–203.

Brummett, B.H. et al. (2001) Characteristics of socially isolated patients with coronary artery disease who are at elevated risk for mortality. *Psychosomatic Medicine*, *63*: 67–272.

Bryere J. (2014) Socioeconomic environment and cancer incidence: A French population-based study in Normandy. *BMC Cancer*, *14*: 87.

Buckley, B.S. et al. (2010) Prevalence of urinary incontinence in men, women, and children – current evidence: Findings of the Fourth International Consultation on Incontinence. *Urology*, *76*: 265–270.

Buckman, R. (1992) *How to Break Bad News*. Basingstoke, UK: Papermac.

Buglass, E. (2010) Grief and bereavement theories. *Nursing Standard*, 24(41): 44–47.

Bulik, C.M., Berkman, N.D., Brownley, K.A., Sedway, J.A. & Lohr, K.N. (2007) Anorexia nervosa treatment: A systematic review of randomized controlled trials. *International Journal of Eating Disorders*, *40*: 310–320.

Bulik, C.M., Kleiman, S.C. & Yilmaz, Z. (2016) Genetic epidemiology of eating disorders. *Current Opinion in Psychiatry*, *29*: 383–388.

Burger, J.M. (1999) The foot-in-the-door compliance procedure: A multiple-process analysis and review. *Personality and Social Psychology Review*, *3*: 303–325.

Burgess, H., Sharkey, K. & Eastman, C. (2002) Bright light, dark and melatonin can promote circadian adaptation in night shift workers. *Sleep Medicine Reviews*, *6*: 407–420.

Burt, J., Abel, G., Elmore, N., Campbell, J., Roland, M., Benson, J. & Silverman, J. (2014) Assessing communication quality of consultations in primary care: Initial reliability of the Global Consultation Rating Scale, based on the Calgary-Cambridge Guide to the Medical Interview. *BMJ Open*, *4*(3): e004339.

Burton, A., Burgess, C., Dean, S., Koutsopoulou, G.Z. & Hugh-Jones, S. (2017) How effective are mindfulness-based interventions for reducing stress among healthcare professionals? A systematic review and meta-analysis. *Stress Health*, *33*(1): 3–13.

Buske-Kirschbaum, A., von Auer, K., Kreiger, S., Weis, S., Rauh, W. & Hellhammer, D. (2003) Blunted cortisol responses to psychosocial stress in asthmatic children: A general feature of atopic disease? *Psychosomatic Medicine*, *65*: 806–810.

Busse, J.W., Montori, V.M., Krasnik, C., Patelis-Siotis, I. & Guyatt, G.H. (2009) Psychological intervention for premenstrual syndrome: A meta-analysis of randomized controlled trials. *Psychotherapy and Psychosomatics*, *78*: 6–15.

Butler, A.C., Chapman, J.E., Forman, E.M. & Beck, A.T. (2006) The empirical status of cognitive-behavioural therapy: A review of meta-analyses. *Clinical Psychology Review*, *26*: 17–31.

Cameron, D.S., Bertenshaw, E.J. & Sheeran, P. (2015) The impact of positive affect on health cognitions and behaviours: A meta-analysis of the experimental evidence. *Health Psychology Review*, *9*(3): 345–365.

Cameron, E.E., Sedov, I.D. & Tomfohr-Madsen, L.M. (2016) Prevalence of paternal depression in pregnancy and the postpartum: An updated meta-analysis. *Journal of Affective Disorders*, December: 189–203.

Cameron, L.D., Leventhal, E.A. & Leventhal, H. (1993) Symptom representations and affect as determinants of care seeking in a community-dwelling, adult sample population. *Health Psychology*, *12*: 171–179.

Cameron, L.D. & Moss-Morris, R. (2004) Illness-related cognition and behaviour, in A.A. Kaptein & J.A. Weinman (eds), *Health Psychology: An Introduction*. Oxford: Blackwell. pp. 84–110.

Campbell, S.M. & Rowland, M.O. (1996) Why do people consult the doctor? *Family Practice*, *13*: 75–83.

Campbell-Jackson, L. & Horsch, A. (2014) The psychological impact of stillbirth: A systematic review. *Illness, Crisis & Loss*, *22*: 237–256.

Cancer Research UK (2008) *Latest UK Cancer Incidence and Mortality Summary – Rates*. Available at: http://publications.cancerresearchuk.org/WebRoot/crukstoredb/CRUK_PDFs/mortality/IncidenceMortalitySummaryRates.pdf (last accessed 22 July 2009).

Cancer Research UK (2010) *Diet and Cancer: The Evidence*. Available at: http://info.cancer researchuk.org/healthyliving/dietandhealthyeating/howdoweknow/diet-and-cancer-the-evidence (last accessed 2 January 2010).

Cannon, M., Jones, P.B. & Murray, R.M. (2002) Obstetric complications and schizophrenia: Historical and meta-analytic review. *American Journal of Psychiatry*, *159*: 1080–1092.

Cao-Lei, L., Dancause, K.N., Elgbeili, G., Massart, R., Szyf, M., Liu, A., Laplante, D.P. & King S. (2015) DNA methylation mediates the impact of exposure to prenatal maternal stress on BMI and central adiposity in children at age 13½ years: Project Ice. *Storm Epigenetics*, *10*(8): 749–761.

Cao-Lei, L., Elgbeili, G., Massart, R., Laplante, D.P., Szyf, M. & King, S. (2015) Pregnant women's cognitive appraisal of a natural disaster affects DNA methylation in their children 13 years later: Project Ice Storm. *Translational Psychiatry*, *24*(5): e515.

Capellino, S. & Straub, R.H. (2008) Neuroendocrine immune pathways in chronic arthritis. *Best Practice and Research: Clinical Rheumatology, 22*: 285–297.

Capitanio, J.P., Mendoza, S.P., Lerche, N.W. & Mason, W.A. (1998) Social stress results in altered glucocorticoid regulation and shorter survival in simian acquired immune deficiency syndrome. *Procedings of the National Academies of Science, 95*: 4714–4719.

Care Quality Commission (2013) Dignity and nutrition for older people . Newcastle upon Tyne: CQC. Available at: www.cqc.org.uk/content/dignity-and-nutrition-older-people-2 (last accessed 1 August 2017).

Carey, M. et al. (2000) Using information, motivational enhancement, and skills training to reduce the risk of HIV infection. *Health Psychology, 19*: 3–11.

Carlisle, M., Uchino, B.N., Sanbonmatsu, D.M., Smith, T.W., Cribbet, M.R., Birmingham, W., Light, K.C. & Vaughn, A.A. (2012) Subliminal activation of social ties moderates cardiovascular reactivity during acute stress. *Health Psychology, 31*: 217–225.

Carlson, N.R. (2007) *Physiology of Behavior* (9th edition). Boston, MA: Allyn & Bacon.

Carlyle, J. (2007) Psychodynamic psychotherapy, in S. Ayers et al. (eds), *Cambridge Handbook of Psychology, Health and Medicine* (2nd edition). Cambridge: Cambridge University Press. pp. 379–383.

Carney, D.R., Cuddy, A.J. & Yap, A.J. (2010) Power posing: Brief nonverbal displays affect neuroendocrine levels and risk tolerance. *Psychological Science, 21*(10): 1363–1368.

Carpeneter, C. (2010) A meta-analysis of the effectiveness of health belief model variables in predicting behavior. *Health Communication, 25*: 661–669.

Carpentier, M. Y., Fortenberry, J. D., Ott, M. A., Brames, M. J., & Einhorn, L. H. (2011). Perceptions of masculinity and self-image in adolescent and young adult testicular cancer survivors: Implications for romantic and sexual relationships. *Psycho-Oncology, 20*, 738–745.

Carr, C.P. et al. (2013) The role of early life stress in adult psychiatric disorders: A systematic review according to childhood trauma subtypes. *Journal of Nervous and Mental Disease, 201*: 1007–1020.

Carrico, A.W. & Antoni, M.H. (2008) Effects of psychological interventions on neuroendocrine hormone regulation and immune status in HIV-positive persons: A review of randomized controlled trials. *Psychosomatic Medicine, 70*: 575–584.

Carroll, D., Ebrahim, S., Tilling, K., Macleod, J. & Smith, G.D. (2002) Admissions for myocardial infarction and World Cup football: Database survey. *British Medical Journal, 325*: 1439–1442.

Carvajal, R. et al. (2013) Managing obesity in primary care practice: A narrative review. *Annals of the New York Academy of Science, 1281*: 191–206.

Carvalho, C., Caetano, J.M., Cunha, L., Rebouta, P., Kaptchuk, T.J. & Kirsch, I. (2016) Open-label placebo treatment in chronic low back pain: A randomized controlled trial. *Pain, 157*(12): 2766–2772.

Cash, T.F. & Deagle, E.A. (1998) The nature and extent of body-image disturbances in anorexia nervosa and bulimia nervosa: A meta-analysis. *International Journal of Eating Disorders, 22*: 107–126.

Caso, J.R., Leza, J.C. & Menchen, L. (2008) The effects of physical and psychological stress on the gastrointestinal tract. *Current Molecular Medicine*, 8: 299–312.

Catarino, A. (2015) Failing to forget: Inhibitory-control deficits compromise memory suppression in posttraumatic stress disorder. *Psychological Science*, 26: 604–616.

Centers for Disease Control and Prevention (2008) State-specific prevalence of obesity among adults – United States, 2007. *Morbidity & Mortality Weekly Report*, 57: 765–768.

Centers for Disease Control and Prevention (2014) *National Diabetes Statistics Report: Estimates of Diabetes and Its Burden in the United States*. Atlanta, GA: US Department of Health and Human Services.

Chalder, T. & Willis, C. (2017) Medically unexplained symptoms, in C.D. Llewellyn & S. Ayers et al. (eds), *Cambridge Handbook of Psychology, Health and Medicine* (3rd edition). Cambridge: Cambridge University Press.

Champagne, F. & Meaney, M.J. (2001) Like mother, like daughter: Evidence for non-genomic transmission of parental behaviour and stress responsivity. *Progress in Brain Research*, 133: 287–302.

Chan, A.O.O. et al. (2005) Differing coping mechanisms, stress level and anorectal physiology in patients with functional constipation. *World Journal of Gastroenterology*, 11: 5362–5366.

Chang, H.Y. et al. (2015) Depression as a risk factor for overall and hormone-related cancer: The Korean cancer prevention study. *Journal of Affective Disorders*, 173: 1–8.

Chapillon, P., Patin, V., Roy, V., Vincent, A. & Caston, J. (2002) Effects of pre- and postnatal stimulation on developmental, emotional, and cognitive aspects in rodents: A review. *Developmental Psychobiology*, 41: 373–387.

Charles, C., Gafni, A. & Whelan, T. (1997) Shared decision-making in the medical encounter: What does it mean? (Or it takes a least two to tango). *Social Science & Medicine*, 44: 681–692.

Chartrand, T.L, Van Baaren, R.B. & Bargh, J.A. (2006) Linking automatic evaluation to mood and information processing style: Consequences for experienced affect, impression formation, and stereotyping. *Journal of Experimental Psychology: General*, 135: 70–77.

Charuvastra, A. & Cloitre, M. (2008) Social bonds and posttraumatic stress disorder. *Annual Review of Psychology*, 59: 301–328.

Chase, W.G. & Ericsson, K.A. (1982) Skill and working memory, in G.H. Bower (ed.), *The Psychology of Learning and Motivation* (Vol. 16). New York: Academic Press. pp. 1–58.

Chaudhuri, K.R., Healy, D.G. & Schapira, A.H. (2006) Non-motor symptoms of Parkinson's disease: Diagnosis and management. *Lancet Neurology*, 5: 235–245.

Chemerinski, E. & Robinson, R.G. (2000) The neuropsychiatry of stroke. *Psychosomatics*, 41: 5–14.

Chen, R., Cohen, L.G. & Hallett, M. (2002) Nervous system reorganization following injury. *Neuroscience*, 111: 761–773.

Cheok, G., Tan, D., Low, A. & Hewitt, J. (2015) Is Nintendo Wii an Effective Intervention for Individuals With Stroke? A Systematic Review and Meta-Analysis. *Journal of the American Medical Directors Association*, 16(11): 923–32.

Cheong, Y.C. et al. (2014) Non-surgical interventions for the management of chronic pelvic pain. *Cochrane Database of Systematic Reviews*, 3: CD008797.

Cherry, D., Burt, C. & Woodwell, D. (2001) National ambulatory medical care survey: 1999 summary. *Division of Healthcare Statistics*, 204: 322.

Chida, Y. et al. (2008) Do stress-related psychosocial factors contribute to cancer incidence and survival? *Nature Clinical Practice Oncology*, 5: 466–475.

Chida, Y. & Steptoe, A. (2008) Positive psychological well-being and mortality: A quantitative review of prospective observational studies. *Psychosomatic Medine*, 70(7): 741–756.

Chida, Y. & Steptoe, A. (2009) The association of anger and hostility with future coronary heart disease. *Journal of the American College of Cardiology*, 53(11): 936–946.

Chiu, M., Austin, P.C., Manuel, D.G., Shah, B.R. & Tu, J.V. (2011) Deriving ethnic-specific BMI cutoff points for assessing diabetes risk. *Diabetes Care*, 34(8): 1741–1748.

Chomsky, N. (1965) *Aspects of the Theory of Syntax*. Cambridge, MA: MIT Press.

Chong, K. & Unruh, M. (2017) Why does quality of life remain an under-investigated issue in chronic kidney disease and why is it rarely set as an outcome measure in trials in this population? *Nephrology Dialysis Transplantation*, 32(suppl. 2): 47–52.

Christenfeld, N. & Gerin, W. (2000) Social support and cardiovascular reactivity. *Biomedicine & Pharmacotherapy*, 54: 251–257.

Christensen, A.J. & Ehlers, S.L. (2002) Psychological factors in end-stage renal disease: An emerging context for behavioral medicine research. *Journal of Consulting & Clinical Psychology*, 70: 712–724.

Christensen, A.J. et al. (2002) Effect of a behavioral self-regulation intervention on patient adherence in hemodialysis. *Health Psychology*, 21: 393–397.

Christian, L.M., Graham, J.M., Padgett, D.A., Glaser, R. & Kiecolt-Glaser, J.K. (2007) Stress and wound healing. *NeuroImmunoModulation*, 13: 337–346.

Christy, S.M. et al. (2014) Integrating men's health and masculinity theories to explain colorectal cancer screening behavior. *American Journal of Men's Health*, 8: 54–65.

Chu, M.W. et al. (2011) Prospective evaluation of consultant surgeon sleep deprivation and outcomes in more than 4000 consecutive cardiac surgical procedures. *Arch Surgery*, 146(9): 1080–1085.

Church, K. & Mayhew, S.H. (2009) Integration of STI and HIV prevention, care, and treatment into family planning services: A review of the literature. *Studies in Family Planning*, 40: 171–186.

Cialdini, R.B., Schaller, M., Houlihan, D., Arps, K., Fultz, J. & Beaman, A.L. (1987) Empathy-based helping: Is it selflessly or selfishly motivated? *Journal of Personality & Social Psychology*, 52: 749–758.

Cialkowska-Rysz, A. & Dzierzanowski, T. (2013) Personal fear of death affects the proper process of breaking bad news. *Archives of Medical Science*, 9(1): 127–131.

Ciao, A.C., Loth, K. & Neumark-Sztainer, D. (2014) Preventing eating disorder pathology: Common and unique features of successful eating disorders prevention programs. *Current Psychiatry Reports*, 16: 453.

Ciechanowski, P.S., Katon, W.J. & Russo, J.E. (2000) Depression and diabetes: Impact of depressive symptoms on adherence, function, and costs. *Archives of Internal Medicine*, 160: 3278–3285.

Ciesla, J.A. & Roberts, J.E. (2001) Meta-analysis of the relationship between HIV infection and risk for depressive disorders. *American Journal of Psychiatry*, 158: 725–730.

Claar, R.L., Simons, L.E. & Logan, D.E. (2008) Parental response to children's pain: The moderating impact of children's emotional distress on symptoms and disability. *Pain*, *138*(1): 172–179.

Clark, D. & Seymour, J. (1999) *Reflections on Palliative Care*. Buckingham: Open University Press.

Clark, D.M. (1986) A cognitive approach to panic disorder. *Behaviour Research and Therapy*, *24*: 461–470.

Clark, J.E. (2015) Diet, exercise or diet with exercise: Comparing the effectiveness of treatment options for weight-loss and changes in fitness for adults (18–65 years old) who are overfat, or obese: Systematic review and meta-analysis. *Journal of Diabetes and Metabollic Disorders*, *14*: 31.

Clark, K.M. et al. (2006) Breastfeeding and mental and motor development at 5½ years. *Ambulatory Pediatrics*, 6: 65–71.

Clark, M., Kelly, T. & Deighan, C. (2011) A systematic review of the Heart Manual literature. *European Journal of Cardiovascular Nursing*, *10*: 3–13.

Clarke, D.M. & Currie, K.C. (2009) Depression, anxiety and their relationship with chronic diseases: A review of the epidemiology, risk and treatment evidence. *Medical Journal of Australia*, *190*: s54–s60.

Clayton, M.F. & Dudley, W.N. (2009) Patient-centered communication during oncology follow-up visits for breast cancer survivors: Content and temporal structure. *Oncology Nursing Forum*, 36: E68–E79.

Coan, J.A., Schaefer, H.S. & Davidson, R.J. (2006) Lending a hand: Social regulation of the neural response to threat. *Psychological Science*, *17(12)*: 1032–1039.

Cohen, R.D. (2002) The quality of life in patients with Crohn's disease. *Alimentary Pharmacology & Therapeutics*, 16: 1603–1609.

Cohen, S. (2005) The Pittsburgh common cold studies: Psychosocial predictors of susceptibility to respiratory infectious illness. *International Journal of Behavioral Medicine*, 12: 123–131.

Cohen, S., Frank, E., Doyle, W.J., Skoner, D.P., Rabin, B.S. & Gwaltney, J.M. (1998) Types of stressors that increase susceptibility to the common cold in healthy adults. *Health Psychology*, 17: 214–223.

Cohen, S., Kamarck, T. & Mermelstein, R. (1983) A global measure of perceived stress. *Journal of Health and Social Behavior*, 24: 385–396.

Cohen, S. & Rodriguez, M. (2001) Stress, viral respiratory infections, and asthma, in D.P. Skoner (ed.), *Asthma and Respiratory Infections. Lung Biology in Health and Disease* series (Vol. 154). New York: Marcel Dekker. pp. 193–208.

Cohn, L.D., Macfralane, S., Yanez, C. & Imai, W.K. (1995) Risk-perception: Differences between adolescents and adults. *Health Psychology*, 14: 217–222.

Colagiuri, B., Schenk, L.A., Kessler, M.D., Dorsey, S.G. & Colloca, L. (2015) The placebo effect: From concepts to genes. *Neuroscience*, 307: 171–190.

Cole, S.A. & Bird, J. (2000) *The Medical Interview: The Three Function Approach*. St Louis, MO: Mosby.

Colloca, L., Lopiano, L., Lanotte, M. & Benedetti, F. (2004) Overt versus covert treatment for pain, anxiety, and Parkinson's disease. *Lancet Neurology*, *3*(11): 679–84.

Colloca, L. & Miller, F.G. (2011) The nocebo effect and its relevance for clinical practice. *Psychosomatic Medicine*, 73: 598–603.

Colloca, L., Sigaudo, M. & Benedetti, F. (2008) The role of learning in nocebo and placebo effects. *Pain*, 136: 211–218.

Conn, V.S., Enriquez, M., Ruppar , T.M. & Chan K.C. (2016) Meta-analyses of theory use in medication adherence intervention research. *American Journal of Health Behavior*, 40: 155–71.

Conner, M., Povey, R., Sparks, P., James, R. & Shepherd, R. (2003) Moderating role of attitudinal ambivalence within the theory of planned behaviour. *British Journal of Social Psychology*, 42: 75–94.

Connor, J. (2017) Alcohol consumption as a cause of cancer. *Addiction*, 112: 222–228.

Conron, K.J. et al. (2010) A population-based study of sexual orientation identity and gender differences in adult health. *American Journal of Public Health*, 100: 1953–1960.

Conroy, T., Marchal, F. & Blazeby, J.M. (2006) Quality of life in patients with oesophageal and gastric cancer: An overview. *Oncology*, 70: 391–402.

Contrada, R.J. & Goyal, T.M. (2005) Individual differences, health and illness: The role of emotional traits and generalized expectancies, in S. Sutton et al. (eds), *SAGE Handbook of Health Psychology*. London: Sage. pp. 143–168.

Cooke, D., Newman, S., Sacker, A., DeVellis, B., Bebbington, P. & Meltzer, H. (2007) The impact of physical illnesses on non-psychotic psychiatric morbidity. *British Journal of Health Psychology*, 12: 463–471.

Coplan, J.D. & Lydiard, R.B. (1998) Brain circuits in panic disorder. *Biological Psychiatry*, 44: 1264–1276.

Cordoni, A. & Cordoni, L.E. (2001) Eutectic mixture of local anaesthetics reduces pain during intravenous catheter insertion in the paediatric patient. *Clinical Journal of Pain*, 17: 115–118.

Coresh, J. et al. (2007) Prevalence of chronic kidney disease in the United States. *Journal of the American Medical Association*, 298: 2038–2047.

Cornman, D.H. et al. (2008) Clinic-based intervention reduces unprotected sexual behaviour among HIV-infected patients in KwaZulu Natal, South Africa: Results of a pilot study. *Journal of Aquired Immune Deficiency Syndromes*, 48: 553–560.

Coulibaly, R., Séguin, L., Zunzunegui, M.V. & Gauvin, L. (2006) Links between maternal breast-feeding duration and Québec infants' health: A population-based study. Are the effects different for poor children? *Maternal & Child Health Journal*, 10: 537–543.

Courneya, K.S. & Friedenreich, C.M. (1999) Physical exercise and quality of life following cancer diagnosis: A literature review. *Annals of Behavioral Medicine*, 21: 171–179.

Courtenay, W. (2000) Constructions of masculinity and their influence on men's well-being: A theory of gender and health. *Social Science & Medicine*, 50: 1385–1401.

Cox, D.J. et al. (1991) Intensive versus standard glucose awareness training (BGAT) with insulin-dependent diabetes: Mechanisms and ancillary effects. *Psychosomatic Medicine*, 53: 453–462.

Coyne, K.S. et al. (2012) Urinary incontinence and its relationship to mental health and health-related quality of life in men and women in Sweden, the United Kingdom, and the United States. *European Urology*, 61: 88–95.

Crawley, R., Lomax, S. & Ayers, S. (2013) Recovering from stillbirth: The effects of making and sharing memories on maternal mental health. *Journal of Reproductive and Infant Psychology*, *31*(2): 195–207.

Crenshaw, K.W. (1991) Mapping the margins: Intersectionality, identity politics, and violence against women of color. *Stanford Law Review*, *43*: 1241–1299.

Critchley, J. & Capewell, S. (2004) Smoking cessation for the secondary prevention of coronary heart disease. *Cochrane Database of Systematic Reviews*, *1*: Art. CD003041.

Crombez, G., Eccleston, C., Van Damme, S., Vlaeyen, J.W. & Karoly P. (2012) Fear-avoidance model of chronic pain: The next generation. *Clinical Journal of Pain*, *28*(6): 475–483.

Croyle, R.T. & Sande, G.N. (1988) Denial and confirmatory search: Paradoxical consequences of medical diagnosis. *Journal of Applied Social Psychology*, *18*: 473–490.

Cummings, J.H. & Bingham, S.A. (1998) Diet and the prevention of cancer. *British Medical Journal*, *317*: 1636–1640.

Cunningham, A.J. & Watson, K. (2004) How psychological therapy may prolong survival in cancer patients: New evidence and a simple theory. *Integrative Cancer Therapies*, *3*: 214–229.

Currier, J.M., Neimeyer, R.A. & Berman, J.S. (2008) The effectiveness of psychotherapeutic interventions for bereaved persons: A comprehensive quantitative review. *Psychological Bulletin*, *134*(5): 648–661.

Cushing, H.W. (1932) The basophil adenomas of the pituitary body and their clinical manifestations. *Bulletin of Johns Hopkins Hospital*, *50*: 137–195.

Czarnocka, J. & Slade, P. (2000) Prevalence and predictors of post-traumatic stress symptoms following childbirth. *British Journal of Clinical Psychology*, *39*: 35–51.

D'Agostino, T.A. et al. (2017) Promoting patient participation in healthcare interactions through communication skills training: A systematic review. *Patient Education and Counselling*. doi: 10.1016/j.pec.2017.02.016. [Epub ahead of print].

Dalgard, F.J. et al. (2015) The psychological burden of skin diseases: A cross-sectional multi-center study among dermatological out-patients in 13 European countries. *Journal of Investigative Dermatology*, *135*: 984–991.

Danhauer, S.C. et al. (2009) A longitudinal investigation of coping strategies and quality of life among younger women with breast cancer. *Journal of Behavioral Medicine*, *32*: 371–379.

Daniels, H. (ed.) (1996) *An Introduction to Vygotsky*. London: Routledge.

Dannemiller, J.L. & Stephens, B.R. (1988) A critical test of infant pattern preference models. *Child Development*, *59*: 210–216.

Dante, G., Pedrielli, G., Annessi, E. & Facchinetti, F. (2013) Herb remedies during pregnancy: A systematic review of controlled clinical trials. *Journal of Maternal-Fetal & Neonatal Medicine*, *26*(3): 306–312.

Daugirdaitė, V., van den Akker, O. & Purewal, S. (2015) Posttraumatic stress and posttraumatic stress disorder after termination of pregnancy and reproductive loss: A systematic review. *Journal of Pregnancy*, 646345.

Davies, J., Hey, E., Reid, W. & Young, G. (1996) Prospective regional study of planned home births. Home Birth Study Steering Group. *British Medical Journal*, *313*(7068): 1302–1306.

Davis, C. (1939) Results of the self-selection of diets by young children. *Canadian Medical Association Journal*, *41*: 257–261.

Davis, C., Kleinman, J.T., Newhart, M., Gingis, L., Pawlak, M. & Hillis, A.E. (2008) Speech and language functions that require a functioning Broca's area. *Brain & Language*, *105*: 50–58.

Davison, G.C. & Garcia, L.M. (2018). Behaviour therapy, in C.D. Llewellyn, et al. (eds), *The Cambridge Handbook of Psychology, Health and Medicine* (3rd edition). Cambridge: Cambridge University Press.

de Brouwer, S.J. (2010) Experimental stress in inflammatory rheumatic diseases: A review of psychophysiological stress responses. *Arthritis Research & Therapy*, 12: r89.

de Groot, M., Anderson, R.J., Freedland, K.E., Clouse, R.E. & Lustman, P.J. (2001) Association of depression and diabetes complications: A meta-analysis. *Psychosomatic Medicine*, 63: 619–630.

de Haas, S. et al. (2012) Prevalence and characteristics of sexual violence in the Netherlands, the risk of revictimization and pregnancy: Results from a national population survey. *Violence and Victims*, 27: 592–608.

de Moor, C. et al. (2002) A pilot study of the side effects of expressive writing on psychological and behavioural adjustment in patients in a phase II trial of vaccine therapy for metastatic renal cell carcinoma. *Health Psychology*, 21: 615–619.

de Sanjosé, S. et al. (2007) Worldwide prevalence and genotype distribution of cervical human papillomavirus DNA in women with normal cytology: A meta-analysis. *Lancet Infectious Diseases*, 7: 453–459.

de Sousa, A. et al. (2012) Psychological aspects of prostate cancer: a clinical review. *Prostate Cancer and Prostatic Diseases*, 15: 120–127.

de Visser, R.O. (2015) Personalized feedback based on a drink-pouring exercise may improve knowledge of, and adherence to, government guidelines for alcohol consumption. *Alcoholism: Clinical and Experimental Research*, 39: 317–323.

de Visser, R.O. et al. (2014a) Attitudes toward sex and relationships: The Second Australian Study of Health and Relationships. *Sex Health*, *11*(5): 397–405.

de Visser, R.O. et al. (2014b) Experiences of sexual coercion in a representative sample of adults: The Second Australian Study of Health and Relationships. *Sex Health*, *11*(5): 472–480.

de Visser, R.O. et al. (2014c) Safer sex and condom use: Findings from the Second Australian Study of Health and Relationships. *Sex Health*, *11*(5): 495–504.

de Visser, R.O., Brown, C.E., Cooke, R., Cooper, G. & Memon, A. (2017a) Using alcohol unit-marked glasses enhances capacity to monitor intake: Evidence from a mixed-method intervention trial. *Alcohol and Alcoholism*, 52: 206–212.

de Visser, R.O., Richters, J., Yeung, A., Rissel, C.E. & Simpson, J.M. (2017b) Sexual difficulties: Prevalence, impact, and help-seeking in a population-representative sample. Paper presented at the 19th Congress of the European Society for Sexual Medicine, Nice, France.

de Visser, R.O. & McDonnell, E.J. (2008) Correlates of parents' reports of acceptability of human Papilloma virus vaccination for their school-aged children. *Sexual Health*, 5, 331–338.

de Visser, R.O. & McDonnell, E.J. (2013) 'Man points': Masculine capital and men's health behaviour. *Health Psychology*, *32*: 5–14.

de Visser, R.O. & O'Neill, N. (2013) Identifying and understanding barriers to sexually transmissible infection testing among young people. *Sex Health*, 10: 553–558.

de Visser, R.O., Rissel, C., Richters, J. & Smith, A. (2007) The impact of sexual coercion on psychological, physical, and sexual well-being. *Archives of Sexual Behavior*, 36: 676–686.

de Visser, R.O., Rissel, C., Smith, A. & Richters, J. (2006) Sociodemographic correlates of smoking, drinking, injecting drug use, and sexual risk behaviour. *International Journal of Behavioral Medicine*, 13: 153–162.

de Visser, R.O. & Smith, A. (2001) Relationship between sexual partners influences rates and correlates of condom use. *AIDS Education and Prevention*, 13: 413–427.

de Visser, R.O., Smith, A., Rissel, C., Richters, J. & Grulich, A. (2003) Sex in Australia: Safer sex and condom use. *Australian and New Zealand Journal of Public Health*, 27: 223–29.

de Visser, R.O. & Smith, J. (2007) Alcohol consumption and masculine identity among young men. *Psychology & Health*, 22: 595–614.

De Vries, A.M. et al. (2014) Clinician characteristics, communication, and patient outcome in oncology: A systematic review. *Psychooncology*, 23: 375–381.

Debiec, J. & Sullivan, R.M. (2016) The neurobiology of safety and threat learning in infancy. *Neurobiology of Learning and Memory*, pii: S1074–7427(16)30285–4. (doi: 10.1016/j.nlm.2016.10.015) [Epub ahead of print].

DeBruine, L., Jones, B.C., Frederick, D.A., Haselton, M.G., Penton-Voak, I.S. & Perrett, D.I. (2010) Evidence for menstrual cycle shifts in women's preferences for masculinity: A response to Harris (in press) 'Menstrual cycle and facial preferences reconsidered'. *Evolutionary Psychology*, 8(4): 768–775.

Deecher, D., Andree, T.H., Sloan, D. & Schechter, L.E. (2008) From menarche to menopause: Exploring the underlying biology of depression in women experiencing hormonal changes. *Psychoneuroendocrinology*, 33: 3–17.

Dejong, H., Broadbent, H. & Schmidt U. (2012) A systematic review of dropout from treatment in outpatients with anorexia nervosa. *International Journal of Eating Disorders*, 45: 635–647.

Del Giudice, M., Ellis, B.J. & Shirtcliff, E.A. (2011) The adaptive calibration model of stress responsivity. *Neuroscience and Biobehavioral Review*, 35(7): 1562–1592.

Del Piccolo, L. et al. (2014) How psychiatrist's communication skills and patient's diagnosis affect emotions disclosure during first diagnostic consultations. *Patient Education and Counselling*, 96: 151–158.

Delicate, A., Ayers, S., Easter, A. & McMullen, S. (2018) The impact of childbirth-related post-traumatic stress on a couple's relationship: A systematic review and meta-synthesis. *Journal of Reproductive and Infant Psychology*.

Delvaux, N., Razavi, D., Marchal, S., Bredart, A., Farvacques, C. & Slachmuylder, J.L. (2004) Effects of a 105 hour psychological training program on attitudes, communication skills and occupational stress in oncology: A randomised study. *British Journal of Cancer*, 90: 106–114.

Dempster, M., Howell, D. & McCorry, N.K. (2015) Illness perceptions and coping in physical health conditions: A meta-analysis. *Journal of Psychosomatic Research*, 79(6): 506–513.

Demyttenaere, K. (2001) Compliance and acceptance in antidepressant treatment. *International Journal of Psychiatry in Clinical Practice*, 5(Suppl. 1): s29–s35.

Dennerstein, L., Guthrie, J.R., Clark, M., Lehert, P. & Henderson, V.W. (2004) A population-based study of negative mood in middle-aged, Australian-born women. *Menopause*, 11: 563–568.

Department of Health (2001) *Treatment Choice in Psychological Therapies and Counselling: Evidence Based Clinical Practice Guidelines*. London: Department of Health.

Department of Health & Human Services (1990) *The Health Benefits of Smoking Cessation: A Report of the Surgeon General*. Washington, DC: DHHS.

Descartes, R. (1637) *Discours de la Méthode*. Leiden, NL: Elsevier.

Devonport, T.J. et al. (2017) A systematic review of the association between emotions and eating behaviour in normal and overweight adult populations. *Journal of Health Psychology* (in press).

Dhabhar, F.S. (2013) Psychological stress and immunoprotection versus immunopathology in the skin. *Clinical Dermatology*, 31: 18–30.

Dhar, A.K. & Barton, D.A. (2016) Depression and the link with cardiovascular disease. *Frontiers in Psychiatry*, 7: 33.

Dickens, C., McGowan, L., Clark-Carter, D. & Creed, F. (2002) Depression in rheumatoid arthritis: A systematic review of the literature with meta-analysis. *Psychosomatic Medicine*, 64: 52–60.

Dick-Read, G. (1933) *Natural Childbirth*. London: Pinter & Martin.

Dick-Read, G. (2004) *Childbirth without Fear: The Principles and Practice of Natural Childbirth*. London: Pinter & Martin.

DiMatteo, M.R. (2004a) Variations in patients' adherence to medical recommendations: A quantitative review of 50 years of research. *Medical Care*, 42: 200–209.

DiMatteo, M.R. (2004b) Social support and patient adherence to medical treatment: A meta analysis. *Health Psychology*, 23: 207–218.

DiMatteo, M.R., Giordani, P.J., Lepper, H.S. & Croghan, T.W. (2002) Patient adherence and medical treatment outcomes: A meta-analysis. *Medical Care*, 40: 794–811.

DiMatteo, M.R., Haskard, K.B. & Williams, S.L. (2007) Health beliefs, disease severity, and patient adherence: A meta-analysis. *Medical Care*, 45: 521–528.

DiMatteo, M.R., Lepper, H.S. & Croghan, T.W. (2000) Depression is a risk factor for noncompliance with medical treatment: Meta-analysis of the effects of anxiety and depression on patient adherence. *Archives of Internal Medicine*, 160: 2101–2107.

Dimidjian, S., Arch, J.J., Schneider, R.L., Desormeau, P., Felder, J.N. & Segal, Z.V. (2016) Considering meta-analysis, meaning, and metaphor: A systematic review and critical examination of 'third wave' cognitive and behavioral therapies. *Behavior Therapy*, 47(6): 886–905.

Ding, X.X., Wu, Y.L., Xu, S.J., Zhu, R.P., Jia, X.M., Zhang, S.F., Huang, K., Zhu, P., Hao, J.H. & Tao, F.B. (2014) Maternal anxiety during pregnancy and adverse birth outcomes: A systematic review and meta-analysis of prospective cohort studies. *Journal of Affective Disorders*, 159: 103–110.

Dinges, D.F. et al. (1997) Cumulative sleepiness, mood disturbance, and psychomotor vigilance performance decrements during a week of sleep restricted to 4–5 hours per night. *Sleep*, 20: 267–277.

Dixon, R.P., Roberts, L.M., Lawrie, S., Jones, L.A. & Humphreys, M.S. (2008) Medical students' attitudes to psychiatric illness in primary care. *Medical Education*, 42: 1080–1087.

Djernes, J.K. (2006) Prevalence and predictors of depression in populations of elderly: A review. *Acta Psychiatrica Scandinavica*, 113: 372–387.

Dockx, K., Bekkers, E.M., Van den Bergh, V., Ginis, P., Rochester, L., Hausdorff, J.M., Mirelman, A. & Nieuwboer, A. (2016) Virtual reality for rehabilitation in Parkinson's disease. *Cochrane Database of Systematic Review*, 21(12). Art. CD010760.

Dolin, D.J. & Booth-Butterfield, S. (1995) Foot-in-the-door and cancer prevention. *Health Communication*, 7: 55–66.

Douglas, R.M., Hemilä, H., Chalker, E. & Treacy, B. (2007) Vitamin C for preventing and treating the common cold. *Cochrane Database of Systematic Reviews*, 3 (Art. sCD000980).

Doyle, C., Lennox, L. & Bell, D. (2013) A systematic review of evidence on the links between patient experience and clinical safety and effectiveness. *BMJ Open*, 3(1). pii: e001570.

Dragioti, E., Karathanos, V., Gerdle, B. & Evangelou, E. (2017) Does psychotherapy work? An umbrella review of meta-analyses of randomized controlled trials. *Acta Psychiatrica Scandinavica*, 27 February: 1–11. (doi: 10.1111/acps.12713).

Dray-Spira, R., Lert, F., Marimoutou, C., Bouhnik, A.-D. & Obadia, Y. (2003) Socio-economic conditions, health status and employment among persons living with HIV/AIDS in France in 2001. *AIDS Care*, 15: 739–748.

Dresler, T. et al. (2013) Revise the revised? New dimensions of the neuroanatomical hypothesis of panic disorder. *Journal of Neural Transmission*, 120: 3–29.

Driessen, E., Hegelmaier, L.M., Abbass, A.A., Barber, J.P., Dekker, J.J., Van, H.L., Jansma, E.P. & Cuijpers, P. (2015) The efficacy of short-term psychodynamic psychotherapy for depression: A meta-analysis update. *Clinical Psychology Review*, 42: 1–15.

Driver, H.S. & Taylor, S.R. (2000) Exercise and sleep. *Sleep Medicine Reviews*, 4: 387–402.

Driver, H.S., Werth, E., Dijk, D.J. & Borbely, A.A. (2008) The menstrual cycle effects on sleep. *Sleep Medicine Clinics*, 3(1): 1–11.

Drossman, D.A., Camilleri, M., Mayer, E.A. & Whitehead, W.E. (2002) AGA technical review on irritable bowel syndrome, *Gastroenterology*, 123: 2108–2131.

Dumoulin, C. et al. (2014) Pelvic floor muscle training versus no treatment, or inactive control treatments, for urinary incontinence in women. *Cochrane Database of Systematic Reviews*, 5: CD005654.

Duncan, R.E., Vandeleur, M., Derks, A. & Sawyer, S. (2011) Confidentiality with adolescents in the medical setting: What do parents think? *Journal of Adolescent Health*, 49: 428–430.

Dunn, E.C., Brown, R.C., Dai, Y., Rosand, J., Nugent, N.R., Amstadter, A.B., & Smoller, J.W. (2015) Genetic determinants of depression: recent findings and future directions. *Harvard Review of Psychiatry*, 23, 1–18.

Eagle, A. & Worrell, M. (2018) Cognitive behaviour therapy, in Llewellyn, C.D. et al. (eds) *The Cambridge Handbook of Psychology, Health and Medicine* (3rd edition). Cambridge: Cambridge University Press.

Eagley, A. & Chaiken, S. (1993) *The Psychology of Attitudes*. Fort Worth, TX: Harcourt Brace.

Eaker, E.D., Sullivan, L.M., Kelly-Hayes, M., D'Agostino, R.B. & Benjamin, E.J. (2007) Marital status, marital strain, and risk of coronary heart disease or total mortality: The Framingham offspring study. *Psychosomatic Medicine*, 69: 509–513.

Eastridge, B.J. et al. (2003) Effect of sleep deprivation on the performance of simulated laparoscopic surgical skill. *American Journal of Surgery*, 186: 169–174.

Edgcumbe, D.P., Silverman, J. & Benson, J. (2012) An examination of the validity of EPSCALE using factor analysis. *Patient Education and Counselling*, 87(1): 120–124.

Edmondson, D., Omarson, S., Falzon, L., Davidson, K.W., Mills, M.A. & Neria, Y. (2012) Posttraumatic stress disorder prevalence and risk of recurrence in acute coronary syndrome patients: A meta-analytic review. *PLoS One*, 7(6): e38915.

Edwards, A., Elwyn, G. & Mulley, A. (2002) Explaining risks: Turning numerical data into meaningful pictures. *British Medical Journal*, 324: 827–830.

Egede, L.E. (2007) Major depression in individuals with chronic medical disorders: Prevalence, correlates and association with health resource utilization, lost productivity and functional disability. *General Hospital Psychiatry*, 29: 409–416.

Ehlers, A. & Clark, D.M. (2000) A cognitive model of posttraumatic stress disorder. *Behaviour Research and Therapy*, 38: 319–345.

Ehlers, A., Stangier, U. & Geiler, U. (1995) Treatment of atopic dermatitis: A comparison of psychological and dermatological approaches to relapse prevention. *Journal of Consulting and Clinical Psychology*, 63: 624–635.

Ein-Dor, T. & Hirschberger, G. (2016) Rethinking attachment theory from a theory of relationships to a theory of individual and group survival. *Current Directions in Psychological Science*, 25: 2237

Ekman, P. (1992) An argument for basic emotions. *Cognition and Emotion*, 6: 169–200.

Ekman, P. (1999) Basic emotions, in T. Dalgleish & T. Power (eds), *Handbook of Cognition and Emotion*. Chichester, UK: Wiley. pp. 45–60.

Elkind, D. (1967) Egocentrism in adolescence. *Child Development*, 38: 1025–1034.

Elnegaard, S., Andersen, R.S., Pedersen, A.F., Larsen, P.V., Søndergaard, J., Rasmussen, S., Balasubramaniam, K., Svendsen, R.P., Vedsted, P. & Jarbøl, D.E. (2015) Self-reported symptoms and healthcare seeking in the general population – exploring 'The Symptom Iceberg'. *BMC Public Health*, 15: 685.

El-Salhy, M. (2012) Irritable bowel syndrome: Diagnosis and pathogenesis. *World Journal of Gastroenterology*, 18: 5151–5163.

El-Salhy, M. (2015) Recent developments in the pathophysiology of irritable bowel syndrome. *World Journal of Gastroenterology*, 21: 7621–7636.

El-Sayed, A.M., Scarborough, P. & Galea, S. (2011) Ethnic inequalities in obesity among children and adults in the UK: A systematic review of the literature. *Obesity Reviews*, 12(5): e516–534.

Elsenbruch, S. et al. (2005) Effects of mind-body therapy on quality of life and neuroendocrine and cellular immune functions in patients with ulcerative colitis. *Psychotherapy and Psychosomatics*, 74: 277–287.

Emdin, C.A., Odutayo, A., Wong, C.X., Tran, J., Hsiao, A.J. & Hunn, B.H. (2016) Meta-analysis of anxiety as a risk factor for cardiovascular disease. *American Journal of Cardiology*, 118(4): 511–519.

Emens, J.S. & Burgess, H.J. (2015) Effect of light and melatonin and other melatonin receptor agonists on human circadian physiology. *Sleep Medicine Clinics*, 10: 435–453.

Emery, C.F., Kiecolt-Glaser, J.K., Glaser, R., Malarkey, W.B. & Frid, D.J. (2005) Exercise accelerates wound healing among healthy older adults: A preliminary investigation. *Journals of Gerontology, Series A*, 60: 1432–1436.

Engel, G. (1977) The need for a new medical model: The challenge for biomedicine. *Science*, 196: 129–136.

Engelhard, I.M., van den Hout, M.A. & Arntz, A. (2001) Posttraumatic stress disorder after pregnancy loss. *General Hospital Psychiatry*, 23: 62–66.

Englar, R.E., Williams, M. & Weingand, K. (2016) Applicability of the Calgary-Cambridge Guide to Dog and Cat Owners for teaching veterinary clinical communications. *Journal of Veterinary Medical Education*, 43(2): 143–169.

Ericsson, K.A. (2004) Deliberate practice and the acquisition and maintenance of expert performance in medicine and related domains. *Academic Medicine*, 79: s70–s81.

Erikson, E.H. (1950) *Childhood and Society*. New York: W.W. Norton.

Erikson, E.H. (1968) *Identity: Youth and Crisis*. New York: W.W. Norton.

Erin, C. Dunn et al. (2015) Genetic determinants of depression: Recent findings and future directions. *Harvard Review of Psychiatry*, 23: 1–18.

Ernst, E. (2009) Massage therapy for cancer palliation and supportive care: A systematic review of randomised clinical trials. *Support Care Cancer*, 17: 333–337.

Escobar, J.I., Cook, B., Chen, C.N., Gara, M.A., Alegría, M., Interian, A. & Diaz, E. (2010) Whether medically unexplained or not, three or more concurrent somatic symptoms predict psychopathology and service use in community populations. *Journal of Psychosomatic Research*, 69(1): 1–8.

Esgate, A. & Groome, D. (2005) *An Introduction to Applied Cognitive Psychology*. Hove: Psychology Press.

Espejo, E.P. et al. (2012) Elevated appraisals of the negative impact of naturally occurring life events: A risk factor for depressive and anxiety disorders. *Journal of Abnormal Child Psychology*, 40: 303–315.

Essex, H. & Pickett, K. (2008) Mothers without companionship during childbirth: Analysis within Millennium cohort study. *Birth*, 35: 266–276.

European Centre for Disease Prevention and Control (2009) *HIV/AIDS Surveillance in Europe 2008*. WHO Regional Office for Europe. Stockholm: European CDPC.

European Centre for Disease Prevention and Control (2015) *Sexually Transmitted Infections in Europe 2013*. Stockholm: European CDPC.

European Centre for Disease Prevention and Control (2016) *HIV/AIDS Surveillance in Europe 2015*. WHO Regional Office for Europe. Stockholm: European CDPC.

Evans, G.W., Wener, R.E. & Phillips, D. (2002) The morning rush hour: Predictability and commuter stress. *Environment and Behavior*, 34: 521–530.

Everson-Rose, S.A., House, J.S. & Mero, R.P. (2004) Depressive symptoms and mortality risk in a national sample: Confounding effects of health status. *Psychosomatic Medicine*, 66(6): 823–830.

Evidence Development and Standards Branch, Health Quality Ontario (2014) Arthroscopic debridement of the knee: An evidence update. *Ontario Health Technology Assessment Series*, 14(13): 1–43.

Eysenck, M.W. (2000) *Psychology: A Student's Handbook*. Hove: Psychology Press.

Ezzati, M., Obermeyer, Z., Tzoulaki, I., Mayosi, B.M., Elliott, P. & Leon, D.A. (2015) The contributions of risk factor trends and medical care to cardiovascular mortality trends. *Nature Reviews Cardiology*, 12: 508–530.

Ezzy, D. (2000) Illness narratives: Time, hope, and HIV. *Social Science & Medicine*, 50: 605–617.

Ezzy, D., de Visser, R. & Bartos, M. (1999) Poverty, disease progression and employment among people living with HIV/AIDS in Australia. *AIDS Care*, 11: 405–414.

Fabbro, F. & Crescentini, C. (2014) Facing the experience of pain: A neuropsychological perspective. *Physics of Life Reviews*, 11(3): 540–552.

Fagan, J., Galea, S., Ahern, J., Bonner, S. & Vlahov, D. (2003) Relationship of self-reported asthma severity and urgent health care utilization to psychological sequelae of the September 11, 2001 terrorist attacks on the World Trade Center among New York City area residents. *Psychosomatic Medicine*, 65: 993–996.

Fahrenkopf, A.M., Sectish, T.C., Barger, L.K., Sharek, P.J., Lewin, D., Chiang, V.W., Edwards, S., Wiedermann, B.L. & Landrigan, C.P. (2008) Rates of medication errors among depressed and burnt out residents: Prospective cohort study. *BMJ*, 336(7642): 488–491. (doi: 10.1136/bmj.39469.763218.BE.)

Fairbrother, N. & Abramowitz, J.S. (2016) Obsessions and compulsions during pregnancy and the postpartum period, in A. Wenzel (ed.), *The Oxford Handbook of Perinatal Psychology*. New York and Oxford: Oxford University Press. pp. 167–181.

Fallowfield, L. & Jenkins, V. (2004) Communicating sad, bad, and difficult news in medicine. *Lancet*, 363(9405): 312–319.

Fandrew, J.R. et al. (2009) Treatment for depression after traumatic brain injury: A systematic review. *Journal of Neurotrauma*, 26: 2383–2402.

Fang, J.Y. & Tolleson, C. (2017) The role of deep brain stimulation in Parkinson's disease: An overview and update on new developments. *Neuropsychiatric Disease and Treatment*, 13: 23–32.

Farroni, T., Csibra, G., Simion, F. & Johnson, M.H. (2002) Eye contact detection in humans from birth. *Proceedings of the National Academy of Science*, 99: 9602–9605.

Farsides, T. (2009) What counseling is, in B. Alder, C. Abraham, E. van Teijlingen & M. Porter (eds), *Psychology and Sociology Applied to Medicine* (3rd edition). Edinburgh: Elsevier Science. pp. 132–133.

Fässler, M., Meissner, K., Schneider, A. & Linde, K. (2010) Frequency and circumstances of placebo use in clinical practice: A systematic review of empirical studies. *BMC Medicine*, 8: 15.

Faunce, G.J. (2002) Eating disorders and attentional bias: A review. *Eating Disorders*, 10: 125–139.

Fei, K. et al. (2016) Prevalence of depression among stroke survivors: Racial-ethnic differences. *Stroke*, 47: 512–515.

Feinstein, A. (2011) Multiple sclerosis and depression. *Multiple Sclerosis*, 17: 1276–1281.

Feinstein, R.E., Blumenfield, M., Orlowski, B., Frishman, W.H. & Ovanessian, S. (2006) A national survey of cardiovascular physicians' beliefs and clinical care practices when diagnosing and treating depression in patients with cardiovascular disease. *Cardiology in Review*, 14: 164–169.

Fennel, M.J.V. (1998) Low self-esteem, in N. Tarrier, A. Wells & G. Haddock (eds), *Treating Complex Cases: The Cognitive Therapy Approach*. Chichester, UK: Wiley. pp. 217–240.

Fenton, K. et al. (2001) Sexual behaviour in Britain: Reported sexually transmitted infections. *Lancet*, 358: 1851–1854.

Fenton, K. et al. (2004) Recent trends in the epidemiology of sexually transmitted infections in the European Union. *Sexually Transmitted Infections*, 80: 255–263.

Ferner, R.E. & McDowell, S. E. (2006) Doctors charged with manslaughter in the course of medical practice, 1795–2005: A literature review. *Journal of the Royal Society of Medicine*, 99: 309–314.

Ferri, C.P. et al. (2005) Global prevalence of dementia. *Lancet*, *366*: 2112–2117.

Festinger, L. (1957) *A Theory of Cognitive Dissonance*. Evanston, IL: Row, Peterson.

Fiedorowicz, J.G. (2014) Depression and cardiovascular disease: An update on how course of illness may influence risk. *Current Psychiatry Reports*, *16*(10): 492.

Field, T., Diego, M. & Hernandez-Reif, M. (2007) Massage therapy research. *Developmental Review*, *27*: 75–89.

Finan, P.H., Quartana, P.J. & Smith, M.T. (2015) The effects of sleep continuity disruption on positive mood and sleep architecture in healthy adults. *Sleep*, *38*: 1735–1742.

Finch, S.J. (2003) Pregnancy during residency: A literature review. *Academic Medicine*, *78*: 418–428.

Fink, G. (2011) Stress controversies: Post-traumatic stress disorder, hippocampal volume, gastroduodenal ulceration. *Journal of Neuroendocrinology*, *23*: 107–117.

Finlay, I.G. et al. (2002) Palliative care in hospital, hospice, at home: Results from a systematic review. *Annals of Oncology*, *13*(Suppl. 4): 257–264.

Firth-Cozens, J. (2001) Medical student stress. *Medical Education*, *35*: 6–7.

Fischer, P., Krueger, J.I., Greitemeyer, T., Vogrincic, C., Kastenmüller, A., Frey, D., Heene, M., Wicher, M. & Kainbacher, M. (2011) The bystander-effect: A meta-analytic review on bystander intervention in dangerous and non-dangerous emergencies. *Psychological Bulletin*, *137*: 517–37.

Fisher, C.A., Hetrick, S.E. & Rushford, N. (2010) Family therapy for anorexia nervosa. *Cochrane Database of Systematic Reviews*, 2010, 14(4):CD004780.

Fitts, S.S., Guthrie, M.R. & Blagg, C.R. (1999) Exercise coaching and rehabilitation counseling improve quality of life for predialysis and dialysis patients. *Nephron*, *82*: 115–121.

Fitzsimmons-Craft, E.E. (2011) Social psychological theories of disordered eating in college women: Review and integration. *Clinical Psychology Review*, *31*: 1224–1237.

Flaherty, D.K. (2011) The vaccine-autism connection: A public health crisis caused by unethical medical practices and fraudulent science. *Annals of Pharmacotherapy*, *45*: 1302–1304.

Flaherty, R.J. (2007) *Medical Myths: Evidence-based Medicine for Student Health Services*. Available at: www.montana.edu/wwwebm/myths.htm (last accessed 31/08/07).

Flickinger, T.E., Saha, S., Roter, D., Korthuis, P.T., Sharp, V., Cohn, J., Moore, R.D., Ingersoll, K.S. & Beach, M.C. (2016) Respecting patients is associated with more patient-centered communication behaviors in clinical encounters. *Patient Education and Counselling*, *99*(2): 250–255.

Flocke, S.A., Miller, W.L. & Crabtree, B.F. (2002) Relationships between physician practice style, patient satisfaction, and attributes of primary care. *Journal of Family Practice*, *51*: 835–840.

Floud, S., Balkwill, A., Canoy, D., Wright, F.L., Reeves, G.K., Green, J., Beral, V. & Cairns, B.J. (2014) Million Women Study Collaborators. Marital status and ischemic heart disease incidence and mortality in women: A large prospective study. *BMC Medicine*, *12*: 42.

Floyd, D.L., Prentice-Dunn, S. & Rogers, R.W. (2000) A meta-analysis of research on protection motivation theory. *Journal of Applied Social Psychology*, *30*: 407–429.

Folstein, M.F., Folstein, S.E. & McHugh, P.R. (1975) 'Mini-mental state': A practical method for grading the cognitive state of patients for the clinician. *Journal of Psychiatric Research*, *12*: 189–198.

Forcier, K. et al. (2006) Links between physical fitness and cardiovascular reactivity and recovery to psychological stressors: A meta-analysis. *Health Psychology*, *25*: 723–739.

Ford, A.C. et al. (2014) Effect of antidepressants and psychological therapies, including hypnotherapy, in irritable bowel syndrome: Systematic review and meta-analysis. *American Journal of Gastroenterology*, *109*: 1350–1365. (doi: 10.1038/ajg.2014.148)

Ford, A.C., Talley, N.J., Schoenfeld, P.S., Quigley, E.M.M. & Moayyedi, P. (2009) Efficacy of antidepressants and psychological therapies in irritable bowel syndrome: Systematic review and meta-analysis. *Gut*, *58*: 367–378.

Ford, O., Lethaby, A., Mol, B. & Roberts, H. (2006) Progesterone for premenstrual syndrome. *Cochrane Database of Systematic Reviews*, *4*: CD003415.

Fordyce, W.E., Fowler, R.S. Jr, Lehmann, J.F., Delateur, B.J., Sand, P.L. & Trieschmann, R.B. (1973) Operant conditioning in the treatment of chronic pain. *Archives of Physical Medicine and Rehabilitation*, *54*(9): 399–408.

Foroushani, P.S., Schneider, J. & Assareh, N. (2011) Meta-review of the effectiveness of computerised CBT in treating depression. *BMC Psychiatry*, *11*: 131.

Fortner, B.V. & Neimeyer, R.A. (1999) Death anxiety in older adults: A quantitative review. *Death Studies*, *23*: 387–411.

Foster, M.C. et al. (2008) Overweight, obesity, and the development of stage 3 CKD: The Framingham Heart Study. *American Journal of Kidney Disease*, *52*: 39–48.

Frank, M.G. & Benington, J.H. (2006) The role of sleep in memory consolidation and brain plasticity: Dream or reality? *Neuroscientist*, *12*: 477–488.

Frankel, R.M. & Sherman, H.B. (2015) The secret of the care of the patient is in knowing and applying the evidence about effective clinical communication. *Oral Diseases*, *21*(8): 919–26.

Frankel, R.M. & Stein, T. (1999) Getting the most out of the clinical encounter: the four habits model. *Perm Journal*, *3*: 79–88.

Franks, H.M. & Roesch, S.C. (2006) Appraisals and coping in people living with cancer: A meta-analysis. *Psycho-Oncology*, *15*: 1027–1037.

Frasure-Smith, N. et al. (2000) Depression and health-care costs during the first year following myocardial infarction. *Journal of Pychosomatic Research*, *36*: 471–478.

Frattaroli, J. (2006) Experimental disclosure and its moderators: A meta-analysis. *Psychological Bulletin*, *132*: 823–865.

Fredrickson, B.L. (2004) The broaden-and-build theory of positive emotions. *Philosophical Transactions Royal Society of London Series B. Biological Sciences*, *359*: 1367–1378.

Freeman, E.W. & Sherif, K. (2007) Prevalence of hot flushes and night sweats around the world: A systematic review. *Climacteric*, *10*: 197–214.

Freitas, D.A., Holloway, E.A., Bruno, S.S., Chaves, G.S., Fregonezi, G.A. & Mendonça, K.P. (2013) Breathing exercises for adults with asthma. *Cochrane Database of Systematic Reviews*, *10*: CD001277.

French, D.P., Cooper, A. & Weinman, J. (2006) Illness perceptions predict attendance at cardiac rehabilitation following acute myocardial infarction: A systematic review with meta-analysis. *Journal of Psychosomatic Research*, *61*: 757–67.

French, S.A., Leffert, N., Story, M., Neumark-Sztainer, D., Hannan, P. & Benson, P.L. (2001) Adolescent binge/purge and weight loss behaviors: Associations with developmental assets. *Journal of Adolescent Health*, *28*: 211–221.

Freud, S. (1999 [1900]) *The Interpretation of Dreams* (translator: J. Crick). Oxford: Oxford University Press.

Friebel, U., Eickhoff, S.B. & Lotze, M. (2011) Coordinate-based meta-analysis of experimentally induced and chronic persistent neuropathic pain. *Neuroimage, 58*(4): 1070–1080.

Friedman, H.S. & Booth-Kewley, S. (1987) The 'disease-prone' personality: A meta-analytic view of the construct. *American Psychologist, 42*: 539–555.

Friedman, M. et al. (1986) Alteration of Type A behaviour and its effect on cardiac recurrences in post myocardial infarction patients. *American Heart Journal, 112*: 653–665.

Friedman, T. & Gath, D. (1989) The psychiatric consequences of spontaneous abortion. *British Journal of Psychiatry, 155*: 810–813.

Fries, J.F., Green, L.W. & Levine, S. (1989) Health promotion and the compression of morbidity. *Lancet, 333*: 481–483.

Frijda, N.H. (1986) *The Emotions: Studies in Emotion and Social Interaction.* New York: Cambridge University Press.

Frisina, P.G., Borod, J.C. & Lepore, S.J. (2004) A meta-analysis of the effects of written emotional disclosure on the health outcomes of clinical populations. *Journal of Nervous and Mental Disease, 192*(9): 629–634.

Furnham, A., Petrides, K.V., Sisterson, G. & Baluch, B. (2003) Repressive coping style and positive self-presentation. *British Journal of Health Psychology, 8*: 223–249.

Gage, S.H. et al. (2016) Association between cannabis and psychosis: Epidemiologic evidence. *Biological Psychiatry, 79*: 549–556.

Gagnon, A.J. & Sandall, J. (2007) Individual or group antenatal education for childbirth or parenthood, or both. *Cochrane Database of Systematic Reviews, 3*: CD002869.

Gale, C.R., Batty, G.D. & Deary, I.J. (2008) Locus of control at age 10 years and health outcomes and behaviors at age 30 years. *Psychosomatic Medicine, 70*: 397–403.

Gallicchio, L. & Kalesan, B. (2009) Sleep duration and mortality: A systematic review and meta-analysis. *Journal of Sleep Research, 18*: 148–158.

Gamble, J. & Creedy, D. (2001) Women's preference for a caesarean section: Incidence and associated factors. *Birth, 28*: 101–110.

Gandaglia, G. et al. (2014) A systematic review of the association between erectile dysfunction and cardiovascular disease. *European Urology, 65*: 968–978.

Gangestad, S.W. & Cousins, A.J. (2001) Adaptive design, female mate preferences, and shifts across the menstrual cycle. *Annual Review of Sex Research, 12*: 145–185.

Gangestad, S.W. & Thornhill, R. (2008) Human oestrus. *Proceedings of the Royal Society B: Biological Sciences, 275*(1638): 991–1000.

Gao, W., Ho, Y.K., Verne, J., Gordon, E. & Higginson, I.J. (2014) *Geographical and Temporal Understanding in Place of Death in England (1984–2010): Analysis of Trends and Associated Factors to Improve End-of-life Care (GUIDE_Care) – Primary Research.* Southampton, UK: NIHR Journals Library.

Garakani, A. et al. (2003) Comorbidity of irritable bowel syndrome in psychiatric patients: A review. *American Journal of Therapeutics, 10*: 61–67.

Garcia-Retamero, R. et al. (2012) Using visual aids to improve communication of risks about health: A review. *Scientific World Journal, 2012*: 62637.

Gardner, M. & Steinberg, L. (2005) Peer influence on risk taking, risk preference, and risky decision making in adolescence and adulthood: An experimental study. *Developmental Psychology, 41*: 625–635.

Garrett, V.D., Brantley, P.J., Jones, G.H. & McKnight, G.T. (1991) The relation between daily stress and Crohns disease. *Journal of Behavioral Medicine, 14:* 87–96.

Garssen, B. (2004) Psychological factors and cancer development: Evidence after 30 years of research. *Clinical Psychology Review, 24:* 315–338.

Gathright, E.C., Goldstein, C.M., Josephson, R.A. & Hughes, J.W. (2017) Depression increases the risk of mortality in patients with heart failure: A meta-analysis. *Journal of Psychosomatic Research, 94:* 82–89.

Gavin, L. et al. (2009) Sexual and reproductive health of persons aged 10–24 years – United States, 2002–2007. *Morbidity & Mortality Weekly Report Surveillance Summary, 58*(6): 1–58.

Gdalevich, M., Mimouni, D. & Mimouni, M. (2001a) Breast-feeding and the risk of bronchial asthma in childhood: A systematic review with meta-analysis of prospective studies. *Journal of Pediatrics, 139:* 261–266.

Gdalevich, M., Mimouni, D., David, M. & Mimouni, M. (2001b) Breast-feeding and the onset of atopic dermatitis in childhood: A systematic review and meta-analysis of prospective studies. *Journal of the American Academy of Dermatology, 45:* 520–527.

Geen, R.G. & O'Neal, E.C. (1969) Activation of cue-elicited aggression by general arousal. *Journal of Personality and Social Psychology, 11:* 289–292.

Geenen, R., van Middendorp, H. & Bijlsma, J.W.J. (2006) The impact of stressors on health status and hypothalamic-pituitary-adrenal axis and autonomic nervous system responsiveness in rheumatoid arthritis. *Annals of the New York Academy of Sciences, 1069:* 77–97.

Geeraerts, B. et al. (2005) Influence of experimentally induced anxiety on gastric sensorimotor function in humans. *Gastroenterology, 129:* 1437–1444.

Gehlert, S., Song, I.H., Chang, C.-H. & Hartlage, S.A. (2008) The prevalence of premenstrual dysphoric disorder in a randomly selected group of urban and rural women. *Psychological Medicine, 39:* 129–136.

Gelb, P. (1982) The experience of nonerotic contact in traditional psychotherapy: A critical investigation of the taboo against touch. *Dissertation Abstracts, 43:* 1–13.

Gelder, M. et al. (2012) *Psychiatry* (4th edition) Oxford: Oxford University Press.

Gelder, M., Mayou, R. & Geddes, J. (2005) *Psychiatry* (3rd edition). Oxford: Oxford University Press.

Gellad, W.F. et al. (2011) A systematic review of barriers to medication adherence in the elderly: Looking beyond cost and regimen complexity. *American Journal of Geriatric Pharmacotherapy, 9:* 11–23.

General Medical Council (2009) *Tomorrow's Doctors.* London: General Medical Council.

Georgescu, A.L., Kuzmanovic, B., Roth, D., Bente, G. & Vogeley, K. (2014) The use of virtual characters to assess and train non-verbal communication in high-functioning autism. *Frontiers in Human Neuroscience, 15*(8): 807.

Gerhardt, S. (2004) *Why Love Matters: How Affection Shapes a Baby's Brain.* New York: Brunner-Routledge.

Ghosh, S. & Mitchell, R. (2007) Impact of inflammatory bowel disease on quality of life. *Journal of Crohn's and Colitis, 1:* 10–20.

Gielissen, M., Verhagen, C. & Bleijenberg, G. (2007) Cognitive behaviour therapy for fatigued cancer survivors: Long-term follow-up. *British Journal of Cancer, 97:* 612–618.

Gigerenzer, G., Gaissmaier, W., Kurz-Milcke, E., Schwartz, L.M. & Woloshin, S. (2008) Helping doctors and patients to make sense of health statistics. *Psychological Science in the Public Interest*, 8: 53–96.

Gil, K.M., Somerville, A.M., Cichowski, S. & Savitski, J.L. (2009) Distress and quality of life characteristics associated with seeking surgical treatment for stress urinary incontinence. *Health and Quality of Life Outcomes*, 7(8).

Gilbert, P. (2000) *Overcoming Depression: A Self-Help Guide Using Cognitive Behavioural Techniques*. London: Robinson.

GINA: Global Initiative for Asthma (2001) *Global Strategy for Asthma Management and Prevention*. Bethesda, MD: NIH NHLBI.

Girón, M., Manjón-Arce, P., Puerto-Barber, J., Sánchez-García, E. & Gómez-Beneyto, M. (1998) Clinical interview skills and identification of emotional disorders in primary care. *American Journal of Psychiatry*, 155: 530–535.

Glaser, B. & Strauss, A. (1966) *Awareness of Dying*. Chicago, IL: Aldine.

Glaser, R. & Kiecolt-Glaser, J.K. (2005) Stress-induced immune dysfunction: Implications for health. *Nature Reviews: Immunology*, 5: 243–251.

Glaser, R. et al. (1987) Stress-related immune suppression: Health implications. *Brain, Behavior & Immunity*, 1: 7–20.

Global Initiative for Asthma (2017) *Global Strategy for Asthma Management and Prevention, 2017*. Available at: http://ginasthma.org/2017-gina-report-global-strategy-for-asthma-man agement-and-prevention (last accessed 25 February 2017).

Glover, V. (2016) Maternal stress during pregnancy and infant and child outcomes, in A. Wenzel (ed.), *The Oxford Handbook of Perinatal Psychology*. New York and Oxford: Oxford University Press.

Goebel, M.U., Neykadeh, N., Kou, W., Schedlowski, M. & Hengge, U.R. (2008) Behavioral conditioning of antihistamine effects in patients with allergic rhinitis. *Psychotherapy & Psychosomatics*, 77: 227–234.

Goel, N., Basner, M., Rao, H. & Dinges, D.F. (2013) Circadian rhythms, sleep deprivation, and human performance. *Progress in Molecular Biology and Translational Science*, 119: 155–190.

Goffman, E. (1959) *The Presentation of Self in Everyday Life*. New York: Doubleday.

Goitein, L., Shanafelt, T.D., Wipf, J.E., Slatore, C.G. & Back, A.L. (2005) The effects of work-hour limitations on resident well-being, patient care, and education in an internal medicine residency program. *Archives of Internal Medicine*, 165(22): 2601–2606.

Goldberg, C. (2001) Cognitive processes in panic disorder: an extension of current models. *Psychological Reports*, 88(1): 139–159.

Goldstein, C.M., Gathright, E.C., Gunstad, J., Dolansky, M., Redle, J.D., Josephson, R., Moore, S.M. & Hughes, J.W. (2017) Depressive symptoms moderate the relationship between medication regimen complexity and objectively measured medication adherence in adults with heart failure. *Journal of Behavioral Medicine*, 40(4): 602–611.

Goldstein, L.H. & Leigh, P.N. (1999) Motor neurone disease: A review of its emotional and cognitive consequences for patients and its impact on carers. *British Journal of Health Psychology*, 4: 193–208.

Gonzalez, J.S. (2008) Depression and diabetes treatment nonadherence: A meta-analysis. *Diabetes Care, 31*: 2398–2403.

Gonzalez, J.S. et al. (2011) Depression and HIV/AIDS treatment nonadherence: A review and meta-analysis. *Journal of Acquired Immune Deficiency Syndromes, 58*: 181–187.

Goodwin, R.D., Cox, B.J. & Clara, I. (2006) Neuroticism and physical disorders among adults in the community: Results from the national comorbidity survey. *Journal of Behavioural Medicine, 29*: 229–238.

Gorman, J.M., Kent, J.M., Sullivan, G.M. & Coplan, J.D. (2000) Neuroanatomical hypothesis of panic disorder, revised. *American Journal of Psychiatry, 157*: 493–505.

Gott, M. (2006) Sexual health and the new ageing. *Age & Ageing, 35*: 106–107.

Gott, M. et al. (2004) 'Opening a can of worms': GP and practice nurse barriers to talking about sexual health in primary care. *Journal of Family Practice, 21*: 528–536.

Gottlieb, B. (2007) Social support interventions, in S. Ayers et al. (eds), *Cambridge Handbook of Psychology, Health and Medicine* (2nd edition). Cambridge: Cambridge University Press. pp. 397–402.

Gottlieb, B. & Wachala, E. (2007) Cancer support groups: A critical review of empirical studies. *Psycho-Oncology, 16*: 379–400.

Gough, B. & Conner, M.T. (2006) Barriers to healthy eating among men: A qualitative analysis. *Social Science & Medicine, 62*: 387–395.

Gouin, J.P., Kiecolt-Glaser, J.K., Malarky, W.B. & Glaser, R. (2008) The influence of anger expression on wound healing. *Brain, Behaviour and Immunity, 22*: 699–708.

Gould, N. & Kendall, T. (2007) Developing the NICE/SCIE guidelines for dementia care: The challenges of enhancing the evidence base for social and health care. *British Journal of Social Work, 37*: 475–490.

Government Office for Science (2007) *Tackling Obesities: Future Choices – Project Report* (2nd edition). London: Government Office for Science.

Goyal, M., Singh, S., Sibinga, E.M., Gould, N.F., Rowland-Seymour, A., Sharma, R., Berger, Z., Sleicher, D., Maron, D.D., Shihab, H.M., Ranasinghe, P.D., Linn, S., Saha, S., Bass, E.B. & Haythornthwaite, J.A. (2014) Meditation programs for psychological stress and well-being: A systematic review and meta-analysis. *JAMA Internal Medicine, 174*(3): 357–368.

Goyal, R.K. & Hirano, I. (1996) The enteric nervous system. *New England Journal of Medicine, 334*: 1106–1115.

Gracely, R.H. et al. (2004) Pain catastrophizing and neural responses to pain among persons with fibromyalgia. *Brain, 127*: 835–843.

Grandner, M.A., Jackson, N.J., Izci-Balserak, B., Gallagher, R.A., Murray-Bachmann, R., Williams, N.J., Patel, N.P. & Jean-Louis, G. (2015) Social and behavioral determinants of perceived insufficient sleep. *Frontiers in Neurology, 6*: 112.

Grant, B.F. et al. (2006) The epidemiology of DSM-IV panic disorder and agoraphobia in the United States. *Journal of Clinical Psychiatry, 67*: 363–374.

Grave, J., Soares, S.C., Morais, S., Rodrigues, P. & Madeira, N. (2017) The effects of perceptual load in processing emotional facial expression in psychotic disorders. *Psychiatry Research, 250*: 121–128.

Gravely-Witte, S., Stewart, D.E., Suskin, N., Higginson, L., Alter, D.A. & Grace, S.L. (2008) Cardiologists' charting varied by risk factor, and was often discordant with patient report. *Journal of Clinical Epidemiology*, 61: 1073–1079.

Green, J.M., Coupland, V.A. & Kitzinger, J.V. (1998) *Great Expectations: A Prospective Study of Women's Expectations and Experiences of Childbirth*. Hale, Cheshire: Books for Midwives Press.

Greenhalgh, T. (2006) *How to Read a Paper: The Basics of Evidence-Based Medicine* (3rd edition). Oxford: Blackwell.

Greenhalgh, T. (2014) *How to Read a Paper: The Basics of Evidence-Based Medicine* (5th edition). Oxford: Blackwell.

Greenhalgh, T. (2016) *Cultural Contexts of Health: The Use of Narrative Research in the Health Sector* [Internet]. Copenhagen: WHO Regional Office for Europe. Available at: www.ncbi.nlm.nih.gov/books/NBK391066/.

Greenhalgh, T. & Hurwitz, B. (eds) (1998) *Narrative Based Medicine: Dialogue and Discourse in Clinical Practice*. London: British Medical Journal Books.

Greenhill, N., Anderson, C., Avery, A. & Pilnick, A. (2011) Analysis of pharmacist–patient communication using the Calgary–Cambridge guide. *Patient Education and Counselling*, 83(3): 423–431.

Greer, S., Morris, T. & Pettingale, K.W. (1979) Psychological responses to breast cancer: Effect on outcome. *Lancet*, 393: 785–787.

Greitemeyer, T. & Mügge, D.O. (2014) Video games do affect social outcomes: A meta-analytic review of the effects of violent and prosocial video game play. *Personality and Social Psychology Bulletin*, 40: 578–589.

Grenard, J.L. et al. (2011) Depression and medication adherence in the treatment of chronic diseases in the United States: A meta-analysis. *Journal of General Internal Medicine*, 26: 1175–1182.

Griffin, J.E. & Ojeda, S.R. (2004) *Textbook of Endocrine Physiology* (5th edition). Oxford: Oxford University Press.

Griffin, J.E. & Ojeda, S.R. (2011) *Textbook of Endocrine Physiology* (6th edition). Oxford: Oxford University Press.

Griffiths, K.M., Calear, A.L. & Banfield, M. (2009) Systematic review on Internet Support Groups (ISGs) and depression (1): Do ISGs reduce depressive symptoms? *Journal of Medical Internet Research*, 11(3): e40.

Grilo, C.M., Masheb, R.M. & Wilson, G.T. (2005) Efficacy of cognitive behavioral therapy and fluoxetine for the treatment of binge eating disorder: A randomized double-blind placebo controlled comparison. *Biological Psychology*, 57: 301–309.

Grodzinsky, E. et al. (2015) More negative self-esteem and inferior coping strategies among patients diagnosed with IBS compared with patients without IBS: A case-control study in primary care. *BMC Family Practice*, 16: 6.

Groeger, J.A., Zijlstra, FR.H. & Dijk, D.-J. (2004) Sleep quantity, sleep difficulties and their perceived consequences in a representative sample of some 2000 British adults. *Journal of Sleep Research*, 13: 359–371.

Groome, D. & Eysenck, M. (2016) *An Introduction to Applied Cognitive Psychology* (2nd edition). Hove: Psychology Press.

Gross, A.L. et al. (2010) Depression and cancer risk: 24 years of follow-up of the Baltimore Epidemiologic Catchment Area sample. *Cancer Causes Control*, 21: 191–199.

Gross, J.J. & Thompson, R.A. (2007) Emotion regulation: Conceptual foundations, in J.J. Gross (ed.), *Handbook of Emotion Regulation*. London: Guilford Press. pp. 3–24.

Groß, M. et al. (2016) Unemployment, health, and education of HIV-infected males in Germany. *International Journal of Public Health*, 61: 593–602.

Grover, A.K. & Samson, S.E. (2014) Antioxidants and vision health: facts and fiction. *Molecular and Cellular Biochemistry*, 388(1–2): 173–183.

Grover, S.A. et al. (2006) The prevalence of erectile dysfunction in the primary care setting: Importance of risk factors for diabetes and vascular disease. *Archives of Internal Medicine*, 166: 213–219.

Gruber, A.J. & Pope, H.G. (2000) Psychiatric and medical effects of anabolic-androgenic steroid use in women. *Psychotherapy & Psychosomatics*, 69: 19–26.

Grulich, A.E. et al. (2014) Knowledge about and experience of sexually transmissible infections in a representative sample of adults: The Second Australian Study of Health and Relationships. *Sexual Health*, 11: 481–494.

Grulich, A. et al. (2003) Sex in Australia: Sexually transmissible infection. *Australian and New Zealand Journal of Public Health*, 27: 234–241.

Guéguen, N., Silone, F. & David, M. (2016) The effect of the two feet-in-the-door technique on tobacco deprivation. *Psychology & Health*, 31: 768–775.

Guillaumie, L., Boiral, O. & Champagne, J. (2016) A mixed-methods systematic review of the effects of mindfulness on nurses. *Journal of Advanced Nursing*, 73(5): 1017–1034.

Guinjoan, S.M. et al. (2004) Cardiac parasympathetic dysfunction related to depression in older adults with acute coronary symptoms. *Journal of Psychosomatic Research*, 56: 83–88.

Gullette, E.C.D. et al. (1997) Effects of mental stress on myocardial ischaemia in daily life. *Journal of the American Medical Association*, 277: 1521–1526.

Gupton, A., Beaton, J., Sloan, J. & Bramadat, I. (1991) The development of a scale to measure childbirth expectations. *Canadian Journal of Nursing Research*, 23(2): 35–47.

Gurevich, M., Bishop, S., Bower, J., Malka, M. & Nyhof-Young, J. (2004) (Dis)embodying gender and sexuality in testicular cancer. *Social Science & Medicine*, 58: 1597–1607.

Gustafson, J. & Welling, D. (2009) 'No acid, no ulcer' – 100 years later: A review of the history of peptic ulcer disease. *Journal of American College of Surgeons*, 210: 110–116.

Gustafsson, P.A., Duchén, K., Birberg, U. & Karlsson, T. (2004) Breastfeeding, very long polyunsaturated fatty acids and IQ at 6½ years of age. *Acta Paediatrica*, 93: 1280–1287.

Gutman, D.A. & Nemeroff, C.B. (2003) Persistent central nervous system effects of an adverse early environment: Clinical and preclinical studies. *Physiology & Behaviour*, 79: 471–478.

Haas, J.S. et al. (2004) Changes in the health status of women during and after pregnancy. *Journal of General Internal Medicine*, 20: 45–51.

Hagedoorn, M., Kuijer, E.F., Buunk, V.P., DeJong, G., Wobbes, T. & Sanderman, R. (2000) Marital satisfaction in patients with cancer: Does support from intimate partners benefit those who need it the most? *Health Psychology*, 19: 274–282.

Hägele, C. et al. (2014) How do we 'learn' addiction? Risk factors and mechanisms getting addicted to alcohol. *Neuropsychobiology*, 70: 67–76.

Hahn, S. et al. (2008) Patient and visitor violence in general hospitals: A systematic review of the literature. *Aggression & Violent Behavior*, 13: 431–441.

Hall, E.T. (1966) *The Hidden Dimension*. Garden City, NY: Doubleday.

Hall, J.A. & Roter, D.L. (2002) Do patients talk differently to male and female physicians? A meta-analytic review. *Patient Education & Counseling*, 48: 217–224.

Hall, W.J., Chapman, M.V., Lee, K.M., Merino, Y.M., Thomas, T.W., Payne, B.K., Eng, E., Day, S.H. & Coyne-Beasley, T. (2015) Implicit racial/ethnic bias among health care professionals and its influence on health care outcomes: A systematic review. *American Journal of Public Health*, 105: e60–e76.

Halvorsen, L., Nerum, H., Øian, P. & Sørlie, T. (2008) Is there an association between psychological stress and request for caesarean section? *Tidsskrift for den Norske Laegeforening*, 12: 1388–1391.

Hamer, M., Chida, Y. & Molloy, G.J. (2009) Psychological distress and cancer mortality. *Journal of Psychosomatic Research*, 66: 255–258.

Han, M.H., Lee, E.H. & Koh, S.H. (2016) Current opinion on the role of neurogenesis in the therapeutic strategies for Alzheimer disease, Parkinson disease, and ischemic stroke: Considering neuronal voiding function, *International Neurourology Journal*, 20: 276–287.

Hanauer, S.B. (2008) Review article: Evolving concepts in treatment and disease modification in ulcerative colitis. *Alimentary Pharmacology & Therapeutics*, 27: 15–21.

Hancock, L., Windsor, A.C. & Mortensen, N.J. (2006) Inflammatory bowel disease: The view of the surgeon. *Colorectal Disease*, 8: 10–14.

Hann, K.E. & McCracken, L.M. (2014) A systematic review of randomized controlled trials of Acceptance and Commitment Therapy for adults with chronic pain: Outcome domains, design quality. and efficacy. *Journal of Contextual Behavioral Science*, 3(4): 217–227.

Harcourt, D. (2017) Disfigurement, in C.D. Llewellyn et al. (eds), *Cambridge Handbook of Psychology, Health and Medicine* (3rd edition). Cambridge: Cambridge University Press.

Hardeman, W. et al. (2002) Application of the Theory of Planned Behaviour in behaviour change interventions: A systematic review. *Psychology of Health*, 17: 123–158.

Harlow, H.F. (1958) The nature of love. *American Psychologist*, 13: 673–685.

Harrigan, J.A., Oxman, T.E. & Rosenthal, R. (1985) Rapport expressed through nonverbal behaviour. *Journal of Nonverbal Behaviour*, 9: 95–110.

Harrington, P. & Ayers, S. (2008) *Systematic Review of Depression in People with Neurological Disease*. Falmer: Brighton & Sussex Medical School (unpublished).

Harris, A.H. (2006) Does expressive writing reduce health care utilization? A meta-analysis of randomized trials. *Journal of Consulting and Clinical Psychology*, 74(2): 243–252.

Harris, R. (2006) Embracing your demons: An overview of acceptance and commitment therapy. *Psychotherapy in Australia*, 12(4): 2–8.

Harrison, J.A., Mullen, P.D. & Green, L.W. (1992) A meta-analysis of studies of the Health Belief Model with adults. *Health Education Research*, 7: 107–116.

Harrison, S.L., Lee, A., Janaudis-Ferreira, T., Goldstein, R.S. & Brooks, D. (2016) Mindfulness in people with a respiratory diagnosis: A systematic review. *Patient Education and Counselling*, 99(3): 348–355.

Hart, A. & Kamm, M.A. (2002) Review article: Mechanisms of initiation and perpetuation of gut inflammation by stress. *Alimentary Pharmacology & Therapeutics*, 16: 2017–2028.

Harvey, A. et al. (2004) *Cognitive Behavioural Processes across Psychological Disorders: A Transdiagnostic Approach to Research and Treatment.* Oxford: Oxford University Press.

Hashash, J. et al. (2008) Clinical trial: A randomized controlled cross-over study of flupenthixol & melitracen in functional dyspepsia. *Alimentary Pharmacology & Therapeutics*, 27: 1148–1155.

Haslam, N., Loughnan, S. & Perry, G. (2014) Meta-Milgram: An empirical synthesis of the obedience experiments. *PLoS One*, 9(4): e93927.

Hatipoglu, E. et al. (2014) Impact of exercise on quality of life and body-self perception of patients with acromegaly. *Pituitary*, 17: 38–43.

Hauser, G., Pletikosic, S. & Tkalcic, M. (2014) Cognitive behavioral approach to understanding irritable bowel syndrome. *World Journal of Gastroenterology*, 20(22): 6744–6758.

Hawks, S.R., Madanat, H.N. & Christley, H.S. (2008) Psychosocial associations of dietary restraint: Implications for healthy weight promotion. *Ecology of Food and Nutrition*, 47: 450–483.

Hay, P.P. et al. (2009) Psychological treatments for bulimia nervosa and binging. *Cochrane Database of Systematic Reviews*, 7: CD000562.

Hayes, S.C. (2004) Acceptance and commitment therapy and the new behaviour therapies: Mindfulness, acceptance, and relationship, in S.C. Hayes, V.M. Follette & M.M. Linehan (eds), *Mindfulness and Acceptance: Expanding the Cognitive Behavioural Tradition*. New York: Guilford Press. pp. 1–29.

Hayes, S.C., Strosahl, K.D. & Wilson, N.G. (1999) *Acceptance and Commitment Therapy: An Experimental Approach to Behaviour Change*. New York: Guilford Press.

Hay-Smith, J. & Dumoulin, C. (2006) Pelvic floor muscle training versus no treatment, or inactive control treatments, for urinary incontinence in women. *Cochrane Database of Systematic Reviews*, 1 (Art. CD005654).

Healthcare Commission (2007) *Caring for Dignity*. London: Healthcare Commission.

Heber, E., Ebert, D.D., Lehr, D., Cuijpers, P., Berking, M., Nobis, S. & Riper, H. (2017) The benefit of web- and computer-based interventions for stress: A systematic review and meta-analysis. *Journal of Medical Internet Research*, 19(2): e32.

Heilmayr, D. & Friedman, H. (2018) Personality and health, in C.D. Llewellyn et al. (eds), *The Cambridge Handbook of Psychology, Health and Medicine* (3rd edition). Cambridge: Cambridge University Press.

Heim, C. & Binder, E.B. (2012) Current research trends in early life stress and depression: Review of human studies on sensitive periods, gene-environment interactions, and epigenetics. *Experimental Neurology*, 233: 102–111.

Heinrichs, N., Hoffman, E.C. & Hofmann, S.G. (2001) Cognitive-behavioral treatment for social phobia in Parkinson's disease: A single-case study. *Cognitive & Behavioral Practice*, 8: 328–335.

Heiwe, S. & Jacobson, S.H. (2011) Exercise training for adults with chronic kidney disease. *Cochrane Database of Systematic Reviews*, 10 (Art. CD003236).

Hemilä, H. & Chalker, E. (2013) Vitamin C for preventing and treating the common cold. *Cochrane Database of Systematic Reviews*, 1 (Art. CD000980).

Hennessy, M.B., Kaiser, S. & Sachser, N. (2009) Social buffering of the stress response: Diversity, mechanisms, and functions. *Frontiers in Neuroendocrinology*, 30(4): 470–482.

Henry, S.G. et al. (2012) Association between nonverbal communication during clinical interactions and outcomes: A systematic review and meta-analysis. *Patient Education and Counselling*, 86: 297–315.

Herbert, T.B. & Cohen, S. (1993) Depression and immunity: A meta-analytic review. *Psychological Bulletin*, 113: 472–486.

Heron, M.P. (2007) *Deaths: Leading Causes for 2004*. Hyattsville, MD: National Center for Health Data and Methods.

Herzog, D.B. et al. (2000) Mortality in eating disorders: A descriptive study. *International Journal of Eating Disorders*, 28: 20–26.

Hettema, J., Neale, M.C. & Kendler, K.S. (2001) A review and meta-analysis of the genetic epidemiology of anxiety disorders. *American Journal of Psychiatry*, 158: 1568–1578.

Hettema, J., Steele, J. & Miller, W.R. (2005) Motivational interviewing, *Annual Review of Clinical Psychology*, 1: 91–111.

Hewitt, J.K. & Turner, J.R. (1995) Behavior genetic studies of cardiovascular responses to stress, in J.R. Turner, L.R. Cardon & J.K. Hewitt (eds), *Behavior Genetic Approaches in Behavioral Medicine*. New York: Plenum. pp. 87–103.

Heyn, P., Abreu, B.C. & Ottenbacher, K.J. (2004) The effects of exercise training on elderly persons with cognitive impairment and dementia: A meta-analysis. *Archives of Physical Medicine and Rehabilitation*, 85: 1694–1704.

Higgins, E.T. (1987) Self-discrepancy: A theory relating self and affect. *Psychological Review*, 94: 319–340.

Hill, C., Abraham, C. & Wright, D.B. (2007) Can theory-based messages in combination with cognitive prompts promote exercise in classroom settings? *Social Science & Medicine*, 65: 1049–1058.

Hilton, L., Hempel, S., Ewing, B.A., Apaydin, E., Xenakis, L., Newberry, S., Colaiaco, B., Maher, A.R., Shanman, R.M., Sorbero, M.E. & Maglione, M.A. (2016) Mindfulness meditation for chronic pain: Systematic review and meta-analysis. *Annals of Behavioral Medicine*, 51(2): 199–213.

Hinchliff, S. & Gott, M. (2011) Seeking medical help for sexual concerns in mid- and later life: A review of the literature. *Journal of Sex Research*, 48: 106–117.

Hing, E. & Albert, M. (2016) *State Variation in Preventive Care Visits, by Patient Characteristics, 2012*. NCHS data brief, no. 234. Hyattsville, MD: National Center for Health Statistics.

Hiscock, R., Bauld, L., Amos, A., Fidler, J.A. & Munafò, M. (2012) Socioeconomic status and smoking: A review. *Annals of the New York Academy of Science*, 1248: 107–123.

Hobson, J.A. (2009) REM sleep and dreaming: Toward a theory of protoconsciousness. *Nature Reviews Neuroscience*, 10: 803–813.

Hobson, J.A. & McCarley, R.W. (1977) The brain as a dream state generator: An activation-synthesis hypothesis of the dream process. *American Journal of Psychiatry*, 134: 1335–1348.

Hodnett, E.D., Gates, S., Hofmeyr, G.J. & Sakala, C. (2013) Continuous support for women during childbirth. *Cochrane Database of Systematic Reviews*, 7 (Art. CD003766).

Hoey, L.M., Ieropoli, S.C., White, V.M. & Jefford, M. (2008) Systematic review of peer-support programs for people with cancer. *Patient Education and Counselling*, 70: 315–337.

Hofling, C.K., Brotzman, E., Dalrymple, S., Graves, N. & Pierce, C.M. (1966) An experimental study of nurse–physician relationships. *Journal of Nervous and Mental Disease*, *143*: 171–180.

Hofmann, M., Dack, C., Barker, C. & Murray, E. (2016) The impact of an internet-based self-management intervention (HeLP-Diabetes) on the psychological well-being of adults with Type 2 diabetes: A mixed-method cohort study. *Journal of Diabetes Research*, Epub 2015 Nov 22.

Hogg, M.A. & Vaughan, G.M. (2008) *Social Psychology* (5th edition). Harlow: Pearson Prentice-Hall.

Hohman, Z.P., Crano, W.D., Siegel, J.T. & Alvaro, E.M. (2014) Attitude ambivalence, friend norms, and adolescent drug use. *Prevention Science*, *15*: 65–74.

Holman, E.A., Silver, R.C., Poulin, M., Andersen, J., Gil-Rivas, V. & McIntosh, D.N. (2008) Terrorism, acute stress, and cardiovascular health: A 3-year national study following the September 11th attacks. *Archives of General Psychiatry*, *65*: 73–80.

Holt-Lunstad, J., Smith, T.B., Baker, M., Harris, T. & Stephenson, D. (2015) Loneliness and social isolation as risk factors for mortality: A meta-analytic review. *Perspectives on Psychological Science*, *10*(2): 227–237.

Holt-Lunstad, J., Smith, T.B. & Layton, J.B. (2010) Social relationships and mortality risk: A meta-analytic review. *PLoS Medicine*, *27*;7(7): e1000316.

Hong, C.C.H. et al. (1996) Language in dreaming and regional EEG alpha power. *Sleep*, *19*: 232–235.

Hong, Y., Peña-Purcell, N.C. & Ory, M.G. (2012) Outcomes of online support and resources for cancer survivors: A systematic literature review. *Patient Education and Counselling*, *86*: 288–296.

Hood, M. et al. (2016) What do we know about mobile applications for diabetes self-management? A review of reviews. *Journal of Behavioral Medicine*, *39*: 981–994.

Hormes, J.M. & Rozin, P. (2009) Perimenstrual chocolate craving: What happens after menopause. *Appetite*, *53*(2): 256–259.

Horn, S.R., Charney, D.S. & Feder, A. (2016) Understanding resilience: New approaches for preventing and treating PTSD. *Experimental Neurology*, *284* (Pt B): 119–132.

Horne, R. et al. (2013) Understanding patients' adherence-related beliefs about medicines prescribed for long-term conditions: A meta-analytic review of the Necessity-Concerns Framework. *PLoS One*, *8*(12): e80633.

Horowitz, M.J., Duff, D.F. & Stratton, L.O. (1969) Body-buffer zones. *Archives of General Psychiatry*, *11*: 651–656.

Horta, B.L., Loret de Mola, C. & Victora, C.G. (2015) Breastfeeding and intelligence: A systematic review and meta-analysis. *Acta Paediatrica*, *104*: 14–19.

Houts, P.S., Doak, C.C., Doak, L.G. & Loscalzo, M.J. (2006) The role of pictures in improving health communication: A review of research on attention, comprehension, recall, and adherence. *Patient Education and Counseling*, *61*: 173–190.

Howard, F.M. (2003) Chronic pelvic pain. *Obstetrics & Gynecology*, *101*: 594–611.

Howren, M.B. et al. (2013) Advances in patient adherence to medical treatment regimens: The emerging role of technology in adherence monitoring and management. *Social and Personality Psychology Compass*, *7*: 427–443.

Hsieh, S. et al. (2013) Validation of the Addenbrooke's Cognitive Examination III in frontotemporal dementia and Alzheimer's disease. *Dementia and Geriatric Cognitive Disorders*, 36: 242–250.

Huang, C.-J., Webb, H.E., Zourdos, M.C. & Acevedo, E.O. (2013) Cardiovascular reactivity, stress, and physical activity. *Frontier in Physiology*, 4: 314.

Huang, C.Y. et al. (2010) Mediating roles of social support on post stroke depression and quality of life in patients with ischemic stroke. *Journal of Clinical Nursing*, 19: 2752–2762.

Huang, T. & Hu, F.B. (2015) Gene-environment interactions and obesity: Recent developments and future directions. *BMC Medical Genomics*, 8(Suppl. 1): S2.

Huddart, R.A. et al. (2005) Fertility, gonadal and sexual function in survivors of testicular cancer. *British Journal of Cancer*, 93: 200–207.

Hudson, J.I., Hiripi, E., Pope, H.G. & Kessler, R.C. (2007) The prevalence and correlates of eating disorders in the National Comorbidity Survey Replication. *Biological Psychiatry*, 61: 348–358.

Hudson, J.L., Bundy, C., Coventry, P.A. & Dickens, C. (2014) Exploring the relationship between cognitive illness representations and poor emotional health and their combined association with diabetes self-care: A systematic review with meta-analysis. *Journal of Psychosomatic Research*, 76(4): 265–274.

Hughes, T.L. (2016) The influence of gender and sexual orientation on alcohol use and alcohol-related problems: Toward a global perspective. *Alcohol Research*, 38: 121–132.

Hui, W.M., Shiu, L.P. & Lam, S.K. (1999) The perception of life events and daily stress in nonulcer dyspepsia. *American Journal of Gastroenterology*, 86: 292–296.

Hull, K.L. & Harvey, S. (2003) Growth hormone therapy and quality of life: Possibilities, pitfalls and mechanisms. *Journal of Endocrinology*, 179: 311–333.

Hunot, V., Moore, T.H., Caldwell, D.M., Furukawa, T.A., Davies, P., Jones, H., Honyashiki, M., Chen, P., Lewis, G. & Churchill, R. (2013) 'Third wave' cognitive and behavioural therapies versus other psychological therapies for depression. *Cochrane Database of Systematic Reviews*, 10 (Art. CD008704).

Hunt, P.J. et al. (2000) Improvement in mood and fatigue after dehydroepiandrosterone replacement in Addison's disease in a randomized, double blind trial. *Journal of Clinical Endocrinology and Metabolism*, 85: 4650–4656.

Hunter, M., Ussher, J., Cariss, M., Browne, S. & Jelly, R. (2002a) A randomised comparison of psychological (cognitive behaviour therapy, CBT), medical (fluoxetine) and combined treatment for women with Premenstrual Dysphoric Disorder. *Journal of Psychosomatic Obstetrics and Gynaecology*, 23: 193–199.

Hunter, M.S., Ussher, J.M., Cariss, M., Browne, S., Jelley, R. & Katz, M. (2002b) Medical (fluoxetine) and psychological (cognitive-behavioural therapy) treatment for premenstrual dysphoric disorder: A study of treatment processes. *Journal of Psychosomatic Research*, 53(3): 811–817.

Huntley, A., White, A. & Ernst, E. (2002) Relaxation therapies for asthma: A systematic review. *Thorax*, 57: 127–131.

Huppertz-Hauss, G. et al. (2015) Health-related quality of life in inflammatory bowel disease in a European-wide population-based cohort 10 years after diagnosis. *Inflammatory Bowel Disease*, 21: 337–344.

Hydén, L.C. (1997) Illness and narrative. *Sociology of Health and Illness, 19*: 48–69.

Ilic, D. et al. (2013) Screening for prostate cancer. *Cochrane Database of Systematic Reviews*, 1: CD004720.

Imai, H., Nakao, H., Tsuchiya, M., Kuroda, Y. & Katoh, T. (2004) Burnout and work environments of public health nurses involved in mental health care. *Occupational and Environmental Medicine, 61*(9): 764–768.

Ingersoll, K.S. & Jessye Cohen, J. (2008) The impact of medication regimen factors on adherence to chronic treatment: A review of literature. *Journal of Behavioural Medicine, 31*: 213–224.

Institute of Medicine (2005) *Estimating the Contributions of Lifestyle-Related Factors to Preventable Death: A Workshop Summary*. Washington, DC: National Academies Press.

Institute of Medicine (2011) *Relieving Pain in America: A Blueprint for Transforming Prevention, Care, Education, and Research*. Washington, DC: National Academies Press.

International Committee of Medical Journal Editors (2017) *Recommendations for the Conduct, Reporting, Editing, and Publication of Scholarly Work in Medical Journals*. Available online at: www.icmje.org (accessed 22 March 2017).

Iravani, M., Zarean, E., Janghorbani, M. & Bahrami, M. (2015) Women's needs and expectations during normal labor and delivery. *Journal of Education and Health Promotion, 4*: 6.

Ishigami, T. (1919) The influence of psychic acts on the progress of pulmonary tuberculosis. *American Review of Tuberculosis, 2*: 470–484.

Izard, C.E. (1991) *The Psychology of Emotions*. New York: Plenum.

Jackson, L.A. & Ervin, K.S. (1992) Height stereotypes of women and men: The liabilities of shortness for both sexes. *Journal of Social Psychology, 132*: 433–445.

Jackson, M., Dahlen, H. & Schmied, V. (2012) Birthing outside the system: Perceptions of risk amongst Australian women who have freebirths and high risk homebirths. *Midwifery, 28*(5): 561–567.

Jackson, T., Wang, Y. & Fan, H. (2014) Associations between pain appraisals and pain outcomes: Meta-analyses of laboratory pain and chronic pain literatures. *Journal of Pain, 15*(6): 586–601.

Jacobsen, P.B., Bovbjerg, D.J. & Redd, W.H. (1993) Anticipatory anxiety in patients receiving cancer chemotherapy. *Health Psychology, 12*: 469–475.

Jané-Llopis, E. & Matytsina, I. (2006) Mental health and alcohol, drugs and tobacco: A review of the comorbidity between mental disorders and the use of alcohol, tobacco and illicit drugs. *Drug and Alcohol Review, 25*: 515–536.

Janicki Deverts, D., Cohen, S. & Doyle, W.J. (2016) Dispositional affect moderates the stress-buffering effect of social support on risk for developing the common cold. *Journal of Personality*, Epub ahead of print.

Janis, I.L. & Mann, L. (1977) *Decision Making: A Psychological Analysis of Conflict, Choice, and Commitment*. New York: Free Press.

Jankowska, M. (2011) Sexual functioning of testicular cancer survivors and their partners: A review of literature. *Reports of Practical Oncology and Radiotherapy, 17*(1): 54–62.

Janssen, V., De Gucht, V., Dusseldorp, E. & Maes, S. (2013) Lifestyle modification programmes for patients with coronary heart disease: A systematic review and meta-analysis of randomized controlled trials. *European Journal of Preventive Cardiology, 20*: 620–640.

Janz, N.K. & Becker, M.H. (1984) The Health Belief Model: A decade later. *Health Education Quarterly*, *11*: 1–47.

Jefferson, L. et al. (2013) Effect of physicians' gender on communication and consultation length: A systematic review and meta-analysis. *Journal of Health Services Research & Policy*, *18*: 242–248.

Jeffery, R.W., Adlis, S.A. & Forster, J.L. (1991) Prevalence of dieting among working men and women: The healthy worker project. *Health Psychology*, *10*: 274–281.

Jennings, E.M. et al. (2014) Stress-induced hyperalgesia. *Progress in Neurobiology*, 121: 1–18.

Jensen, P.M., Trollope-Kumar, K., Waters, H. & Everson, J. (2008) Building physician resilience. *Canadian Family Physician*, *54*(5): 722–729.

Jeongseon, K. et al. (2014) Gene-diet interactions in gastric cancer risk: A systematic review. *World Journal of Gastroenterology*, *20*(28): 9600–9610.

Jessberger, S. & Gage, F.H. (2014) Adult neurogenesis: Bridging the gap between mice and humans. *Trends in Cell Biology*, *24*: 558–563.

Jessop, D.C., Craig, L. & Ayers, S. (2014) Applying Leventhal's self-regulatory model to pregnancy: Evidence that pregnancy-related beliefs and emotional responses are associated with maternal health outcomes. *Journal of Health Psychology*, *19*(9): 1091–1102.

Jha, V. et al. (2013) Chronic kidney disease: Global dimension and perspectives. *Lancet*, *382*: 260–272.

Jin, J., Sklar, G.E., Oh, V.M.S. & Li, S.C. (2008) Factors affecting therapeutic compliance: A review from the patient's perspective. *Therapeutics & Clinical Risk Management*, *4*: 269–286.

Joekes, K. (2018) Breaking bad news, in C.D. Llewellyn et al. (eds), *The Cambridge Handbook of Psychology, Health and Medicine* (3rd edition). Cambridge: Cambridge University Press.

Johansen, M.L. & Risor, M.B. (2017) What is the problem with medically unexplained symptoms for GPs? A meta-synthesis of qualitative studies. *Patient Education and Counselling*, *100*(4): 647–654.

Johns, E. & Tracey, I. (2009) Neuroimaging of visceral pain. *Reviews in Pain*, *3*: 2–5.

Johnson, W.D. et al. (2008) Behavioral interventions to reduce risk for sexual transmission of HIV among men who have sex with men. *Cochrane Database of Systematic Reviews*, *3* (Art. CD001230).

Johnston, M. & Vogele, C. (1993) Benefits of psychological preparation for surgery: A meta-analysis. *Annals of Behavioral Medicine*, *15*: 245–256.

Jones, B.C., DeBruine, L.M., Perrett, D.I., Little, A.C., Feinberg, D.R. & Law Smith, M.J. (2008) Effects of menstrual cycle phase on face preferences. *Archives of Sexual Behavior*, *37*(1): 78–84.

Jonker-Pool, G. et al. (2001) Sexual functioning after treatment for testicular cancer: Review and meta-analysis of 36 empirical studies between 1975–2000. *Archives of Sexual Behavior*, *30*: 55–74.

Jopson, N. & Moss-Morris, R. (2003) The role of illness severity and illness representations in adjusting to multiple sclerosis. *Journal of Psychosomatic Research*, *54*: 503–511.

Jordan, B. (1993) *Birth in Four Cultures: A Crosscultural Investigation of Childbirth in Yucatan, Holland, Sweden and the United States*. Long Grove, IL: Waveland Press.

Jordan, J. & Neimeyer, R. (2003) Does grief counselling work? *Death Studies*, *27*: 765–786.

Juárez, S.P., Goodman, A. & Koupil, I. (2016) From cradle to grave: tracking socioeconomic inequalities in mortality in a cohort of 11,868 men and women born in Uppsala, Sweden, 1915–1929. *Journal of Epidemiology and Community Health*, 70(6): 569–75.

Jung, X.T. & Newton, R. (2009) Cochrane Reviews of non-medication-based psychotherapeutic and other interventions for schizophrenia, psychosis, and bipolar disorder: A systematic literature review. *International Journal of Mental Health Nursing*, 18: 239–249.

Kabat-Zinn, J. (1990) *Full Catastrophe Living*. New York: Delacorte.

Kadden, R.M. & Litt, M.D. (2011) The role of self-efficacy in the treatment of substance use disorders. *Addictive Behaviors*, 36: 1120–1126.

Kajikawa, N., Maeno, T. & Maeno, T. (2014) Does a child's fear of needles decrease through a learning event with needles? *Issues in Comprehensive Pediatric Nursing*, 37: 183–194.

Kamen, C. et al. (2014) Anticipatory nausea and vomiting due to chemotherapy. *European Journal of Pharmacology*, 722: 172–179.

Kanayama, G., Hudson, J.I. & Pope, H.G. (2008) Long-term psychiatric and medical consequences of anabolic-androgenic steroid abuse: A looming public health concern? *Drug & Alcohol Dependence*, 98: 1–12.

Kangas, M., Henry, J.L. & Bryant, R.A. (2002) Posttraumatic stress disorder following cancer: A conceptual and empirical review. *Clinical Psychology Review*, 22: 499–524.

Kaplan, G.A. & Reynolds, P. (1988) Depression and cancer mortality and morbidity: Prospective evidence from the Alameda County Study. *Journal of Behavioral Medicine*, 11: 1–13.

Kaplan, G.A., Seeman, T.E., Cohen, R.D., Knudsen, L.P. & Garulnik, J. (1987) Mortality among the elderly in the Alameda County Study: Behavioral and demographic risk factors. *American Journal of Public Health*, 77: 307–312.

Kaplan, K.A. & Harvey, A.G. (2009) Hypersomnia across mood disorders: A review and synthesis. *Sleep Medicine Reviews*, 13: 275–285.

Kaplan, R. (1990) Behavior as the central outcome in health care. *American Psychologist*, 70: 1211–1220.

Kaptein, A.A. et al. (2010) Behavioural research in patients with end-stage renal disease: A review and research agenda. *Patient Education and Counselling*, 81: 23–29.

Kapur, S. & Remington, G. (1996) Serotonin-dopamine interaction and its relevance to schizophrenia. *American Journal of Psychiatry*, 153: 466–476.

Kardas, P. et al. (2013) Determinants of patient adherence: A review of systematic reviews. *Frontiers in Pharmacology*, 4: 91.

Karyotaki, E. et al. (2017) Efficacy of self-guided internet-based cognitive behavioral therapy in the treatment of depressive symptoms: A meta-analysis of individual participant data. *JAMA Psychiatry*, doi: 10.1001/jamapsychiatry.2017.0044 [Epub ahead of print].

Kato, P.M. & Mann, T. (1999) A synthesis of psychological interventions for the bereaved. *Clinical Psychology Review*, 19: 275–296.

Katon, W.J. & Walker, E.A. (1998) Medically unexplained symptoms in primary care. *Journal of Clinical Psychiatry*, 59(suppl. 20): s15–s21.

Katz, M.L. et al. (2012) Patient–provider discussions about colorectal cancer screening: Who initiates elements of informed decision making? *Journal of General Internal Medicine*, 27: 1135–1141.

Kaye, J.A. & Jick, H. (2003) Incidence of erectile dysfunction and characteristics of patients before and after the introduction of sildenafil in the United Kingdom: Cross-sectional study with comparison patients. *British Medical Journal*, *326*: 424–425.

Keegan, T.H.M., Gomez, S.L., Clarke, C.A., Chan, J.K. & Glaser, S.L. (2007) Recent trends in breast cancer incidence among 6 Asian groups in the Greater Bay Area of Northern California. *International Journal of Cancer*, *120*: 1324–1329.

Keightley, P.C. (2015) Pathways in gut-brain communication: Evidence for distinct gut-to-brain and brain-to-gut syndromes. *Australian and New Zealand Journal of Psychiatry*, *49*: 207–214.

Keller, V.F. & Caroll, J.G. (1994) A new model for physician-patient communication. *Patient Education and Counselling*, *35*: 121–140.

Kellett, S. & Gilbert, P. (2001) Acne: A biopsychosocial and evolutionary perspective with a focus on shame. *British Journal of Health Psychology*, *6*: 1–24.

Kendrick, A.H., Higgs, C.M.B., Whitfield, M.J. & Laszlo, G. (1993) Accuracy of perception of severity of asthma: Patients treated in general practice. *British Medical Journal*, *307*: 422–424.

Kennedy, R.M., Luhmann, J. & Zempsky, W.T. (2008) Clinical implications of unmanaged needle-insertion pain and distress in children. *Pediatrics*, *122*: 130–133.

Kennedy, T.M. et al. (2006) Cognitive behavioural therapy in addition to antispasmodic therapy for irritable bowel syndrome in primary care: Randomised controlled trial. *British Medical Journal*, *331*: 435–440.

Kenny, D.T. (2007) Stress management, in S. Ayers et al. (eds), *Cambridge Handbook of Psychology, Health and Medicine* (2nd edition). Cambridge: Cambridge University Press. pp. 403–407.

Kessels, R.P.C. (2003) Patients' memory for medical information. *Journal of the Royal Society of Medicine*, *96*: 219–222.

Kew, K.M., Nashed, M., Dulay, V. & Yorke, J. (2016) Cognitive behavioural therapy (CBT) for adults and adolescents with asthma. *Cochrane Database of Systematic Reviews*, *9* (Art. CD011818).

Khakbazan, Z., Taghipour, A., Latifnejad Roudsari, R. & Mohammadi, E. (2014) Help seeking behavior of women with self-discovered breast cancer symptoms: A meta-ethnographic synthesis of patient delay. *PLoS One*, 3;9(12): e110262.

Khan, L. (2015) *Falling through the Gaps: Perinatal Mental Health and General Practice*. London: Royal College of General Practitioners and Centre for Mental Health.

Khan, N., Afaq, F. & Mukhtar, H. (2010) Lifestyle as risk factor for cancer: Evidence from human studies. *Cancer Letters*, *293*: 133–143.

Khaw, K.T., Wareham, N., Bingham, S., Welch, A., Luben, R. & Day, N. (2008) Combined impact of health behaviours and mortality in men and women: The EPIC-Norfolk prospective population study. *PLoS Medicine*, *5*: e12.

Kiecolt-Glaser, J.K. & Glaser, R. (2002) Depression and immune function: Central pathways to morbidity and mortality. *Journal of Psychosomatic Research*, *53*: 873– 876.

Kiecolt-Glaser, J.K., McGuire, L., Robles, T.F. & Glaser, R. (2002a) Psychoneuroimmunology: Psychological influences on immune function and health. *Journal of Consulting and Clinical Psychology*, *70*: 537–547.

Kiecolt-Glaser, J.K., McGuire, L., Robles, T.F. & Glaser, R. (2002b) Emotions, morbidity, and mortality: New perspectives from psychoneuroimmunology. *Annual Review of Psychology*, 53: 83–107.

Kiernan, J. (2002) The experience of therapeutic touch in the lives of five postpartum women. *The American Journal of Maternal Child Nursing*, 27: 47–53.

Killgore, W.D. (2010) Effects of sleep deprivation on cognition. *Progress in Brain Research*, 185: 105–129.

Kim, S. et al. (2008) Self-reported experience and outcomes of care among stomach cancer patients at a median follow-up time of 27 months from diagnosis. *Supportive Care in Cancer*, 16: 831–839.

Kim, S.H. & Lee, A. (2016) Health-literacy-sensitive diabetes self-management interventions: A systematic review and meta-analysis. *Worldviews on Evidence-Based Nursing*, 13(4): 324–333.

Kinsman, R.A., Dirks, J.F. & Jones, N.F. (1982) Psychomaintenance of chronic physical illness, in T. Millon, C. Green & R. Meagher (eds), *Handbook of Clinical Health Psychology*. New York: Plenum. pp. 435–466.

Kirby, D. (2006) Can fear arousal in public health campaigns contribute to the decline of HIV prevalence? *Journal of Health Communication*, 11: 262–266.

Kirsch, I. (2007) Placebos, in S. Ayers et al. (eds), *Cambridge Handbook of Psychology, Health and Medicine* (2nd edition). Cambridge: Cambridge University Press. pp. 161–167.

Kirsch, I. (2018) Placebo and nocebo, in C.D. Llewellyn et al. (eds), *The Cambridge Handbook of Psychology, Health and Medicine* (3rd edition). Cambridge: Cambridge University Press.

Kirsch, I., Deacon, B.J., Huedo-Medina, T.B., Scoboria, A., Moore, T.J. & Johnson, B.T. (2008) Initial severity and antidepressant benefits: A meta-analysis of data submitted to the Food and Drug Administration. *PLoS Medicine*, 5: 260–268.

Kirschner-Hermanns, R. & Jakse, G. (2002) Quality of life following radical prostatectomy. *Critical Reviews in Oncology and Hematology*, 43: 141–151.

Kisely, S., Goldberg, D. & Simon, G. (1997) A comparison between somatic symptoms with and without clear organic cause: Results of an international study. *Psychological Medicine*, 27: 1011–1019.

Kishi, T. et al. (2012) Are antipsychotics effective for the treatment of anorexia nervosa? Results from a systematic review and meta-analysis. *Journal of Clinical Psychiatry*, 73: e757–e66.

Kivlighan, D.M. III, Goldberg, S.B., Abbas, M., Pace, B.T., Yulish, N.E., Thomas, J.G., Cullen, M.M., Flückiger, C. & Wampold, B.E. (2015) The enduring effects of psychodynamic treatments vis-à-vis alternative treatments: A multilevel longitudinal meta-analysis. *Clinical Psychology Review*, 40: 1–14.

Klein, C.T.F. & Helweg-Larsen, M. (2002) Perceived control and the optimistic bias: A meta-analytic review. *Psychology and Health*, 17: 437–446.

Knight, M., Kenyon, S., Brocklehurst, P., Neilson, J., Shakespeare, J. & Kurinczuk, J.J. (eds) on behalf of MBRRACE-UK (2014) *Saving Lives, Improving Mothers' Care: Lessons Learned to Inform Future Maternity Care from the UK and Ireland Confidential Enquiries into Maternal Deaths and Morbidity 2009–12*. Oxford: National Perinatal Epidemiology Unit, University of Oxford.

Knowles, S.R., Monshat, K. & Castle, D.J. (2013) The efficacy and methodological challenges of psychotherapy for adults with inflammatory bowel disease: A review. *Inflammatory Bowel Diseases*, *19*: 2704–2715.

Knutson, K.L. (2012) Does inadequate sleep play a role in vulnerability to obesity? *American Journal of Human Biology*, *24*: 361–371.

Ko, W.F. & Sawatzky, J.A. (2008) Understanding urinary incontinence after radical prostatectomy. *Clinical Journal of Oncology Nursing*, *12*: 647–654.

Kok, G. (2007) Health promotion, in S. Ayers et al. (eds), *Cambridge Handbook of Psychology, Health and Medicine* (2nd edition). Cambridge: Cambridge University Press. pp. 355–359.

Koob, G.F. (2006) The neurobiology of addiction: A neuroadaptational view relevant for diagnosis. *Addiction*, *101*(suppl.1): s23–s30.

Koob, G.F. & Volkow, N.D. (2016) Neurobiology of addiction: A neurocircuitry analysis. *Lancet Psychiatry*, *3*: 760–773.

Koutrouli, N. (2012) Posttraumatic stress disorder and posttraumatic growth in breast cancer patients: A systematic review. *Women Health*, *52*(5): 503–516.

Kraaij, V., Arensman, E. & Spinhoven, P. (2002) Negative life events and depression in elderly persons: A meta-analysis. *Journals of Gerontology: Series B: Psychological Sciences & Social Sciences*, *57B*: 87–94.

Kraft, T.L. & Pressman, S.D. (2012) Grin and bear it: The influence of manipulated facial expression on the stress response. *Psychological Science*, *23*: 1372–1378.

Krakower, D.S. et al. (2015) Antiretrovirals for primary HIV prevention: the current status of pre- and post-exposure prophylaxis. *Current HIV/AIDS Reports*, *12*: 127–138.

Kramer, M.S. & Kakuma, R. (2012) Optimal duration of exclusive breastfeeding. *Cochrane Database of Systematic Reviews*, *8* (Art. CD003517).

Kramer, M.S. et al. (2008) Breastfeeding and child cognitive development: New evidence from a large randomized trial. *Archives of General Psychiatry*, *65*: 578–584.

Krantz, D.S., Helmers, K.F., Bairey, N., Nebel, L.E., Hedges, S.M. & Rozanski, A. (1991) Cardiovascular reactivity and mental stress-induced myocardial ischaemia in patients with coronary artery disease. *Psychosomatic Medicine*, *53*: 1–12.

Krantz, D.S. & McCeney, M.K. (2002) Effects of psychological and social factors on organic disease: A critical assessment of research on coronary heart disease. *Annual Review of Psychology*, *53*: 341–369.

Kristeller, J. (2018). Cognitive behaviour therapy, in Llewellyn, C.D. et al. (eds) *The Cambridge Handbook of Psychology, Health and Medicine* (3rd edition). Cambridge: Cambridge University Press.

Kroenke, K. (2003a) Patients presenting with somatic complaints: Epidemiology, psychiatric comorbidity and management. *International Journal of Methods in Psychiatric Research*, *12*: 34–43.

Kroenke, K. (2003b) The interface between physical and psychological symptoms. *Journal of Clinical Psychiatry*, *5*(suppl.7): s11–s18.

Krueger, R.F. & Eaton, N.R. (2015) Transdiagnostic factors of mental disorders. *World Psychiatry*, *14*: 27–29.

Ksir, C. & Hart, C.L. (2016) Cannabis and psychosis: A critical overview of the relationship. *Current Psychiatry Reports*, *18*: 12.

Kübler-Ross, E. (1969) *On Death and Dying*. New York: Macmillan.

Kundakovic, M. & Champagne, F.A. (2015) Early-life experience, epigenetics, and the developing brain. *Neuropsychopharmacology*, *40*: 141–153.

Kunkel, E.J., Bakker, J.R., Myers, R.E., Oyesanmi, O. & Gomella, L.G. (2000) Biopsychosocial aspects of prostate cancer. *Psychosomatics*, *41*: 85–94.

Kurihara, H., Maeno, T. & Maeno, T. (2014) Importance of physicians' attire: Factors influencing the impression it makes on patients, a cross-sectional study. *Asia Pacific Family Medicine*, *13*(1): 2.

Kurtz, S.M. & Silverman, J.D. (1996) The Calgary-Cambridge observation guides: An aid to defining the curriculum and organizing the teaching in communication training programmes. *Medical Education*, *30*: 83–89.

Kwekkeboom, K.L. & Gretarsdottir, E. (2006) Systematic review of relaxation interventions for pain. *Journal of Nursing Scholarship*, *38*: 269–277.

Lackner, J.M. et al. (2004) Psychological treatments for irritable bowel syndrome: A systematic review and meta-analysis. *Journal of Consulting and Clinical Psychology*, *72*: 1100–1113.

Lacy, B.E. et al. (2016) Bowel disorders. *Gastroenterology*, *150*: 1393–1407.

Ladomenou, F., Kafatos, A. & Galanakis, E. (2007) Risk factors related to intention to breastfeed, early weaning and suboptimal duration of breastfeeding. *Acta Paediatrica*, *96*: 1441–1444.

Laessle, R.G. & Schulz, S. (2009) Stress-induced laboratory eating behavior in obese women with binge eating disorder. *International Journal of Eating Disorders*, *42*: 505–510.

LaFrance, M. & Ickes, W. (1981) Posture mirroring and interactional involvement: Sex and sex typing effects. *Journal of Nonverbal Behaviour*, *5*: 139–154.

Lahtinen, V., Lonka, K. & Lindblom-Ylänne, S. (1997) Spontaneous study strategies and the quality of knowledge construction. *British Journal of Educational Psychology*, *67*: 13–24.

Lai, H., Lai, S., Krongrad, A., Trapido, E., Page, J.B. & McCoy, C.B. (1999) The effect of marital status on survival in late-stage cancer patients. *International Journal of Behavioral Medicine*, *6*: 150–176.

Lam, T.P., Lam, K.F., Lam, E.W.W. & Sun, K.S. (2015) Does postgraduate training in community mental health make a difference to primary care physicians' attitudes to depression and schizophrenia? *Community Mental Health Journal*, *51*: 641–646.

Lameris, A.I. et al. (2015) The impact of formative testing on study behaviour and study performance of (bio)medical students: A smartphone application intervention study. *BMC Medical Education*, *15*: 72.

Lamont, S. et al. (2013) Assessing patient capacity to consent to treatment: an integrative review of instruments and tools. *Journal of Clinical Nursing*, *22*: 2387–2403.

Lang, P.J. & Bradley, M.M. (2010) Emotion and the motivational brain. *Biological Psychology*, *84*(3): 437–450.

Lang, P.J. & Davis, M. (2006) Emotion, motivation, and the brain: Reflex foundations in animal and human research. *Progress in Brain Research*, *156*: 3–29.

Langa, K.M. et al. (2008) Trends in the prevalence and mortality of cognitive impairment in the United States: Is there evidence of a compression of cognitive morbidity? *Alzheimer's & Dementia*, *4*: 134–144.

Langius-Eklöf, A. et al. (2009) Health-related quality of life in relation to sense of coherence in a Swedish group of HIV-infected patients over a two-year follow-up. *AIDS Patient Care STDS*, 23: 59–64.

Laplante, D.P., Brunet, A. & King, S. (2016) The effects of maternal stress and illness during pregnancy on infant temperament: Project Ice Storm. *Pediatric Research*, 79(1–1): 107–113.

Laplante, D.P., Brunet, A., Schmitz, N., Ciampi, A. & King, S. (2008) Project Ice Storm: Prenatal maternal stress affects cognitive and linguistic functioning in 5½-year-old children. *Journal of the American Academy of Child and Adolescent Psychiatry*, 47(9): 1063–1072.

Large, M.M., Ryan, C.J., Singh, S.P., Paton, M.B. & Nielssen, O.B. (2011) The predictive value of risk categorization in schizophrenia. *Harvard Review of Psychiatry*, 19(1): 25–33.

Larkin, M., Clifton, E. & de Visser, R. (2009) Making sense of 'consent' in a constrained environment. *International Journal of Law & Psychiatry*, 32: 176–183.

Larson, R.W., Richards, M.H., Moneta, G. & Holmbeck, G.C. (1996) Changes in adolescents' daily interactions with their families from ages 10 to 18: Disengagement and transformation. *Developmental Psychology*, 32: 744–754.

Larsson, S.C. & Wolk, A. (2006) Meat consumption and risk of colorectal cancer: A meta-analysis of prospective studies. *International Journal of Cancer*, 119: 2657–2664.

Larsson, S.C. & Wolk, A. (2007) Obesity and colon and rectal cancer risk: A meta-analysis of prospective studies. *American Journal of Clinical Nutrition*, 86: 556–565.

Lassen, B. et al. (2013) A systematic review of physical impairments following radical prostatectomy: Effect of psychoeducational interventions. *Journal of Advanced Nursing*, 69: 2602–2612.

Latané, B. & Darley, J.M. (1970) *The Unresponsive Bystander*. New York: Appleton Century Crofts.

Laumann, E.O., Gagnon, J.H., Michael, R.T. & Michaels, S. (1994) *The Social Organization of Sexuality: Sexual Practices in the United States*. Chicago, IL: University of Chicago Press.

Laumann, E.O., Paik, A. & Rosen, R.C. (1999) Sexual dysfunction in the United States: Prevalence and predictors. *Journal of the American Medical Association*, 281: 537–544.

Laupattarakasem, W., Laopaiboon, M., Laupattarakasem, P. & Sumananont, C. (2008) Arthroscopic debridement for knee osteoarthritis. *Cochrane Database of Systematic Reviews*, 1 (Art. CD005118).

Laureati, M. et al. (2014) School-based intervention with children: Peer-modeling, reward and repeated exposure reduce food neophobia and increase liking of fruits and vegetables. *Appetite*, 83: 26–32.

Laursen, T.M., Munk-Olsen, T., Nordentoft, M. & Mortensen, P.B. (2007) Increased mortality among patients admitted with major psychiatric disorders: A register-based study comparing mortality in unipolar depressive disorder, bipolar affective disorder, schizoaffective disorder, and schizophrenia. *Journal of Clinical Psychiatry*, 68(6): 899–907.

Laursen, M., Johansen, C. & Hedegaard, M. (2009) Fear of childbirth and risk for birth complications in nulliparous women in the Danish National Birth Cohort. *British Journal of Obstetrics & Gynaecology*, 116: 1350–1355.

Laver, K.E., George, S., Thomas, S., Deutsch, J.E. & Crotty. M. (2015) Virtual reality for stroke rehabilitation. *Cochrane Database of Systematic Reviews*, 2 (Art. CD008349).

Lavie, P. (2001) Sleep-wake as a biological rhythm. *Annual Review of Psychology*, *52*: 277–303.

Lawler, M. & Nixon, E. (2010) Body dissatisfaction among adolescent boys and girls: The effects of body mass, peer appearance culture and internalization of appearance ideals. *Journal of Youth & Adolescence* [Epub ahead of print].

Lawrie, S.M. et al. (1998) General practitioners' attitudes to psychiatric and medical illness. *Psychological Medicine*, *28*: 1463–1467.

Layard, R. (2006) *The Depression Report: A New Deal for Depression and Anxiety Disorders*. London: London School of Economics.

Lazarus, R.S. & Folkman, S. (1984) *Stress, Appraisal and Coping*. New York: Springer.

Lazarus, R.S., Opton, E.M., Nomikos, S.M. & Rankin, N.O. (1965) The principle of short-circuiting of threat: Further evidence. *Journal of Personality*, *33*: 622–635.

Le Doux, J.E. (1996) *The Emotional Brain*. New York: Simon & Schuster.

Leach, L.S., Poyser, C., Cooklin, A.R. & Giallo, R. (2016) Prevalence and course of anxiety disorders (and symptom levels) in men across the perinatal period: A systematic review. *Journal of Affective* Disorders, *190*: 675–686.

Lee, I.S., Yoon, S.S., Lee, S.H., Lee, H., Park, H.J., Wallraven, C. et al. (2013) An amplification of feedback from facial muscles strengthened sympathetic activations to emotional facial cues. *Autonomic Neuroscience*, *179*: 37–42.

Lee, J.H. (2016) The effects of music on pain: A meta-analysis. *Journal of Music Therapy*, *53*(4): 430–477.

Lee, R.T., Seo, B., Hladkyj, S., Lovell, B.L. & Schwartzmann, L. (2013) Correlates of physician burnout across regions and specialties: A meta-analysis. *Human Resouces for Health*, *11*: 48.

Lefler, L.L. & Bondy, K.N. (2004) Women's delay in seeking treatment with myocardial infarction: A meta-synthesis. *Journal of Cardiovascular Nursing*, *19*(4): 251–268.

Lefroy, J., Thomas, A., Harrison, C., Williams, S., O'Mahony, F., Gay, S., Kinston, R. & McKinley, R.K. (2014) Development and face validation of strategies for improving consultation skills. *Advances in Health Sciences Education: Theory & Practice*, *5*: 661–685.

Leichsenring, F. (2005) Are psychodynamic and psychoanalytic psychotherapies effective? A review of empirical data. *International Journal of Psychoanalysis*, *86*: 841–868.

Leichsenring, F. & Rabung, S. (2011) Long-term psychodynamic psychotherapy in complex mental disorders: Update of a meta-analysis. *British Journal of Psychiatry*, *199*: 15–22.

Leiter, M.P. & Maslach, C. (2000) Burnout and health, in A. Baum, T. Revenson & J. Singer (eds), *Handbook of Health Psychology*. Hillsdale, NJ: Lawrence Erlbaum. pp. 415–426.

Leiter, M.P. & Maslach, C. (2004) Areas of worklife: A structured approach to organizational predictors of job burnout, in P.L. Perrewe & D.C. Ganster (eds), *Research in Occupational Stress and Well-Being* (Vol. 3). Oxford: Elsevier. pp. 91–134.

Lenz, A.S., Taylor, R., Fleming, M. & Serman, N. (2014) Effectiveness of dialectical behavior therapy for treating eating disorders. *Journal of Counseling & Development*, *2*: 26–35.

Leonhardt, C., Margraf-Stiksrud, J., Badners, L., Szerencsi, A. & Maier, R.F. (2014) Does the 'Teddy Bear Hospital' enhance preschool children's knowledge? A pilot study with a pre/post-case control design in Germany. *Journal of Health Psychology*, *19*: 1250–1260.

Lepore, S.J., Helgeson, V.S., Eton, D.T. & Schulz, R. (2003) Improving quality of life in men with prostate cancer: A randomized controlled trial of group education interventions. *Health Psychology*, *22*: 443–452.

Leserman, J. (2008) Role of depression, stress, and trauma in HIV disease progression. *Psychosomatic Medicine*, 70: 539–545.

Leserman, J. et al. (1999) Progression to AIDS: The effects of stress, depressive symptoms, and social support. *Psychosomatic Medicine*, 61: 397–406.

Lett, H.S. et al. (2004) Depression as a risk factor for coronary artery disease: Evidence, mechanisms, and treatment. *Psychosomatic Medicine*, 66: 305–315.

Levav, I. et al. (2000) Cancer incidence and survival following bereavement. *American Journal of Public Health*, 90: 1601–1607.

Levenstein, S. (2000) The very model of a modern etiology: A biopsychosocial view of peptic ulcer. *Psychosomatic Medicine*, 62: 176–185.

Levenstein, S. et al. (2015) Psychological stress increases risk for peptic ulcer, regardless of Helicobacter pylori infection or use of nonsteroidal anti-inflammatory drugs. *Clinical Gastroenterology and Hepatology*, 13: 498–506.e1.

Leventhal, H. et al. (2016) The common-sense model of self-regulation (CSM): A dynamic framework for understanding illness self-management. *Journal of Behavioral Medicine*, 39: 935–936.

Leventhal, H., Brissette, I. & Leventhal, E.A. (2003) The common-sense model of self-regulation of health and illness, in L.D. Cameron & H. Leventhal (eds), *The Self-Regulation of Health and Illness Behaviour*. London: Routledge. pp. 42–65.

Leventhal, H., Nerenz, D.R. & Steele, D.J. (1984) Illness representations and coping with health threats, in A. Baum et al. (eds), *Handbook of Psychology and Health*. Hillsdale, NJ: Lawrence Erlbaum. pp. 219–252.

Levinson, C.A. et al. (2017) The core symptoms of bulimia nervosa, anxiety, and depression: A network analysis. *Journal of Abnormal Psychology* (in press). (doi: 10.1037/abn0000254.)

Levinson, W., Hudak, P. & Tricco, A.C. (2013) A systematic review of surgeon–patient communication: Strengths and opportunities for improvement. *Patient Education and Counselling*, 93(1): 3–17.

Lewin, B. (2007) Coronary heart disease: Rehabilitation, in S. Ayers et al. (eds), *Cambridge Handbook of Psychology, Health and Medicine* (2nd edition). Cambridge: Cambridge University Press. pp. 656–659.

Lewin, B. et al. (1992) Effects of self-help post myocardial infarction rehabilitation on psychological adjustment and use of health services. *Lancet*, 339: 1036–1040.

Lewis, E. & Casement, P. (1986) The inhibition of mourning by pregnancy: A case study. *Psychoanalytic Psychotherapy*, 2: 45–52.

Lewis, G. & Wesseley, S. (1992) The epidemiology of fatigue: More questions than answers. *Journal of Epidemiology and Community Health*, 46: 92–97.

Lexchin, J. (2006) Bigger and better: How Pfizer redefined erectile dysfunction. *PLoS Medicine*, 3(4): e132.

Ley, P. (1997) Recall by patients, in A. Baum et al. (eds), *Cambridge Handbook of Psychology Health & Medicine*. Cambridge: Cambridge University Press. pp. 315–317.

Leza, J.C. & Menchen, L. (2008) Editorial [Hot topic: Stress-induced deleterious consequences in the gastrointestinal tract]. *Current Molecular Medicine*, 8: 244–246.

Lichtman, J.H. et al. (2008) Depression and coronary heart disease: Recommendations for screening, referral, and treatment. *Circulation*, 118: 1768–1775.

Lichtman, J.H., Froelicher, E.S., Blumenthal, J.A., Carney, R.M., Doering, L.V., Frasure-Smith, N. et al. (2014) Depression as a risk factor for poor prognosis among patients with acute coronary syndrome: Systematic review and recommendations: A scientific statement from the American Heart Association. *Circulation*, 129(12): 1350–1369.

Lieb, K. (2012) Psychological therapies for people with borderline personality disorder. *Cochrane Database of Systematic Reviews*, 8 (Art. CD005652).

Lietzén, R., Virtanen, P., Kivimäki, M., Sillanmäki, L., Vahtera, J. & Koskenvuo, M. (2011) Stressful life events and the onset of asthma. *European Respiratory Journal*, 37: 1360–1365.

Lightener, J.M. (1980) Competition of external and internal information in an exercise setting. *Journal of Personality and Social Psychology*, 39: 165–174.

Lill, M.M. & Wilkinson, T.J. (2005) Judging a book by its cover: Descriptive survey of patients' preferences for doctors' appearance and mode of address. *British Medical Journal*, 331: 524–1527.

Lim, M.M. & Young, L.J. (2006) Neuropeptidergic regulation of affiliative behavior and social bonding in animals. *Hormones and Behavior*, 50(4): 506–517. Review. Erratum in: *Hormones and Behaviour*, 51(2): 292–293.

Lin, H.R. & Bauer-Wu, S.M. (2003) Psycho-spiritual well-being in patients with advanced cancer: An integrative review of the literature. *Journal of Advanced Nursing*, 44: 69–80.

Linehan, M.M. (2014) *Skills Training Manual for Treating Borderline Personality Disorder* (2nd edition). New York: Guilford Press.

Linkins, R.W. & Comstock, G.W. (1990) Depressed mood and development of cancer. *American Journal of Epidemiology*, 132: 962–972.

Lins, S., Hayder-Beichel, D., Rücker, G., Motschall, E., Antes, G., Meyer, G. & Langer, G. (2014) Efficacy and experiences of telephone counselling for informal carers of people with dementia. *Cochrane Database of Systematic Reviews*, 9 (Art. CD009126).

Linton, S.J. (2013) A transdiagnostic approach to pain and emotion. *Journal of Applied Biobehavioral Research*, 18: 82–103.

Lintz, K. et al. (2003) Prostate cancer patients' support and psychological care needs: Survey from a non-surgical oncology clinic. *Psycho-Oncology*, 12: 769–783.

Lipp, M.R. (1986) *Respectful Treatment: A Practical Handbook of Patient-Care*. New York: Elsevier.

Lipsitt, D.R., Joseph, R., Meyer, D. & Notman, M.T. (2015) Medically unexplained symptoms: Barriers to effective treatment when nothing is the matter. *Harvard Review of Psychiatry*, 23(6): 438–448.

Little, A.C. & Jones, B.C. (2012) Variation in facial masculinity and symmetry preferences across the menstrual cycle is moderated by relationship context. *Psychoneuroendocrinology*, 37(7): 999–1008.

Little, A.C., Jones, B.C. & Burriss, R.P. (2007) Preferences for masculinity in male bodies changes across the menstrual cycle. *Hormones and Behavior*, 51: 633–639.

Liu, X., Olsen, J., Agerbo, E., Yuan, W., Cnattingius, S., Gissler, M. & Li, J. (2013) Psychological stress and hospitalization for childhood asthma: A nationwide cohort study in two Nordic countries. *PLoS One, 8*(10): e78816.

Llewellyn, C.D. (2018) Motivational interviewing, in C.D. Llewellyn et al. (eds), *The Cambridge Handbook of Psychology, Health and Medicine* (3rd edition). Cambridge: Cambridge University Press.

Lloyd, M. & Bor, R. (2004) *Communication Skills for Medicine* (2nd edition). Edinburgh: Churchill Livingstone.

Lloyd, M. & Bor, R. (2009) *Communication Skills for Medicine* (3rd edition). Edinburgh: Churchill Livingstone.

Lodge, C.J., Tan, D.J., Lau, M.X.Z., Dai, X., Tham, R., Lowe, A.J., Bowatte, G., Allen, K.J. & Dharmage, S.C. (2015) Breastfeeding and asthma and allergies: A systematic review and meta-analysis. *Acta Paediatrica, 104*: 38–53

Lok, I.H. & Neugebauer, R. (2007) Psychological morbidity following miscarriage. *Best Practice & Research in Clinical Obstetrics & Gynaecology, 21*: 229–247.

Longe, S.E., Wise, R., Bantick, S., Lloyd, D., Johansen-Berg, H., McGlone, F. & Tracey, I. (2001) Counter-stimulatory effects on pain perception and processing are significantly altered by attention: an fMRI study. *Neuroreport, 12*(9): 2021–2025.

Lorber, W., Mazzoni, G. & Kirsch, I. (2007) Illness by suggestion: Expectancy, modeling, and gender in the production of psychosomatic symptoms. *Annals of Behavioral Medicine, 33*: 112–116.

Lorig, K.R. & Holman, H. (2003) Self-management education: History, definition, outcomes, and mechanisms. *Annals of Behavioral Medicine, 26*(1): 1–7.

Lorig, K.R., Ritter, P., Stewart, A.L. et al. (2001) Chronic disease self-management program: 2-year health status and health care utilization outcomes. *Medical Care, 39*: 1217–1223.

Lovallo, W.R. (2004) *Stress & Health: Biological and Psychological Interactions*. Thousand Oaks, CA: Sage.

Lowe, M.R. et al. (2013) Dieting and restrained eating as prospective predictors of weight gain. *Frontiers in Psychology, 4*: 577.

Lowe, C.F., Dowey, A. & Horne, P. (1998) Changing what children eat, in A. Murcott (ed.), *The Nation's Diet: The Social Science of Food Choice*. Harlow: Addison Wesley Longman. pp. 57–80.

Luebbert, K., Dahme, B. & Hasenbring, M. (2001) The effectiveness of relaxation training in reducing treatment-related symptoms and improving emotional adjustment in acute non-surgical cancer treatment: A meta-analytical review. *Psycho-Oncology, 10*: 490–502.

Lundholm, L. et al. (2015) Anabolic androgenic steroids and violent offending: confounding by polysubstance abuse among 10,365 general population men. *Addiction, 110*: 100–108.

Luppa, M., Sikorski, C., Luck, T., Ehreke, L., Konnopka, A., Wiese, B., Weyerer, S., König, H.H. & Riedel-Heller, S.G. (2012) Age- and gender-specific prevalence of depression in latest-life: Systematic review and meta-analysis. *Journal of Affective Disorders, 136*: 212–221.

Luria, A.R. (1963 [1948]) *Restoration of Function after Brain Injury*. New York: Macmillan.

Lustman, P.J., Anderson, R.J., Freedland, K.E., de Groot, M., Carney, R.M. & Clouse, R.E. (2000) Depression and poor glycemic control: A meta-analytic review of the literature. *Diabetes Care*, 23: 934–942.

Lutgendorf, S.K. & Sood, A.K. (2011) Biobehavioral factors and cancer progression: Physiological pathways and mechanisms. *Psychosomatic Medicine*, 73: 724–730.

Lynch, J.W., Kaplan, G.A., Cohen, R.D., Tuomilehto, J. & Solonen, J.T. (1996) Do cardiovascular risk factors explain the relation between socioeconomic status, risk of all-cause mortality, cardiovascular mortality, and acute myocardial infarction? *American Journal of Epidemiology*, 144: 934–942.

Lyons, A.C. & Willott, S.A. (2008) Alcohol consumption, gender identities and women's changing social positions. *Sex Roles*, 59: 694–712.

Ma, N., Dinges, D.F., Basner, M. & Rao, H. (2015) How acute total sleep loss affects the attending brain: a meta-analysis of neuroimaging studies. *Sleep*, 38: 233–240.

Ma, Y. et al. (2013) Obesity and risk of colorectal cancer: A systematic review of prospective studies. *PLoS One*, 8: e53916.

MacDonald, G.M., Higgins, J.P., Ramchandani, P., Valentine, J.C., Bronger, L.P., Klein, P., O'Daniel, R., Pickering, M., Rademaker, B., Richardson, G. & Taylor, M. (2012) Cognitive-behavioural interventions for children who have been sexually abused. *Cochrane Database of Systematic Reviews*, 5 (Art. CD001930).

MacDonald, G.M., Higgins, J.P.T. & Ramchandani, P. (2006) Cognitive-behavioural interventions for children who have been sexually abused. *Cochrane Database of Systematic Reviews*, 4 (Art. CD001930).

Macêdo, T.M., Freitas, D.A., Chaves, G.S., Holloway, E.A. & Mendonça, K.M. (2016) Breathing exercises for children with asthma. *Cochrane Database of Systematic Review*, 4 (Art. CD011017).

Macer, B.J., Prady, S.L. & Mikocka-Walus, A. (2017) Antidepressants in inflammatory bowel disease: A systematic review. *Inflammatory Bowel Diseases*, 23: 534–550.

Madey, S.F. & Gomez, R. (2003) Reduced optimism for perceived age-related medical conditions. *Basic and Applied Social Psychology*, 25: 213–219.

Maglione, M.A., Maher, A.R., Ewing, B., Colaiaco, B., Newberry, S., Kandrack, R., Shanman, R.M., Sorbero, M.E. & Hempel, S. (2017) Efficacy of mindfulness meditation for smoking cessation: A systematic review and meta-analysis. *Addictive Behaviors*, 69: 27–34.

Magos, A.L. & Studd, J.W.W. (1988) A simple method for the diagnosis of the premenstrual syndrome by use of a self-assessment disk. *American Journal of Obstetrics and Gynecology*, 158: 1024–1028.

Mahajan, N.N. et al. (2009) Adjustment to infertility: The role of interpersonal and intrapersonal resources/vulnerabilities. *Human Reproduction*, 24: 906–912.

Mahalik, J.R. et al. (2006) Masculinity and perceived normative health behaviours as predictors of men's health behaviours. *Social Science & Medicine*, 64: 2201–2209.

Mahoney, L., Ayers, S. & Seddon, P. (2010) The association between parents' and healthcare professional's behavior and children's coping and distress during venipuncture. *Journal of Pediatric Psychology*, 35(9): 985–995.

Mainio, A., Hakko, H. Niemelä, A., Koivukangas, J. & Räsänen, P. (2005) Depression and functional outcome in patients with brain tumors: A population-based 1-year follow-up study. *Journal of Neurosurgery, 103*: 841–847.

Makoul, G. (2001) The SEGUE Framework for teaching and assessing communication skills. *Patient Education and Counselling, 45*(1): 23–34.

Malacrida, C. & Boulton, T. (2012) Women's perceptions of childbirth 'choices'. *Competing Discourses of Motherhood, Sexuality and Selflessness, 26*(5): 748–772.

Mancia, M. (ed.) (2006) *Psychoanalysis and Neuroscience.* New York: Springer.

Manfredini, R., De Giorgi, A., Tiseo, R., Boari, B., Cappadona, R., Salmi, R., Gallerani, M., Signani, F., Manfredini, F., Mikhailidis, D.P. & Fabbian, F. (2017) Marital status, cardiovascular diseases, and cardiovascular risk factors: A review of the evidence. *Journal of Women's Health* (in press). (doi: 10.1089/jwh.2016.6103).

Manuck, S.B., Harvey, A., Lecheiter, S. & Neil, K. (1978) Effects of coping on blood pressure responses to threat of aversive stimulation. *Psychophysiology, 15*: 544–549.

Mapes, D.L. et al. (2004) Health-related quality of life in the Dialysis Outcomes and Practice Patterns Study (DOPPS). *American Journal of Kidney Disease, 44*(Suppl 2): 54–60.

Margaretten, M. et al. (2011) Depression in patients with rheumatoid arthritis: Description, causes and mechanisms. *International Journal of Clinical Rheumtology, 6*(6): 617–623.

Margison, F.R et al. (2000) Measurement and psychotherapy: Evidence-based practice and practice-based evidence. *British Journal of Psychiatry, 177*: 123–130.

Marsh, A.A. & Blair, R.J. (2008) Deficits in facial affect recognition among antisocial populations: A meta-analysis, *Neuroscience and Biobehavioral Reviews, 32*: 454–465.

Marsland, A.L., Cohen, S. & Bachen, E. (2007) Cold, common, in S. Ayers et al. (eds), *Cambridge Handbook of Psychology, Health and Medicine* (2nd edition). Cambridge: Cambridge University Press. pp. 637–638.

Marteau, T.M. & Weinman, J. (2004) Communicating about health threats and treatments, in S. Sutton et al. (eds), *The SAGE Handbook of Health Psychology.* London: Sage. pp. 270–298.

Martinez Devesa, P., Waddell, A., Perera, R. & Theodoulou, M. (2007) Cognitive behavioural therapy for tinnitus. *Cochrane Database of Systematic Reviews, 1* (Art. CD005233).

Marucha, P.T., Kiecolt-Glaser, J.K. & Favagehi, M. (1998) Mucosal wound healing is impaired by examination stress. *Psychosomatic Medicine, 60*: 362–365.

Maslach, C. (2007) Burnout in health professionals, in S. Ayers et al. (eds), *Cambridge Handbook of Psychology, Health and Medicine* (2nd edition). Cambridge: Cambridge University Press. pp. 427–430.

Mastellos, N., Gunn, L.H., Felix, L.M., Car, J. & Majeed, A. (2014) Transtheoretical model stages of change for dietary and physical exercise modification in weight loss management for overweight and obese adults. *Cochrane Database of Systematic Reviews, 2* (Art. CD008066).

Matarazzo, J. (1980) Behavioral health and behavioural medicine: Frontiers of a new health psychology. *American Psychologist, 35*: 807–817.

Matteson, M.L. & Russell, C. (2010) Interventions to improve hemodialysis adherence: A systematic review of randomized-controlled trials. *Hemodialysis International, 14*: 370–382.

Matthey, S. (2016) Anxiety and stress during pregnancy and the postpartum period, in A. Wenzel (ed.), *The Oxford Handbook of Perinatal Psychology.* New York and Oxford: Oxford University Press. pp. 167–181.

Maxson, P.J., Edwards, S.E., Valentiner, E.M. & Miranda, M.L. (2016) A multidimensional approach to characterizing psychosocial health during pregnancy. *Maternal and Child Health Journal*, 6: 1103–1113.

May, A.M. et al. (2009) Long-term effects on cancer survivors' quality of life of physical training versus physical training combined with cognitive-behavioral therapy: Results from a randomized trial. *Support Care Cancer*, 17: 653–663.

Mayo-Wilson, E. & Montgomery, P. (2013) Media-delivered cognitive behavioural therapy and behavioural therapy (self-help) for anxiety disorders in adults. *Cochrane Database of Systematic Reviews*, 9 (Art. CD005330).

Mayr, M. & Schmid, R.M. (2010) Pancreatic cancer and depression: myth and truth. *BMC Cancer*, 10: 569.

Mazzeo, S.E., Mitchell, K.S., Bulik, C.M., Reichborn-Kjennerud, T., Kendler, K.S. & Neale, M.C. (2009) Assessing the heritability of anorexia nervosa symptoms using a marginal maximal likelihood approach. *Psychological Medicine*, 39: 463–473.

Mazzi, M.A., Rimondini, M., Deveugele, M., Zimmermann, C., Moretti, F., van Vliet, L., Deledda, G., Fletcher, I. & Bensing, J. (2015) What do people appreciate in physicians' communication? An international study with focus groups using videotaped medical consultations. *Health Expectations*, 18(5): 1215–1226.

Mbuagbaw, L. et al. (2015) Interventions for enhancing Adherence to Antiretroviral Therapy (ART): A systematic review of high quality studies. *AIDS Patient Care STDS*, 29: 248–266.

McAndrew, F., Thompson, J., Fellows, L., Large, A., Speed, M. & Renfrew, M.J. (2012) *Infant Feeding Survey 2010*. Leeds, UK: Health and Social Care Information Centre

McBride, C.M. & Koehly, L.M. (2017) Imagining roles for epigenetics in health promotion research. *Journal of Behavioral Medicine*, 40: 229–238.

McCaffery, J.M. et al. (2006) Common genetic vulnerability to depressive symptoms and coronary artery disease: A review and development of candidate genes related to inflammation and serotonin. *Psychosomatic Medicine*, 68: 187–200.

McClenahan, C., Shevlin, M., Adamson, G., Bennett, C. & O'Neill, B. (2007) Testicular self-examination: A test of the health belief model and the theory of planned behaviour. *Health Education Research*, 22: 272–284.

McCombie, A. et al. (2014) Preferences of inflammatory bowel disease patients for computerised versus face-to-face psychological interventions. *Journal of Crohn's and Colitis*, 8: 536–542.

McCourt, C., Weaver, J., Statham, H., Beake, S., Gamble, J. & Creedy, D.K. (2007) Elective cesarean section and decision making: A critical review of the literature. *Birth*, 34(1): 65–79.

McCrae, R.R. & Costa, P.T. (2003) *Personality in Adulthood: A Five-Factor Theory Perspective* (2nd edition). New York: Guilford Press.

McCracken, L.M. & Morley, S. (2014) The psychological flexibility model: a basis for integration and progress in psychological approaches to chronic pain management. *Journal of Pain*, 15(3):221–34.

McDonald, H.P., Garg, A.X. & Haynes, R.B. (2002) Interventions to enhance patient adherence to medication prescriptions: Scientific review. *Journal of the American Medical Association*, 288: 2868–2879.

McEachan, R.R.C., Conner, M., Taylor, N.J. & Lawton, R.J (2011) Prospective prediction of health-related behaviours with the theory of planned behaviour: A meta-analysis. *Health Psychology Review, 5*(2): 97–144.

McEwen, B.S. (1998a) Stress, adaptation, and disease: Allostasis and allostatic load. *Annals of the New York Academy of Science, 840*: 33–44.

McEwen, B.S. (1998b) Protective and damaging effects of stress mediators. *New England Journal of Medicine, 338*: 171–179.

McGinty, H.L. et al. (2014) Cognitive functioning in men receiving androgen deprivation therapy for prostate cancer: A systematic review and meta-analysis. *Support Care Cancer, 22*: 2271–2280.

McGrath, J. et al. (2008) Schizophrenia: A concise overview of incidence, prevalence, and mortality. *Epidemiology Review, 30*: 67–76.

McGregor, B.A. & Antoni, M.H. (2009) Psychological intervention and health outcomes among women treated for breast cancer: A review of stress pathways and biological mediators. *Brain, Behaviour & Immunity, 23*: 159–166.

McKinstry, B. (2000) Do patients wish to be involved in decision-making in the consultation? A cross-sectional survey with video vignettes. *British Medical Journal, 321*: 867–871.

McManus, F., Sacadura, C. & Clark, D.M. (2008) Why social anxiety persists: An experimental investigation of the role of safety behaviours as a maintaining factor. *Journal of Behavior Therapy & Experimental Psychiatry, 39*: 147–161.

McManus, I.C., Keeling, A. & Paice, E. (2004) Stress, burnout and doctors' attitudes to work are determined by personality and learning style: A twelve year longitudinal study of UK medical graduates. *BMC Medicine, 2*: 1–12.

McNair, L., Woodrow, C. & Hare, D. (2016) Dialectical Behaviour Therapy (DBT) with people with intellectual disabilities: A systematic review and narrative analysis. *Journal of Applied Research in Intellectual Disabilities*, July 26.

McWhinney, I. (1989) The need for a transformed clinical method, in M. Stewart & D. Roter (eds), *Communicating with Medical Patients*. Newbury Park, CA: Sage. pp. 25–40.

Meads, C. & Nouwen, A. (2005) Does emotional disclosure have any effects? A systematic review of the literature with meta-analyses. *International Journal of Technology Assessment in Health Care, 21*(2): 153–164.

Meechan, G., Collins, J. & Petrie, K.J. (2003) The relationship of symptoms and psychological factors to delay in seeking medical care for breast symptoms. *Preventive Medicine, 36*: 374–378.

Meissner, K. (2009). Effects of placebo interventions on gastric motility and general autonomic activity. *Journal of Psychosomatic Research, 66*, 391–398.

Meissner, C.A. & Brigham, J.C. (2001) Thirty years of investigating the own-race bias in memory for faces: A meta-analytic review. *Psychology, Public Policy & Law, 7*: 3–35.

Melby, M.K., Lock, M. & Kaufert, P. (2005) Culture and symptom reporting at menopause. *Human Reproduction Update, 11*: 495–512.

Melendez-Torres, G.J. et al. (2015) A systematic review and critical appraisal of qualitative meta-synthetic practice in public health to develop a taxonomy of operations of reciprocal translation. *Research Synthesis Methods, 6*: 357–371.

Meltzoff, A.N. & Moore, M.K. (1977) Imitation of facial and manual gestures by human neonates. *Science*, *198*: 75–78.

Melzack, R. (1999) From the gate to the neuromatrix. *Pain*, 6: S121–S126.

Melzack, R. & Wall, P. (1965) Pain mechanisms: A new theory. *Science*, *150*: 971–979.

Meman, J., van Ijzendoom, M.H. & Bakermans-Kranenberg, M.J. (2009) The many faces of the Still-Face Paradigm: A review and meta-analysis. *Development Review*, *29*: 120–162

Memon, A. et al. (2016) Perceived barriers to accessing mental health services among black and minority ethnic (BME) communities: A qualitative study in Southeast England. *BMJ Open*, 6(11): e012337.

Mendell, L.M. (2014) Constructing and deconstructing the gate theory of pain. *Pain*, *155*(2): 210–216.

Mendes-Silva, A.P. et al. (2016) Shared biologic pathways between Alzheimer's disease and major depression: A systematic review of microRNA expression studies. *American Journal of Geriatric Psychiatry*, *24*: 903–912.

Mendle, J., Turkheimer, E. & Emery, R.E. (2007) Detrimental psychological outcomes associated with early pubertal timing in adolescent girls. *Developmental Review*, *27*: 151–171.

Menz, R. & Al-Roubaie, A. (2008) Interruptions, status, and gender in medical interviews: The harder you brake the longer it takes. *Discourse Society*, *19*: 645–666.

Mercer, C. et al. (2005) Who reports sexual function problems? *Sexually Transmitted Infections*, *81*: 394–399.

Mereish, E.H. & Bradford, J.B. (2014) Intersecting identities and substance use problems: Sexual orientation, gender, race, and lifetime substance use problems. *Journal of Studies on Alcohol and Drugs*, *75*: 179–188.

Merel, S.E., McKinney, C.M., Ufkes, P., Kwan, A.C. & White, A.A. (2016) Sitting at patients' bedsides may improve patients' perceptions of physician communication skills. *British Journal of Hospital Medicine*, *11*(12): 865–868.

Merikangas, K.R. et al. (2011) Prevalence and correlates of bipolar spectrum disorder in the world mental health survey initiative. *Archives of General Psychiatry*, *68*: 241–251.

Mesmer-Magnus, J. & DeChurch, L. (2009) Information sharing and team performance: A meta-analysis. *Journal of Applied Psychology*, *94*: 535–546.

Meyer, D., Levental, H. & Guttman, M. (1985) Common-sense models of illness: The example of hypertension. *Health Psychology*, *4*: 115–135.

Michie, S., van Stralen, M.M. & West, R. (2011) The behaviour change wheel: A new method for characterising and designing behaviour change interventions. *Implementation Science*, 6: 42.

Michie, S., Wood, C.E., Johnston, M., Abraham, C., Francis, J.J. & Hardeman, W. (2015) Behaviour change techniques: The development and evaluation of a taxonomic method for reporting and describing behaviour change interventions. *Health Technology Assessment*, *19*: 1–188.

Milgram, S. (1974) *Obedience to Authority*. New York: Harper & Row.

Millar, K., Purushotham, A.D., McLatchie, E., George, W.D. & Murray, G.D. (2005) A 1-year prospective study of individual variation in distress and illness perceptions, after treatment for breast cancer. *Journal of Psychosomatic Research*, *58*: 335–342.

Miller, A.C. & Shriver, T.E. (2012) Women's childbirth preferences and practices in the United States. *Social Science & Medicine*, 75(4): 709–716.

Miller, G.A. (1956) The magic number seven, plus or minus two: Some limits on our capacity for processing information. *Psychological Review*, 63: 81–93.

Miller, G.E. & Cohen, S. (2000) Psychological interventions and the immune system: A meta-analytic review and critique. *Health Psychology*, 20: 47–63.

Miller, K.J. (2003) The other side of estrogen replacement therapy: Outcome study results of mood improvement in estrogen users and nonusers. *Current Psychiatry Reports*, 5(6): 439–444.

Miller, M., Mangano, C., Park, Y., Goel, R., Plotnick, G.D. & Vogel, R.A. (2006) Impact of cinematic viewing on endothelial function. *Heart*, 92: 261–262.

Miller, T.Q., Smith, T.W., Turner, C.W., Guijarro, M.L. & Hallet, A.J. (1996) A meta-analytic review of research on hostility and physical health. *Psychological Bulletin*, 119: 322–348.

Miller, W.C. & Zenilman, J.M. (2005) Epidemiology of chlamydial infection, gonorrhea, and trichomoniasis in the United States – 2005. *Infectious Disease Clinics of North America*, 19: 281–296.

Miller, W.R. (1995) *Motivational Enhancement Therapy with Drug Abusers*. Albuquerque, NM: University of New Mexico.

Miller, W.R. & Rollnick, S. (2002) *Motivational Interviewing: Preparing People for Change*. New York: Guilford Press.

Miller, W.R. & Rollnick, S. (2013) *Motivational Interviewing: Helping People Change*. New York: Guilford Press.

Mioshi, E., Dawson, K., Mitchell, J., Arnold, R. & Hodges, J.R. (2006) Addenbrooke's Cognitive Examination Revised (ACE-R). *International Journal of Geriatric Psychiatry*, 21: 1078–1085.

Miskovic, D. et al. (2008) Randomized controlled trial investigating the effect of music on the virtual reality laparoscopic learning performance of novice surgeons. *Surgical Endoscopy*, 22: 2416–2420.

Mitchell, J.T., Zylowska, L. & Kollins, S.H. (2015) Mindfulness meditation training for Attention-Deficit/Hyperactivity Disorder in adulthood: Current empirical support, treatment overview, and future directions. *Cognitive and Behavioral Practice*, 22(2):172–191.

Mitchell, K.R. et al. (2016) Estimating the prevalence of sexual function problems: The impact of morbidity criteria. *Journal of Sex Research*, 53: 955–967.

Mitte, K. (2005) Meta-analysis of cognitive-behavioral treatments for generalized anxiety disorder: A comparison with pharmacotherapy, *Psychological Bulletin*, 131: 785–795.

Mjaaland, T.A. & Finset, A. (2009) Frequency of GP communication addressing the patient's resources and coping strategies in medical interviews: A video-based observational study. *BMC Family Practice*, 10: 49.

Mo, D. et al. (2014) Ten-year change in quality of life in adults on growth hormone replacement for growth hormone deficiency: An analysis of the hypopituitary control and complications study. *Journal of Clinical Endocrinology and Metabolism*, 99: 4581–4588.

Mogk, C., Otte, S., Reinhold-Hurley, B. & Kroner-Herwig, B. (2006) Health effects of expressive writing on stressful or traumatic experiences: A meta-analysis. *Psycho-Social Medicine*, 16(3): Doc06.

Mohr, D.C. & Cox, D. (2001) Multiple sclerosis: Empirical literature for the clinical health psychologist. *Journal of Clinical Psychology*, 57: 479–499.

Mojaverian, T. & Kim, H.S. (2013) Interpreting a helping hand: Cultural variation in the effectiveness of solicited and unsolicited social support. *Personality and Social Psychology Bulletin*, 39(1): 88–99.

Möller-Leimkuhler, A.M. (2002) Barriers to help seeking in men: A review of sociocultural and clinical literature with particular reference to depression. *Journal of Affective Disorders*, 71: 1–9.

Molloy, G.J., Stamatakis, E., Randall, G. & Hamer, M. (2009) Marital status, gender and cardiovascular mortality: Behavioural, psychological distress and metabolic explanations. *Social Science & Medicine*, 69: 223–228.

Monahan, J.L., Murphy, S.T. & Zajonc, R.B. (2000) Subliminal mere exposure: Specific, general and diffuse effects. *Psychological Science*, 11: 462–467.

Montgomery, A. & Maslach, C. (2018) Burnout in health professionals, in C.D. Llewellyn et al. (eds), *The Cambridge Handbook of Psychology, Health and Medicine* (3rd edition). Cambridge: Cambridge University Press.

Montgomery, P. & Dennis, J. (2002) Cognitive behavioural interventions for sleep problems in adults aged 60+. *Cochrane Database of Systematic Reviews*, 2 (Art. CD003161).

Monz, B. et al. (2005) Patient-reported impact of urinary incontinence – results from treatment seeking women in 14 European countries. *Maturitas*, 52(suppl. 2): s24–s34.

Mooney, C.J., Elliot, A.J., Douthit, K.Z., Marquis, A. & Seplaki, C.L. (2016) Perceived control mediates effects of socioeconomic status and chronic stress on physical frailty: Findings from the health and retirement study. *Journal of Gerontology B: Psychological Sciences and Social Sciences*, Epub ahead of print.

Moore, P.J., Sickel, A.E., Malat, J., Williams, D., Jackson, J. & Adler, N.E. (2004) Psychosocial factors in medical and psychological treatment avoidance: The role of the doctor-patient relationship. *Journal of Health Psychology*, 9: 421–433.

Moos, R.H. & Schaefer, J.A. (1984) The crisis of physical illness: An overview and conceptual approach, in R.H. Moos (ed.), *Coping with Physical Illness: Vol 2: New Perspectives*. New York: Plenum. pp. 3–25.

Moreau, C. et al. (2016) Sexual dysfunction among youth: An overlooked sexual health concern. *BMC Public Health*, 16: 1170.

Moreira, J.F.G. & Telzer, E.H. (2016) Mother still knows best: Maternal influence uniquely modulates adolescent reward sensitivity during risk taking. *Developmental Science*, 4 November (doi: 10.1111/desc.12484).

Morey, M.C., Pieper, C.F., Crowley, G.M., Sullivan, R.J. & Puglisi, C.M. (2002) Exercise adherence and 10-year mortality in chronically ill older adults. *Journal of the American Geriatric Society*, 50: 2089–2091.

Morgan, N. et al. (2014) The effects of mind–body therapies on the immune system: Meta-analysis. *PLoS One*, 9(7): e100903.

Morina, N., Ijntema, H., Meyerbröker, K. & Emmelkamp, P.M. (2015) Can virtual reality exposure therapy gains be generalized to real-life? A meta-analysis of studies applying behavioral assessments. *Behaviour Research and Therapy*, 74: 18–24.

Morley, S. (2007) Pain management, in S. Ayers et al. (eds), *Cambridge Handbook of Psychology, Health and Medicine* (2nd edition). Cambridge: Cambridge University Press. pp. 370–374.

Morley, S., Eccleston, C. & Williams, A. (1999) Systematic review and meta-analysis of randomized controlled trials of cognitive behaviour therapy and behaviour therapy for chronic pain in adults, excluding headache. *Pain, 80*: 1–13.

Morroni, C. et al. (2014) The impact of oral contraceptive initiation on young women's condom use in three American cities: Missed opportunities for intervention. *PLoS One, 9*(7): e101804.

Mortensen, E.L., Michaelsen, K.F., Sanders, S.A. & Reinisch, J.M. (2002) The association between duration of breastfeeding and adult intelligence. *Journal of the American Medical Association, 287*: 2365–2371.

Moseley, J.B. et al. (2002) A controlled trial of arthroscopic surgery for osteoarthritis of the knee. *New England Journal of Medicine, 347*: 81–88.

Moser, G. et al. (1993) Inflamatory bowel disease: Patients' beliefs about the etiology of their disease. *Psychosomatic Medicine, 55*: 131.

Moulton, C.D., Pickup, J.C. & Ismail, K. (2015) The link between depression and diabetes: The search for shared mechanisms. *Lancet Diabetes & Endocrinology, 3*: 461–471.

Mozurkewich, E.L., Luke, B., Avni, M. & Wolf, F.M. (2000) Working conditions and adverse pregnancy outcome: A meta-analysis. *Obstetrics and Gynecology, 95*: 623–635.

Mulligan, K. & Newman, S. (2018) Self-management interventions, in C.D. Llewellyn et al. (eds), *The Cambridge Handbook of Psychology, Health and Medicine* (3rd edition). Cambridge: Cambridge University Press.

Mullington, J.M., Haack, M., Toth, M., Serrador, J.M. & Meier-Ewert, H.K. (2009) Cardiovascular, inflammatory, and metabolic consequences of sleep deprivation. *Progress in Cardiovascular Diseases, 51*: 294–302.

Murphy, C.C., Schei, B., Myhr, T.L. & Du Mont, J. (2001) Abuse: A risk factor for low birth weight? A systematic review and meta-analysis. *Canadian Medical Association Journal, 164*: 1567–1572.

Murray E. (2012) Web-based interventions for behavior change and self-management: Potential, pitfalls, and progress. *Medicine 2.0, 1*(2):e3.

Murray, E., Charles, C. & Gafni, A. (2006) Shared decision-making in primary care: Tailoring the Charles et al. model to fit the context of general practice. *Patient Education & Counseling, 62*: 205–211.

Murray, L., Halligan, S.L. & Cooper, P.J. (2010) Effects of postnatal depression on mother–infant interactions, and child development, in G. Bremner & T. Wachs (eds), *Handbook of Infant Development* (2nd edition, Vol. 2). Chichester, UK: Wiley-Blackwell. pp. 192–220.

Murray, M.A., Fiset, V., Young, S. & Kryworuchko, J. (2009) Where the dying live: A systematic review of determinants of place of end-of-life cancer care. *Oncology Nursing Forum, 36*: 69–77.

Muscatello, M.R. et al. (2014) Role of negative affects in pathophysiology and clinical expression of irritable bowel syndrome. *World Journal of Gastroenterology, 20*: 7570–7586.

Mustian, K.M. et al. (2017) Comparison of pharmaceutical, psychological, and exercise treatments for cancer-related fatigue: A meta-analysis. *JAMA Oncology* (doi: 10.1001/jama oncol.2016.6914).

Myers, L.B. (2010) The importance of the repressive coping style: Findings from 30 years of research. *Anxiety Stress Coping*, *23*(1): 3–17.

Myers, L.B. & Midence, K. (1998) Concepts and issues in adherence, in L.B. Myers & K. Midence (eds), *Adherence to Treatment in Medical Conditions*. Amsterdam: Harwood. pp. 1–24.

Nahon, S. et al. (2012) Risk factors of anxiety and depression in inflammatory bowel disease. *Inflammatory Bowel Diseases*, *18*: 2086–2091.

Naliboff, B.D. et al. (1997) Evidence for two distinct perceptual alterations in irritable bowel syndrome. *Gut*, *41*: 505–512.

Nanni, M.G. et al. (2015) Depression in HIV infected patients: A review. *Current Psychiatry Reports*, 17: 530.

Nasreddine, Z.S., Phillips, N.A., Bedirian, V., Charbonneau, S., Whitehead, V., Collin, I. et al. (2005) The Montreal Cognitive Assessment (MoCA): A brief screening tool for mild cognitive impairment. *Journal of the American Geriatric Society*, *53*(4): 695–699.

National Center for Health Statistics (NCHS) (2007) *Health, United States, 2007*. Hyattsville, MD: NCHS.

National Institute for Clinical Excellence (NICE) (2005) *Post-Traumatic Stress Disorder (PTSD): The Management of PTSD in Adults and Children in Primary and Secondary Care*. Clinical Guidelines 26. London: NICE.

National Institute for Health and Clinical Excellence (NICE) (2006) *Urinary Incontinence: The Management of Urinary Incontinence in Women*. Clinical Guidelines 40. London: RCOG Press.

National Institute for Health and Care Excellence (NICE) (2011) *Common Mental Health Problems: Identification and Pathways to Care*. Clinical Guidelines 123. London: NICE.

National Institute for Clinical Excellence (NICE) (2014) *Antenatal and Postnatal Mental Health: Clinical Management and Service Guidance*. Clinical Guidelines 192. London: NICE.

National Institute of Allergy and Infectious Diseases (NIAID) (2006) *The Common Cold*. London: NIAID. Avilable at: www3.niaid.nih.gov/healthscience/healthtopics/colds/ (last accessed 18 September 2009).

Nausheen, B., Gidron, Y., Peveler, R. & Moss-Morris, R. (2009) Social support and cancer progression: A systematic review. *Journal of Psychosomatic Research*, *67*: 403–415.

Navarro, X., Vivó, M. & Valero-Cabré, A. (2007) Neural plasticity after peripheral nerve injury and regeneration. *Progress in Neurobiology*, *82*: 163–201.

Naylor, C., Parsonage, M., McDaid, D., Knapp, M., Fossey, M. & Galea, A. (2012) *Long-term Conditions and Mental Health: The Cost of Co-morbidities*. London: The Kings Fund and Centre for Mental Health.

Neimeyer, R.A., Wittkowski, J. & Moser, R.P. (2004) Psychological research on death attitudes: An overview and evaluation. *Death Studies*, *28*(4): 309–340.

Nelson, C.J., Lee, J.S., Gamboa, M.C. & Roth, A.J. (2008) Cognitive effects of hormone therapy in men with prostate cancer: A review. *Cancer*, *115*: 1097–1106.

Nelson, J.E. (1999) Saving lives and saving deaths. *Annals of Internal Medicine*, *130(9)*: 776–777.

Nelson, L.D. & Morrison, E.L. (2005) The symptoms of resource scarcity: Judgements of food and finances influence preferences for potential partners. *Psychological Science*, *16*: 167–173.

Nelson, M.D., Saykin, A.J., Flashman, L.A. & Riordan, H.J. (1998) Hippocampal volume reduction in schizophrenia as assessed by Magnetic Resonance Imaging: A meta-analytic study. *Archives of General Psychiatry*, *55*: 433–440.

Neumann, M., Edelhäuser, F., Tauschel, D., Fischer, M.R., Wirtz, M., Woopen, C., Haramati, A. & Scheffer, C. (2011) Empathy decline and its reasons: A systematic review of studies with medical students and residents. *Academic Medicine*, *86*(8): 996–1009.

Neumark-Sztainer, D. et al. (2011) Dieting and disordered eating behaviors from adolescence to young adulthood: Findings from a 10-year longitudinal study. *Journal of the American Diet Association*, *111*: 1004–1011.

Newby, J.M., Twomey, C., Yuan Li, S.S. & Andrews, G. (2016) Transdiagnostic computerised cognitive behavioural therapy for depression and anxiety: A systematic review and meta-analysis. *Journal of Affective Disorders*, *199*: 30–41.

Newton, T.L. (2009) Cardiovascular functioning, personality, and the social world: The domain of hierarchical power. *Neuroscience and Biobehavioral Reviews*, *33*: 145–159.

Nexø, M.A. et al. (2015) Exploring the experiences of people with hypo- and hyperthyroidism. *Qualitative Health Research*, *25*: 945–953.

Niedenthal, P.M. (2007) Embodying emotion. *Science*, *316*(5827): 1002–1005.

Nieminen, K., Stephansson, O. & Ryding, E.L. (2009) Women's fear of childbirth and preference for cesarean section: A cross-sectional study at various stages of pregnancy in Sweden. *Acta Obstetricia et Gynecologica Scandinavica*, *88*(7): 807–813.

Nieuwlaat, R. et al. (2014) Interventions for enhancing medication adherence. *Cochrane Database of Systematic Reviews*, *11* (Art. CD000011).

Nimnuan, C., Hotopf, M. & Wessely, S. (2001) Medically unexplained symptoms: an epidemiological study in seven specialities. *Journal of Psychosomatic Research*, *51*(1):361–7.

Nishino, S. (2007) Narcolepsy: Pathophysiology and pharmacology. *Journal of Clinical Psychiatry*, *68*(Suppl 13): 9–15.

Nishino, S., Ripley, B., Overeem, S., Lammers, G.J. & Mignot, E. (2000) Hypocretin (orexin) deficiency in human narcolepsy. *Lancet*, *355*: 39–40.

Nitti, V.W. (2001) The prevalence of urinary incontinence. *Reviews in Urology*, *3*(Suppl. 1): s2–s6.

Nitzan, U. & Lichtenberg, P. (2004) Questionnaire survey on use of placebo. *British Medical Journal*, *329*: 944–946.

Noble, L.M. (1998) Doctor–patient communication and adherence to treatment, in L.B. Myers & K. Midence (eds), *Adherence to Treatment in Medical Conditions*. Amsterdam: Harwood. pp. 51–82.

Nolan, K., Shope, C.B., Citrome, L. & Volavka, J. (2009) Staff and patient views of the reasons for aggressive incidents. *Psychiatric Quarterly*, *80*: 167–172.

Nykamp, K., Rosenthal, L., Folkerts, M., Roehrs, T., Guido, P. & Roth, T. (1998) The effects of REM sleep deprivation on the level of sleepiness/alertness. *Sleep*, *21*: 609–614.

O'Brien, K.H.M. et al. (2016) Sexual and gender minority youth suicide: Understanding subgroup differences to inform interventions. *LGBT Health*, *3*: 248–251.

O'Connor, T.G. et al. (2000) The effects of global severe privation on cognitive competence. *Child Development*, *71*: 376–390.

O'Connor, T.G., Heron, J., Golding, J., Beveridge, M. & Glover, V. (2002) Maternal antenatal anxiety and children's behavioural/emotional problems at 4 years. *British Journal of Psychiatry*, 180: 502–508.

O'Donovan, D. (2008) *The Atlas of Health: Mapping the Challenges and Causes of Disease*. London: Earthscan.

O'Farrell, T.J. & Clements, K. (2012) Review of outcome research on marital and family therapy in treatment for alcoholism. *Journal of Marital and Family Therapy*, 38(1): 122–144.

Ocañez, K.L., McHugh, R.K. & Otto, M.W. (2010) A meta-analytic review of the association between anxiety sensitivity and pain. *Depression and Anxiety*, 27(8): 760–767.

Ochsner, K.N. & Gross, J.J. (2005) The cognitive control of emotion. *Trends in Cognitive Science*, 9(5): 242–249.

Oddens, B.J., den Tonkelaar, I. & Nieuwenhuyse, H. (1999) Psychosocial experiences in women facing fertility problems: A comparative survey. *Human Reproduction*, 14, 255–261.

Odegård, S., Finset, A., Mowinckel, P., Kvien, T.K. & Uhlig, T. (2007) Pain and psychological health status over a 10-year period in patients with recent onset rheumatoid arthritis. *Annals of Rheumatic Disease*, 66: 1195–1201.

Oerlemans, M.E.J., van den Akker, M., Schuurman, A.G., Kellen, E. & Buntinx, R. (2007) A meta-analysis on depression and subsequent cancer risk. *Clinical Practice and Epidemiology in Mental Health*, 3: 1–11.

Office for National Statistics (2000) *Key Health Statistics from General Practice 1998*. Series MB6, No. 2. London: ONS.

Office for National Statistics (2002a) *Tobacco, Alcohol and Drug Use and Mental Health*. London: ONS.

Office for National Statistics (2002b) *Households in Receipt of Benefit: By Type of Benefit, 2001/02: Regional Trends 38*. London: ONS. Available at: www.statistics.gov.uk/STATBASE/ssdataset.asp?vlnk=7755 (last accessed 1 August 2009).

Office for National Statistics (2008) *Birth Statistics*. Newport, UK: ONS.

Office for National Statistics (2015) *Provisional Analysis of Death Registrations, 2015*. London: ONS. Available at: www.ons.gov.uk/peoplepopulationandcommunity/birthsdeathsandmarriages/deaths/articles/provisionalanalysisofdeathregistrations/2015 (last accessed 26 March 2017).

Office of the Surgeon General (2004) *The Health Consequences of Smoking*. London: OSG. Available at www.surgeongeneral.gov/library/smokingconsequences (last accessed 29 September 2009).

Ogden, J., Reynolds, R. & Smith, A. (2006) Expanding the concept of parental control: A role for overt and covert control in children's snacking behaviour. *Appetite*, 47: 100–106.

Ogutmen, B. et al. (2006) Health-related quality of life after kidney transplantation in comparison to intermittent hemodialysis, peritoneal dialysis, and normal controls. *Transplantation Proceedings*, 38: 419–421.

Okano, H. & Sawamoto, K. (2008) Neural stem cells: Involvement in adult neurogenesis and CNS repair. *Philosophical Transactions of the Royal Society B*, 363: 2111–2122.

Olander, E.K., Darwin, Z.J., Atkinson, L., Smith, D.M. & Gardner, B. (2016) Beyond the 'teachable moment': A conceptual analysis of women's perinatal behaviour change. *Women and Birth*, 29(3): e67–71.

Olatunji, B.O., Cisler, J.M. & Deacon, B.J. (2010) Efficacy of cognitive behavioral therapy for anxiety disorders: A review of meta-analytic findings. *Psychiatric Clinics of North America*, 33(3): 557–577.

Oliveira, V.C. et al. (2012) Communication that values patient autonomy is associated with satisfaction with care: A systematic review. *Journal of Physiotherapy*, 58: 215–229.

Olthuis, J.V., Watt, M.C., Bailey, K., Hayden, J.A. & Stewart, S.H. (2016) Therapist-supported internet cognitive behavioural therapy for anxiety disorders in adults. *Cochrane Database of Systematic Reviews*, 3 (Art. CD011565).

Onakomaiya, M.M. & Henderson, L.P. (2016) Mad men, women and steroid cocktails: A review of the impact of sex and other factors on anabolic androgenic steroids effects on affective behaviors. *Psychopharmacology*, 233: 549–569.

Ong, L.M.L., de Haes, J.C.J.M., Hoos, A.M. & Lammes, F.B. (1995) Doctor–patient communication: A review of the literature. *Social Science & Medicine*, 40: 903–918.

Ost, L.G. (2014) The efficacy of Acceptance and Commitment Therapy: An updated systematic review and meta-analysis. *Behaviour Research and Therapy*, 61: 105–121.

Osterberg, L. & Blaschke, T. (2005) Adherence to medication. *New England Journal of Medicine*, 353: 487–497.

Ott, M. et al. (2002) The trade-off between hormonal contraceptives and condoms. *Perspectives on Sexual & Reproductive Health*, 34: 6–14.

Ott, M.J., Norris, R.L. & Bauer-Wu, S.M. (2009) Mindfulness meditation for oncology patients: A discussion and critical review. *Integrative Cancer Therapies*, 5: 98–108.

Ougrin D. (2011) Efficacy of exposure versus cognitive therapy in anxiety disorders: Systematic review and meta-analysis. *BMC Psychiatry*, 20(11): 200.

Ouimet, A.J., Gawronski, B. & Dozois, D.J.A. (2009) Cognitive vulnerability to anxiety: A review and an integrative model. *Clinical Psychology Review*, 29: 459–470.

Pae, C.U., Masand, P.S., Ajwani, N., Lee, C. & Patkar, A.A. (2007) Irritable bowel syndrome in psychiatric perspectives: A comprehensive review. *International Journal of Clinical Practice*, 61: 1708–1718.

Palma, J.A., Urrestarazu, E. & Iriarte, J. (2013) Sleep loss as risk factor for neurologic disorders: A review. *Sleep Medicine* , 14: 229–236.

Palmeira, L., Pinto-Gouveia, J. & Cunha, M. (2016) The role of weight self-stigma on the quality of life of women with overweight and obesity: A multi-group comparison between binge eaters and non-binge eaters. *Appetite*, 105: 782–789.

Palmer, S. et al. (2013) Prevalence of depression in chronic kidney disease: Systematic review and meta-analysis of observational studies. *Kidney International*, 84: 179–191.

Palmer, W.L., Bottle, A. & Aylin, P. (2015) Association between day of delivery and obstetric outcomes: Observational study. *British Medical Journal*, 351: h5774.

Paniagua, F.A. (1999) Commentary on the possibility that Viagra may contribute to transmission of HIV and other sexual diseases among older adults. *Psychological Reports*, 85: 942–944.

Pantanetti, P., Sonino, N., Arnaldi, G. & Boscaro, M. (2002) Self image and quality of life in acromegaly. *Pituitary*, *5*: 17–19.

Panza, F., Frisardi, V., Capurso, C., D'Introno, A., Colacicco, A.M, Imbimbo, B.P., Santamato, A., Vendemiale, G., Seripa, D., Pilotto, A., Capurso, A. & Solfrizzi, V. (2010) Late-life depression, mild cognitive impairment, and dementia: Possible continuum? *American Journal of Geriatric Psychiatry*, *18*: 98–116.

Park, N.W. & Ingles, J.L. (2000) Effectiveness of attention training after an acquired brain injury: A meta-analysis of rehabilitation studies. *Brain and Cognition* (Special Issue), *44*: 5–9.

Park, S.H. et al. (2008) Self-reported health-related quality of life predicts survival for patients with advanced gastric cancer treated with first-line chemotherapy. *Quality of Life Research*, *17*: 207–214.

Parry, C.H. (1825) *Collections from the Unpublished Writings of the Late C.H. Parry* (Vol 2). London: Underwoods.

Parsons, T. (1975) The sick role and the role of the physician reconsidered. *Millbank Memorial Fund Quarterly*, *53*: 257–278.

Pascoe, L. & Edvardsson, D. (2013) Benefit finding in cancer: A review of influencing factors and health outcomes. *European Journal of Oncology Nursing*, *17*(6): 760–766.

Paulsen, J.S. et al. (2005) Depression and stages of Huntington's disease. *Journal of Neuropsychiatry & Clinical Neuroscience*, *17*: 496–502.

Paulson, J.F. & Bazemore, S.D. (2010) Prenatal and postpartum depression in fathers and its association with maternal depression: A meta-analysis. *JAMA*, *303*(19): 1961–1969.

Payne, H.E., Lister, C., West, J.H. & Bernhardt, J.M. (2015) Behavioral functionality of mobile apps in health interventions: A systematic review of the literature. *JMIR mHealth uHealth*, *3*(1): e20.

Payne, S., Horn, S. & Relf, M. (1999) *Loss and Bereavement*. Buckingham: Open University Press.

Pearl, S.B. & Norton, P.J. (2017) Transdiagnostic versus diagnosis specific cognitive behavioural therapies for anxiety: A meta-analysis. *Journal of Anxiety Disorders*, *46*: 11–24.

Pearson, R.M., Cooper, R.M., Penton-Voak, I.S., Lightman, S.L. & Evans, J. (2009) Depressive symptoms in early pregnancy disrupt attentional processing of infant emotion. *Psychological Medicine*, *40*: 621–631.

Peat, C.M., Peyerl, N.L. & Muehlenkamp, J.J. (2008) Body image and eating disorders in older adults: A review. *Journal of General Psychology*, *135*: 343–358. (doi: 10.3200/GENP.135.4.343-358.)

Peltzer, K. & Pengpid, S. (2015) Trying to lose weight among non-overweight university students from 22 low, middle and emerging economy countries. *Asia Pacific Journal of Clinical Nutrition*, *24*: 177–183.

Pennant, M.E., Loucas, C.E., Whittington, C., Creswell, C., Fonagy, P., Fuggle, P., Kelvin, R., Naqvi, S., Stockton, S. & Kendall, T. (2015) Expert Advisory Group. Computerised therapies for anxiety and depression in children and young people: A systematic review and meta-analysis. *Behaviour Research and Therapy*, *67*: 1–18.

Perkins-Porras, L., Whitehead, D.L., Strike, P.C. & Steptoe, A. (2009) Pre-hospital delay in patients with acute coronary syndrome: Factors associated with patient decision time and home-to-hospital delay. *European Journal of Cardiovascular Nursing*, *8*: 26–33.

Perlman, R.L. et al. (2005) Quality of life in chronic kidney disease (CKD). *American Journal of Kidney Disease*, 45: 658–666.

Peters, S.A.E., Huxley, R.R. & Woodward, M. (2014) Diabetes as risk factor for incident coronary heart disease in women compared with men: A systematic review and meta-analysis of 64 cohorts including 858,507 individuals and 28,203 coronary events. *Diabetologia*, 57: 1542.

Petersen, S., Taube, K., Lehmann, K., Van den Bergh, O. & von Leupoldt, A. (2012) Social comparison and anxious mood in pulmonary rehabilitation: The role of cognitive focus. *British Journal of Health Psychology*, 17: 463–476.

Petrie, K.J. et al. (2012) A text message programme designed to modify patients' illness and treatment beliefs improves self-reported adherence to asthma preventer medication. *British Journal of Health Psychology*, 17: 74–84.

Petrie, K.J., Broadbent, E. & Meechan, G. (2003) Self-regulatory interventions for improving the self management of chronic illness, in L.D. Cameron & H. Leventhal (eds), *The Self-Regulation of Health and Illness Behaviour*. London: Routledge. pp. 257–277.

Petrie, K.J., Buick, D.L., Weinman, J. & Booth, R.J. (1999) Positive effects of illness reported by myocardial infarction and breast cancer patients. *Journal of Psychosomatic Research*, 47: 537–543.

Petrie, K.J., Cameron, L.D., Ellis, C.J., Buick, D. & Weinman, J. (2002) Changing illness perceptions after myocardial infarction: An early intervention randomized controlled trial. *Psychosomatic Medicine*, 64: 580–586.

Petrie, K.J., Faasse, K., Crichton, F. & Grey, A. (2014) How common are symptoms? Evidence from a New Zealand national telephone survey. *BMJ Open*, 4(6): e005374.

Petrie, K.J., Moss-Morris, R., Grey, C. & Shaw, M. (2004) The relationship of negative affect and perceived sensitivity to symptom reporting following vaccination. *British Journal of Health Psychology*, 9: 101–111.

Petrie, K.J. & Pennebaker, J.W. (2004) Health-related cognitions, in S. Sutton et al. (eds), *The SAGE Handbook of Health Psychology*. London: Sage. pp. 127–142.

Petrie, K.J., Weinman, J., Sharpe, N. & Buckley, J. (1996) Role of patients' view of their illness in predicting return to work and functioning after myocardial infarction: Longitudinal study. *British Medical Journal*, 312: 1191–1194.

Petrilli, C.M., Mack, M., Petrilli, J.J., Hickner, A., Saint, S. & Chopra, V. (2015) Understanding the role of physician attire on patient perceptions: A systematic review of the literature – targeting attire to improve likelihood of rapport (TAILOR) investigators. *BMJ Open*, 5(1): e006578.

Petscher, E.S., Rey, C. & Bailey, J.S. (2009) A review of empirical support for differential reinforcement of alternative behaviour. *Research in Developmental Disabilities*, 30: 409–425.

Petticrew, M., Bell, R. & Hunter, D. (2002) Influence of psychological coping on survival and recurrence in people with cancer: Systematic review. *British Medical Journal*, 325: 1–10.

Phillips, A.C., Gallagher, S. & Carroll, D. (2009) Social support, social intimacy, and cardiovascular reactions to acute psychological stress. *Annals of Behavioral Medicine*, 37: 38–45.

Piaget, J. (1954) *The Construction of Reality in the Child*. New York: Basic Books.

Picardi, A. & Abeni, D. (2001) Stressful life events and skin diseases: Disentangling evidence from myth. *Psychotherapy and Psychosomatics*, 70: 118–136.

Picardi, A., Abeni, D., Melchi, C.F., Puddu, P. & Paquini, P. (2000) Psychiatric morbidity in dermatological outpatients: An issue to be recognized. *British Journal of Dermatology*, *143*: 920–921.

Picchioni, M.M. et al. (2017) Familial and environmental influences on brain volumes in twins with schizophrenia. *Journal of Psychiatry Neuroscience*, *42*: 122–130.

Pierce, T.W., Grim, R.D. & King, J.S. (2005) Cardiovascular reactivity and family history. *Psychophysiology*, *42*: 125–131.

Piliavin, I.M., Rodin, J. & Piliavin, J.A. (1969) Good Samaritanism: An underground phenomenon? *Journal of Personality and Social Psychology*, *1*: 289–299.

Pilver, C.E., Kasl, S., Desai, R. & Levy, B.R. (2011) Exposure to American culture is associated with premenstrual dysphoric disorder among ethnic minority women. *Journal of Affective Disorders*, *130*(1–2): 334–341.

Pincus, T., Griffith, J., Pearce, S. & Isenberg, D. (1996) Prevalence of self-reported depression in patients with rheumatoid arthritis. *British Journal of Rheumatology*, *35*: 879–883.

Pinel, J.P.J. (2007) *Biopsychology* (7th edition). Boston, MA: Pearson.

Pinel, J.P.J. (2014) *Biopsychology* (9th edition). Boston, MA: Pearson.

Pinquart, M. & Duberstein, P.R. (2010) Associations of social networks with cancer mortality: A meta-analysis. *Oncology Hematology*, *75*: 122–137.

Plotsky, P.M., Owens, M.J. & Nemeroff, C.B. (1998) Psychoneuroendocrinology of depression: Hypothalamic-pituitary-adrenal axis. *Psychiatric Clinics of North America*, *21*: 293–307.

Poncet, M.C., Toullic, P., Papazian, L., Kentish-Barnes, N., Timsit, J.F., Pochard, F., Chevret, S., Schlemmer, B. & Azoulay, E. (2007) Burnout syndrome in critical care nursing staff. *American Journal of Respiratory and Critical Care Medicine*, *175*(7): 698–704.

Ponsford, J. (2004) Rehabilitation following traumatic brain injury and cerebrovascular accident, in J. Ponsford (ed.), *Cognitive and Behavioral Rehabilitation*. New York: Guilford Press. pp. 299–342.

Pope, H.G. et al. (2006) Binge eating disorder: A stable syndrome. *American Journal of Psychology*, *163*: 2181–2183.

Popham, F. & Mitchell, R. (2006) Leisure time exercise and personal circumstances in the working age population. *Journal of Epidemiology and Community Health*, *60*: 270–274.

Porcelli, P., Leoci, C., Guerra, V., Taylor, G.J. & Bagby, R.M. (1996) A longitudinal study of alexithymia and psychological distress in inflammatory bowel disease. *Journal of Psychosomatic Research*, *41*: 569–573.

Porter, A.C. et al. (2016) Predictors and outcomes of health-related quality of life in adults with CKD. *Clinical Journal of the American Society of Nephrology*, *11*: 1154–1162.

Posner, M.I. & Petersen, S.E. (1990) The attention system of the human brain. *Annual Review of Neuroscience*, *13*: 25–42.

Powell, R. et al. (2016) Psychological preparation and postoperative outcomes for adults undergoing surgery under general anaesthesia. *Cochrane Database of Systematic Reviews*, *5* (Art. CD008646).

Powers, M.B., Vedel, E. & Emmelkamp, P.M.G. (2008) Behavioural couples therapy (BCT) for alcohol and drug use disorders: A meta-analysis. *Clincial Psychology Review*, *28*: 952–962.

Pressman, S.D. & Black, L. (2012) *The Oxford Handbook of Psychoneuroimmunology*. Oxford: Oxford Univesrsity Press.

Pressman, S.D. & Cohen, S. (2005) Does positive affect influence health? *Psychological Bulletin*, *131*: 925–971.

Presson, P.K. & Benassi, V.A. (1996) Locus of control orientation and depressive symptomatology: A meta-analysis. *Journal of Social Behavior & Personality*, *11*: 201–212.

Price, D.D. et al. (2007) Placebo analgesia is accompanied by large reductions in pain-related brain activity in irritable bowel syndrome patients. *Pain*, *127*: 63–72.

Price, J. et al. (2006) Attitudes of women with chronic pelvic pain to the gynaecological consultation. *British Journal of Obsetrics & Gynaecology*, *113*: 446–452.

Price, J.R. & Couper, J. (2000) Cognitive behaviour therapy for chronic fatigue syndrome in adults. *Cochrane Database of Systematic Reviews*, *1* (Art. CD001027).

Price, J.R., Mitchell, E., Tidy, E. & Hunot, V. (2008) Cognitive behaviour therapy for chronic fatigue syndrome in adults. *Cochrane Database of Systematic Reviews*, *3* (Art. CD001027).

Priest, R.G., Vize, C., Roberts, A., Roberts, M. & Tylee, A. (1996) Lay people's attitudes to treatment of depression: Results of opinion poll for Defeat Depression Campaign just before its launch. *British Medical Journal*, *313*: 858–859.

Prigatano, G.P. (1999) *Principles of Neuropsychological Rehabilitation*. Oxford: Oxford University Press.

Pritchard, S.E. et al. (2015) Effect of experimental stress on the small bowel and colon in healthy humans. *Neurogastroenterology & Motility*, *27*: 542–549.

Prochaska, J.O. & DiClemente, C.C. (1983) Stages and processes of self-change of smoking: Toward an integrative model of change. *Journal of Consulting and Clinical Psychology*, *51*: 390–395.

Prochaska, J.O., Velicer, W.F., Fava, J.L., Rossi, J.S. & Tsoh, J.Y. (2001) Evaluating a population-based recruitment approach and a stage-based expert system intervention for smoking cessation. *Addictive Behaviors*, *26*: 583–602.

Proudfoot, J. et al. (2004) Clinical efficacy of computerised cognitive-behavioural therapy for anxiety and depression in primary care: Randomised controlled trial. *British Journal of Psychiatry*, *185*: 46–54.

Proudfoot, J., Goldberg, D.P., Mann, A. et al. (2003) Computerised, interactive, multimedia cognitive behaviour therapy for anxiety and depression in general practice. *Psychological Medicine*, *33*: 217–227.

Purnell, T.S. et al. (2013) Comparison of life participation activities among adults treated by hemodialysis, peritoneal dialysis, and kidney transplantation: A systematic review. *American Journal of Kidney Disease*, *62*: 953–973.

Pyett, P. et al. (2005) Using hormone treatment to reduce the adult height of tall girls: Are women satisfied with the decision in later years? *Social Science & Medicine*, *61*: 1629–1639.

Qamar, N., Pappalardo, A.A., Arora, V.M. & Press, V.G. (2011) Patient-centered care and its effect on outcomes in the treatment of asthma. *Patient Related Outcome Measures*, *2*: 81–109.

Quirk, S.E. et al. (2016) Population prevalence of personality disorder and associations with physical health comorbidities and health care service utilization: A review. *Personal Disorders*, *7*: 136–146.

Rajaratnam, S.M.W. et al. (2009) Melatonin agonist tasimelteon (VEC-162) for transient insomnia after sleep-time shift: Two randomised controlled multicentre trials. *Lancet, 373*: 482–491.

Ramchand, R., Marshall, G.N., Schell, T.L. & Jaycox, L.H. (2008) Posttraumatic distress and physical functioning: A longitudinal study of injured survivors of community violence. *Journal of Consulting and Clinical Psychology, 76*: 668–676.

Ramirez, A.J. et al. (1996) Mental health of hospital consultants: The effects of stress and satisfaction at work. *Lancet, 347*: 724–728.

Ranson, K.E. & Urichuk, L.J. (2008) The effect of parent-child attachment relationships on child biopsychosocial outcomes: A review. *Early Child Development and Care, 178*: 129–152.

Rao, J.K., Anderson, L.A., Inui, T.S. & Frankel, R.M. (2007) Communication interventions make a difference in conversations between physicians and patients: A systematic review of the evidence. *Medical Care, 45*: 340–349.

Rapkin, A. (2003) A review of treatment of premenstrual syndrome and premenstrual dysphoric disorder. *Psychoneuroendocrinology, 28*: 39–53.

Rapkin, A.J. & Lewis, E.I. (2013) Treatment of premenstrual dysphoric disorder. *Women's Health, 9*(6): 537–56.

Rasmussen, H.N., Scheier, M.F. & Greenhouse, J.B. (2009) Optimism and physical health: A meta-analytic review. *Annals of Behavioral Medicine, 37*(3): 239–256.

Raven, B.H. (1965) Social influence and power, in I.D. Steiner & M. Fishbein (eds), *Current Studies in Social Psychology*. New York: Holt, Reinhart & Winston. pp. 399–444.

Ravi, D.K., Kumar, N. & Singhi, P. (2016) Effectiveness of virtual reality rehabilitation for children and adolescents with cerebral palsy: An updated evidence-based systematic review. *Physiotherapy*, 26 September. http://dx.doi.org/10.1016/j.physio.2016.08. [Epub ahead of print].

Rayan, A. & Ahmad, M. (2017) Mindfulness and parenting distress among parents of children with disabilities: A literature review. *Perspectives on Psychiatric Care*, March. doi: 10.1111/ppc.12217. [Epub ahead of print].

Read, J., van Os, J., Morrison, A.P. & Ross, C.A. (2005) Childhood trauma, psychosis and schizophrenia: A literature review with theoretical and clinical implications. *Acta Psychiatrica Scandinavica, 112*: 330–350.

Rees, K., Bennett, P., West, R., Davey, S.G. & Ebrahim, S. (2004) Psychological interventions for coronary heart disease. *Cochrane Database of Systematic Reviews, 2* (Art. CD002902).

Rehm, J. et al. (2017) The relationship between different dimensions of alcohol use and the burden of disease – an update. *Addiction, 112*(6): 968–1001. doi: 10.1111/add.13757.

Rehman, S.U., Neater, P.J., Cope, D.W. & Kilpatrick, A.O. (2005) What to wear today? Effect of doctor's attire on the trust and confidence of patients. *American Journal of Medicine, 118*: 1279–1286.

Reiche, E.M.V., Nunes, S.O.V. & Morimoto, H.K. (2004) Stress, depression, the immune system, and cancer. *Lancet Oncology, 5*: 617–625.

Reiner, M., Niermann, C., Jekauc, D. & Woll, A. (2013) Long-term health benefits of physical activity: A systematic review of longitudinal studies. *BMC Public Health, 13*: 813.

Reiss, S., Peterson, R.A., Gursky, D.M. & McNally, R.J. (1986) Anxiety sensitivity, anxiety frequency and the prediction of fearfulness. *Behaviour Research & Therapy, 24*: 1–8.

Ren, Y., Yang, H., Browning, C., Thomas, S. & Liu, M. (2015) Performance of screening tools in detecting major depressive disorder among patients with coronary heart disease: A systematic review. *Medical Science Monitor, 21*: 646–653.

Rennung, M. & Göritz, A.S. (2016) Prosocial consequences of interpersonal synchrony: A meta-analysis. *Z Psychology, 224*(3): 168–189.

Revol, O., Milliez, N. & Gerard, D. (2015) Psychological impact of acne on 21st-century adolescents: Decoding for better care. *British Journal of Dermatology, 172*(Suppl. 1): 52–58.

Rey, E. & Talley, N.J. (2009) Irritable bowel syndrome: Novel views on the epidemiology and potential risk factors. *Digestive and Liver Disease, 41*: 772–780.

Reyna, V.F. et al. (2009) How numeracy influences risk comprehension and medical decision making. *Psychological Bulletin, 135*: 943–973.

Reynolds, A.C. & Banks, S. (2010) Total sleep deprivation, chronic sleep restriction and sleep disruption. *Progress in Brain Research, 185*: 91–103.

Reynolds, C.F., Kupfer, D.J., Hoch, C.C., Stack, J.A., Houck, P.R. & Berman, S.R. (1986) Sleep deprivation in healthy elderly men and women: Effects on mood and on sleep during recovery. *Sleep, 9*: 492–501.

Rhudy, J.L. & Meagher, M.W. (2000) Fear and anxiety: Divergent effects on human pain thresholds. *Pain, 84*: 65–75.

Ricciardi, R., & Tommaso de Paolis, L. (2014) A comprehensive review of serious games in health professions. *International Journal of Computer Games Technology*, Article ID 787968, 11 pages. http://dx.doi.org/10.1155/2014/787968

Rice, F., Jones, I. & Thapar, A. (2007) The impact of gestational stress and prenatal growth on emotional problems in offspring: A review. *Acta Psychiatrica Scandinavica, 115*: 171–183.

Richardson, E.M., Schüz, N., Sanderson, K., Scott, J.L. & Schüz, B. (2016) Illness representations, coping, and illness outcomes in people with cancer: A systematic review and meta-analysis. *Psycho-Oncology*, July. doi: 10.1002/pon.4213.

Richardson, P. (2006) National Clinical Practice Guidelines (NICE Guidelines on Depression) – Core interventions in the management of depression in primary & secondary care. *APP Newsletter, 34*: 2–5.

Richters, J. et al. (2003a) Sexual difficulties. *Australian and New Zealand Journal of Public Health, 27*: 164–170.

Richters, J. et al. (2003b) Sexual and emotional satisfaction in regular relationships. *Australian and New Zealand Journal of Public Health, 27*: 171–179.

Ridsdale, L. et al. (2001) Chronic fatigue in general practice: Is counselling as good as cognitive behaviour therapy? A UK randomised trial. *British Journal of General Practice, 51*: 19–24.

Riebl, S.K. et al. (2015) A systematic literature review and meta-analysis: The Theory of Planned Behavior's application to understand and predict nutrition-related behaviors in youth. *Eating Behaviors, 18*: 160–178.

Rimondini, M. (2015) How do national cultures influence lay people's preferences toward doctors' style of communication? A comparison of 35 focus groups from an European cross national research. *BMC Public Health, 15*: 1239.

Rissel, C.E., Richters, J., Grulich, A.E., de Visser, R.O. & Smith A.M.A. (2003) Attitudes toward sex in a representative sample of adults. *Australian & New Zealand Journal of Public Health, 27*: 118–123.

Ritz, T. & Roth, W.T. (2003) Behavioral interventions in asthma. *Behavior Modification, 27*: 710–730.

Roalf, D.R. et al. (2013) Comparative accuracies of two common screening instruments for classification of Alzheimer's disease, mild cognitive impairment, and healthy aging. *Alzheimer's and Dementia*, *3*(9): 529–537.

Roberts, A.R. (2005) *Crisis Intervention Handbook: Assessment, Treatment, and Research* (3rd edition). Oxford: Oxford University Press.

Robertson, I.M., Jordan, J.M. & Whitlock, F.A. (1975) Emotions and skin (II): The conditioning of scratch responses in cases of lichen simplex. *British Journal of Dermatology*, *92*: 407–412.

Robine, J.M. et al. (2007) Who will care for the oldest people in our ageing society? *British Medical Journal*, *334*: 570–571.

Robinson, J. et al. (2009) Self-medication of anxiety disorders with alcohol and drugs: Results from a nationally representative sample. *Journal of Anxiety Disorders*, *23*: 38–45.

Robles, T.F., Slatcher, R.B., Trombello, J.M. & McGinn, M.M. (2014) Marital quality and health: A meta-analytic review. *Psychological Bulletin*, *140*: 140–187.

Rodenburg, G. et al. (2014) Associations of parental feeding styles with child snacking behaviour and weight in the context of general parenting. *Public Health Nutrition*, *17*: 960–969.

Roerecke, M. & Rehm, J. (2014a) Alcohol consumption drinking patterns and ischaemic heart disease: A narrative review of meta-analyses and a systematic review and meta-analysis of the impact of heavy drinking occasions on risk for moderate drinkers. *BMC Medicine*, *12*: 182.

Roerecke, M. & Rehm, J. (2014b) Chronic heavy drinking and ischaemic heart disease: A systematic review and meta-analysis. *Open Heart*, *1*: e000135.

Rogers, C. (1951) *Client-centered Therapy: Its Current Practice, Implications and Theory*. London: Constable.

Rohling, M.L., Faust, M.E., Beverly, B. & Demakis, G. (2009) Effectiveness of cognitive rehabilitation following acquired brain injury: A meta-analytic re-examination of Cicerone et al. 's (2000, 2005) systematic reviews. *Neuropsychology*, *23*(1): 20–39.

Rohrer, J.M., Egloff, B. & Schmukle, S.C. (2015) Examining the effects of birth order on personality. *Proceedings of the National Academy of Science USA*, *112*(46): 14224–14229.

Roig, E., Castaner, A., Simmons, B., Patel, R., Ford, E. & Cooper, R. (1987) In-hospital mortality rates from acute myocardial infarction by race in US hospitals: Findings from the National Hospital Discharge Survey. *Circulation*, *76*: 280–288.

Ropacki, S.A. & Jeste, D.V. (2005) Epidemiology of and risk factors for psychosis of Alzheimer's Disease. *American Journal of Psychiatry*, *162*: 2022–2030.

Rosen, M.I., Ryan, C. & Rigsby, M. (2002) Motivational enhancement and MEMS review to improve medication adherence. *Behaviour Change*, *19*: 183–190.

Rosenblatt, A. & Leroi, I. (2000) Neuropsychiatry of Huntington's Disease and other basal ganglia disorders. *Psychosomatics*, *41*: 24–30.

Rosendal, M., Olde Hartman, T.C., Aamland, A., van der Horst, H., Lucassen, P., Budtz-Lilly, A. & Burton, C. (2017) 'Medically unexplained' symptoms and symptom disorders in primary care: prognosis-based recognition and classification. *BMC Family Practice*,18(1):18.

Rosenstock, I.M. (1974) Historical origins of the Health Belief Model. *Health Education Monographs*, *2*: 1–8.

Rosenzweig, J., Blaizot, A., Cougot, N., Pegon-Machat, E., Hamel, O., Apelian, N., Bedos, C., Munoz-Sastre, M.T. & Vergnes, J.N. (2016) Effect of a person-centered course on the empathic ability of dental students. *Journal of Dental Education*, 80(11): 1337–1348.

Ross, L. (1977) The intuitive psychologist and his shortcomings, in L. Berkowitz (ed.), *Advances in Experimental Social Psychology* (Vol. 10). Orlando, FL: Academic Press. pp. 173–240.

Ross L.E. & McLean, L.M. (2006) Anxiety disorders during pregnancy and the postpartum period: A systematic review. *Journal of Clinical Psychiatry*, 67: 1285–98.

Roter, D.L. & Hall, J.A. (2004) Physician gender and patient-centered communication: A critical review of empirical research. *Annual Review of Public Health*, 25: 497–519.

Roter, D.L., Hall, J.A. & Katz, N.R. (1988) Patient-physician communication: A descriptive summary of the literature. *Patient Education & Counseling*, 12: 99–119.

Roth, A. & Fonagy, P. (2004) *What Works for Whom? A Critical Review of Psychotherapy Research* (2nd edition). New York: Guilford Press.

Rothman, A.J. & Salovey, P. (1997) Shaping perceptions to motivate healthy behavior: The role of message framing. *Psychological Bulletin*, 121: 3–19.

Rouhe, H., Salmela-Aro, K., Halmesmäki, E. & Saisto, T. (2009) Fear of childbirth according to parity, gestational age, and obstetric history. *British Journal of Obstetrics & Gynaecology*, 116(1): 67–73.

Rouleau, C.R., Garland, S.N. & Carlson, L.E. (2015) The impact of mindfulness-based interventions on symptom burden, positive psychological outcomes, and biomarkers in cancer patients. *Cancer Management and Research*, 7: 121–131.

Rovito, M.J. et al. (2015) Interventions promoting testicular self-examination (TSE) performance: A systematic review. *American Journal of Men's Health*, 9: 506–518.

Rowles, S.V., Prieto, L., Badia, X., Shalet, S.M., Webb, S.M. & Trainer, P.J. (2005) Quality of Life (QOL) in patients with acromegaly is severely impaired. *Journal of Clinical Endocrinology & Metabolism*, 90: 3337–3341.

Roy, T. & Lloyd, C.E. (2012) Epidemiology of depression and diabetes: A systematic review. *Journal of Affective Disorders*, 142: s8–s21.

Rozin, P., Haidt, J. & McCauley, C.R. (2000) Disgust, in M. Lewis & J.M. Haviland Jones (eds), *Handbook of Emotions* (2nd edition). New York: Guilford. pp. 637–652.

Rudberg, L., Nilsson, S., Wikblad, K. & Carlsson, M. (2005) Testicular cancer and testicular self-examination: Knowledge and attitudes of adolescent Swedish men. *Cancer Nursing*, 28: 256–262.

Ruffault, A., Czernichow, S., Hagger, M.S., Ferrand, M., Erichot, N., Carette, C., Boujut, E. & Flahault, C. (2016) The effects of mindfulness training on weight-loss and health-related behaviours in adults with overweight and obesity: A systematic review and meta-analysis. *Obesity Research & Clinical Practice*, 19 September, pii: S1871-403X(16)30083-7. doi: 10.1016/j.orcp.2016.09.002. [Epub ahead of print].

Ruiter, R.A. et al. (2014) Sixty years of fear appeal research: Current state of the evidence. *International Journal of Psychology*, 49(2): 63–70.

Ruotsalainen, J.H., Verbeek, J.H., Mariné, A. & Serra, C. (2015) Preventing occupational stress in healthcare workers. *Cochrane Database of Systematic Reviews*, 7(4) (Art. CD002892).

Russell, S.L. et al. (2017) An experimental analysis of the affect regulation model of binge eating. *Appetite*, 110: 44–50. (doi: 10.1016/j.appet.2016.12.007)

Ruta, D.A., Garratt, A.M., Leng, M., Russell, I.T. & MacDonald, L.M. (1994) A new approach to the measurement of quality of life: The Patient-Generated Index. *Medical Care*, 32(11): 1109–1126.

Rutishauser, C., Esslinger, A., Bond, L. & Sennhauser, F.H. (2003) Consultations with adolescents: The gap between their expectations and their experiences. *Acta Pædiatrica*, 92: 1322–1326.

Ryback, R.S. & Lewis, O.F. (1971) Effects of prolonged bed rest on EEG sleep patterns in young, healthy volunteers. *Electroencephalography & Clinical Neurophysiology*, 31: 395–399.

Ryding, E.L., Lukasse, M., Parys, A.S., Wangel, A.M., Karro, H., Kristjansdottir, H., Schroll, A.M., Schei, B. & Bidens Group (2015) Fear of childbirth and risk of cesarean delivery: A cohort study in six European countries. *Birth*, 42(1): 48–55.

Ryu, E. et al. (2016) Quantifying the impact of chronic conditions on a diagnosis of major depressive disorder in adults: A cohort study using linked electronic medical records. *BMC Psychiatry*, 16: 114.

Saab, M.M. et al. (2016) Testicular cancer awareness and screening practices: A systematic review. *Oncology Nursing Forum*, 43: E8–E23.

Sabini, J. & Silver, M. (2005) Ekman's basic emotions: Why not love and jealousy? *Cognition & Emotion*, 19: 693–712.

Sackett, D.L., Rosenberg, W.M.C., Gray, J.A.M., Haynes, R.B. & Richardson, W.S. (1996) Evidence based medicine: What it is and what it isn't. *British Medical Journal*, 312: 71–72.

Sajadinejad, M.S. et al. (2012) Psychological issues in inflammatory bowel disease: An overview. *Gastroenterology Research and Practice*, Art. 106502 (11 pages). doi: 10.1155/2012/106502.

Salkovskis, P.M., Hackmann, A., Wells, A., Gelder, M.G. & Clark, D.M. (2006) Belief disconfirmation versus habituation processes to situational exposure in panic disorder with agoraphobia: A pilot study. *Behaviour Research and Therapy*, 45: 877–885.

Salomonsson, B., Gullberg, M.T., Alehagen, S. & Wijma, K. (2013) Self-efficacy beliefs and fear of childbirth in nulliparous women. *Journal of Psychosomatic Obstetrics and Gynaecology*, 34(3): 116–121.

Sanada, K., Alda Díez, M., Salas Valero, M., Pérez-Yus, M.C., Demarzo, M.M., Montero-Marín, J., García-Toro, M. & García-Campayo, J. (2017) Effects of mindfulness-based interventions on biomarkers in healthy and cancer populations: A systematic review. *BMC Complementary and Alternative Medicine*, 17(1): 125.

Sanada, K., Montero-Marin, J., Alda Díez, M., Salas-Valero, M., Pérez-Yus, M.C., Morillo, H., Demarzo, M.M., García-Toro, M. & García-Campayo, J. (2016) Effects of mindfulness-based interventions on salivary cortisol in healthy adults: A meta-analytical review. *Frontiers in Physiology*, 7: 471.

Sandberg, S. et al. (2000) The role of acute and chronic stress in asthma attacks in children. *Lancet*, 356: 982–987.

Sanders, S. & Reinisch, J. (1999) Would you say you 'had sex' if…? *Journal of the American Medical Association*, 281: 275–277.

Sandhu, H. et al. (2009) The impact of gender dyads on doctor-patient communication: A systematic review. *Patient Education and Counselling*, 76: 348–355.

Sansom-Daly, U.M., Peate, M., Wakefield, C.E., Bryant, R.A. & Cohn, R.J. (2012) A systematic review of psychological interventions for adolescents and young adults living with chronic illness. *Health Psychology*, 31(3): 380–393.

Santos, J., Alonso, C., Vicario, M., Ramos, L., Lobo, B. & Malagelada, J.R. (2008) Neuropharmacology of stress-induced mucosal inflammation: Implications for inflammatory bowel disease and irritable bowel syndrome. *Current Molecular Medicine*, 8: 258–273.

Saracci, R. (1997) The World Health Organisation needs to reconsider its definition of health. *British Medical Journal*, 314: 1409.

Sarafino, E.P. (2002) *Health Psychology: Biopsychosocial Interactions* (5th edition). Hoboken, NJ: Wiley.

Saunders, K.A. & Hawton, K. (2006) Suicidal behaviour and the menstrual cycle. *Psychological Medicine*, 36: 901–912.

Savage, L.J. (1954) *The Foundations of Statistics*. New York: Wiley.

Sawyer, A., Ayers, S. & Field, A. (2010) Posttraumatic growth and adjustment among individuals with cancer or HIV/AIDS: A meta-analysis. *Clinical Psychology Review*, 30 (4): 436–447.

Saxby, D.E. (2017) Birth of a new perspective? A call for biopsychosocial research on childbirth. *Current Directions in Psychological Science*, 26(1): 81–86.

Sayette, M.A. (2007) Alcohol abuse, in S. Ayers et al. (eds) *Cambridge Handbook of Psychology, Health and Medicine* (2nd edition). Cambridge: Cambridge University Press. pp. 534–537.

Sayin, A., Mutluay, R. & Sindel, S. (2007) Quality of life in hemodialysis, peritoneal dialysis, and transplantation patients. *Transplantation Proceedings*, 39: 3047–3053.

Schablon, A., Zeh, A., Wendeler, D. et al., (2012) Frequency and consequences of violence and aggression toward employees in the German healthcare and welfare system: a cross-sectional study. *BMJ Open*, 2: e001420.

Scharloo, M., Kaptein, A.A., Weinman, J., Hazes, J.M., Breedveld, F.C. & Rooijmans, H.G.M. (1999) Predicting functional status in patients with rheumatoid arthritis. *Journal of Rheumatology*, 26: 1686–1693.

Schaumberg, K. et al. (2016) Dietary restraint: What's the harm? A review of the relationship between dietary restraint, weight trajectory and the development of eating pathology. *Clinical Obesity*, 6: 89–100.

Schedlowski, M. & Tewes, U. (1992) Physiological arousal and perception of bodily state during parachute jumping. *Psychophysiology*, 29: 95–103.

Scheier, M.F., Carver, C.S. & Bridges, M.W. (1994) Distinguishing optimism from neuroticism (and trait anxiety, self-mastery, and self-esteem): A re-evaluation of the Life Orientation Test. *Journal of Personality and Social Psychology*, 67: 1063–1078.

Schenker, Y. et al. (2011) Interventions to improve patient comprehension in informed consent for medical and surgical procedures: a systematic review. *Medical Decision Making*, 31: 151–173.

Schiavone, S. et al. (2015) Impact of early life stress on the pathogenesis of mental disorders: Relation to brain oxidative stress. *Current Pharmaceutical Design*, 21: 1404–1412.

Schneider, M.L., Moore, C.F., Roberts, A.D. & Dejesus, O. (2001) Prenatal stress alters early neurobehavior, stress reactivity and learning in non-human primates: A brief review. *Stress*, 4: 183–193.

Schomerus, G., Schwahn, C., Holzinger, A., Corrigan, P.W., Grabe, H.J., Carta, M.G. & Angermeyer, M.C. (2012) Evolution of public attitudes about mental illness: A systematic review and meta-analysis. *Acta Psychiatrica Scandinavica*, 125: 440–452.

Schoretsanitis, G., Kutynia A., Stegmayer, K., Strik, W. & Walther, S. (2016) Keep at bay! Abnormal personal space regulation as marker of paranoia in schizophrenia. *European Psychiatry*, *31*: 1–7.

Schout, B.M.A., Hendrikx, A.J.M., Scheele, F., Bemelmans, B.M.H. & Scherpbier, A.J.J.A. (2010) Validation and implementation of surgical simulators: A critical review of present, past, and future. *Surgery & Endoscopy*, *24*: 536–546.

Schouten, B.C. & Meeuwesen, L. (2006) Cultural differences in medical communication: A review of the literature. *Patient Education and Counselling*, *64*: 21–34.

Schreiner, P.J. (2016) Emerging cardiovascular risk research: Impact of pets on cardiovascular risk prevention. *Current Cardiovascular Risk Reports*, *10*(2).

Schrimpf, M. et al. (2015) The effect of sleep deprivation on pain perception in healthy subjects: A meta-analysis. *Sleep Medicine*, *16*: 1313–1320.

Schuster, R., Bornovalova, M. & Hunt, E. (2012) The influence of depression on the progression of HIV: Direct and indirect effects. *Behavior Modification*, *36*: 123–45.

Schwartz, G. (1982) Testing the biopsychosocial model: The ultimate challenge facing behavioural medicine? *Journal of Consulting and Clinical Psychology*, *50*: 1040–1053.

Schwarz, J.K. (2004) Responding to persistent requests for assistance in dying: A phenomenological inquiry. *International Journal of Palliative Nursing*, *10*: 225–235.

Scott, W. & McCracken, L.M. (2018) Chronic pain, in C.D. Llewellyn et al. (eds), *The Cambridge Handbook of Psychology, Health and Medicine* (3rd edition). Cambridge: Cambridge University Press.

Scottish Intercollegiate Guidelines Network (SIGN) (2012) *Management of Perinatal Mood Disorders*. SIGN publication no. 127. Edinburgh: SIGN, www.sign.ac.uk/guidelines/full text/127/.

Seale, C. (2008) *Constructing Death: The Sociology of Dying and Bereavement* (2nd edition). Cambridge: Cambridge University Press.

Sechrest, L. & Wallace, J. (1964) Figure drawings and naturally occurring events: Elimination of the expansive euphoria hypothesis. *Journal of Educational Psychology*, *55*: 42–44.

Sedgh, G., Finer, L.B., Bankole, A., Eilers, M.A. & Singh, S. (2015) Adolescent pregnancy, birth, and abortion rates across countries: Levels and recent trends. *Journal of Adolescent Health*, *56*: 223–230.

Segal, Z.V., Williams, J.M.G. & Teasdale, J.D. (2002) *Mindfulness-Based Cognitive Therapy for Depression: A New Approach for Preventing Relapse*. New York: Guilford Press.

Segerstrom, S.C. (2005) Optimism and immunity: Do positive thoughts always lead to positive effects? *Brain, Behavior, and Immunity*, *19*: 195–200.

Segerstrom, S.C. & Miller, G.E. (2004) Psychological stress and the human immune system: A meta-analytic study of 30 years of inquiry. *Psychological Bulletin*, *130*(4): 601–630.

Segerstrom, S.C., Taylor, S.E., Kemeny, M.E. & Fahey, J.L. (1998) Optimism is associated with mood, coping, and immune change in response to stress. *Journal of Personality and Social Psychology*, *74*: 1646–1655.

Seibt, B., Häfner, M. & Deutsch, R. (2007) Prepared to eat: How immediate affective and motivational responses to food cues are influenced by food deprivation. *European Journal of Social Psychology*, *37*: 359–379.

Selic, P. et al. (2011) What factors affect patients' recall of general practitioners' advice? *BMC Family Practice*, 12: 141.

Seligman, M.E.P. (1975) *Helplessness: On Depression, Development, and Death*. San Francisco, CA: W.H. Freeman.

Selye, H. (1956) *The Stress of Life*. New York: McGraw-Hill.

Sep, M.S. (2014) The power of clinicians' affective communication: How reassurance about non-abandonment can reduce patients' physiological arousal and increase information recall in bad news consultations: An experimental study using analogue patients. *Patient Education and Counselling*, 95: 45–52.

Shack, L. et al. (2008) Variation in incidence of breast, lung and cervical cancer and malignant melanoma of the skin by socioeconomic group in England. *BMC Cancer*, 8: 1–10.

Shanafelt, T.D., Boone, S., Tan, L., Dyrbye, L.N., Sotile, W., Satele, D., West, C.P., Sloan, J. & Oreskovich, M.R. (2012) Burnout and satisfaction with work-life balance among US physicians relative to the general US population. *Archives of Internal Medicine*, 8, 1377–1385.

Shand, L.K., Cowlishaw, S., Brooker, J.E., Burney, S. & Ricciardelli, L.A. (2015) Correlates of post-traumatic stress symptoms and growth in cancer patients: A systematic review and meta-analysis. *Psycho-Oncology*, 24(6): 624–634.

Shapiro, D.E., Boggs, S.R, Melamed, B.G. & Graham-Pole, J. (1992) The effect of varied physician affect on recall, anxiety, and perceptions in women at risk for breast cancer: An analogue study. *Health Psychology*, 11, 61–66.

Sharma, N., Classen, J. & Cohen, L.G. (2013) Neural plasticity and its contribution to functional recovery. *Handbook of Clinical Neurology*, 110: 3–12.

Sharpe, M. (2013) Somatic symptoms: Beyond 'medically unexplained'. *British Journal of Psychiatry*, 203: 320–321.

Sharpley, C.F., Halat, J., Rabinowicz, T., Weiland, B. & Stafford, J. (2001) Standard posture, postural mirroring, and client-perceived rapport. *Counselling Psychology Quarterly*, 14: 267–280.

Sheeran, P. et al. (1999) Psychosocial correlates of condom use. *Psychological Bulletin*, 125: 90–132.

Shenefelt, P.D. (2010) Psychological interventions in the management of common skin conditions. *Psychology Research and Behavior Management*, 3: 51–63.

Shenefelt, P.D. (2011) Psychodermatological disorders: Recognition and treatment. *International Journal of Dermatology*, 50: 1309–1322.

Sheps, D.S. et al. (2002) Mental stress-induced ischemia and all-cause mortality in patients with coronary artery disease: Results from the psychophysiological investigations of myocardial ischemia study. *Circulation*, 105: 1780–1784.

Shields, C.G. et al. (2009) Patient-centered communication and prognosis discussions with cancer patients. *Patient Education and Counseling*, 77: 437–442.

Shimada-Sugimoto, M. et al. (2015) Genetics of anxiety disorders: Genetic epidemiological and molecular studies in humans. *Psychiatry and Clinical Neurosciences*, 69: 388–401.

Shin, H. & Kim, K. (2015) Virtual reality for cognitive rehabilitation after brain injury: A systematic review. *Journal of Physical Therapy Science*, 27(9): 2999–3002.

Shin, J.K. et al. (2011) Schizophrenia: A systematic review of the disease state, current therapeutics and their molecular mechanisms of action. *Current Medical Chemistry*, 18: 1380–1404.

Shraim, M., Mallen, C.D. & Dunn, K.M. (2013) GP consultations for medically unexplained physical symptoms in parents and their children: a systematic review. *British Journal of General Practice*, *63*(610): e318–e325.

Siegfried, N. et al. (2011) Antiretrovirals for reducing the risk of mother-to-child transmission of HIV infection. *Cochrane Database of Systematic Reviews*, *7* (Art. CD003510).

Silva, A.C., Dos Santos Ferreira, S., Alves, R.C., Follador, L. & Da Silva, S.G. (2016) Effect of music tempo on attentional focus and perceived exertion during self-selected paced walking. *International Journal of Exercise Science*, *9*(4): 536–544.

Silverman, D.H.S., Munakata, J.A., Ennes, H., Mandelkern, M.A., Hoh, C.K. & Mayer, E.A. (1997) Regional cerebral activity in normal and pathological perception of visceral pain. *Gastroenterology*, *112*: 64–72.

Silverman, J., Kurtz, S. & Draper, J. (2013) *Skills for Communicating with Patients* (3rd edition). Oxford: Radcliff Medical Press.

Simoni, J.M., Pearson, C.R., Pantalone, D.W., Marks, G. & Crepaz, N. (2006) Efficacy of interventions in improving highly active antiretroviral therapy adherence and HIV-1 RNA viral load: A meta-analytic review of randomized controlled trials. *Journal of Acquired Immune Deficiency Syndromes*, *43*: s23–s35.

Simons, G., Mallen, C.D., Kumar, K., Stack, R.J. & Raza, K. (2015) A qualitative investigation of the barriers to help-seeking among members of the public presented with symptoms of new-onset rheumatoid arthritis. *Journal of Rheumatology*, *42*(4): 585–592.

Singh, S., Graff, L.A. & Bernstein, C.N. (2009) Do NSAIDs, antibiotics, infections, or stress trigger flares in IBD? *American Journal of Gastroenterology*, *104*: 1298–1313.

Sinha, B., Chowdhury, R., Sankar, M.J., Martines, J., Taneja, S., Mazumder, S., Rollins, N., Bahl, R. & Bhandari, N. (2015) Interventions to improve breastfeeding outcomes: A systematic review and meta-analysis. *Acta Paediatrica*, *104*: 114–134

Sirois, F. (1992) Denial in coronary heart disease. *Canadian Medical Association Journal*, *147*: 315–321.

Skinner, B.F. (1957) *Verbal Behaviour*. Acton, MA: Copley.

Skokou, M., Soubasi, E. & Gourzis, P. (2012) Depression in multiple sclerosis: A review of assessment and treatment approaches in adult and pediatric populations. *ISRN Neurology*, Art. 427102 (6 pages). doi: 10.5402/2012/427102.

Sloboda, J.A., Davidson, J.W. & Howe, M.J.A. (1994) Is everyone musical? *The Psychologist*, *7*: 349–354.

Smedslund, G., Dalsb, T.K., Steiro, A.K., Winsvold, A. & Clench-Aas, J. (2007) Cognitive behavioural therapy for men who physically abuse their female partner. *Cochrane Database of Systematic Reviews*, *3* (Art. CD006048).

Smink, F.R., van Hoeken, D. & Hoek, H.W. (2012) Epidemiology of eating disorders: Incidence, prevalence and mortality rates. *Current Psychiatry Reports*, *14*: 406–414.

Smith, J. (2007) From base evidence through to evidence base: A consideration of the NICE guidelines. *Psychoanalytic Psychotherapy*, *21*: 40–60.

Smith, T.P., Kennedy, S.L. & Fleshner, M. (2004) Influence of age and physical activity on the primary in vivo antibody and T cell–mediated responses in men, *Journal of Applied Physiology*, *97*: 491–498.

Smith, T.W. & MacKenzie, J. (2006) Personality and risk of physical illness. *Annual Review of Clinical Psychology*, *2*: 435–467.

Soler, J.K., Yaman, H., Esteva, M., Dobbs, F., Asenova, R.S., Katic, M., Ozvacic, Z., Desgranges, J.P., Moreau, A., Lionis, C., Kotányi, P., Carelli, F., Nowak, P.R., de Aguiar Sá Azeredo, Z., Marklund, E., Churchill, D. & Ungan, M. (2008) European General Practice Research Network Burnout Study Group. Burnout in European family doctors: The EGPRN study. *Journal of Family Practice*, 25(4): 245–265.

Sommer, J., Lanier, C., Perron, N.J., Nendaz, M., Clavet, D. & Audétat, M.C. (2016) A teaching skills assessment tool inspired by the Calgary-Cambridge model and the patient-centered approach. *Patient Education and Counselling*, 99(4): 600–609.

Sonino, N. et al. (2004) Persistent psychological distress in patients treated for endocrine disease. *Psychotherapy and Psychosomatics*, 73: 78–83.

Sonino, N. et al. (2007) Psychosocial approach to endocrine disease. *Advanced Psychosomatic Medicine*, 28: 21–33.

Sonino, N. & Fava, G.A. (2001) Psychiatric disorders associated with Cushing's syndrome: Epidemiology, pathophysiology and treatment. *CNS Drugs*, 15: 361–373.

Sonino, N. & Fava, G.A. (2012) Improving the concept of recovery in endocrine disease by consideration of psychosocial issues. *Journal of Clinical Endocrinology and Metabolism*, 97: 2614–2616.

Sonnenberg, P. et al. (2013) Prevalence, risk factors and uptake of interventions for sexually transmitted infections: Findings from the British National Surveys of Sexual Attitudes and Lifestyles (Natsal). *Lancet*, 382: 1795–1806.

Soo, C. & Tate, R. (2007) Psychological treatment for anxiety in people with traumatic brain injury. *Cochrane Database of Systematic Reviews*, 3 (Art. CD005239).

Speigel, D. & Giese-Davis, J. (2003) Depression and cancer: mechanisms and disease progression. *Biological Psychiatry*, 54: 269–282.

Spence Laschinger, H.K., Leiter, M.P., Day, A., Gilin-Oore, D. & Mackinnon, S.P. (2012) Building empowering work environments that foster civility and organizational trust: Testing an intervention. *Nursing Research*, 61(5): 316–325.

Sperber, A.D. et al. (2016) The global prevalence of IBS in adults remains elusive due to the heterogeneity of studies: A Rome Foundation working team literature review. *Gut*, 27 January [online]. doi: 10.1136/gutjnl-2015-311240.

Spiegel, B., Schoenfeld, P. & Naliboff, B. (2007) Systematic review: The prevalence of suicidal behaviour in patients with chronic abdominal pain and irritable bowel syndrome. *Alimentary Pharmacology & Therapeutics*, 26: 183–193.

Spiegel, D., Bloom, J.R., Kraemer, H.C. & Gottheil, E. (1989) Effect of psychosocial treatment on survival of patients with metastatic breast cancer. *Lancet*, 334: 888–891.

Squier, R.W. (1990) A model of empathic understanding and adherence to treatment regimens in practitioner-patient relationships. *Social Science & Medicine*, 30: 325–339.

Stabler, B. et al. (1996) Links between growth hormone deficiency, adaptation and social phobia. *Hormone Research*, 45: 30–33.

Stahl, S.M. (2000) *Essential Psychopharmacology of Depression and Bipolar Disorder*. Cambridge: Cambridge University Press.

Stamps, A.E. (2011) Distance mitigates perceived threat. *Perceptual and Motor Skills*, 113(3): 751–763.

Stangier, U. (2007) Skin disorders, in S. Ayers et al. (eds) *Cambridge Handbook of Psychology, Health and Medicine* (2nd edition). Cambridge: Cambridge University Press. pp. 880–883.

Stangier, U. & Ehlers, A. (2000) Stress and anxiety in dermatological disorders, in D.I. Mostofsky & D.H. Barlow (eds), *The Management of Stress and Anxiety in Medical Disorders*. Needham Heights, MA: Allyn & Bacon. pp. 304–333.

Stapleton, A.B., Lating, J., Kirkhart, M. & Everly, G.S. (2006) Effects of medical crisis intervention on anxiety, depression, and posttraumatic stress symptoms: A meta-analysis. *Psychiatric Quarterly*, 77: 231–238.

Starkweather, A. et al. (2011) A biobehavioral perspective on depressive symptoms in patients with a cerebral astrocytoma. *Journal of Neuroscience Nursing*, 43: 17–28.

Stead, L.F., Buitrago, D., Preciado, N., Sanchez, G., Hartmann-Boyce, J. & Lancaster, T. (2013) Physician advice for smoking cessation. *Cochrane Database of Systematic Reviews*, 5 (Art. CD000165).

Steadman, L. & Quine, L. (2004) Encouraging young males to perform testicular self-examination: A simple, but effective, implementation intentions intervention. *British Journal of Health Psychology*, 9: 479–487.

Steinberg, L. & Silverberg, S. (1986) The vicissitudes of autonomy in early adolescence. *Child Development*, 57: 841–851.

Steinmetz, H., Knappstein, M., Ajzen, I., Schmidt, P. & Kabst, R. (2016) How effective are behavior change interventions based on the theory of planned behavior? A three-level meta-analysis. *Zeitschrift für Psychologie*, 224: 216–233.

Stepanovic, J., Ostojic, M., Beleslin, B., Vukovic, O., Djordjevic-Dikic, A., Giga, V., Nedeljkovic, I., Nedeljkovic, M., Stojkovic, S., Vukcevic, V., Dobric, M., Petrasinovic, Z., Marinkovic, J. & Lecic-Tosevski, D. (2012) Mental stress-induced ischemia in patients with coronary artery disease: Echocardiographic characteristics and relation to exercise-induced ischemia. *Psychosomatic Medicine*, 74: 766–772.

Steptoe, A. (2006) *Depression and Physical Illness*. Oxford: Oxford University Press.

Steptoe, A. & Ayers, S. (2005) Stress, health and illness, in S. Sutton et al. (eds), *SAGE Handbook of Health Psychology*. London: Sage. pp. 169–196.

Steptoe, A. & Brydon, L. (2009) Emotional triggering of cardiac events. *Neuroscience and Biobehavioral Reviews*, 33: 63–70.

Steptoe, A. & Kivimäki, M. (2013) Stress and cardiovascular disease: An update on current knowledge. *Annual Review of Public Health*, 34: 337–354.

Steptoe, A. & Vogele, C. (1986) Are stress responses influenced by cognitive appraisal? An experimental comparison of coping strategies. *British Journal of Psychology*, 77: 243–255.

Stevens, L. & Rodin, I. (2001) *Psychiatry*. Edinburgh: Churchill Livingstone.

Stevens, L. & Rodin, I. (2010) *Psychiatry: An Illustrated Colour Text* (2nd edition). Edinburgh: Churchill Livingstone.

Stevenson, F.A., Barry, C.A., Britten, N., Barber, N. & Bradley, C.P. (2000) Doctor–patient communication about drugs: The evidence for shared decision making. *Social Science & Medicine*, 50: 829–840.

Stewart, B.W. & Wild, C.P. (eds) (2014) *World Cancer Report 2014*. Lyon: International Agency for Research on Cancer.

Stewart, M., Belle Brown, J., McWhinney, I.R., *et al.* (1995). *Patient-centred Medicine: Transforming the Clinical Method*. Thousand Oaks, CA: Sage.

Stewart, M., Brown, J.B., Donner, A., McWhinney, I.R., Oates, J., Weston, W.W. & Jordan, J. (2000) The impact of patient-centered care on outcomes. *Journal of Family Practice*, 49(9): 796–804.

Stewart, M.A. et al. (1997) *The Impact of Patient-centred Care on Patient Outcomes in Family Practice*. London, ON: University of Western Ontario.

Stice, E. & Shaw, H. (2007) Eating disorders, in S. Ayers et al. (eds), *Cambridge Handbook of Psychology, Health and Medicine* (2nd edition). Cambridge: Cambridge University Press. pp. 690–693.

Stice, E., Shaw, H. & Marti, C.N. (2008) A meta-analytic review of eating disorder prevention programs. *Annual Review of Clinical Psychology*, 3: 207–231.

Stickgold, R., Hobson, J.A., Fosse, R. & Fosse, M. (2001) Sleep, learning, and dreams: Off-line memory reprocessing. *Science*, 294: 1052–1057.

Stiles, W.B., Barkham, M., Mellor-Clark, J. & Connell, J. (2008) Effectiveness of cognitive-behavioural, person-centred, and psychodynamic therapies in UK primary-care routine practice: Replication in a larger sample. *Psychological Medicine*, 38(5): 677–688.

Stiles, W.B., Barkam, M., Twigg, E., Mellor-Clark, J. & Cooper, M. (2006) Effectiveness of cognitive-behavioural, person-centred and psychodynamic therapies as practised in the UK National Health Service settings. *Psychological Medicine*, 36: 555–566.

Stiles-Shields, C. & Keefer, L. (2015) Web-based interventions for ulcerative colitis and Crohn's disease: Systematic review and future directions. *Clinical and Experimental Gastroenterology*, 8: 149–157.

Stinson, J., Connelly, M., Kamper, S.J., Herlin, T. & Toupin April, K. (2016) Models of care for addressing chronic musculoskeletal pain and health in children and adolescents. *Best Practice & Research: Clinical Rheumatology*, 3: 468–482.

Stockhorst, U. et al. (1998) Effects of overshadowing on conditioned nausea in cancer patients: An experimental study. *Physiology & Behaviour*, 64: 743–753.

Stockhorst, U., Steingrueber, H.J., Enck, P. & Klosterhalfen, S. (2006) Pavlovian conditioning of nausea and vomiting. *Autonomic Neuroscience: Basic & Clinical*, 129: 50–57.

Stoffers, J.M., Völlm, B.A., Rücker, G., Timmer, A., Huband, N., & Lieb, K. (2012). Psychological therapies for people with borderline personality disorder. *Cochrane Database of Systematic Reviews*. 2012 Aug 15;(8):CD005652.

Stone, A.A., Neale, J.M., Cox, D.S., Napoli, A., Valdimarsdottir, H. & Kennedy-Moore, E. (1994) Daily events are associated with a secretory immune response to an oral antigen in men. *Health Psychology*, 13: 440–446.

Stone, N. & Ingham, R. (2003) When and why do young people in the United Kingdom first use sexual health services? *Perspectives on Sexual & Reproductive Health*, 35: 114–120.

Stone, S.V. & McCrae, R.R. (2007) Personality and health, in S. Ayers et al. (eds), *Cambridge Handbook of Psychology, Health and Medicine* (2nd edition). Cambridge: Cambridge University Press. pp. 151–155.

Stones, W., Cheong, Y.C. & Howard, F.M. (2005) Interventions for treating chronic pelvic pain in women. *Cochrane Database of Systematic Reviews*, 2 (Art. CD000387).

Størksen, H.T., Garthus-Niegel, S., Vangen, S. & Eberhard-Gran, M. (2013) The impact of previous birth experiences on maternal fear of childbirth. *Acta Obstetricia et Gynecologica Scandinavica*, 92(3): 318–324.

Stramrood, C., Paarlberg, K.M., Huis In 't Veld, E.M., Berger, L.W., Vingerhoets, A.J., Schultz, W.C. & van Pampus, M.G. (2011) Post-traumatic stress disorder following childbirth in home-like and hospital settings. *Journal of Psychosomatic Obstetrics and Gynaecology*, 32(2): 88–97.

Stranges, S., Tigbe, W., Gómez-Olivé, F.X., Thorogood, M. & Kandala, N.B. (2012) Sleep problems: An emerging global epidemic? Findings from the INDEPTH WHO-SAGE study among more than 40,000 older adults from eight countries across Africa and Asia. *Sleep*, 35: 1173–1181.

Straus, S.E., Richardson, W.S., Glasziou, P. & Haynes, R.B. (2010) *Evidence-Based Medicine: How to Practice and Teach it* (4th edition). London: Elsevier.

Strecher, V.J., Chapion, V.L. & Rosenstock, I.M. (1997) The Health Belief Model and health behaviour, in D.S. Gochman (ed.), *Handbook of Health Behavior Research I: Personal and Social Determinants*. New York: Plenum Press. pp. 71–91.

Street, R.L., Makoul, G., Arora, N.K. & Epstein, R.M. (2009) How does communication heal? Pathways linking clinician–patient communication to health outcomes. *Patient Education & Counseling*, 74: 295–301.

Striegel-Moore, R.H. & Franko, D.L. (2008) Should binge eating disorder be included in the DSM-V? A critical review of the state of the evidence. *Annual Review of Clinical Psychology*, 4: 305–324.

Stroebe, M., Schut, H. & Stroebe, W. (2007) Coping with bereavement, in S. Ayers et al. (eds), *Cambridge Handbook of Psychology, Health and Medicine* (2nd edition). Cambridge: Cambridge University Press. pp. 41–46.

Ströhle, A. et al. (2015) Drug and exercise treatment of Alzheimer disease and mild cognitive impairment: A systematic review and meta-analysis of effects on cognition in randomized controlled trials. *American Journal of Geriatric Psychiatry*, 23(12): 1234–1249. doi: 10.1016/j.jagp.2015.07.007.

Sturm, L.A., Mays, R.M. & Zimet, G.D. (2005) Parental beliefs and decision making about child and adolescent immunization: from polio to sexually transmitted infections. *Journal of Developmental & Behavioral Pediatrics*, 26: 441–452.

Subramanian, S.W., Elwert, F. & Christakis, N. (2008) Widowhood and mortality among the elderly: The modifying role of neighborhood concentration of widowed individuals. *Social Science & Medicine*, 66: 873–884.

Sullivan, P.F., Kendler, K. & Neale, M. (2003) Schizophrenia as a complex trait: Evidence from a meta-analysis of twin studies. *Archives of General Psychiatry*, 60: 1187–1192.

Sullivan, P.F., Neale, M.C. & Kendler, K.S. (2000) Genetic epidemiology of major depression: Review and meta-analysis. *American Journal of Psychiatry*, 157: 1552–1562.

Suls, J., Martin, R. & Wheeler, L. (2002) Social comparison: Why, with whom and with what effect? *Current Directions in Psychological Science*, 11: 159–163.

Suls, J. & Rothman, A. (2004) Evolution of the biopsychosocial model: Prospects and challenges for health psychology. *Health Psychology*, 23(2): 119–125.

Surtees, P.G., Wainwright, N.W.J., Luben, R.N., Wareham, N.J., Bingham, S.A. & Khaw, K.T. (2008) Depression and ischemic heart disease mortality: Evidence from the EPIC-Norfolk United Kingdom prospective cohort study. *American Journal of Psychiatry*, *165*: 515–523.

Suskind, A.M. et al. (2013) The prevalence and overlap of interstitial cystitis/bladder pain syndrome and chronic prostatitis/chronic pelvic pain syndrome in men: results of the RAND Interstitial Cystitis Epidemiology male study. *Journal of Urology*, *189*: 141–145.

Sutton, S. (2007) Transtheoretical model of behaviour change, in S. Ayers et al. (eds), *Cambridge Handbook of Psychology, Health and Medicine* (2nd edition). Cambridge: Cambridge University Press. pp. 228–232.

Swamia, V. et al. (2008) Factors influencing preferences for height: A replication and extension. *Personality and Individual Differences*, *45*: 395–400.

Swami, V. & Tovee, M.J. (2006) Does hunger influence judgements of female physical attractiveness? *British Journal of Psychology*, *97*: 353–363.

Swayden, K.J., Anderson, K.K., Connelly, L.M., Moran, J.S., McMahon, J.K. & Arnold, P.M. (2012) Effect of sitting vs. standing on perception of provider time at bedside: A pilot study. *Patient Education and Counselling*, *86*(2): 166–171.

Taddio, A. et al. (2009) Inadequate pain management during childhood immunizations: The nerve of it. *Clinical Therapy*, *31*(Suppl 2): s152–s67.

Tajfel, H. & Turner, J. (1986) An integrative theory of intergroup conflict, in S. Worchel & W. Austin (eds), *Psychology of Intergroup Relations*. Chicago, IL: Nelson-Hall. pp. 2–24.

Tak, H. et al. (2015) The association between patient-centered attributes of care and patient satisfaction. *Patient*, *8*: 187–197.

Talge, N.M., Neal, C. & Glover, V. (2007) Antenatal maternal stress and long-term effects on child neurodevelopment: How and why? *Journal of Child Psychology and Psychiatry*, *48*: 245–261.

Tallis, R.C. (1996) Burying Freud. *The Lancet*, *347*: 669–671.

Talsma, D., Senkowski, D., Soto-Faraco, S. & Woldorff, M.G. (2010) The multifaceted interplay between attention and multisensory integration. *Trends in Cognitive Science*, *14*: 400–410.

Tan, C.C., Cheng, K.K. & Wang, W. (2015) Self-care management programme for older adults with diabetes: An integrative literature review. *International Journal of Nursing Practice*, *21* (Suppl. 2): 115–124.

Tanofsky-Kraff, M. et al. (2007) Laboratory-based studies of eating among children and adolescents. *Current Nutrition & Food Science*, *3*: 55–74.

Taylor, C.B., Miller, N.H., Smith, P.M. & DeBusk, R.F. (1997) The effect of a home-based, case-managed, multifactorial risk-reduction program on reducing psychological distress in patients with cardiovascular disease. *Journal of Cardiopulmonary Rehabilitation*, *17*: 157–162.

Taylor, R.S. et al. (2004) Exercise-based rehabilitation for patients with coronary heart disease: Systematic review and meta-analysis of randomized controlled trials. *American Journal of Medicine*, *116*: 682–692.

Taylor, S., Pinnock, H., Epiphanou, E., Pearce, G., Parke, H., Schwappach, A., Purushotham, N., Jacob, S., Griffiths, C., Greenhalgh, T. & Sheikh, A. (2014) A rapid synthesis of the evidence on interventions supporting self-management for people with long-term conditions:

PRISMS – Practical systematic Review of Self-Management Support for long-term conditions. *Health Services and Delivery Research*, 4/2(53).

Taylor, S.E. (2006) Tend and befriend: Biobehavioral bases of affiliation under stress. *Current Directions in Psychological Science*, 15(6): 273–277.

Taylor, S.E. (2007) Social support, in H.S. Friedman and R.C. Silver (eds), *Foundations of Health Psychology*. New York: Oxford University Press. pp. 145–171.

Taylor, S.E. (2010) Affiliation and stress, in S. Folkman (ed.), *The Oxford Handbook of Stress, Health, and Coping*. Oxford: Oxford University Press.

Taylor, S.E. (2012) Tend and befriend theory, in P.A.M. van Lange, A.W. Kruglanski & E.T. Higgins (eds), *Handbook of Theories of Social Psychology* (Vol. 1). London: Sage. pp. 32–94.

Taylor, S.E., Cousino Klein, L., Lewis, B.P., Gruenewald, T.L., Gurung, R.A.R. & Updegraff, J.A. (2000) Biobehavioral responses to stress in females: Tend-and-befriend, not fight-or-flight. *Psychological Review*, 107: 411–429.

Taylor, S. E., Saphire-Bernstein, S., & Seeman, T. E. (2009). Plasma oxytocin in women and plasma vasopressin in men are markers of distress in primary relationships. *Psychological Science*, 21 (1): 3–7.

Taylor, S.E., Saphire-Bernstein, S. & Seeman, T.E. (2010) Are plasma oxytocin in women and plasma vasopressin in men biomarkers of distressed pair-bond relationships? *Psychological Science*, 21(1): 3–7.

Taylor, S.E., Welch, W.T., Kim, H.S. & Sherman, D.K. (2007) Cultural differences in the impact of social support on psychological and biological stress responses. *Psychological Science*, 18: 831–837.

Tedeshi, R.G. & Calhoun, L.G. (2004) *Posttraumatic Growth: Conceptual Foundation and Empirical Evidence*. Philadelphia, PA: Lawrence Erlbaum Associates.

Tedstone, J.E. & Tarrier, N. (2003) Posttraumatic stress disorder following medical illness and treatment. *Clinical Psychology Review*, 23: 409–448.

Tekampe, J. et al. (2017) Conditioning immune and endocrine parameters in humans: A systematic review. *Psychotherapy and Psychosomatics*, 86(2): 99–107.

Teri, L. et al. (1999) Anxiety of Alzheimer's disease: Prevalence, and comorbidity. *Journals of Gerontology Series A*, 54: 348–352.

Teutsch, C. (2003) Patient-doctor communication. *Medical Clinics of North America*, 87: 1115–1145.

The, A.M., Hak, T., Koeter, G. & van der Wal, G. (2000) Collusion in doctor-patient communication about imminent death: An ethnographic study. *British Medical Journal*, 321: 1376–1381.

Thiblin, I. & Petersson, A. (2004) Pharmacoepidemiology of anabolic androgenic steroids: A review. *Fundamental & Clinical Pharmacology*, 19: 27–44.

Thier, S.L. et al. (2008) In chronic disease, nationwide data show poor adherence by patients to medication and by physicians to guidelines. *American Journal of Managed Care*, 17: 48–57.

Thomas, K., Hevey, D., Pertl M., Ní Chuinneagáin, S., Craig, A. & Maher, L. (2011) Appearance matters: The frame and focus of health messages influences beliefs about skin cancer. *British Journal of Health Psychology*, 16(Pt 2): 418–429.

Thomas, P.W., Thomas, S., Hillier, C., Galvin, K. & Baker, R. (2006) Psychological interventions for multiple sclerosis. *Cochrane Database of Systematic Reviews*, 1 (Art. CD004431).

Thompson, R.J. et al. (2010) Maladaptive coping, adaptive coping, and depressive symptoms: Variations across age and depressive state. *Behaviour Research and Therapy*, 48: 459–466.

Thorburn, A.W. (2005) Prevalence of obesity in Australia. *Obesity Review*, 6: 187–189.

Thorlund, J.B., Juhl, C.B., Roos, E.M. & Lohmander, L.S. (2015) Arthroscopic surgery for degenerative knee: Systematic review and meta-analysis of benefits and harms. *British Medical Journal*, 350: h2747. (doi: 10.1136/bmj.h2747.)

Thorn, B.E., Ward, L.C., Sullivan, M.J. & Boothby, J.L. (2003) Communal coping model of catastrophizing: Conceptual model building. *Pain*, 107(3): 280.

Thümmler, K. et al. (2009) *Data and Information on Women's Health in the European Union*. Brussels: European Commission.

Tian, J., Chen, Z.C. & Hang, L.F. (2009) Effects of nutritional and psychological status of the patients with advanced stomach cancer on physical performance status. *Support Care Cancer*, 17: 1263–1268.

Timmons, B.H. & Ley, R. (1994) *Behavioral and Psychological Approaches to Breathing Disorders*. New York: Plenum.

Tobin, E.T. et al. (2015) Naturalistically observed conflict and youth asthma symptoms. *Health Psychology*, 34: 622–631.

Tomlinson, J. (ed.) (2004) *ABC of Sexual Health* (2nd edition). London: Wiley.

Torquato Lopes, A.P. & Decesaro, M. (2014) The adjustments experienced by persons with an ostomy: An integrative review of the literature. *Ostomy Wound Manage*, 60: 34–42.

Towle, A., Godolphin, W. & van Staalduinen, S. (2006) Enhancing the relationship and improving communication between adolescents and their health care providers: A school based intervention by medical students. *Patient Education & Counseling*, 62: 189–192.

Treiber, F.A., Kamarck, T., Schneiderman, N., Sheffield, D., Kapuku, G. & Taylor, T. (2003) Cardiovascular reactivity and development of preclinical and clinical disease states. *Psychosomatic Medicine*, 65: 46–62.

Trenholm, C. et al. (2008) Impacts of abstinence education on teen sexual activity, risk of pregnancy, and risk of sexually transmitted diseases. *Journal of Policy Analysis and Management*, 27: 255–276.

Trojian, T.H., Mody, K. & Chain, P. (2007) Exercise and colon cancer: Primary and secondary prevention. *Current Sports Medicine Reports*, 6: 120–124.

Trufelli, D.C. et al. (2008) Burnout in cancer professionals: A systematic review and meta-analysis. *European Journal of Cancer Care*, 17: 524–531.

Trzepacz, P.T. & Baker, R.W. (1993) *The Psychiatric Mental Status Examination*. Oxford: Oxford University Press.

Tsai, Y.-C. et al. (2017, in press) Quality of life predicts risks of end-stage renal disease and mortality in patients with chronic kidney disease. *Nephrology Dialysis Transplantation*.

Tsakanikos, E. (2006) Perceptual biases and positive schizotypy: The role of perceptual load. *Personality and Individual Differences*, 41: 951–958.

Tsugane, S. (2005) Salt, salted food intake, and risk of gastric cancer: Epidemiological evidence. *Cancer Science*, 96: 1–6.

Tucker, L.A. & Bates, L. (2009) Restrained eating and risk of gaining weight and body fat in middle-aged women: A 3-year prospective study. *American Journal of Health Promotion*, *23*: 187–194.

Turiano, N.A., Chapman, B.P., Agrigoroaei, S., Infurna, F.J. & Lachman, M. (2014) Perceived control reduces mortality risk at low, not high, education levels. *Health Psychology*, *33*(8): 883–890.

Turk Charles, S., Gatz, M., Kato, K. & Pedersen, N.L. (2008) Physical health 25 years later: The predictive ability of neuroticism. *Health Psychology*, *27*: 369–378.

Turner, J.S., Pettit, K.E., Buente, B.B., Humbert, A.J., Perkins, A.J. & Kline, J.A. (2016) Medical student use of communication elements and association with patient satisfaction: A prospective observational pilot study. *BMC Medical Education*, *21*(16): 150.

Turner-Cobb, J.M. & Katsampouris, E. (2018) Stress, in C.D. Llewellyn et al. (eds), *The Cambridge Handbook of Psychology, Health and Medicine* (3rd edition). Cambridge: Cambridge University Press.

Turton, P., Hughes, P., Evans, C.D.H. & Fainman, D. (2001) Incidence, correlates, and predictors of post-traumatic stress disorder in the pregnancy after stillbirth. *British Journal of Psychiatry*, *178*: 556–560.

Tversky, A. & Kahneman, D. (1974) Judgment under uncertainty: Heuristics and biases. *Science*, *185*: 1124–1130.

Tzelepis, F. et al. (2014) Are we missing the Institute of Medicine's mark? A systematic review of patient-reported outcome measures assessing quality of patient-centred cancer care. *BMC Cancer*, *14*: 41.

Uchino, B.N., Kent de Grey, R.G., Cronan, S. & Trettevik, R. (2018) Social relationships, in C.D. Llewellyn et al. (eds), *The Cambridge Handbook of Psychology, Health and Medicine* (3rd edition). Cambridge: Cambridge University Press.

UK ECT Review Group (2003) Efficacy and safety of electroconvulsive therapy in depressive disorders: A systemic review and meta-analysis. *Lancet*, *361*: 799–808.

UNAIDS/WHO (2009) *AIDS Epidemic Update*. Geneva: UNAIDS.

Ünal, B., Critchley, J.A., Fidan, D. & Capewell, S. (2005) Life-years gained from modern cardiological treatments and population risk factor changes in England and Wales, 1981–2000. *American Journal of Public Health*, *95*: 103–108.

UNICEF (2001) *A League Table of Teenage Births in Rich Nations*. Florence: UNICEF, Innocenti Research Centre.

Ussher, J.M. (2010) Are we medicalizing women's misery? A critical review of women's higher rates of reported depression. *Feminism & Psychology*, *20*(1): 9–35.

Ussher, J.M. (2018) Premenstrual syndrome, in C.D. Llewellyn et al. (eds), *The Cambridge Handbook of Psychology, Health and Medicine* (3rd edition). Cambridge: Cambridge University Press.

Ussher, J.M., Hunter, M. & Cariss, M. (2002) A woman-centred psychological intervention for premenstrual symptoms, drawing on cognitive-behavioural and narrative therapy. *Clinical Psychology and Psychotherapy*, *9*: 319–331.

Valentiner, D.P., Holahan, C.J. & Moos, R.H. (1994) Social support, appraisals of event controllability, and coping: An integrative model. *Journal of Personality and Social Psychology*, *66*: 1094–1102.

van Amsterdam, J. et al. (2010) Adverse health effects of anabolic-androgenic steroids. *Regulatory Toxicology and Pharmacology*, 57: 117–123.

van den Dries, L., Juffer, F., van Ijzendoorn, M.H. & Bakermans-Kranenburg, M.J. (2009) Fostering security? A meta-analysis of attachment in adopted children. *Children and Youth Services Review*, 31: 410–421.

van der Bruggen, C.O., Stams, G.J. & Bogels, S.M. (2008) Research review: The relation between child and parent anxiety and parental control. *Journal of Child Psychology and Psychiatry, and Allied Disciplines*, 49: 1257–1269.

van der Klink, J.J.L., Blonk, R.W.B., Schene, A.H. & van Dijk, F.J.H. (2001) The benefits of interventions for work-related stress. *American Journal of Public Health*, 91: 270–276.

van Dessel, N., den Boeft, M., van der Wouden, J.C., Kleinstäuber, M., Leone, S.S., Terluin, B., Numans, M.E., van der Horst, H.E. & van Marwijk, H. (2014) Non-pharmacological interventions for somatoform disorders and medically unexplained physical symptoms (MUPS) in adults. *Cochrane Database of Systematic Reviews*, 11 (Art. CD011142).

van Dixhoorn, J. & White, A. (2005) Relaxation therapy for rehabilitation and prevention in ischaemic heart disease: A systematic review and meta-analysis. *European Journal of Cardiovascular Prevention and Rehabilitation*, 12: 193–202.

van Duijn, E. et al. (2014) Course of irritability, depression and apathy in Huntington's disease in relation to motor symptoms during a two-year follow-up period. *Neurodegenerative Diseases*, 13: 9–16.

van Emmerik, A.A., Reijntjes, A. & Kamphuis, J.H. (2013) Writing therapy for posttraumatic stress: A meta-analysis. *Psychotherapy and Psychosomatics*, 82(2): 82–88.

van Gils, A., Schoevers, R.A., Bonvanie, I.J., Gelauff, J.M., Roest, A.M. & Rosmalen, J.G. (2016) Self-help for medically unexplained symptoms: A systematic review and meta-analysis. *Psychosomatic Medicine*, 78(6): 728–739.

van Groenestijn, A.C. et al. (2016) Associations between psychological factors and health-related quality of life and global quality of life in patients with ALS: A systematic review. *Health and Quality of Life Outcomes*, 14: 107.

van Ijzendoorn, M.H. & Kroonenberg, P.M. (1988) Cross-cultural patterns of attachment: A meta-analysis of the Strange Situation. *Child Development*, 59: 147–156.

van Londen, W.M., Juffer, F. & van Izendoorn, M.H. (2007) Attachment, cognitive and motor development in adopted children: Short-term outcomes after international adoption. *Journal of Pediatric Psychology*, 32: 1259–1263.

van Oudenhove, L. & Aziz, Q. (2009) Recent insights on central processing and psychological processes in functional gastrointestinal disorders. *Digestive and Liver Disease*, 41: 781–787.

van Oudenhove, L. & Aziz, Q. (2013) The role of psychosocial factors and psychiatric disorders in functional dyspepsia. *Nature Reviews: Gastroenterology and Hepatology*, 10: 158–167.

van Parys, A., Ryding, E.L., Schei, B., Lukasse, M. & Temmerman, M. (2012) Fear of childbirth and mode of delivery in six European countries: The BIDENS study. *22nd European Congress of Obstetrics and Gynaecology*, Book of Abstracts (S14.4). Ghent: Ghent University.

Vancampfort, D. et al. (2014) A systematic review of physical therapy interventions for patients with anorexia and bulimia nervosa. *Disability and Rehabilitation*, 36: 628–634.

Veehof, M.M., Trompetter, H.R., Bohlmeijer, E.T. & Schreurs, K.M. (2016) Acceptance- and mindfulness-based interventions for the treatment of chronic pain: A meta-analytic review. *Cognitive Behaviour Therapy*, 5(1): 5–31.

Venn, A. et al. (2004) The use of oestrogen to reduce the adult height of tall girls: Long-term effects on fertility. *Lancet*, 364: 1513–1518.

Vercellini, P. et al. (2009) Chronic pelvic pain in women: Etiology, pathogenesis and diagnostic approach. *Gynecological Endocrinology*, 25: 149–158.

Vertes, R.P. & Eastman, K.E. (2000) The case against memory consolidation in REM sleep. *Behavioral and Brain Sciences*, 23: 867–876.

Vetter, M.L. et al. (2010) Behavioral and pharmacologic therapies for obesity. *Nature Reviews: Endocrinology*, 6: 578–588.

Villanacci, V. et al. (2008) Enteric nervous system abnormalities in inflammatory bowel diseases. *Neurogastroenterology & Motility*, 20: 1009–1016.

Vingeliene, S. et al. (2016) An update of the WCRF/AICR systematic literature review on esophageal and gastric cancers and citrus fruits intake. *Cancer Causes Control*, 27: 837–851.

Vogel, T., Brechat, P.H., Leprêtre, P.M., Kaltenbach, G., Berthel, M. & Lonsdorfer, J. (2009) Health benefits of physical activity in older patients: A review. *International Journal of Clinical Practice*, 63: 203–320.

Vogeley, K. & Bente, G. (2010) 'Artificial humans': Psychology and neuroscience perspectives on embodiment and nonverbal communication. *Neural Networks*, 23(8–9): 1077–1090.

Vos, M.S. & de Haes, J.C.J.M. (2007) Denial in cancer patients: An explorative review. *Psycho-Oncology*, 16: 12–25.

Voth, J. & Sirois, F.M. (2009) The role of self-blame and responsibility in adjustment to inflammatory bowel disease. *Rehabilitation Psychology*, 54: 99–108.

Vuilleumier, P. (2005) How brains beware: Neural mechanisms of emotional attention. *Trends in Cognitive Sciences*, 9: 585–594.

Vuilleumier, P. & Huang, Y.M. (2009) Emotional attention: Uncovering the mechanisms of affective biases in perception. *Current Directions in Psychological Science*, 18: 148–152.

Wadhwa, P.D., Buss, C., Entringer, S. & Swanson, J.M. (2009) Developmental origins of health and disease: Brief history of the approach and current focus on epigenetic mechanisms. *Seminars in Reproductive Medicine*, 27(5): 358–368.

Walburn, J. et al. (2009) Psychological stress and wound healing in humans: A systematic review and meta-analysis. *Journal of Psychosomatic Research*, 67: 253–271.

Wali, S.O. et al. (2013) Effect of on-call-related sleep deprivation on physicians' mood and alertness. *Annals of Thoracic Medicine*, 8: 22–27.

Walker, J. (2001) *Control and the Psychology of Health*. Buckingham: Open University Press.

Wallston, K.A. (2007) Perceived control, in S. Ayers et al. (eds), *Cambridge Handbook of Psychology, Health and Medicine* (2nd edition). Cambridge: Cambridge University Press. pp. 148–150.

Wallston, K.A., Wallson, B.S. & DeVellis, R. (1978) Development of the multidimensional health locus of control (MHLC) scales. *Health Education Monographs*, 6: 160–170.

Walsh, J.C., Lynch, M., Murphy, A.W. & Daly, K. (2004) Factors influencing the decision to seek treatment for symptoms of acute myocardial infarction: An evaluation of the Self-Regulatory Model of illness behaviour. *Journal of Psychosomatic Research*, 56: 67–73.

Wampold, B.E., Minami, T., Tierney, S.C., Baskin, T.W. & Bhati, D.S. (2005) The placebo is powerful: Estimating placebo effects in medicine and psychotherapy from randomised clinical trials. *Journal of Clinical Psychology*, 61: 835–854.

Wang, Y. & Beydoun, M.A. (2007) The obesity epidemic in the United States – gender, age, socioeconomic, racial/ethnic, and geographic characteristics: A systematic review and meta-regression analysis. *Epidemiologic Reviews*, 29: 6–28.

Wardle, J., Griffith, J., Johnson, F. & Rapoport, L. (2000) Intentional weight control and food choice habits in a national representative sample of adults in the UK. *International Journal of Obesity*, 24: 534–540.

Wardle, J., Steptoe, A., Burckhardt, R., Vögele, C., Vila, J. & Zarczynski, Z. (1994) Testicular self-examination: Attitudes and practices among young men in Europe. *Preventive Medicine*, 23: 206–210.

Wardle, J., Steptoe, A., Oliver, G. & Lipsey, Z. (2000) Stress, dietary restraint and food intake. *Journal of Psychosomatic Research*, 48: 195–202.

Watson, D. & Tellegen, A. (1985) Toward a consensual structure of mood. *Psychological Bulletin*, 98: 219–223.

Watson, P.W.B. & McKinstry, B. (2009) A systematic review of interventions to improve recall of medical advice in healthcare consultations. *Journal of the Royal Society of Medicine*, 102: 235–243.

Watts, S. et al. (2014) Depression and anxiety in prostate cancer: A systematic review and meta-analysis of prevalence rates. *BMJ Open*, 4(3): e003901.

Way, B.M. & Taylor, S.E. (2009) Genetic factors in social pain, in G. MacDonald & L.A. Jensen-Campbell (eds), *Social Pain: A Neuroscientific, Social, Clinical, and Developmental Analysis*. Washington, DC: American Psychological Association.

Webb, E., Ashton, C.H., Kelly, P. & Kamali, F. (1996) Alcohol and drug use in university students. *Lancet*, 348: 922–925.

Webb, R. & Ayers, S. (2015) Cognitive biases in processing infant emotion by women with depression, anxiety and post-traumatic stress disorder in pregnancy or after birth: A systematic review. *Cognition & Emotion*, 29: 1278–1294.

Webb, S.M. & Badia, X. (2016) Quality of life in acromegaly. *Neuroendocrinology*, 103: 106–111.

Wegner, D.M. (2003) The mind's best trick: How we experience conscious will. *TRENDS in Cognitive Science*, 7: 65–69.

Weinman, J., Ebrecht, M., Scott, S., Walburn, J. & Dyson, M. (2008) Enhanced wound healing after emotional disclosure intervention. *British Journal of Health Psychology*, 13: 95–102.

Weinstein, N.D. (1987) Unrealistic optimism about susceptibility to health problems: Conclusions from a community-wide sample. *Journal of Behavioral Medicine*, 10: 481–500.

Weiser, E.B. (2007) The prevalence of anxiety disorders among adults with asthma: A meta-analytic review. *Journal of Clinical Psychology in Medical Settings*, 14: 297–307.

Weisz, G. & Knaapen, L. (2009) Diagnosing and treating premenstrual syndrome in five western nations. *Social Science & Medicine*, 68: 1498–1505.

Weiten, W. (2004) *Psychology Themes and Variations* (6th edition). Belmont, CA: Wadsworth/Thomson Learning.

Welch, J.L. et al. (2013) Using a mobile application to self-monitor diet and fluid intake among adults receiving hemodialysis. *Research in Nursing & Health*, 36: 284–298. doi: 10.1002/nur.21539

Welch, J.L. & Thomas-Hawkins, C. (2005) Psycho-educational strategies to promote fluid adherence in adult hemodialysis patients: A review of intervention studies. *International Journal of Nursing Studies*, 42: 597–608.

Wells, A. (1997) *Cognitive Therapy of Anxiety Disorders: A Practice Manual and Conceptual Guide*. New York: Wiley.

Wells, A. (2010) Metacognitive theory and therapy for worry and generalized anxiety disorder: Review and status. *Journal of Experimental Psychopathology*, 1(1): 133–145.

Wengreen, H.J. et al. (2013) Incentivizing children's fruit and vegetable consumption: Results of a United States pilot study of the Food Dudes Program. *Journal of Nutrition Education and Behaviour*, 45: 54–59.

West, C. & Zimmerman, D. (1987) Doing gender. *Gender & Society*, 1: 125–151.

West, R. (2006) *Theory of Addiction*. Oxford: Blackwell.

West, R. & Brown, J. (2013) *Theory of Addiction* (2nd edition). Oxford: Wiley Blackwell Press.

West, R. & Hardy, A. (2007) Tobacco use, in S. Ayers et al. (eds), *Cambridge Handbook of Health Psychology* (2nd edition). Cambridge: Cambridge University Press. pp. 908–912.

Wettergren, L., Kettis-Lindblad, A., Sprangers, M. & Ring, L. (2009) The use, feasibility and psychometric properties of an individualised quality-of-life instrument: A systematic review of the SEIQoL-DW. *Quality of Life Research*, 18: 737–746.

Wexler, T. et al. (2009) Growth hormone deficiency is associated with decreased quality of life in patients with prior acromegaly. *Journal of Clinical Endocrinology and Metabolism*, 94: 2471–2477.

Whalley, B., Rees, K., Davies, P., Bennett, P., Ebrahim, S., Liu, Z., West, R., Moxham, T., Thompson, D.R. & Taylor, R.S. (2011) Psychological interventions for coronary heart disease. *Cochrane Database of Systematic Reviews*, 8 (Art. CD002902).

White, A. et al. (2011) *The State of Men's Health in Europe*. Brussels: European Commission.

White, J., Levinson, W. & Roter, D. (1994) 'Oh by the way' – the closing moments of the medical interview. *Journal of General Internal Medicine*, 9: 24–28.

White, K.M. et al. (2012) An extended theory of planned behaviour intervention for older adults with Type 2 diabetes and cardiovascular disease. *Journal of Aging and Physical Activity*, 20: 281–299.

Whitten, C.E., Donovan, M. & Cristobal, K. (2005) Treating chronic pain: New knowledge, more choices. *The Permanente Journal*, 9: 9–18.

Wiklund, I., Edman, G. & Andolf, E. (2007) Cesarean section on maternal request: Reasons for the request, self-estimated health, expectations, experience of birth and signs of depression among first-time mothers. *Acta Obstetricia et Gynecologica Scandinavica*, 86: 451–456.

Wilbert-Lampen, U. et al. (2008) Cardiovascular events during World Cup soccer. *New England Journal of Medicine*, 358: 475–483.

Wilcher, R. (2013) Integration of family planning into HIV services: A synthesis of recent evidence. *AIDS*, 27(Suppl. 1): S65–S75.

Wilfley, D.E., Wilson, G.T. & Agras, W.S. (2003) The clinical significance of binge eating disorder. *International Journal of Eating Disorders*, 34(Suppl. 1): s96–s106.

Wilhelmsen, I. (2000) Brain-gut axis as an example of the bio-psycho-social model. *Gut, 47* (Suppl. IV)*: iv5–iv7.

Williams, A. (2014) Central nervous system regeneration – where are we? *QJM, 107*: 335–339

Williams, A.C. & Craig, K.D. (2016) Updating the definition of pain. *Pain, 157*(11): 2420–2423.

Williams, A.C., Eccleston, C. & Morley, S. (2012) Psychological therapies for the management of chronic pain (excluding headache) in adults. *Cochrane Database of Systematic Reviews, 11* (Art. CD007407).

Williams, J.M. & Binnie, L.M. (2002) Children's concepts of illness: An intervention to improve knowledge. *British Journal of Health Psychology, 7*: 129–147.

Williams, S., Weinman, J. & Dale, J. (1998) Doctor-patient communication and patient satisfaction: A review. *Journal of Family Practice, 15*: 480–492.

Wilson, B.A. (2007) Neuropsychological rehabilitation, in S. Ayers et al. (eds), *Cambridge Handbook of Psychology, Health and Medicine* (2nd edition). Cambridge: Cambridge University Press. pp. 367–369.

Wilson, B.A. et al. (eds) (2009) *Neuropsychological rehabilitation: Theory, Models, Therapy and Outcome*. Cambridge: Cambridge University Press.

Winstanley, S. (2005) Cognitive model of patient aggression towards health care staff: The patient's perspective. *Work & Stress, 19*: 340–350.

Winterich, J.A. et al. (2009) Masculinity and the body: How African American and white men experience cancer screening exams involving the rectum. *American Journal of Men's Health, 3*: 300–309.

Witte, K. & Allen, M. (2000) A meta-analysis of fear appeals: Implications for effective public health campaigns. *Health Education & Behavior, 27*: 591–615.

Wolchik, S.A., Sandler, I.N., Millsap, R.E., Plummer, B.A., Greene, S.M., Anderson, E.R., Dawson-McClure, S.R., Hipke, K. & Haine, R.A. (2002) Six-year follow-up of preventive interventions for children of divorce: A randomized controlled trial. *JAMA, 288*(15): 1874–1881.

Wolf, F.M., Guevera, J.P., Grum, C.M., Clark, N.M. & Cates, C.J. (2003) Educational interventions for asthma in children. *Cochrane Database of Systematic Reviews, 2* (Art. CD000326).

Wolitzky-Taylor, K.B., Horowitz, J.D., Powers, M.B. & Telch, M.J. (2008) Psychological approaches in the treatment of specific phobias: A meta-analysis. *Clinical Psychology Review, 28*: 1021–1037.

Women's Health Initiative (2009) *Postmenopausal Hormone Therapy Trials*. Available at www.nhlbi.nih.gov/whi/index.html (last accessed 21 July 2009).

Wong, J.G., Clare, I.C.H., Gunn, M.J. & Holland, A.J. (1999) Capacity to make health care decisions: Its importance in clinical practice. *Psychological Medicine, 29*: 437–446.

Worden, J.W. (1991) *Grief Counselling and Grief Therapy: A Handbook for the Mental Health Practitioner* (2nd edition). New York: Springer.

Worden, J.W. (2009) *Grief Counselling and Grief Therapy: A Handbook for the Mental Health Practitioner* (4th edition). New York: Springer.

World Alliance for Patient Safety (2008) *World Health Organization Surgical Safety Checklist and Implementation Manual*. Geneva: WHO.

World Association for Sexual Health (2007) *Definitions Accepted by the WAS General Assembly, 17 April 2007, Sydney Australia.* Available at: www.worldsexology.org/doc/definitions-of-specialties.pdf (last accessed 17 July 2017).

World Bank (2017) *Fertility Rate, Total (Births per Woman).* Washington, DC: World Bank. Available at: http://data.worldbank.org/indicator/SP.DYN.TFRT.IN? (last accesed 29 January 2017).

World Health Organisation (1992) *Basic Documents* (39th edition). Geneva: WHO.

World Health Organisation (1996) *Diagnostic and Management Guidelines for Mental Disorders in Primary Care. ICD-10 Chapter V Primary Care Version.* Geneva: WHO.

World Health Organisation (2002) *Global Strategy on Infant and Young Child Feeding.* Geneva: WHO.

World Health Organisation (2004) *International Statistical Classification of Diseases and Health Related Problems (The) ICD-10* (2nd edition). Geneva: WHO.

World Health Organisation (2005) *Gender, Health & Alcohol Use.* Geneva: WHO.

World Health Organisation (2006) *Report of a Technical Consultation on Sexual Health, 28–31 January 2002.* Geneva: WHO.

World Health Organization (2007). *Global Surveillance, Prevention and Control of Chronic Respiratory Diseases. A comprehensive approach.* Geneva: WHO

World Health Organisation (2008a) *The Top Ten Causes of Death: Fact Sheet Number 310.* Geneva: WHO.

World Health Organisation (2008b) *Closing the Gap in a Generation: Health Equity through Action on the Social Determinants of Health.* Geneva: WHO, Commission on Social Determinants of Health.

World Health Organisation (2008c) *The Global Burden of Disease: 2004 Update.* Geneva: WHO. 2008. Available at:www.who.int/healthinfo/global_burden_disease/GBD_report_2004update_full.pdf?ua=1 (last accessed 22 March 2017).

World Health Organisation (2009a) *Mortality Database.* Available at: http://apps.who.int/whosis/database/mort/table1.cfm (last accessed 17 July 2017).

World Health Organisation (2009b) *Global Health Risks: Mortality and Burden of Disease Attributable to Selected Major Risks.* Geneva: WHO.

World Health Organisation (2009c) *Surgical Safety Checklist.* Available at: http://www.who.int/patientsafety/safesurgery/checklist/en/ (last accessed 1 August 2017)

World Health Organisation (2012) *Dementia: A Public Health Priority.* Geneva: WHO.

World Health Organisation (2013) *Long-term Effects of Breastfeeding: A Systematic Review.* Geneva: WHO.

World Health Organisation (2014a) *New WHO Safe and Dignified Burial Protocol: Key to Reducing Ebola Transmission.* Geneva: WHO. Available at: www.who.int/mediacentre/news/notes/2014/ebola-burial-protocol/en/ (last accessed 20 March 2017).

World Health Organisation (2014b) *Global Status Report on Alcohol and Health.* Geneva: WHO. Available at: www.who.int/substance_abuse/publications/global_alcohol_report/msb_gsr_2014_1.pdf?ua=1 (last accessed 22 March 2017).

World Health Organisation (2014c) *Global Status Report on Noncommunicable Diseases 2014.* Geneva: WHO.

World Health Organisation (2015) *Caesarean Sections Should be Performed Only when Necessary, News Release*. Geneva: WHO. Available at: www.who.int/mediacentre/news/releases/2015/caesarean-sections/en/ (last accessed 11 January 2017).

World Health Organisation (2016a) *Global Health Estimates 2015: Deaths by Cause, Age, Sex, by Country and by Region, 2000–2015*. Geneva: WHO.

World Health Organisation (2016b) *World Health Statistics 2016: Monitoring Health for the SDGs (Sustainable Development Goals)*. Geneva: WHO. Available at: www.who.int/gho/publications/world_health_statistics/2016/en/ (last accessed 17 July 2017).

World Health Organisation (2017a) *Depression and Other Common Mental Disorders: Global Health Estimates*. Geneva: WHO. Available at: http://apps.who.int/iris/bitstream/10665/254610/1/WHO-MSD-MER-2017.2-eng.pdf?ua=1 (last accessed 9 March 2017).

World Health Organisation (2017b) *Top 10 Causes of Death. Global Health Observatory (GHO) Data*. Geneva: WHO. Available at: www.who.int/gho/mortality_burden_disease/causes_death/top_10/en/ (lat accessed 5 April 2017).

World Health Organisation (2017c) *HIV Progress Report 2016*. Geneva: WHO. Available at: www.who.int/hiv/data/en (last accessed 27 March 2017).

World Health Organisation (2017d) *Life Expectancy: Data by WHO Region*. Geneva: WHO. Available at: http://apps.who.int/gho/data/view.main.SDG2016LEXREGv?lang=en (last accessed 29 January 2017).

Wright, D.B. & Loftus, E.F. (2008) Eyewitness memory, in G. Cohen & M. Conway (eds), *Memory in the Real World* (3rd edition). New York: Psychology. pp. 91–105.

Wright, R.J. et al. (2004) Community violence and asthma morbidity. *American Journal of Public Health*, 94: 625–632.

Wyatt, K., Dimmock, P., Jones, P., Obhrai, M. & O'Brien, S. (2001) Efficacy of progesterone and progestogens in management of premenstrual syndrome: Systematic review. *British Medical Journal*, 323: 776–780.

Wyatt, K.M., Dimmock, P.W. & O'Brien, P.M. (2002) Selective serotonin reuptake inhibitors for premenstrual syndrome. *Cochrane Database of Systematic Reviews*, 4 (Art. CD001396).

Xi, J. & Zhang, S.-C. (2008) Stem cells in development of therapeutics for Parkinson's disease: A perspective. *Journal of Cellular Biochemistry*, 105: 1153–1160.

Yabroff, K.R. & Mandelblatt, J.S. (1999) Interventions targeted toward patients to increase mammography use. *Cancer Epidemiology Biomarkers and Prevention*, 8: 749–775.

Yamamoto T. (2013) Nutrition and diet in inflammatory bowel disease. *Current Opinion in Gastroenterology*, 29: 216–221. (doi: 10.1097/MOG.0b013e32835b9a40)

Yamamoto, T., Nakahigashi, M. & Saniabadi, A.R. (2009) Diet and inflammatory bowel disease – epidemiology and treatment. *Alimentary Pharmacology & Therapeutics*, 30: 99–112.

Yarzebski, J., Goldberg, R.J., Gore, J.M. & Alpert, J.S. (1994) Temporal trends and factors associated with extent of delay to hospital arrival in patients with acute myocardial infarction. *American Heart Journal*, 128: 255–263.

Yedidia, M.J. et al. (2003) Effect of communications training on medical student performance. *Journal of the American Medical Association*, 290: 1157–1165.

Yorke, J., Fleming, S.L. & Shuldham, C.M. (2004) Psychological interventions for adults with asthma. *Cochrane Database of Systematic Reviews*, 1 (Art. CD002982).

Yoshida, F. & Hori, H. (1989) Personal space as a function of eye-contact and spatial arrangements of a group. *Japanese Journal of Psychology*, 60: 53–56.

Young, H.N. et al. (2016) How does patient-provider communication influence adherence to asthma medications? *Patient Education and Counselling*, 100(4): 696–702.

Young, J., Angevaren, M., Rusted, J. & Tabet, N. (2015) Aerobic exercise to improve cognitive function in older people without known cognitive impairment. *Cochrane Database of Systematic Reviews*, 4 (Art. CD005381).

Young, J.E., Klosko, J.S. & Weishaar, M.E. (2004) Cognitive therapy of borderline personality disorder. *Bipolar Disorders*, 5: 14–21.

Young, K.D. (2005) Pediatric procedural pain. *Annals of Emergency Medicine*, 45: 160–171.

Young, Q.R. et al. (2007) Brief screen to identify five of the most common forms of psychosocial distress in cardiac patients: Validation of the screening tool for psychological distress (STOP-D). *Journal of Cardiovascular Nursing*, 22: 525–534.

Yovell, Y. et al. (2015) The case for neuropsychoanalysis: Why a dialogue with neuroscience is necessary but not sufficient for psychoanalysis. *International Journal of Psychoanalysis*, 96: 1515–1553.

Zachariae, R. & O'Toole, M.S. (2015) The effect of expressive writing intervention on psychological and physical health outcomes in cancer patients: A systematic review and meta-analysis. *Psycho-Oncology*, 24(11): 1349–1359.

Zaki, J. & Williams, W.C. (2013) Interpersonal emotion regulation. *Emotion*, 13(5): 803–810.

Zautra, A.J. & Reich, J.W. (2010) Resilience: The meanings, methods, and measures of a fundamental characteristic of human adaptation, in S. Folkman (ed.), *The Oxford Handbook of Stress, Health, and Coping*. Oxford: Oxford University Press.

Zellner, D.A., Garriga-Trillo, A., Centeno, S. & Wadsworth, E. (2004) Chocolate craving and the menstrual cycle. *Appetite*, 42: 119–121.

Zhang, J., Xu, R., Wang, B. & Wang, J. (2016) Effects of mindfulness-based therapy for patients with breast cancer: A systematic review and meta-analysis. *Complementary Therapies in Medicine*, 26: 1–10.

Zhang, Q.-L. & Rothenbacher, D. (2008) Prevalence of chronic kidney disease in population-based studies: Systematic review. *BMC Public Health*, 8: 117.

Zillmer, E.A., Spiers, M.V. & Culbertson, W.C. (2008) *Principles of Neuropsychology* (2nd edition). Belmont, CA: Wadsworth.

Zondervan, K.T. et al. (2001) The community prevalence of chronic pelvic pain in women and associated illness behaviour. *British Journal of General Practice*, 51: 541–547.

Zorrilla, E.P. et al. (2001) The relationship of depression and stressors to immunological assays: A meta-analytic review. *Brain, Behavior, and Immunity*, 15: 199–226.

Zvolensky, M.J. & Eifert, G.H. (2001) A review of psychological factors/processes affecting anxious responding during voluntary hyperventilation and inhalations of carbon dioxide-enriched air. *Clinical Psychology Review*, 21: 375–400.

Zweifel, J.E. & O'Brien, W.H. (1997) A meta-analysis of the effect of hormone replacement therapy upon depressed mood. *Psychoneuroendocrinology*, 22: 189–212.

Zweyer, K., Velker, B. & Willibald, R. (2004) Do cheerfulness, exhilaration, and humor production moderate pain tolerance? *Humor: International Journal of Humor Research*, 17: 85–119.

Zwikker, H.E. et al. (2014) Psychosocial predictors of non-adherence to chronic medication: Systematic review of longitudinal studies. *Patient Preference and Adherence*, 8: 519–563.

INDEX

Page numbers in *italics* refer to figures and tables, those in **bold** indicate boxes.

BMA LIBRARY
WITHDRAWN
FROM LIBRARY
BRITISH MEDICAL ASSOCIATION